Executive Editor: Richard A. Weimer
Production Editor: Janis K. Oppelt
Art Director: Don Sellers, AMI
Illustrators: Bernard Vervin; Joe Vitek
Cover Design by: Don Sellers
Text Designer: Janis K. Oppelt
Typesetting: Prestige Editorial and Graphics Services, Inc.
      Washington, D.C.
Typeface: Optima (text); Palatino (display)
Printed by: Fairfield Graphics, Fairfield, Pennsylvania

Assessment & Intervention in Emergency Nursing, 2nd Edition

Library of Congress Cataloging in Publication Data

Lanros, Nedell E., date
    Assessment & intervention in emergency nursing.

    Includes bibliographies and index.
    1. Emergency nursing.   I. Title.
RT120.E4L35   1982   610.73'6   83-12920
ISBN 0-89303-114-3

Prentice-Hall International, Inc., London
Prentice-Hall Canada, Inc., Scarborough, Ontario
Prentice-Hall of Australia, Pty., Ltd., Sydney
Prentice-Hall of India Private Limited, New Delhi
Prentice-Hall of Japan, Inc., Tokyo
Prentice-Hall of Southeast Asia Pte. Ltd., Singapore
Whitehall Books, Limited, Petone, New Zealand

Printed in the United States of America

83 84 85 86 87 88 89 90 91 92 93   10 9 8 7 6 5 4 3 2

ASSESSMENT & INTERVENTION
IN
EMERGENCY NURSING

2nd Edition

NEDELL E. LANROS, R.N.
Education Coordinator
Oregon EDNA
Portland, Oregon

Robert J. Brady Co. • **Bowie, Maryland 20715**
A Prentice-Hall Publishing and Communications Company

CONTENTS

FOREWORD TO THE 1ST EDITION

When I was a boy growing up in the Pacific Northwest, emergency department nurses were not exactly a common element in our lives. In the occasional circumstance that one of us made a visit to the "ambulance entrance" of the hospital (usually tearful and trailing twigs of the tree from which we had just departed somewhat abruptly), we would catch a rare glimpse of our local emergency department nurse. She sat behind a small desk in the "first-aid station." She was very kind, a little chubby, starched, and gray-haired. I remember that the room itself had white steel cabinets, windows full of arcane instruments, pale blue walls, a single exam table, and a very prominent phone. I think I remember the phone best because it was the only tool (other than a thermometer) I ever saw the kind nurse use. It was simple then—an emergency department nurse just smiled, consoled you, took your temperature, and telephoned your doctor. It made some sense, in an era when families had a close relationship with family doctors, when cars didn't go quite so fast, and when nurses were the designated handmaidens of the American health care delivery system.

However, as you have undoubtedly heard if you spend any time at cocktail parties, *times have changed*. Fortunately for all of us, so have emergency departments and emergency department nurses. The delivery of medical services to the United States' patient community has been dramatically altered from the Hippocratic-age standard of one doctor to one patient. The age of specialization is, and has been, here for 30 years. The wonderful doctor who fixed your broken arm last year is clearly tongue-tied when asked to stop Johnny's bloody nose or deal with your spouse's asthma. The kindly obstetrician who delivered your kids doesn't know a plaster cast from a pacemaker and thinks an ocular foreign body is an Italian car design. The age of the "clinic concept" is here too, and surprisingly few Americans seem able to answer the simple question, "Who is your family doctor?", except perhaps in the plural. The age of the telephone answering service is here, with most physicians trying to sleep at night like ordinary folk. And the age of the ambulance service. And the age of paramedics and radio communications. And television shows like "Emergency." And everyone sensitized to the concept of urgent health care. And CPR training in public schools. And eight-lane freeways, whip-lash, hunting accidents, drowning, drug overdoses, 911, and Mr. Yuk.

Throughout the 50s, 60s and 70s, more and more Americans have been visiting their local emergency department, seeking urgent health care in the increasingly complicated delivery system of the mid-twentieth century. These patients represent a wide spectrum of urgent health problems, ranging from recent minor injuries, pains, and medical problems to the assorted casualties of major auto accidents, myocardial infarctions, respiratory failure, and high-speed urban anxiety. In 1974, it was estimated that there were 65 million visits to metropolitan emergency departments in the United States.

These 65 million Americans had at least three things in common: 1) They all felt the need for urgent medical care; 2) they all sought it in a hospital emergency department; and 3) in each instance, a significant part of their care would be delivered by an emergency nurse.

Since 1978, the emergency department nurse has clearly emerged as a new breed of nursing specialist, who daily greets, assesses, triages, stabilizes, evaluates, initially treats, helps diagnose, therapizes, educates, transports, and waves goodbye to this amazing batch of patients. The evolution of this kind of nursing specialist has not been very easy. The wave of patient arrivals far antedated the existence of adequate training programs, political support for emergency nursing, or a body of literature dealing with the precise skills and knowledge necessary to perform this complicated new role. In responding to these needs for training, politics and appropriate literature, practicing emergency department nurses have, themselves, been the biggest single contributors—not universities, not nursing schools, not legislators, and not physicians.

Nedell Lanros' new book *Assessment & Intervention in Emergency Nursing* is a particularly good example of this kind of contribution. Ms. Lanros is from Portland, Oregon. In the early 1970s, I saw her and other Oregonian nurses at educational conferences throughout the Pacific Northwest. Like many emergency nurses, they were faced with the awful prospect of going to work each day to confront a great variety of acute medical problems, but without any prior formal training and without much nursing literature to read at night to prepare for the next day's onslaught. Like a few other emergency nurses in the United States confronted with this dilemma, Ms. Lanros and her peers realized that the only way out was to do something about it themselves.

That "something" in Oregon was the REN Program (Registered Emergency Nurse). In 1973, a group of emergency department nurses in the Portland area began to develop a formal educational program for practicing emergency nurses like themselves. Initially assisted by 1973-74 DHEW grant monies, the program has grown to a remarkable 108 hours of didactic and laboratory teaching specifically designed to solve the educational needs of this new branch of nursing.

Ms. Lanros has been the Educational Coordinator of the REN Program since its inception. Under her guidance and with her great energy, the program has now been presented in its entirety some 16 times in the Northwest. As it has evolved, the course syllabus material was gradually collated, edited, and compiled to form a manual of emergency nursing. In the past several years, Ms. Lanros, in addition to her responsibilities as course director, has taken on the burden of further developing the manual to become this readable and eminently useful textbook of emergency nursing.

Because of its origin as a practical course manual, *Assessment & Intervention in Emergency Nursing* is full of those "pearls" of nursing practice which rarely occur in printed form. Throughout Ms. Lanros' extensive writing, rewriting, editing, and amplifying, the book has acquired considerable depth and a perspective unique to the needs of the professional emergency nurse. My own favorite chapters are those on triage (for its development of the role and guidelines of nursing triage), physical assessment (for the unusually full analysis of vital signs and the nurses' role in pain management), respiratory emergencies, and the medical examiner. I think the reader will find numerous other areas of interest.

Educators will find the "Key Concepts" and "Review," which precede and follow each chapter respectively, a pleasant addition. Nursing instructors and in-service directors will find many of the chapters organized along didactic lecture outlines and, therefore, useful in preparing their own lesson plans. Nursing and other health profession students will find the material clearly developed and logically explained. Most of all, I think, professional nurses who spend their practice hours on the firing line of our nation's emergency departments will appreciate this unique contribution to the growing literature of their new specialty.

Howard L. Kirz, M.D.
Director, Medical Education
Group Health Cooperative of Puget Sound
Seattle, Washington

FOREWORD TO THE 2ND EDITION

The 2nd Edition of *Assessment & Intervention in Emergency Nursing* is a unique book that offers vital information for the effective diagnosis and treatment of emergency disorders; it is a succinct and understandable volume designed to quickly dispense clinical knowledge. But this book is more. The anatomic and physiologic orientation provides a crisp framework for understanding current medications and new concepts. The multidisciplinary and clinically-oriented approach makes this an important reference.

This volume is the linchpin for the movement of emergency nursing education in expanding the capability of emergency nurses in their role of assessment and intervention; as the interdisciplinary team approach has evolved in patient care, it has become apparent that the nursing function must and does extend beyond traditionally accepted boundaries.

To function with competency and confidence in these newer settings requires a broad foundation of clinical knowledge. These areas are emphasized in Ms. Lanros' contribution to emergency nursing literature. Moreover, the concise outline and organization, in conjunction with its accompanying workbook, make this two-volume offering an indispensable resource for those who plan to complete the certification examination in emergency nursing.

Ms. Lanros has developed a pragmatic resource consolidating a great deal of knowledge not found in standard reference; a major goal of this text is dispersal of this information in a form that is most readily available and useful to the working emergency nurse. The text offers a presentation of applied clinical knowledge to be assimilated and utilized not only in the setting of quiet armchair contemplation but in the very heat of battle as well. I do not know of a better source book for emergency nurses and other members of the emergency care team.

Finally, a description of this book and its outstanding contribution in the field of emergency nursing would not be complete without a mention of its author. Nedell Lanros' commitment to the development of emergency nursing as a specialty within her field is without peer. She is a stimulating lecturer and her involvement with emergency nursing, nationally and internationally, has planted seeds that will allow this increasingly important patient care specialty to realize its full potential.

Gideon Bosker, M.D.
Department of Emergency Medicine
Good Samaritan Hospital/Medical Center
Portland, Oregon

PREFACE

As this work goes into its 2nd edition, it is deeply rewarding to realize how many emergency nurses are utilizing it, not only on a day-to-day basis, but as a study guide and a source book for the national EDNA certified emergency nurse (CEN) examination. Experienced practitioners and beginners alike have found the key concepts and learning objectives outlined at the beginning of each chapter to be helpful in facilitating reader selection of appropriate study/ review areas; specific needs of all who are concerned with capable response and quality care are met. It has been extremely gratifying from an author's standpoint to hear such positive outcome and to realize that emergency nurses continue to grow and develop their full potential.

Emergency nurses in Oregon have been participating since 1974 in a statewide effort to educate and certify Registered Emergency Nurses (REN); this book is not only the outgrowth of that program but a resource in its continuation.

All those who participated so graciously in the beginning and shared their time, efforts, and knowledge with lecture presentations are acknowledged specifically at the start of each chapter; we have tried earnestly to credit all contributors and sources in this very large undertaking and express again our lasting gratitude to *all* who have participated and contributed in any way!

Again, we are most grateful for the steady backing by those who were initial motivating forces of the Oregon movement: Myra Lee, R.N., Joan Henkel, R.N., Sherry Heying, R.N., Terry Lepley Moldanado, R.N., Terry Gough Warrington, R.N., Joan Schlesky, R.N., Barbara Thompson, R.N., Ellie Herreid, R.N., Rita Lusby, E.N., Belle Slesh, R.N., Agnes Haugen, R.N., Diane Rushing, R.N., Alice Sumida, R.N., Ida Jesson, R.N., and Terry Lepley, R.N. A special acknowledgment is made to members of the Education Committee who spent long hours evaluating and providing constructive critique on course format and content including Myra Lee, R.N., Sherry Heying, R.N., Diane Rushing, R.N., and our special educational consultant, Sarah Rich, R.N.

With the publication of this expanded 2nd Edition and its companion, *Review Manual for Certification in Emergency Nursing,* emergency nurses will have access to a complete and comprehensive resource. Text and manual utilized in tandom offer a clear route to rounding out clinical "savvy" and competency, achieving certification in the process.

It is exciting to be in emergency nursing today; the challenge continues to beckon us and strengthens our belief that all emergency nurses should strive for certification through pursuit of expanded clinical knowledge and demonstrated competencies practicing with awareness, integrity, and accountability.

Nedell E. Lanros
Summer, 1982

SECTION I

ASSESSMENT AND TRIAGE

TRIAGE

1

KEY CONCEPTS

The key concepts of this chapter are to promote an understanding of various and versatile types of triage possible and the adaptability of the Triage Nurse System, as well as to outline the criteria required and advantages to be realized in developing a system suitable to the needs of each emergency department. Additionally, information is presented to reinforce guidelines needed for interhospital transfer of critical patients and aeromedical transport considerations and resources. Contributions on these topics are acknowledged from Belle Slesh, R.N., Sue Kelly, R.N., Donna Richardson, R.N. and Pat Roberg, R.N., all of Portland, Oregon.

After reading and studying this chapter, you should be able to:

- Define "triage."
- Describe the function of an emergency medical technician in prehospital triage.
- Outline the criteria for establishing a triage nurse system.
- List at least six purposes served by having a triage nurse.
- List at least six major advantages to the triage nurse system.
- Describe three well-recognized types of formal triage.
- Identify areas of highest priority, secondary priority, and caution indicators in trauma victims.
- Identify a reliable source of guidelines for critical patient evaluation and transfer.
- Outline the major checkpoints to be considered in interhospital patient transfer.
- Describe the major considerations specific to aeromedical transport of the critically ill or injured.
- Describe the safety precautions to be employed around helicopters.
- Define the origin and function of MAST units in aeromedical transport.

Traditionally the practice of medicine has been a contractual agreement between the physician and the patient, with the physician being the point of entry or access to the medical care system. Today, the patient can gain access to the system by way of the emergency department without prior physician contact.

Emergency departments (EDs) have been a distinguishable hospital entity for over 30 years. Although they were generally referred to as trauma centers, receiving wards, or ambulance entrances and functioned as such in varying degrees, they now emerge as fully staffed and equipped departments, many of which provide interdepartmental outpatient facilities and physicians' offices. There has been a good deal of criticism leveled at the ED for treating patients who do not require emergency care; however, few criteria have been developed to limit this practice. Difficult decisions are faced by hospital administrators when they find EDs serving needs traditionally met by the family physician and, consequently, many alternatives have been pondered and initiated. One of the best has been found to be the triage system.

Triage is a continuous and prominent process in the emergency scene today. Although the history of triage is vague in origin, it comes from a French word meaning "choice." Literally, it means to sort out, choose, or place a priority. Its use has come into vogue in recent years although it originally derived from application of the term during World War II battlefield sorting procedures in Europe. Military triage utilized a system of sorting the most viable casualties and giving them priority in care and evacuation to medical facilities. Today, in almost direct contrast to battlefield practice, the triage system is utilized to sort out those patients who are most seriously compromised in their struggle for life. The choosing, sorting out, and placing of priorities has been in practice since patient care began, but triage, as a systematic method to be employed by medical personnel in EDs, has come into its own in recent years only.

PREHOSPITAL TRIAGE

It is essential for the emergency department nurse (EDN) to be knowledgeable about both prehospital and inhospital triage and the importance of its role in the management of effective patient flow and continuity of care in EDs. Emergency medical services systems (EMSs) have been developed all over the United States, providing basic and advanced training for ambulance personnel, procurement and provision of up-to-date ambulances with all the necessary life-support equipment on board, communications equipment to facilitate ambulance to hospital transmissions, and EMS councils functioning in every designated region of every state. This has resulted in a new capability for ambulance personnel enabling them to deliver prehospital care with competence and assurance. Rapid assessment and field triage have become part of that competence. Emergency nurses need to understand and to appreciate the judgments that are called for in the field under unique circumstances, as compared to judgments made on the same patient once inside the ED.

The emergency medical technician (EMT) is taught during training that patients with certain conditions have priority over others and is expected to act accordingly. In the prehospital situation, leadership is the key and the EMT in charge at a given scene must take command, guide what is being done, and have the ability to utilize any help that arrives at the scene, simultaneously deciding how and in what order the ill or injured persons are to be transported to the nearest qualified medical facility. Examination will have determined which patients should be transported immediately and which can receive care at the scene and be allowed to wait. Judgment must also be made about the proper speed of the ambulance to be maintained with a particular patient in transport remembering that excessive speed is rarely necessary and is highly dangerous to both patient and rescuers.

The prehospital emergency care given by EMTs is one facet of the EMS system, and it cannot exist without the hospital ED; the roles of each within the system must be understood.

Disaster drills have become a regular part of EMS preparedness (another facet of the EMS system) and during these actual exercises, on-scene triage is usually carried out by an assigned medical officer or a team of medical officers. These medical officers would respond to actual disaster situations for the purpose of conducting as systematic a triage as possible, dispatching patients to appropriate hospital facilities. In the absence of assigned medical triage officers, the first ambulance EMTs on the scene would assume command responsibility.

INHOSPITAL TRIAGE

Once delivered to the hospital, the patient, optimally, should be able to expect a continuity of care based on an immediate evaluation performed by the nurse who receives him or her from the ambulance stretcher. This is where inhospital triage begins, as well as evaluations that are given patients who arrive by private car, in a wheelchair, or who simply walk into the department and present themselves with moderate distress.

The triage system employed will generally depend upon the size and capabilities of the hospital, the population catchment basin which the hospital serves, and the availability of trained and licensed personnel. Very large hospitals often triage patients directly to trauma units and clinics; medium-sized hospitals do their sorting within the hospital in much the same way routine admissions are categorically assigned. In the small hospital it is often the nurse who screens patients for physicians around the clock and assigns them accordingly.

A formal nurse triage system has many advantages when employed in a hospital of any size, some of which are as follows:

1. Early assessment of the seriously compromised patient
2. Immediate intervention in life-threatening situations
3. Expedition of care for the noncritical patient
4. Alleviating fear and decreasing anxiety and tension levels in patients, with marked benefit to the nursing staff as a result
5. Employment of the team concept

6. Most effective utilization of personnel
7. More effective follow-through on problems
8. Responsibility centered in one person for relating to families, friends, and the public
9. Expedition of requisitioning of preliminary diagnostic studies
10. More effective management resulting in smooth patient flow and traffic patterns.

CRITERIA FOR ESTABLISHING THE EDN TRIAGE SYSTEM

Many triage systems are basically those that have been developed within the individual EDs to meet their needs, while others may have evolved merely as a result of trial and error. As a consequence, there are all too few written systems available to study although there are, in general, certain criteria necessary for setting up an effective nurse triage system as follows:

An *organizational chart,* since triage by its very definition should be an orderly process, defines the functions of doctors, nurses, clerks, and ancillary personnel and places everyone in the appropriate area of responsibility;

A *job description* developed within the ED where the nurse is triaging, dependent on hospital policy as well as departmental identities, and hospital staffing patterns. Specific courses of action to be followed by the triage nurse must be in writing and should probably be included in the job description;

Ongoing *supervision and structured critiques* to provide a continuous check on the effectiveness of the system, with periodic reviews on performance and patient flow rates;

Physician support and participation, which is an essential component of the successful triage system;

Established and ongoing channels of *communication,* both interdepartmental and intradepartmental;

Adequate *orientation* to the responsibilities, policies, and procedures of triaging;

A *patient interview area* that will allow privacy and communication between nurse and patient to establish rapport and confidence and permit accurate evaluations;

Enough *qualified and willing EDNs* within the department to carry out the triage procedure as it is written.

Most EDs using a formal triage system have arrived at the conclusion that the triage person should be a nurse with responsibility for making rapid decisions based on a cursory but accurate assessment of each patient who presents, deciding who needs immediate intervention and where, and who can tolerate a short wait.

The triage nurse, then, becomes the patient's access to the medical care system as we know it today via the ED or outpatient clinic and must direct patient flow in the most expeditious and appropriate manner, utilizing staff and space as effectively as possible. It is self-evident that the position is demanding and one of extreme importance to both patient and staff, requiring a nurse with very special qualities.

Intelligence, the ability to relate to people, a capacity for calm and reasoned judgment in meeting emergencies, and an orientation toward service are essential attributes of the triage nurse, as well as everyone else function ing in the ED for that matter. Other obvious qualifications call for someone experienced in ED nursing and skilled in assessment techniques who can tolerate high stress levels while maintaining a working rapport with coworkers, medical staff, families, and the general public.

In summary, the triage nurse has the primary responsibility to improve patient care by early identification of emergency and urgent problems, early referral of conditions that can effectively be treated elsewhere, reassurance of patients and their families regarding their problems and interpretation of hospital and departmental policies and procedures to patients, their families, and the general public. The secondary and more specific duties of the triage nurse are to improve the quality of care in the department, expedite patient flow, and monitor the overall function of the department. The triage nurse will maintain an overview of the entire departmental situation, assign patients to appropriate treatment teams or areas, and will coordinate activities among clerical, nursing, medical, and laboratory services, expediting patient care, when appropriate, by initiation of preliminary diagnostic studies as allowed by departmental policy.

SOME APPROACHES TO ESTABLISHING A TRIAGE SYSTEM

Probably the most generally employed system is the relatively simple one that has been worked out individually by many moderately sized EDs to meet their own requirements. An excellent example of such a system can be found operating in a Portland, Oregon, hospital, which maintains a large ED as well as a family medical care unit (FMCU). The ED and FMCU function together in a closely related role as the ED handles all emergency and urgent cases while all nonurgent patients are triaged to the FMCU between the hours of 10 A.M. and 10 P.M. All patients presenting between 10 P.M. and 10 A.M. are seen in the ED with priority assigned as indicated.

The usual staffing pattern for this ED is three RNs and one emergency room technician (ERT) on days, three RNs and two ERTs on evenings, and two RNs and one ERT on nights. The department has around-the-clock immediate response on-call personnel from Respiratory Therapy, IV, ECG, Lab, and X-ray, as needed. There is one physician in the department at all times with an on-call roster of all specialty groups and a resident house staff. Generally the EDNs rotate turns at triaging, so that all of them maintain their skills. Consequently, one RN is at the desk triaging incoming patients while the other personnel function as teams in the patient care areas, providing organized, effective care.

Patients who are triaged at the desk and immediately sent to the FMCU are seen by RNs and a full-time staff of general care physicians. Those who qualify as clinic patients may be seen on a continued outpatient basis by the resident staff.

This system has the advantage of being able to provide a full scope of service around the clock to the general public as well as carrying out the wishes of the private physicians where their patients are concerned. It provides a growing and learning experience for each EDN in carrying the responsibility of triage as well as the satisfaction of hands-on patient care interspersed. Systems of this sort are entirely dependent on the physical layout of the department, the services it wishes to provide, and, of course, the availability of qualified personnel.

THE CLINICAL ALGORITHM

The *clinical algorithm* is a triage system being employed in very large hospitals, many of them government-operated and service-related. DeWitt Army Hospital currently employs what it calls a logical algorithmic alternative to a "nonsystem," as it was reported in the May/June issue of The ACEP Journal in 1973. A clinical algorithm is a set of "unambiguous step-by-step instructions for solving a clinical problem." Algorithms are designed to assist the performance of a specific task.

Medical officers at DeWitt have devised clinical algorithms for all types of presenting medical and surgical problems, and these algorithms permit sorting, designating, and assigning of priorities of problems of an entire walk-in patient population by minimally trained volunteers. These volunteers are given eight hours of training—three two-hour classes followed by two hours of on-the-job training—and then they are ready to follow the series of hard and fast *rules* as laid out in the algorithms, which are really substitutes for crash courses in recognition of serious medical problems (Figs. 1.1 and 1.2).

The accuracy of this system is incredibly high in degree and lends itself well to management of great volumes of patients, such as are seen in government-operated medical facilities. There has been an error rate, determined by chart audit, of less than 3% in most institutions where it has been employed.

THE NURSE/SCRIBE SYSTEM

The *nurse/scribe* system is another variation on the triage theme and has been implemented successfully in many large EDs, beginning in a Lansing, Michigan, hospital. This system basically employs four stages of patient care:

1. A *ward clerk* sees the patient and records information necessary for record-keeping and insurance, along with the chief complaint.
2. The *assessment* or *triage* nurse then takes the patient into the ED for a brief evaluation, which includes a short pertinent history, medical information, drugs currently being taken, date of last tetanus booster, and

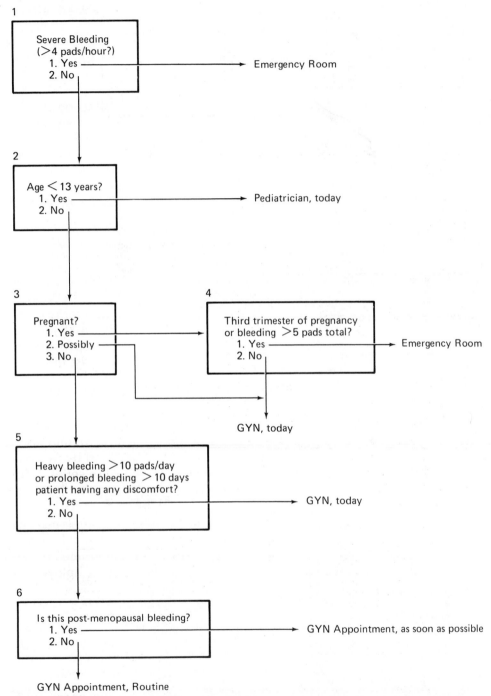

1

Severe Bleeding
(>4 pads/hour?)
  1. Yes ————————————————→ Emergency Room
  2. No

2

Age < 13 years?
  1. Yes ————————————————→ Pediatrician, today
  2. No

3

Pregnant?
  1. Yes
  2. Possibly
  3. No

4

Third trimester of pregnancy
or bleeding >5 pads total?
  1. Yes ————————————→ Emergency Room
  2. No

GYN, today

5

Heavy bleeding >10 pads/day
or prolonged bleeding > 10 days
patient having any discomfort?
  1. Yes ————————————————→ GYN, today
  2. No

6

Is this post-menopausal bleeding?
  1. Yes ————————————————→ GYN Appointment, as soon as possible
  2. No

GYN Appointment, Routine

Figure 1.1. Algorithm in use at DeWitt Army Hospital for vaginal bleeding. (Reprinted with permission of the Journal of the American College of Emergency Physicians. Vol 186, May/June 1973)

allergies. Complete vital signs are taken. The patient is prepped if necessary, gowned for examination if necessary, and equipment is readied for

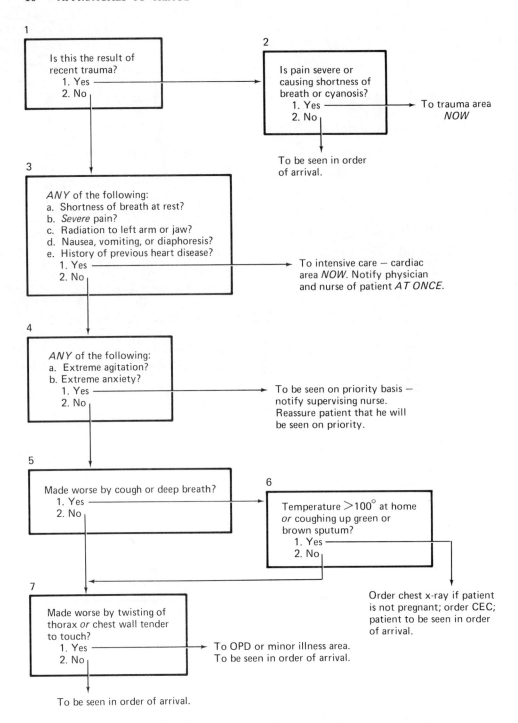

1

Is this the result of recent trauma?
1. Yes
2. No

2

Is pain severe or causing shortness of breath or cyanosis?
1. Yes ⟶ To trauma area *NOW*
2. No

To be seen in order of arrival.

3

ANY of the following:
a. Shortness of breath at rest?
b. *Severe* pain?
c. Radiation to left arm or jaw?
d. Nausea, vomiting, or diaphoresis?
e. History of previous heart disease?
1. Yes ⟶ To intensive care — cardiac area *NOW*. Notify physician and nurse of patient *AT ONCE.*
2. No

4

ANY of the following:
a. Extreme agitation?
b. Extreme anxiety?
1. Yes ⟶ To be seen on priority basis — notify supervising nurse. Reassure patient that he will be seen on priority.
2. No

5

Made worse by cough or deep breath?
1. Yes
2. No

6

Temperature >100° at home *or* coughing up green or brown sputum?
1. Yes
2. No

Order chest x-ray if patient is not pregnant; order CEC; patient to be seen in order of arrival.

7

Made worse by twisting of thorax *or* chest wall tender to touch?
1. Yes ⟶ To OPD or minor illness area. To be seen in order of arrival.
2. No

To be seen in order of arrival.

Figure 1.2. Algorithm for use by an emergency medical technician in management of patient with chest pain. (Reprinted with permission of the Journal of the American College of Emergency Physicians. Vol 186, May/June 1973)

the doctor. The triage nurse then places the concise and legible record of the patient in order of priority on the physician's desk.

3. The *physician* and *nurse/scribe team* review the chart on their way to see the patient. As the physician examines the patient, the nurse/scribe records what he dictates to her regarding positive and negative signs. She writes the appropriate requisitions and prescriptions, which are then presented to the physician for signature.

4. The completed patient record is given to the *medication/discharge* nurse who then administers the necessary medications and/or treatments, explains the instructions for follow-up care to the patient, and completes the discharge procedure.

Some of the many advantages of the nurse/scribe system are:

1. Increased efficiency by organizing patient flow in an orderly manner

2. Inherent educational advantage as the scribe quickly becomes familiar with the physical examination (PE) process, therefore, the scribe role should be rotated.

3. The patient is made aware of physical findings so that follow-up care instructions are documented and clarified before discharge.

4. Charts are completed on the spot in concise legible format. Much pertinent patient information is included that might have been forgotten if time lapse was allowed between examination and completion of the chart.

Implementation of this system requires significant adjustment in the ED by both physicians and nurses. Most have found the team approach is quickly accepted as soon as the patient-flow pattern is established and the ED staff realizes the many advantages and increased productivity of the system. Once adopted, it can improve patient care, further educate nursing personnel, and enable the ED staff to function as a more efficient team.

CONCLUSION

Regardless of hospital size, the development of a triage system to meet specific patient flow needs will have a significant impact on expediting patient care and insuring a higher quality of response from members of the ED staff, with a built-in reassurance to the patient and his family by way of thoughtful and rapidly responsive attention. It is a boon, as well, to efficient use of personnel and certainly well worth the effort involved in developing a system suitable to the department and establishing it officially as departmental policy.

DETERMINING PRIORITIES IN TREATMENT

Problem areas in emergency patient care need to be classified in order to be handled effectively and whether or not an ED utilizes triage as a system, nursing personnel must deal with the whole spectrum of walk-in and wheel-in patients who present with widely varying problems and complaints at any hour of the day or night. Some definitions and relative categorizations have evolved and are generally accepted by most medical personnel who function in the area of emergency care.

These categories provide reliable guidelines for problem management, by and large, although there are certainly exceptions which may crop up and must be dealt with according to priority evaluation. Following are some of the general categorizations which provide triage ground rules.

Emergent

A condition requiring immediate medical attention; time delay would be harmful to the patient; disorder is acute and potentially threatening to life or function. Highest priority is given to these conditions:

- Airway and breathing difficulties
- Cardiac arrest
- Chest pain and acute dyspnea and/or cyanosis
- Seizure states
- Uncontrolled or suspected severe bleeding
- Severe head injuries and/or comatose state
- Severe medical problems, i.e., poisoning, overdose, cardiacs, diabetic complications, etc.
- Open chest or abdominal wounds
- Severe shock
- Obvious multiple injuries
- Excessively high temperature (over 105° F or 40.5° C)
- Emergency childbirth, complications of pregnancy, hemorrhage, or indications of eclampsia

Urgent

A condition requiring medical attention within the period of a few hours; a possible danger exists to the patient if medically unattended. Second priority is given to these conditions:

- Chest pain associated with URI
- Burns
- Major multiple fractures
- Dulled or obtunded level of consciousness (LOC)
- Back injuries with/without spinal cord damage
- Persistent nausea and vomiting and/or diarrhea
- Severe pain
- Temperature of 102° to 105° F or 39° to 40.5° C
- Acute panic states, drug overuse, apparent or suspected poisoning

Nonemergent

A condition which does not require the resources of an ED or emergency service; referral for routine medical care may or may not be needed; disorder is nonacute or minor in severity. Lowest priority is given to conditions such as:

- Chronic backache
- Moderate headache
- Minor fractures or other injuries of a minor nature
- Obviously mortal wounds where death appears reasonably certain (rarely followed criterion)
- Obviously dead (DOA)

EMTs are also taught these orders of priority in their basic training program and follow these guidelines in triaging, loading, and transporting patients to hospital facilities.

TRAUMA VICTIM PRIORITIES

Trauma victims present with some special considerations to which the triage nurse must be alert, and a relative urgency exists with the following associated problems:

1. Progressively increasing respiratory difficulty
2. Incipient shock with progression to be anticipated
3. Rising CVP and decreasing pulse pressure
4. Rapidly deteriorating LOC or sudden coma following lucid period
5. Airway or chest wall problems
6. Sudden hypotension with possibility of occult bleeding
7. Penetrating wounds of chest, abdomen, or head

"RED FLAGS"

There are many danger signals and circumstances that may contribute heavily to disastrous deterioration of a traumatized patient. They are referred to variously as "red flags," "caution indicators," and "axioms" for management. Regardless of what you call them, they are signs of, or contributing circumstances to, serious problems in management of that patient and must be recognized by those observing baselines. They* include but are not limited to:

- Motor vehicle accidents (MVAs) over 35 mph (carry a high probability of ruptured thoracic aorta)
- Forces of deceleration as in falls, explosions, etc.

---

*Any one of these criteria should generally be considered an indication for mandatory admission of the patient for further close observation and intervention if necessary or immediate stabilization and transfer to a larger or more sophisticated facility.

- Loss of consciousness after accident
- Vehement denial of obviously serious injuries with flighty thought and speech patterns and occasionally inappropriate responses
- Chest or abdominal pain after injury
- Fracture of the 1st or 2nd rib (associated with high mortality)
- Fracture of 9th, 10th, 11th ribs or more than three ribs
- Possible aspiration
- Possible extensive lung tissue contusions
- Possible cervical spine trauma in patient with head injury
- Pulse rate over 120/min at rest

In the management of trauma victims the rule of thumb must *always* be to manage as though the most serious problem exists and *be prepared to cope* with it until either treated effectively or ruled out.

INTERHOSPITAL TRANSFER OF PATIENTS

As capabilities for improved initial assessment and stabilization have developed significantly over recent years with the advent of EMS systems, highly trained prehospital personnel, and better standards for patient care, emergency physicians and nurses now have the added responsibility of evaluating, stabilizing, and arranging transfer for critical patients who cannot be managed in the receiving facility.

Although the true emergencies (multiple trauma, severe head injuries, cardiorespiratory problems, burns, shock, etc.) account for a relatively small percentage of patients seen in EDs, these patients frequently have injuries of such multiplicity or life threatening problems of such magnitude that transfer to a larger or more sophisticated facility is in the patient's best interest.

Emergency physicians and, occasionally, nurses find themselves in the position of having to make these determinations. In many areas they are able to follow established transfer patterns; states which have achieved categorization of their hospitals are able to provide resource references to physicians and hospitals when transfer questions arise.

AMERICAN COLLEGE OF SURGEONS STANDARDS FOR TRANSFER*

Through the 1970s the only established standards for advanced life support were those of the American Heart Association; now in the 1980s we have the most welcome standards for Advanced Trauma Life Support (ATLS) which have been developed and disseminated by the American College of Surgeons (ACS) Committee on Trauma. At long last, established guidelines are laid out

---

*Adapted from ATLS Course Manual, Bulletin, ACS, Appendix C-1, pp 195-6, 1980

clearly for patient management in trauma during the initial phase of care. Accompanying the manual on ATLS is a Hospital Resource Document which includes appendices on both interhospital transfer and air ambulance operations, among other things. Appendix C-1 of this document, dealing with interhospital transfer, suggests some long overdue guidelines to be followed which provide for determination of responsibility, accountability, feedback, and documentation.

Checkpoints for Patient Transfer

The following checkpoints are described in the ATLS appendix for patient transfer*:

1. Arrangements for transfer should be by way of direct communication between the referring physician and the receiving physician. Ordinarily this is not relegated to a nurse but if no physician is immediately available in a rural area the responsibility *may* fall to the emergency nurse.

2. The *receiving physician is responsible* for arrangements and details of the transfer, including transportation. The referring physician must oversee details of transfer to ensure optimal management of the patient and should obtain approval for use of local ambulance transport from the receiving physician, unless aeromedical transport is to be employed from the receiving hospital.

3. The patient must be transported with equipment and trained personnel appropriate to his life support needs.

4. The transferring physician should carefully instruct the transfer personnel. Specific instructions on condition and needs during transfer should include, but are not limited to:
   A. Airway management
   B. Fluid volume replacement
   C. Any other special procedures indicated

5. A copy of the written record including the problem, treatment given and status at time of discharge for transfer *must* accompany the patient and should include:
   A. Patient identification, address and next of kin *with* phone numbers
   B. History of injury or illness
   C. Condition on admission
   D. Vital signs from pre-hospital evaluation, during care in ED, and at time of transfer (baseline information)
   E. All treatment given, including medications *with* routes of administration
   F. Laboratory and x-ray findings *including copies of films*
   G. Fluids given by type and volume
   H. Name, address and phone number of referring physician

---

*Adapted from ATLS Course Manual, Bulletin, ACS, Appendix C-1, pp 195-6, 1980

I. Name of physician and hospital to whom patient is being transferred and name of physician at receiving institution who has been contacted for transfer (responsible physician)

J. Management of patient during transport with vital signs, medications, fluids, etc. well documented

Transfer forms and suggested transfer agreement forms have been developed by ACS and further information should be obtained regarding their use and/or availability by contacting the American College of Surgeons, 55 E. Erie Street, Chicago, Illinois 60611.

AEROMEDICAL TRANSPORT

With increasing emphasis being placed on careful evaluation and transfer of patients to institutions which can, minimally, provide safe and effective care for the illness or injury under treatment, the capability for air transport has steadily developed across our country. Although air ambulances have been in operation for many years, mostly of the fixed wing type, they are becoming more sophisticated in equipment and patient care capabilities as each day passes. The advent of medi-evac helicopters with their great versatility has made possible a whole new capability in responding to the needs of critical patients everywhere. Cadres of extremely capable and highly trained flight nurses, paramedics and military pararescuemen (P.J.'s as they are affectionately known) have been developed to meet the needs of patients facing catastrophic illness or injury who require aeromedical evacuation from remote areas and/or smaller community hospitals to larger medical facilities; this in itself opens up a whole new field of interest, responsibility and challenge for emergency nurses preparing patients for transport, accompanying them in flight, or receiving them in critical condition from a heliport or landing strip.

Considerations Specific to Flight

Altitude and Other Factors. A real understanding of the effects of altitude on human physiology is essential in order to knowledgeably prepare a patient for air transport. Careful and adequate preparation on the ground *before* transport can forestall many detrimental and even irreversible adverse effects; intelligent pre-flight assessment and careful attention to otherwise seemingly unimportant details is required when air transfer is being anticipated. Flight personnel arriving to evacuate a critical patient not infrequently have to spend precious minutes rearranging poorly prepared lines, catheters, splints, MAST garments, etc. They will be impressed with your interest and expertise when the patient is "ready to fly." It goes without saying that a great deal of personal satisfaction is gained knowing we have contributed to an expeditious, safe, and efficient patient transfer.

Some significant points to be aware of include the effects of high altitude on oxygen concentration of inspired air, barometric pressure, humidity, temperature, drug potentiation and factors such as noise levels, nausea, G Forces, and the fatigue which results as the sum total of all the stresses involved.

More specifically, let's look closely at each area concerned which results from an increase in altitude.*

1. The partial pressures of atmospheric gases will decrease since barometric pressure (the total pressure of all gases in the air) decreases with increases in altitude. Therefore the amount of inspired oxygen will *decrease* relative to altitude increases.

    A PaO_2 of 100 mmHg at sea level (barometric pressure of 760 mmHg) will decrease to 81 mmHg at 5,000 ft, 61 mmHg at 11,000 ft, and 45 mmHg at 15,000 ft. We seldom need to be concerned with transport altitudes greater than these without the patient being cared for in a well-pressurized cabin where PaO_2 is more normally maintained.

    Flight considerations relating to this *decrease* in PaO_2 include:

    A. ABGs should be done prior to interhospital transfer (if appropriate to patient's condition);
    B. A patient with a hemoglobin of less than 7 Gm should be transfused prior to flight, depending on necessary flight altitude;
    C. Depending on the amount of oxygen the patient will require, determine method of delivery that is adequate (masks that deliver a FiO_2 of near 100% should be available in flight);
    D. Oxygen should be administered to:
        *   *All* patients at altitudes over 5,000 feet
        *   *All* cardiac patients
        *   *All* patients in shock or impending shock
        *   *All* eye injuries (the retina has the highest oxygen need of all body tissue)
        *   *All* head injuries (decreased PaO_2 and a resulting rise in PCO_2 will result in cerebral vasodilation and an increased intracranial pressure);
    E. Suspect hypoxia if anything untoward develops or condition deteriorates;
    F. Obtain good baseline information prior to transport so that LOC and neurological and emotional status changes will be more apparent in your assessment.

2. Altitude increases cause an inversely proportional decrease in barometric pressure (Boyle's law). A mass of gas will expand as altitude increases; a gas volume of 1.0 at sea level will expand to 1.4 at 8,000 ft and 2.1 at 18,000 ft.

    Flight considerations relating to this increase in gas volume include:

    A. *Pneumothorax.* The amount of collapse will increase; this must be evacuated as much as possible prior to transport and during flight, decompression equipment must be available (large gauge angio's, McSwain darts, Heimlich valves, etc.);

---

*Adapted from "Air Transport and the Effects of Altitude," *Emergency Highlights* 1:4 October 1980, compiled and prepared by Pat Robert, RN, Chief Flight Nurse, Emanuel Hospital Life Flight, Portland, Oregon.

B. *Bowel obstruction.* A N/G tube must be placed and kept open to drainage; a danger exists if trapped gas exists within the intestine.

C. *Skull fractures.* X-rays must be checked for presence of free air.

D. *Congested Sinuses.* These patients require slow ascent and descent.

E. *Plugged middle ear.* Have patient awake on descent and instruct to swallow, yawn, tense muscles in throat or perform Valsalva's maneuver (close mouth, pinch nostrils closed, and attempt to blow through nose). Infants and very small children who cannot be instructed should be given a plugged nipple to activate the swallowing response;

F. *Bends.* Nitrogen bubbles present in the blood and extravascular spaces will enlarge with altitude; this patient must be flown under 500 feet, if at all possible;

G. *Blood Pressure.* It is common for BP to decrease slightly as partial pressures of gases decrease;

H. *Airsplints.* Caution must be taken to decrease air volume within splints at altitude and to *closely* reassess the neurovascular status regularly.

I. *MAST garment.* Minimum inflation should be used prior to altitude; the zipper type are not made with pop-off capabilities;

J. *Colostomy.* Gas expansion stimulates GI motility and will cause a greater discharge;

K. *IV bottles.* Air present in the bottle will affect the drip rate so, if possible, change to plastic IV bag. Blood pumps or a Holter pump may be needed; a BP cuff will do in a pinch. The IV will run best with drip chamber at least one-half full;

L. *Stomach contents (gas/secretions).* A N/G tube may be required for safety with the unconscious patient.

3. Humidity will decrease as atmospheric pressure decreases and after an hour at altitude, the relative humidity may get down to less than 0.5 percent. Flight considerations relating to this decrease in humidity include:

A. The intubated patient should have nebulized humidified oxygen during transport;

B. E/T tubes are apt to plug more easily (especially in pediatric patients with small tubes) and should have periodic sterile saline instilled in small amounts);

C. Corneas will dry to air more readily; comatose patients may need liquid tears;

D. Contact lenses may become a problem with drying to cornea.

4. Some drugs are potentiated by altitude.

A. CNS depressants are affected;

B. Antihistamines tend to make the patient more susceptible to hypoxia;

C. Morphine and valium have greater side effects; small incremental doses should be given;

D. Alcohol renders a patient more susceptible to disorientation and hypoxia.

5. Temperature decreases as barometric pressure and humidity decrease; chill factors during winter must also be kept in mind for transport preparation. Patients should be kept warm with mummy wraps with warmed blankets or sleeping bag wraps with velcro closures; hot packs should be available in flight for auxiliary use.

6. Nausea may develop with altitude increases. Some flight considerations which may prove helpful include:

   A. Administration of low flow oxygen (1-2 L unless patient is already receiving oxygen) will frequently help counteract the nausea;

   B. A N/G tube may relieve pressure of gas in stomach and prevent risk of vomiting and aspiration (gravity drainage or intermittent low suction). Always make certain the tube is patent and working;

   C. A strong portable suction source must *always* be available and ready;

   D. Wire cutters should be available for release of repaired jaw fractures if heavy emesis should occur;

   E. Nausea may be diminished or prevented by pre-flight talk with patient to help alleviate fear and anxiety;

   F. Well-accepted antiemetics to be used are Phenergan (promethazine), Compazine (prochlorperazine), Tigan (trimethobenzamide), or Vistaril (hydroxyzine) which also has strong anti-anxiety and anti-spasmodic properties. Dramamine appears to be more effective for sea sickness than altitude sickness.

Other factors which require specific consideration in patient air transport include aircraft vibrations, increases in the noise level, and G Forces on takeoff.

7. Vibrations over a period of time in flight (especially in helicopters) may cause clamps, fittings, screws, and bolts on lines and equipment to loosen; therefore, continual routine checks for patent intact lines, accurate flow rates, and various adjustments are necessary.

8. There will also be an increased noise level in helicopter transport and the following flight consideratins must be observed:

   A. Ear protection is needed for patient and crew (eye pads may be used for infants and small children's ears);

   B. Breath sounds should be checked immediately prior to takeoff and after landing; in infants a doppler may be used for hearing breath sounds. Palpate for adventitious breath sounds. Mark PMI.

   C. Palpate BP or use doppler. Flush method is effective for infants;

   D. Utilize other senses of sight and touch; palpate abdomen for respiratory movement, observe rise and fall of chest, use of accessory muscles, deflations of O_2 reservoir bag, feel over E/T tube for tidal volume force, etc.

9. Problems with G Forces are present in takeoff, although usually not greater than G Force of 1 G. In fixed-wing aircraft transport, the patient should be loaded with feet toward the cockpit and head of stretcher elevated 30 degrees. Positioning the patient in this way accomplishes

several things, e.g., absorption of G Forces through the hip area, prevention of additional increased ICP, and prevention of stagnant hypoxia with
blood rushing toward the feet.

The bottom line consideration as a sum total of all the factors involved in
altitude transport is *fatigue*, which of course increases in illness with lack of rest
and poor or impaired nutrition. This additional bolus of stress for a patient who
is already compromised by trauma or illness takes a significant toll; the
emergency nurse can effectively help in its reduction by knowledgeably preparing the patient for a safer and more comfortable transfer to the next
caring facility.

In many instances the emergency nurse from the small hospital winds up
going along with the critical patient when staffed air ambulances are not available and, generally, on very short notice. It is best, then, to be forearmed with
basic awareness of when air transport involves, both for patient *and* nurse.

SAFETY PRECAUTIONS AROUND HELICOPTERS

Personnel operating in and around helicopters must follow some very real
safety precautions in order to avoid injury to themselves, others, and even the
helicopter. Every hospital ED with a receiving helipad *should* have written
policies and protocols concerning conduct in and around helicopters, with
specific orientation to this area of operation for all department members.
Paramedics, EMTs, nurses, Search and Rescue personnel, firemen, police, and
anyone else participating in rescue and loading efforts with helicopter evacuation in areas other than designated landing pads are at real risk unless made
aware of the important safety rules, which apply generally to *all* activity around
this equipment.

Stated very simply they are:

1. Observe extreme caution during and after the helicopter landing;

2. Approach the helicopter only if necessary, and then only when escorted
   by a crew member or receiving a "thumbs up" signal from the crew;

3. The tail rotor is extremely dangerous; it is practically invisible while the
   engine is running. NEVER APPROACH THE TAIL;

4. Approach or leave the helicopter in the pilot's field of vision, within the
   45 degree angle, as indicated in Figure 1.3;

5. The main rotor blades may droop as low as 5 feet, therefore, *always*
   approach keeping the head down (Fig. 1.4);

6. Always approach and leave DOWNHILL on sloping ground—NEVER UP-
   HILL (Fig. 1.5);

7. If terrain is difficult, wait until skid (landing foot) is firmly on ground and
   pilot signals "OK to Board," as in "thumbs up" (Fig. 1.6);

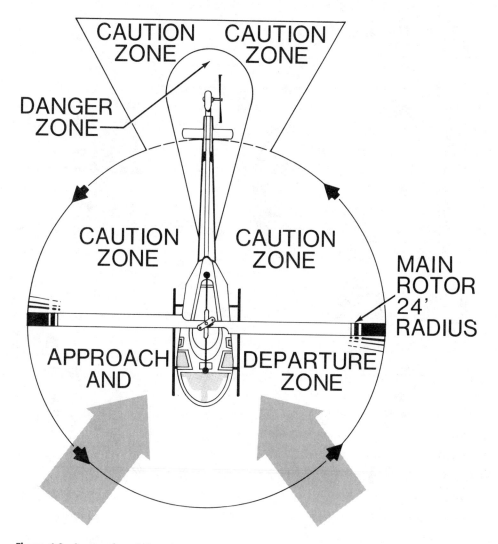

Figure 1.3. Approach and departure zone.

8. Before approaching helicopter with the stretcher, be *certain* that there are no loose objects to be caught up by the tremendous downward and outward rotor wash. Observe the following points:

A. Remove nursing caps and dangling items around neck (stethoscopes)

B. Remove sheet from stretcher pad

C. Tape or tie down stretcher pad

D. Anchor ALL loose items wherever possible

Mishaps happen *very* quickly when downdrafts blow items into the air; main rotor props have been damaged severely when sheets and blankets are swept into their arc and wrapped around the operating mechanisms.

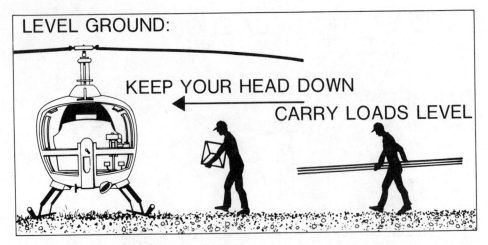

Figure 1.4. Approaching on level ground.

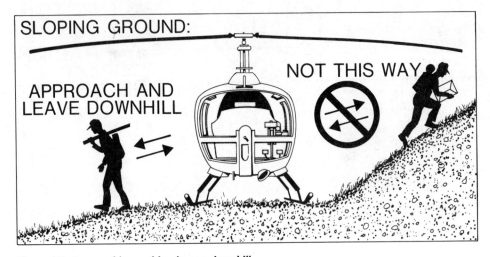

Figure 1.5. Approaching and leaving on downhill.

MAST PROGRAM

Many medical facilities around the country enjoy the support and participation of personnel and equipment from the Military Assistance to Safety and Traffic (MAST) program. In 1970, with the original legislation, and again in 1973 with legislative expansion of MAST, military personnel and aircraft were made available to assist the civilian sector with serious medical emergencies *when other resources could not respond.*

The crews of these aircraft include pararescuemen who are trained in all aspects of rescue as well as emergency medical response. As members of the military, they function under orders issued by their own surgeon general and are subject to Federal regulation in their activities rather than state/county EMS and EMT standards. They are highly trained and have become an

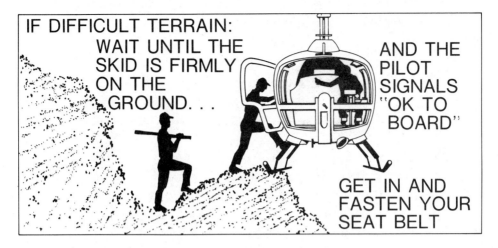

Figure 1.6. Approaching on difficult terrain.

extremely valuable addition to the prehospital and intra-hospital management of critical patients. Because MAST operations are subject to strict rules
and regulations, their participation in medical emergencies must be activated
by someone authorized to do so, acting in their official capacity.

Requests for MAST missions can be originated by law enforcement agencies, state emergency services, physicians, or others in various official federal
capacities. Those requesting MAST participation in medical emergencies must
be ready to provide the following information, at a minimum:

1. Name of party initiating request
2. Nature of request—patient transport, blood or tissue transport, etc.
3. Location
4. If patient transport, name of patient
5. Nature of emergency and patient condition
6. Destination of patient (place and hospital name)
7. Weather conditions and visibility
8. *Call back number*

Make-shift landing sites should be 100 feet in diameter, although a 60 foot
diameter can be used in real emergencies, and should be clear of trees, wires,
etc. Night landings will require some sort of perimeter illumination for the
pilot's assistance; flares or bright flashlights will work, or car headlights pointed
away from the area so that the pilot is not blinded on descent.

MAST units in most areas participate in civilian Search and Rescue (SAR)
activities as well, with some aircraft having hoist capability enabling victim
recovery from water, high peaks, crevasses, etc. Accident victims recovered in
this manner are fortunate to have pararescuemen on the spot giving medical
support.

MAST units benefit from civilian interest and support; they welcome participation in their Civilian Coordinating Councils. All emergency personnel are
encouraged to investigate the activities of their local MAST units, if fortunate

enough to have one, and extend support in whatever way is appropriate to current needs.

REVIEW

1. Give the origin and meaning of the term *triage*.
2. Explain who is in charge at an accident scene, with the responsibility for triaging and transporting multiple victims.
3. Outline at least six criteria for establishing a triage nurse system.
4. List at least six purposes served by having a triage nurse.
5. Name some major advantages of utilizing the triage nurse system.
6. Define an *algorithm*.
7. According to the algorithm given in Figure 1.1, describe the disposition of a pregnant woman in the third trimester with bleeding of less than five saturated pads (total).
8. List at least six conditions which EMTs are taught to accord the highest priority.
9. Define an *emergent* problem and give five examples.
10. Define an *urgent* problem and give five examples.
11. List at least six caution indicators that should be looked for in the traumatized patient.
12. Identify the origin of the ATLS standards and describe the guidelines included which relate to transfer of critical patients.
13. List five major checkpoints to be considered in interhospital transfer.
14. Identify at least eight areas of specific consideration which the EDN should be aware of when preparing a patient for aeromedical transfer.
15. Describe the key safety precautions to be observed around helicopters.
16. Describe a MAST unit's function and capabilities and the circumstances under which one would be employed.

BIBLIOGRAPHY

Barber JM, Dillman PA: Emergency Patient Care. Reston Publishing Co., Reston, Virginia, 1981

Committee on Injuries, American Academy of Orthopedic Surgeons: Emergency Care and Transportation of the Sick and Injured, 3rd ed. Banto Co., Inc., Chicago, Illinois, 1981

Mills J, Webster AL, Wofsy CB, et al: Effectiveness of nurse triage in the emergency department of an urban county hospital. JACEP, Vol 5, No 11, 1976

Roberg P: Air transport and the effects of altitude. Emergency Highlights Vol 1, No 4, Portland, Emanuel Hospital Life Flight, October 1980

Shields J: Making triage work: The experience of an urban emergency department. JACEP Vol 5, No 11, pp 37-41, 1976

Sley LE, Riskin WG: Algorithm: Directed triage in an emergency department. JACEP Vol 5, No 11, 1976

Triage. JACEP Vol 2, pp 185-186, 1973

Vickery DM: Triage: Problem-Oriented Sorting of Patients. The Robert J. Brady Co., Bowie, Maryland, 1975

Warner C: Emergency Care. C.V. Mosby Co., St. Louis, Missouri, 1978

Witt R, Haedtler D: Nurse-scribe system saves time in emergency department. JEN, January/February 1975

PATIENT ASSESSMENT AND VITAL SIGNS 2

KEY CONCEPTS

This chapter provides an overview of the essential steps in obtaining a thorough and accurate clinical nursing assessment of the patient presenting to the emergency department and to promote an understanding of the techniques involved.

After reading and studying this chapter, you should be able to:

- Discuss the importance of an accurate initial assessment.
- Identify some of the problems that are frequently encountered in the initial assessment.
- Describe the mental checklist of areas to be covered on initial inspection.
- Describe the areas to be checked in general assessment.
- Describe the proper techniques for taking temperature, pulse, and respirations and specify some significant variations in pulse rates and characteristics.
- Describe the proper placement of a blood pressure cuff and the techniques that will provide greater intensity of sound.
- Identify the onset and disappearance of arterial sounds and the five phases of sound that are heard.
- Describe the significance of a narrowing pulse pressure and tachycardia in a potential shock candidate.
- Explain the value of obtaining orthostatic vital signs and the criteria applied for significant findings.
- Describe the most effective means of establishing the LOC.
- Explain the components of pain and the factors generally affecting pain.
- Describe the Theory of Specificity and the Gate Control Theory of pain.
- Explain the physiological reactions to pain.
- Describe the recognition and intervention for dealing with anxiety.
- Identify the ways in which the EDN can help in the relief of pain.

INITIAL ASSESSMENT

The initial clinical assessment of the patient who presents to the ED is one of the most important responsibilities of the EDN and frequently exerts a significant influence on the quality of care that the patient receives subsequently. A perceptive EDN is in a key position to recognize physical manifestations of problems that might otherwise be overlooked in a busy department. This initial assessment is essential to evaluate the patient and effectively triage him or her to the appropriate area for treatment, following which there must be further evaluation to determine the diagnosis and institute effective treatment.

Many problems can be encountered with the initial patient assessment. The most important component of effective assessment is the *nurse* who deals with the patient. A nurse without empathy will be unable to adequately and accurately assess the patient and establish the initial working rapport that is so vital to allaying apprehension, stemming anxiety, and building trust in the surroundings. It is extremely important for the EDN to remember that *everything is relative;* this has particular application when attempting to correlate subjective and objective findings in a given situation. Experienced nurses know that what might appear insignificant to the observer may have marked significance to the one being observed.

The nurse is a professional who must demonstrate that status by taking unpleasant situations in stride with the full realization that sick people very often manifest hostility, resentment, anger, and—most frequently—impatience at what is being done (or not done) for them. Frequently, the challenge in emergency nursing is to receive the hostile patient with a calm, warm, and reassuring manner while proceeding quietly and methodically with observations and easy lines of questioning, exhibiting an interest in the patient's comfort and well-being.

Time constraints often hamper efforts to obtain as complete an initial assessment as one would wish ideally in the busy ED. However, the interested and perceptive nurse will learn to obtain key information in a limited period of time and couple it with experienced observations.

The initial steps of assessment of every patient coming to the ED should be based on a mental checklist of observations as follows:

Airway

What is the respiratory status? Is the patient breathing freely and easily? *If not, clear and maintain airway and support respirations as necessary.*

Cardiovascular Status

Do circulation and perfusion appear adequate? *If not, evaluate for CPR.* Is he bleeding heavily? *If so, attempt to control bleeding by direct pressure, arterial pressure points or, as last resort, tourniquet to prevent exsanguination.*

Does he appear to be in shock? *If so, initiate shock position (elevate lower extremities) and large-bore IV line immediately.*

Are there any signs of trauma with the associated possibility of occult bleeding? *If so, exercise special care as precaution against further damage and subsequent bleeding.* (Align and immobilize fractures, etc.)

Level of Consciousness (LOC)

Is he conscious, responsive, and well-oriented as to name, place, and time? *If not, detain and question whoever accompanied the patient.*

Two essential elements to an accurate evaluation in this initial assessment are privacy and good light. Without both, the initial inspection may well fall short of its full yield; good light is essential to determine abnormalities of color, the state of cleanliness, and the condition of the skin and peripheral circulation. It is hoped, too, that the EDN always remains aware of the patient's anxieties and need for privacy with every effort made to provide the position of comfort, a warm blanket, and reassurance while proceeding with the evaluation and vital signs. Frequently, it is helpful to imagine yourself as the patient and anticipate the patient's needs accordingly.

GENERAL ASSESSMENT

In the absence of life-threatening priorities, a general assessment should be carried out in a *systematic* fashion with the following specific areas included in the nurse's general survey of the patient.

General State of Consciousness

Do not confuse the LOC with apprehension or a language barrier. Be very certain that your patient can *hear* you. Use appropriate questions as necessary to elicit response: "Who are you?" "Where are you?" "What is the date, time of day, or season?"

Restlessness

Is the patient developing hypoxemia and restlessness?

Abnormalties of Color

Is there cyanosis, jaundice, pallor, or redness?

Degree of Cooperation

Has the patient been brought to the ED against his will? Is he overcooperative, looking for a disability evaluation or drugs? Is he looking for relief of truly distressing symptoms?

Personal Habits

Observe the state of cleanliness and any deterioration in grooming. Look especially for any variation of the apparent norm. Example: Well-clothed, poorly groomed man or woman obviously neglecting personal hygiene.

State of Nutrition

Note the obese person or the intensely thin person.

Signs of Chronic Illness

Subtle changes such as dull, waxy appearance to face and skin and poor tissue turgor.

Body Size and Shape

Note if grossly larger or smaller than normal.

Posture

Circulatory disease may cause struggle for breath when patient is sitting propped up or is straining forward. Local muscular injuries or pain may cause position which will splint against the pain or reduce its intensity. Example: Patient with fractured rib trying to breathe normally.

Gait

Abnormal gait may be manifestation of CNS involvement. Foot drag, shuffle, limp, scissors gait, steppage gait (raising feet unusually high and planting them down), small-steps gait may be signs.

Speech

It is important to note how the patient says what he says; for example, slurred speech, aphagia, gestures, nods, etc., may indicate vocal cord paralysis or CNS damage.

Odors

Breath: Acetone, ethyl alcohol (ETOH), hydrocyanic acid (resembling bitter almond)

Sputum: Foul sputum emanates from lung abcess or bronchiectasis

Vomitus: Alcohol, phenol; sour smell if fermenting food is retained too long; fecal odor with prolonged violent vomiting from bowel obstruction or peritonitis

Feces: Particularly foul smell is common in pancreatic insufficiency

Urine: Ammonia odor indicates fermentation within the bladder

Pus: Nauseatingly sweet odor is strong indication of pocket of gas gangrene

Skin Lesions

Local skin changes should be noted and described accurately.

Macule: A localized discolored spot on the skin that is not elevated above the surface

Papule: A small circumscribed, superficial, solid elevation of the skin (less than 0.5 cm in diameter)*

Nodule: A small elevated node or area of skin which is solid and can be detected by touch (0.5—1.5 cm in diameter)

Tumor: A morbid enlarged and raised area of skin usually greater than 2.5 cm in diameter

Vesicle: A small blister less than 1 cm in diameter

Bulla: A large vesicle usually 2 cm or more in diameter

Local infection or trauma will often change these primary lesions as described into scale, exudate of serum, blood or pus (which dries and forms a scab), ulcers, hyperpigmentation along the margin of the lesion, and signs of excoriation with varying degrees of healing. It is important to note and *document* the presence of lesions and exudate and to exercise *precautionary techniques* from the outset.

Edema

Presence and character—localized, generalized, dependent, pitting?

Beyond these specific areas of observation the physical examination will, of course, vary with the needs of the patient and the indicated area(s) of assessment. Generally, the review of systems is the responsibility of the physician; however, the nurse would do well to examine and evaluate as a learning tool, comparing findings with those of the physician.

If your observations are of a sick but ambulatory patient, the calm, self-assured, helpful manner of the nurse will help establish an atmosphere of security. If the patient is acutely ill in the ED or the victim of violent trauma, the nurse must remain calm and deliberately proceed with observations despite the surrounding confusion. Even acutely ill patients sense the presence of a calm and deliberate person and may frequently respond by relaxing significantly.

---

*One centimeter = 0.39 inch.

VITAL SIGNS

Vital signs (VS) are those signs necessary to or pertaining to life and represent essential baseline information in the overall evaluation of any patient; they routinely include temperature, pulse rate, respiratory rate, and blood pressure. It is good practice, however, to include the LOC on all patients to provide complete baseline information on arrival in the ED.

Although many nursing personnel find it annoying to obtain complete VS on every patient, there are many good reasons for making this a firm department policy. Not infrequently the patient is running a low-grade temperature, unaware of a chronic focus of infection; not infrequently, the patient's blood pressure far exceeds normal bounds and should be further evaluated; not infrequently, obscure disease processes can be recognized on the basis of VS inconsistent with other findings. It may take just a moment more to obtain complete VS but the patient deserves a full evaluation.

Frequently, deterioration or marked improvement may take place in the patient during the time spent in the ED, but this cannot be accurately confirmed unless *initial baseline data* have been obtained and documented on the ED record. Again, remember that where medical audit and the courtroom are concerned, *VS not documented are VS not taken.* Vital signs written on scratch paper in someone's pocket are of no use to the physician, other nurses, or the patient and must be written on the chart or flow sheet before they are lost in the confusion of a busy department.

TEMPERATURE

Customarily, temperature has been recorded in Fahrenheit (F), but implementation of the metric system will see conversion, throughout the nation, to Celsius (C).

Example: $98.6° F = 37° C$

To convert degrees F to degrees C, subtract 32 from the temperature in F, then multiply by 5/9.

Example: $C = F - 32 \times 5/9$

To convert degrees C to degrees F, multiply by 9/5, then add 32.

Example: $F = C \times 9/5 + 32$

In spite of 1-min directions on thermometers, a true reading may require as long as 5-8 min for an accurate oral temperature. Always check the thermometer before use to be certain the mercury column is below 96° F. (Although disposable thermometers are in wide use, they are not always totally accurate and temperatures should be rechecked with a glass thermometer whenever the clinical picture disagrees with the temperature reading.)

Normal body temperature is somewhere slightly above 98° F and may normally rise to 99-99.5° F. Temperature is usually the lowest in the morning before rising and is referred to as *basal*. As the day's activity progresses, the temperature will rise. This is called the *diurnal variation*. Febrile illness tends to produce the greatest temperature elevation in the afternoon and evening, although it may drop somewhat in the evening. Ovulation and certain other body functions will produce slight but consistent elevations. *Febrile* (with fever) range would be an oral temperature above 99.5° F, a rectal temperature above 100.5° F (1° higher than an oral reading), or an axillary temperature of 98.5° F (at least 1° lower than an oral reading).

Increased Heat Production by the Body

Body heat is produced by chemical reactions in metabolism at the cellular level, and a temperature gradient exists between the higher temperature of internal organs (core temperature) and the lower temperature on the skin surface. Causes of increased temperature are either an impaired heat loss or an increased heat production.

Impaired heat loss is seen in congestive heart failure, heat stroke (from failure of the temperature-regulating mechanism in the brain), temperature climatically higher than that of the body, and in congenital absence of sweat glands when the weather is moderately hot.

Some causes of increased heat production include exercise, thyrotoxicosis, systemic infections, localized infection with accumulation of pus, fractured bones, soft tissue injury from trauma, myocardial infarction, thrombophlebitis, some hematologic disorders such as leukemia and lymphoma.

Signs of Fever

1. Skin may or may not be warm and flushed. Skin temperature may be normal while internal temperature (core temperature) is elevated.
2. Tachycardia is *usually* present (rate of 100 or over).
3. Chills are a manifestation of thermostatic control operation at a higher level with rapid transition from normal to higher as shivering (from involuntary muscle contractions) produces more heat to raise the temperature.
4. Night sweats may be seen with elevated temperature during the night but are also seen in debilitated patients (tuberculosis as a prime example) and in normal children.

Patients with elevated temperatures are more comfortable in a warm room, but clothing should be removed to allow the skin to "breathe off" excess body heat.

PULSE RATE

In taking VS, it is first necessary to determine the presence of a pulse and then to note any abnormalities. The rate normally varies between 60 and 80/

min at rest. Pulse rates below 60 are classified as *bradycardias* although well-conditioned athletes may exhibit a normal heart rate of 60 or less, even in the face of trauma or stress. Slowing of pulse or heart rate is also seen in heart block or as the third component of Cushing's Triad in the patient with severe head injury. Pulse rates over 100 are classified as *tachycardias* although apprehension alone may cause a pulse rate of up to 100/min.

The character of the pulse may be small and barely palpable or full and bounding. Any deviation from a regular pulse rate of good quality should be documented accordingly and the physician advised. The following are some abnormal pulse patterns which may occasionally be recognized:

1. *Water hammer pulse* (Corrigan's pulse) is a jerky pulse with a full expansion followed by a sudden collapse, occurring in aortic regurgitation.

2. *Small late pulse* (almost the opposite of water hammer pulse) is a small hard pulse which rises and falls slowly. It is also described by the Latin words *parvus* (little) *et tardus* (late).

3. *Thready pulse* is usually very rapid and fine so that it is scarcely perceptible.

4. *Pulsus alternans* is the term applied to a variation in the strength of the *regular* pulse contractions. Every other contraction is weak and is caused by a failing myocardium that responds regularly to the sinus-initiated impulses but does not contract with equal strength to each impulse. Some of the myocardial fibers do not recover rapidly enough after a contraction to respond to the next pulse. The degree of *pulsus alternans* will vary with the patient's clinical condition and will usually occur if the patient complains of dyspnea; it will be present if there is cardiac enlargement.

RESPIRATORY RATE*

In the acutely ill patient, the *first* VS to monitor is the respiration. If respiration is imperceptible, impaired, or absent, all else must wait until effective respiration has been reestablished.

In determining respiratory rate the number of breaths per minute is counted, noting character and depth. Respirations *cannot* be counted or guessed at while the patient is talking or moving and should be counted during the pulse evaluation, which usually affords a nonconversant period.

Respirations may be described as regular, irregular, rapid, slow, shallow, deep, labored, easy, sighing, stertorous (like snoring), or barely perceptible.

The rate may be highly indicative. Dyspnea, Kussmaul breathing, orthopnea, or any other deviation from normal, relaxed respiration may be your first index as to the patient's real problem. *Hyperventilation and hypoventilation relate directly to the patient's clinical status.*

---

*Adapted from Ravin A: *The Clinical Significance of the Sounds of Korotkoff.* Merck Sharp & Dohme, West Point, Pennsylvania, 1970

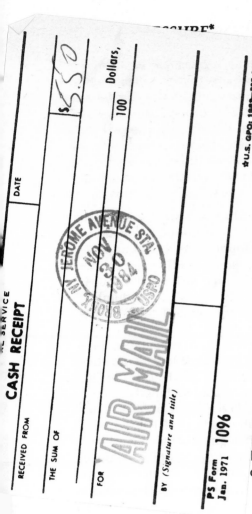

...corded blood pressure (BP) provides one
...line information on an acutely ill patient.
...sists of listening for the onset and disap-
... as the "sounds of Korotkoff," below the
...nsity and character during the procedure,
...nt information. The sounds heard over an
...g deflated, consist of a tapping sound and a
...cter of the tapping sound and the presence
...ounds have been divided into five phases:

...apping sound which gradually increases in

... follows the tap
...d alone, which is loud and high-pitched
...nly becomes lower pitched and less intense

...ce of sound

...ts through the artery beneath the cuff and dis-
...oduces the *systolic pressure,* which is read in
...ometer. The beginning of the fourth phase, or
...related to the occurrence of diastolic pressure.
...er to the true diastolic pressure, but determina-
...epends greatly on technique, level of noise in the
...the changes. Also in some persons there may be
...his may have special significance; therefore, it is
...onset of the fourth and fifth phases be recorded

Technique

The technique used in monitoring BP can influence the quality of the sounds heard; it is important to understand the mechanism by which the sounds are produced. The tapping sound is produced by the sudden distention of the walls of the collapsed artery as the peak of the pulse wave exceeds the cuff pressure, and the blood suddenly enters the collapsed artery. The murmur is produced by the flow of blood from the narrowed artery underneath the cuff into the wider artery distal to the cuff. During a BP determination, the forearm and hand are cut off from the general circulation by the inflated cuff. With the low pressure in the forearm, the tap is louder and the murmur longer and louder.

---

*Adapted from Ravin A: *The Clinical Significance of the Sounds of Korotkoff.* Merck Sharp & Dohme, West Point, Pennsylvania, 1970

While the cuff is being inflated, the venous return is cut off first. If inflation is slow, blood is trapped in the forearm with each beat, therefore, *rapid inflation of the cuff* will decrease the amount of blood in the forearm and louder sounds will be obtained.

A second procedure for decreasing the amount of blood in the forearm is to raise the arm and forearm for several seconds so that the venous blood drains out. The cuff is then inflated while the arm is elevated.

A third technique is to instruct the patient to open and close the fist rapidly 8-10 times after the cuff is inflated above the systolic level (a pressure 20-30 mm higher than needed to block the radial pulse should be obtained). This produces an increase in the blood-holding capacity of the vessels in the forearm and lowers the blood pressure in the forearm.

During inflation, *do not stop* between systolic and diastolic pressure readings and then reinflate to take another systolic reading, this permits the forearm to fill with blood, affecting the intensity and changes in the sounds.

Application of the cuff is important for an accurate result. A deflated cuff is applied evenly and snugly around the arm with the lower edge 1-2 inches above the antecubital space, centered over the artery, anteriorly and medially over the arm. If the cuff is not over the artery, the reading will be too high, and if the cuff is too loose, it results in reduction of the effective width, also resulting in too high a reading. The stethoscope is placed over the brachial artery below the cuff, avoiding too much pressure on the artery as this may compress the artery and a false murmur will be produced.

Cuff Size

Cuff width is important since the pressure of the cuff is best transmitted to the tissues at the center of the cuff and fades off toward the edge.

Adult Cuff: 12 cm wide by 23 cm long (or 5 × 9 inches). This cuff must not be used in obese persons because it may give a high reading and not on children because it may give a low reading.

Obese Cuff: A longer and wider cuff is necessary (14 cm wide × 35 cm long).

Children's Cuff: A narrow cuff is necessary: 5 cm wide cuff, less than 5 years; 7 cm wide cuff, 5-8 years; 9.5 cm wide cuff, 8-14 years; standard cuff, 14 years and over.

Manometers

Mercury manometers should be checked at intervals to be sure that, with no pressure applied, the mercury meniscus (the arc of the crescent-shaped structure appearing at the surface of the mercury column) is at the zero mark.

Normal Ranges of Blood Pressure

Normal BP in adults ranges from 100/60 to 140/90 and represents the pressure of the blood within the systemic arterial system. A *diastolic* pressure *con-*

sistently greater than 95 mm Hg is considered hypertensive and should be given further evaluation.

Normal limits of systolic pressure in children are given in Table 2.1.

Table 2.1 Normal Limits of Systolic Pressure in Children

Age	Normal systolic pressure
Birth to 3 months	60-80 mm
3 months to 1 year	80-100 mm
1 year to 12 years	Add 2 mm for every year + 100

Remember that the emotional and physical status of the patient have an obvious and very direct effect on the BP reading and that BP is very labile (unstable) and may vary from moment to moment. Anxiety, apprehension, anger, pain, frustration, and sudden noises may produce changes of 10-14 mm Hg. If possible, let the patient rest a bit, and if a pressure reading must be double-checked, try to allay the patient's apprehension by explaining that you are trying to get an average reading.

Auscultatory Gap

An *auscultatory gap* is the absence of the second phase (murmur), which results in a silent period between the first and third phases. This occurs when the cuff is inflated above the third phase but *not* above the first phase (See Fig. 2.1). The pulse pressure (which is the difference between the systolic and diastolic pressures and is usually about one-third of the systolic pressure) is low as a result. When this is noted, the procedure should be repeated with cuff inflated to 200 mm Hg or to 30 mm above the disappearance of the radial pulse. Auscultatory gap is likely to occur if inflation is slow (which also gives a false reading).

Impending Shock

A decrease in the intensity of the tap and murmur in a patient who had good sounds previously is an indication of the possibility of a falling cardiac output. This, coupled with a narrowing pulse pressure are ominous signs of a lowering cardiac output due to cardiac failure, shock (hypovolemic) or pulmonary embolus. Since BP is a reflection of cardiac output (CO) times the peripheral vascular resistance (PVR), even a moderate degree of hypovolemia will directly affect the volume return to the right heart and the stroke volume accordingly, reducing the cardiac output. *Tachycardia* occurs rapidly, as one of the body's compensatory mechanisms, and should be recognized as an early warning sign of hypovolemia even before hypotension becomes apparent in a patient who is a candidate for shock.

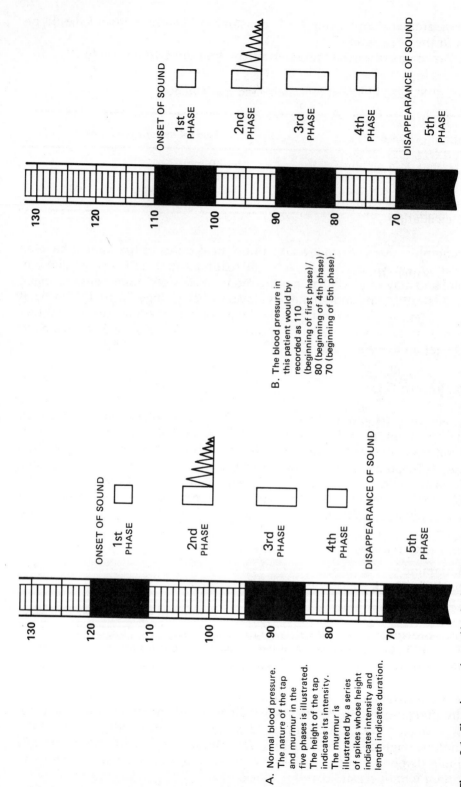

Figure 2.1. Five phases of sound in obtaining blood pressure. (From The Clinical Significance of the Sounds of Korotkoff. Merck Sharp & Dohme, West Point, Pennsylvania, 1970)

Orthostatic Vital Signs

With a narrowing pulse pressure, tachycardia, and the possibility of significant fluid loss, postural or "orthostatic" VS are an effective evaluation when in doubt and frequently lead to early recognition of the volume-depleted patient.

If postural variations in blood pressure and pulse rate are indicated and can be obtained without jeopardy to the patient, they should be done and recorded (Fig. 2.2). A decrease of 20 mm or more in systolic or diastolic pressure or an increase in pulse rate of 20/min or more is considered positive, and if significant changes are elicited during the second phase of evaluation, it should be unnecessary to continue further with the patient standing for the third evaluation.

Patient supine	BP 116/74	Pulse 94
Patient sitting, legs dependent	BP 106/60	Pulse 114
Patient standing	BP 88/52	Pulse 124

Figure 2.2. An example of recording significant changes in pulse and blood pressure which may occur with postural variations in the volume-depleted patient.

LEVEL OF CONSCIOUSNESS

When the level of consciousness (LOC) is being evaluated, it is best to take a comprehensive overall look and determine whether the patient is alert, drowsy, or lethargic. Again, this is frequently a *very* important baseline observation.

Determine whether the patient is oriented to time, place, and if so, whether he or she is confused in other areas. If the patient appears alert and oriented, this should be noted in the Nursing History. Any behavioral deviation from this norm should be recorded in brief but descriptive terms.

PAIN

Pain, by definition, is a sensation of hurting or strong discomfort in some part of the body, caused by injury, disease, or functional disorder; it is a basically unpleasant sensation and is both a *sensory* and *perceptual* experience.

The quality and intensity of pain is influenced by a past history of pain in childhood, the meaning of pain to that person, and the state of mind as related to the *degree of anxiety* and the *degree of pain*. One characteristic of pain is that it enforces *increased preoccupation with the body,* and this is an important concept for the EDN to be aware of. The healthy person generally takes pain-free existence for granted as a way of life. Conversely, when illness strikes and pain becomes a constant companion, that person's body becomes the center of his or her attention.

In evaluating the patient with severe abdominal pain, it is necessary to recognize pain patterns: with irritation of the peritoneum, the patient will lie *very* still, with colic he won't hold still, and with PID the woman will exhibit a "bent" posture to protect the irritated peritoneum as she moves. There are several situations which are recognizable as catastrophic when they cause an immediate stop in activity: ruptured ectopic pregnancy, perforated peptic ulcer, pancreatitis, and ruptured abdominal aneurysm are significant examples.

COMPONENTS OF PAIN

The components of pain are *perception* (the awareness of pain in response to impulses in terms of intensity, frequency, and duration) and *reaction* (the psychological and physiological responses to painful stimuli). The reaction to pain is of three types: 1) *autonomic,* 2) *skeletal muscle,* and 3) *psychic.* The examples in Figure 2.3 portray the three major ways in which man responds to perception of a painful stimulus. All three of these types of responses are called, collectively, the pain reaction.

Pain is a mechanism for self-protection since it warns the organism of internal and/or external threats and continues to warn because there is no sensory adaptation to pain stimulus. It prepares the organism to cope with the threat, and it conditions the organism to avoid previously encountered dangers or threats. Pain reactions may evoke the fight-or-flight response (Fig. 2.4).

PURPOSE OF PAIN

Pain does serve a purpose, then, by warning both of environmental dangers and internal bodily disorders, but at the same time, it is a highly complex entity that manifests itself in many ways and for many reasons. Persons experiencing pain reactions beyond the protective phase may suffer harmful effects if the pain is allowed to persist and should be encouraged to have the cause identified.

VARIABLES IN PERCEPTION OF PAIN

A sociologist named Zubrowski did some studies on the generalities of pain and concluded that 1) there are some strong cultural attitudes toward pain, which influence the individual's response to the pain experience; 2) age has an influence on the acceptance of pain; 3) sensory restrictions, developed in an isolated environment, manifest with a decreased tolerance for pain and an

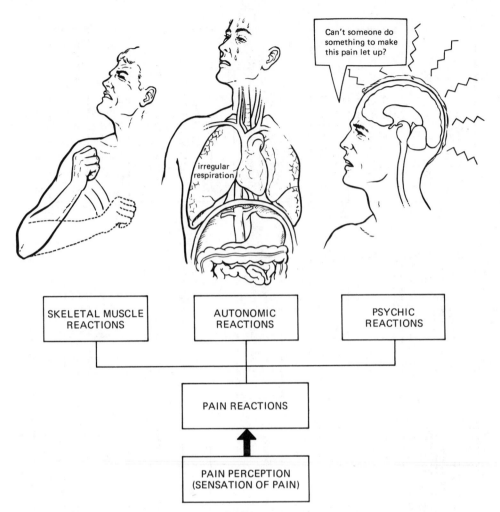

Figure 2.3. Reactions to painful stimuli. (Reproduced with permission from the American Journal of Nursing Co. from the American Journal of Nursing. Vol 66, No 5, May 1966)

increased sensitivity to pain; 4) pain is so complex in nature that there are no absolutes.

Unfortunately, *there are no means of obtaining "blood levels" for pain,* but emergency personnel must accept the description of pain as the patient gives it; pain is real to the person experiencing it, and it must be evaluated objectively and in the context of other signs and symptoms. Many times pain relief may be achieved by such nursing measures as comfortable positioning, use of supportive bolsters and pillows, application of heat or cold, and not infrequently, by listening attentively to the patient and demonstrating an interest in the problem. *Hypothermia* is frequently used to control intractable pain.

Again, all things are relative, and all patients do not *perceive* pain in the same way. One individual may find the pain secondary to injury or trauma intolerable while another individual may appear to totally disregard the pain! Continual assessment of the patient's pain experience is important, noting any

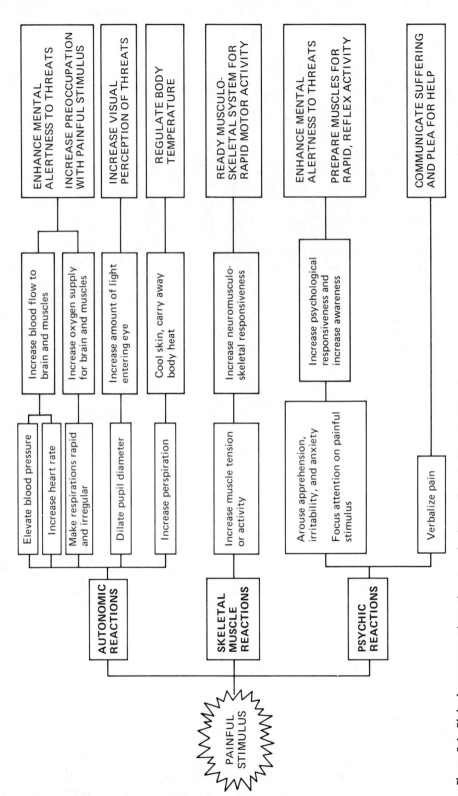

Figure 2.4. Biologic purposes of reactions to pain. (Reproduced with permission from the American Journal of Nursing Co. from the American Journal of Nursing. Vol 66, No 5, May 1966)

changes in character, site, or intensity as well as the modalities of treatment to which the pain responds.

The two leading theories regarding perception of pain, the Theory of Specificity and the Gate Control Theory, are included to help promote an understanding of pain as a reality in patient assessment.

The Theory of Specificity

The *Theory of Specificity* is the traditional theory regarding pain and was developed in 1644. This theory holds that there is the possibility of immediate response to pain and a delayed response to pain. This immediate response can almost be equated to a bell-ringing mechanism, and this theory is also known as the *Bell Ringing Theory* of pain as when someone pulls a rope at the bottom of the tower and rings the bell on top. Basically, what happens with the reflex arc, or the immediate response, is that the stimulus goes to the receptors by way of the afferent nerve to the spinal cord, back by way of the efferent nerve to the muscle, resulting in a muscle contraction. The term *afferent* means to carry toward the spinal cord; the impulses resulting from a painful stimulus are afferent impulses. The term *efferent* means to carry away from the spinal cord; the impulses sent to a muscle to contract it are efferent impulses. The pathway for skeletal muscle reactions to pain is illustrated in Figure 2.5.

The second part of the Specificity Theory involves delayed response: the stimulus from the receptors is sent along the afferent nerve to the spinal cord, the brainstem, the thalamus (where perception occurs), the cerebral cortex (where the interpretation occurs), the hypothalamus, and then back down to the brainstem, and efferent nerve. This response is autonomic, skeletal, and psychic. Figure 2.6 is a representation of the pain pathway and autonomic reactions to pain.

The Gate Control Theory

The *Gate Control Theory* of pain was developed in 1965 by Melzack and Wall* who proposed a theory of pain mechanics that has broadened the view of both the clinical pain experience and its treatment. Their theory challenges the Specificity Theory because the latter does not account for how social, psychological, and cultural factors influence pain.

The Gate Control Theory suggests that there is a spinal cord mechanism that influences the amount of sensory input transmitted from the peripheral nerves. The amount of input received at any one time is dictated by the ratio of activity of large and small peripheral nerve fibers. The small fibers conduct pain while the large fibers conduct sensation or, simply, touch. According to this theory, stimulating the large fibers can, in a sense, "overload" the system and, thus, at the first spinal synapse, inhibit the activity of the smaller pain-conducting fibers. In other words, innocuous sensation carried by the large

---

*Melzack R, Wall PD: Pain mechanisms: A new theory. Science Vol 150, p 971, 1965

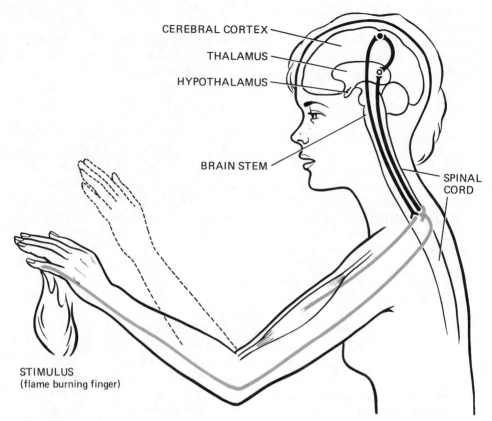

CEREBRAL CORTEX

THALAMUS

HYPOTHALAMUS

BRAIN STEM

SPINAL CORD

STIMULUS
(flame burning finger)

Figure 2.5. Simplified pathway for skeletal muscle reactions to pain. (Reproduced with permission from the American Journal of Nursing Co. from the American Journal of Nursing. Vol 66, No 5, May 1966)

fibers will cause the brain to "close the gate" against the pain being transmitted by the small fibers. The important clinical implication of this theory is the possibility that pain may be relieved or inhibited by stimulating the large nerve fibers.

Transcutaneous Nerve Stimulators (TCNS) work on the basis of gate control and are battery charged to increase the activity of the large fibers and prevent transmission of pain impulses via the small afferent nerves. Three out of five patients suffering chronic pain obtain relief with the use of this type of pain control management.

RESPONSES TO PAIN

Physiological reactions to pain depend upon the duration of the pain. One brief second or so of pain triggers the activation stage and autonomic reaction occurs until the pain is relieved. In the rebound stage, the parasympathetics take over with a drop in pulse rate and BP. In the adaptation state, anxiety decreases; with the stress syndrome, there is an increase of eosinophils from fatigue.

Among the factors that can decrease pain perception are the response of the nurse, patient activity, verbalization or swearing, focusing on the pain site, which is a repetitive and occupying exercise, concentration or visualization, self-hypnosis, and distraction. The EDN can listen and support the patient as much as possible and very often obtain positive results. It is good practice to ask what the *patient* thinks is the cause of the pain, and this may lead to some interesting and beneficial discussion.

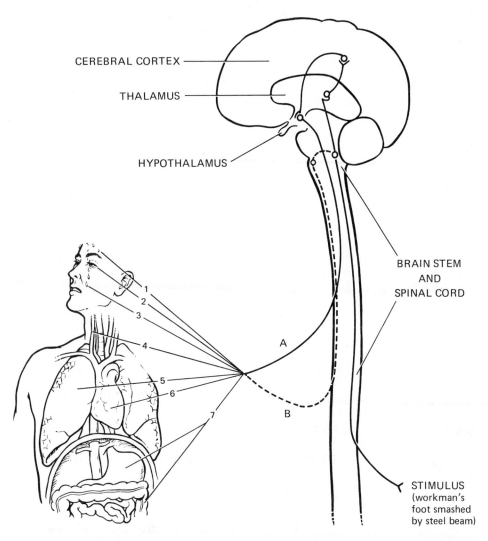

Figure 2.6. Simplified presentation of pain pathway and autonomic reactions to pain. Major pathways mediating impulses that lead to immediate and delayed autonomic reactions to an intensely painful stimulus are shown: 1) sweating; 2) dilation of pupils; 3) lacrimation; 4) increased blood flow to brain; 5) increased respiratory rate; 6) increased heart rate and blood pressure; and 7) gastrointestinal distress (or similar responses). (Reproduced with permission from the American Journal of Nursing Co. from the American Journal of Nursing. Vol 66, No 5, May 1966)

ANXIETY

Severity of pain is affected by distraction and is *increased* with anxiety. Anxiety is frequently associated with three states of mind which threaten the self image: a sense of helplessness (which accompanies the patient into the hospital environment and is most prevalent in men); a sense of isolation (time spent in ICU or CCU); and insecurity (accentuated sharply when the life style is in jeopardy and the prognosis is uncertain).

For the nurse to effectively allay a patient's anxiety, there must be an awareness that the patient is, indeed, anxious. Then the patient is helped to recognize that he or she is anxious, to gain an insight into the anxiety, and to cope with whatever threat he or she is facing, *one step at a time*. The EDN should assess the patient's knowledge of pain, realizing that anxiety increases with ignorance. The attitudes of others toward the patient should be assessed since the relative loss of control will increase the patient's anxiety. The family especially should be reassured in this regard.

THE NURSE'S ROLE IN PAIN MANAGEMENT

A great deal can be accomplished toward allaying anxiety by establishing rapport with the patient by:

1. Touch and eye contact
2. Calling the patient by his/her first name (after requesting permission)
3. Allowing the patient to participate in arranging his/her own comfort
4. Not bargaining with the patient; *give* medication
5. Reassuring the patient about the doctor's availability
6. Reassuring the patient that his/her responses are appropriate (reinforcement)
7. Teaching how to treat pain other than with medication
8. Providing sensory input in the form of distractions
9. Promoting rest and relaxation

Nursing Guidelines for Giving Analgesics

Employ a positive attitude in giving medications. ("You *will* be more comfortable.")

Medicate in the anticipatory stage; stay ahead of pain. If medication is ordered, give it as ordered and do not moralize.

Emphasize the value of nonnarcotic medications for analgesia when possible, e.g., antibiotics. ("This will help the infection and the pain will improve.") Explain when medication is ordered for problems other than pain, but assure the patients that it, too, will help.

Use other pain relief methods and reinforce those behaviors that will reduce pain.

Analgesics which are administered orally should *not* be given on a full stomach, as it interferes with absorption.

Keep medications on schedule as ordered.

Remember to prepare the patient for painful procedures and to tell him when the procedure is terminated. This is an effective means of reducing apprehension.

REVIEW

1. Identify five essential points to be checked in the initial "overview" of the patient.
2. Identify two essential requirements in the physical surroundings when examining a patient.
3. List the important areas to be checked in a general nursing assessment.
4. Describe the correct technique for obtaining temperature, pulse, and respirations (TPR).
5. Identify some specific significant variations in pulse patterns and their characteristics.
6. Describe the proper placement of a BP cuff.
7. List three techniques that will provide a greater intensity of sound in taking the blood pressure.
8. Describe the five phases of sound which are heard when taking a blood pressure.
9. Explain the significance of a narrowing pulse pressure and tachycardia in a potential shock candidate.
10. Convert a temperature reading of 100.8° F to Celsius.
11. Define *febrile*.
12. Explain the value of obtaining orthostatic vital signs.
13. Identify the criteria applied for orthostatic vital sign findings to be considered significant.
14. Describe the method of obtaining and recording orthostatic vital signs.
15. Identify the major indication for obtaining orthostatic vital signs.
16. Describe the best way to evaluate a patient's level of consciousness.
17. Identify the components of pain and the two main factors that influence an individual's reactions to pain.
18. Explain the Specificity Theory and the Gate Control Theory of pain.
19. Describe four autonomic nervous system responses to pain.
20. Describe some signs of anxiety and identify steps which the nurse should take.
21. Describe the nursing guidelines relating to administration of analgesics.

BIBLIOGRAPHY

Assessing Vital Functions Accurately. Nursing 77 Books, Horsham, Pennsylvania, 1977

Bates B: A Guide to Physical Examination, 2nd ed. J. B. Lippincott Co., Philadelphia, Pennsylvania, 1979

Buckingham W, Sparberg M, Brandfonbrener M: A Primer of Clinical Diagnosis, 2nd ed. Harper and Row, New York, 1979

Budassi SA, Barber JM: Emergency Nursing: Principles and Practice. C. V. Mosby Co., St. Louis, Missouri, 1981

DeGowin E, DeGowin R: Bedside Diagnostic Examination: A Comprehensive Pocket Textbook. The Macmillan Co., New York, 1981

Jarvis CM: Vital Signs. Nursing 76, pp 31-37, April 1976

Jarvis CM: Perfecting Physical Assessment, Part 3. Nursing 77, pp 44-53, July 1977

McVan B: Assessment of Odors. Nursing 77, pp 46-49, April 1977

Ravin A: The Clinical Significance of the Sounds of Korotkoff. Merck Sharp and Dohme, West Point, Pennsylvania, 1970

Roach B: Assessment of Color Changes in Dark Skin. Nursing 77, pp 48-51, January 1977

Rudy FB, Gray VR: Handbook of Health Assessment. The Robert J. Brady Co., Bowie, Maryland, 1981

Warner C: Emergency Care: Assessment and Intervention, 2nd ed. C. V. Mosby Co., St. Louis, Missouri, 1978

NURSING HISTORY AND THE INTERVIEW 3

KEY CONCEPTS

This chapter has been prepared to help the EDN understand the importance of formulating a concise and accurate working history from the nursing standpoint and to offer ideas and assistance in methods of dealing with distraught and anxious patients who present themselves for emergency care. After reading and studying this chapter, you should be able to:

- Identify the main components of a nursing history.
- Describe the types of problems that the EDN should be prepared to encounter in documenting a patient history.
- Outline a suggested approach to interviewing.
- Discuss the purpose of a focused interview.
- Identify some guidelines for conducting a patient interview.
- Identify specific areas of questioning that are appropriate for histories on the critically ill patient, motor vehicle accidents, other injuries, illnesses, lacerations, burns, poisonings and overdoses, and vaginal bleeding.
- List the initial laboratory procedures most likely to be anticipated in various situations, including mentation changes, electrolyte imbalances, hemorrhagic states, shock, diabetes mellitus, tetany, renal dysfunction, and respiratory functional deficits.

THE NURSING HISTORY

The nursing history is a distillate of all the observations and parameters that the nurse has evaluated and gathered.

The nursing history must be both *concise* and *accurate* and should contain the age, race or color, sex, mode of admission, chief complaint or "complaints of" (c/o), and the general mental status of the patient on admission. The chief complaint should always be written in quotes in the patient's own words; it is vitally important to record any allergies and current medications.

The VS, although not written as part of the nurse's narrative, must be considered an integral part of the history and a prime responsibility in documentation. Vital signs *not documented* are vital signs *not taken* insofar as medical audit or the courtroom is concerned.

The most difficult aspect of documentation for the nurse is probably the ability to condense and "crystallize" into written form the initial impressions and observations of the patient and the EDN must realize that the history will become a part of permanent medical record of that patient. *Discretion* is strongly advised in the use of descriptions that may be construed later as derogatory; a strong example is written statement that a patient is "drunk" or "smells of alcohol." That same patient can just as easily be described as "staggering" or "uncoordinated" with "slurred speech." This will corroborate the physician's notation (which is the physician's prerogative) indicating that the patient has "ETOH on breath" and will tell the story well enough if it ever becomes a courtroom matter.

The nurse should not be swayed by subjective findings and opinions but must make every effort to document only the *objective* findings in concise, accurate, and meaningful fashion.

THE INTERVIEW

Physicians point out repeatedly that *a good working history on the patient is probably 85% responsible for the formulation of the diagnosis.* The first nurse who receives the patient is in the best position to elicit a short, meaningful, working history before the physician begins his examination. This can prove to be a very valuable asset, not only as a means of expediting treatment but as an area of fulfillment and satisfaction for the nurse who develops this skill. Since the *diagnostic process begins when nurse and patient sight each other,* the interview begins based on essential visual observations that the nurse has already made.

Approach to Interviewing

At the onset, the EDN must be mindful of the fact that when a patient presents at the ED or brings in a member of his or her family, he or she is concerned about a problem. Even though probably 80% of the patients seen in the ED are not true emergencies, but fall somewhere in the less urgent and non-urgent categories, every patient considers their problem an emergency and looks for a fast response as well as efficient care. The EDN is called upon to respond accordingly and to receive the patient in the same way that he/she would wish to be treated and given the level of care which that nurse would expect for his/her own person. The Golden Rule, as always, has an important application here.

The fact that the patient has come to the ED for help gives the nurse a major advantage in obtaining pertinent history. A major drawback, however, is the fear of truth since the patient generally experiences a high level of anxiety about what is *really* wrong. The fastest way to dispel anxiety in the patient is to demonstrate a warm interest and *smile* (no matter how difficult it is sometimes). Employ a polite and positive manner and display confidence as you begin the interview.

The Focused Interview

The initial interview is considered to be *focused* because it concentrates on rapidly defining the nature of the problem from the patient's point of view. The purpose of this focused interview is to maximize accuracy in determining the *real* reason for the patient's presenting to the ED as well as to stimulate the patient in communicating effectively and reducing irrelevancies. The interview should be focused but not rigid.

GUIDELINES FOR CONDUCTING AN INTERVIEW

Some important guidelines for conducting an effective and productive interview are as follows:

1. Greet the person by name if at all possible. Don't be afraid to use first names.
2. Establish and maintain eye contact with the patient throughout the interview.
3. Introduce yourself and *smile!* The exact greeting is not important, but it should convey your sincere question of "What can we do for you?" or "How can we help you?" Although the patient may not respond with the *real* chief complaint, he or she will certainly be assured that the nurse is present to assist. If the patient is bluntly asked why he or she came to the ED, the response is likely (and understandably) to be defensive since the patient has been made to feel that he or she is disturbing the department's tranquility. The interview is bound to start on a negative note under these circumstances!
4. It is important to establish physical contact with the patient for several reasons. The good old "laying on of hands" provides the nurse with a direct evaluation of the warmth and texture of the skin as well as the patient's response to touch. A great deal of reassurance can be given in many instances by the simple gesture of touching, thereby reinforcing the fact that someone is there to be concerned and offer help.

5. Questions should be open-ended, and the EDN should never lose sight of the initial or chief complaint. The patient's response to questions may be affected by a language barrier, fear of embarrassment, or the sheer inability to express himself or herself. An offhand or hostile attitude on the part of the nurse or the physician may cause the patient to retreat into a defensive silence. Remember that most patients do not possess what can be referred to as an organized knowledge of diseases and that symptoms may be described in an unconnected and disorganized manner as they come to mind. An ability to see the problems from the patient's point of view, however, can make your questions meaningful. You must use terms that can be understood but at the same time will not sound as though you are speaking down to the patient. Imagine yourself in the patient's place and experience the symptoms and events as they are related.

6. Reinforcing cues can be given in nonverbal fashion by facial expression and body postures, exhibiting a sympathetic attitude and encouraging the patient to continue talking, although aimless rambling must not be allowed. Paraphrasing the meaning may help to clarify the story as understood by you. It indicates that you understand the patient's statements, that meanings can be corrected as necessary, and it finishes the point. It also gives the patient an idea of your evaluation and assurance that something will be done. There may be occasions when silence is indicated, allowing the patient to ventilate, during which time the pertinent information can be sorted out and then paraphrased back for a condensed confirmation.

7. Know your own hang-ups and avoid, at all costs, being judgmental. The patient may well have reservations about some of your questions if your attitude seems hostile or judicial. This results in the anticipated negative answer and will close up the patient's responses, impeding the free flow of information. Be careful not to jump to conclusions that may lead to a trap and jeopardize patient welfare! Try to use your knowledge of human motivations and respect your patients as individuals, just as you would wish to be treated.

8. Explain to your patient what will be happening next after you have obtained your information. Remember the importance of realizing that anxiety and apprehension walk in side by side with the patient, and the EDN is in the best position to calm the patient by reassuringly explaining what is going to happen next and why.

9. During this brief interview, use your background of experience to formulate a nursing judgment concerning priorities of treatment.

10. Listen closely to responses on past illnesses and surgeries.

11. Document carefully and concisely the essentials of what the patient has communicated to you, both verbally and visually. Remember to *use your eyes* when talking with your patient and be as observant as possible when the patient is responding to questions. Very often the patient's own statement is a highly reliable index to his acutal condition.

Perhaps this is the place to reiterate the old warning to *watch your talk,* even with unconscious patients! All too often a patient who is apparently unconscious regains consciousness and has entirely too much recall about what was said in the room. Many experienced EDNs make it a practice to talk directly *to* the unconscious patient as though he or she is indeed conscious. Every now and then an unexpected response will be elicited.

SPECIFIC AREAS OF ATTENTION IN HISTORY TAKING

LOCATIONS OF PAIN

Pain is a classic universal symptom which leads to a *preoccupation with the body,* although some patients with serious or even fatal disease may not necessarily experience pain. When pain is a symptom, the nurse should use a gentle cross-examination technique to determine the following features of the pain:

- Location (have the patient point with one finger to *where* pain is worst *now*)
- Chronology (sequence of development of symptoms from onset)
- Severity (usually in terms of its effect on pertinent functions, and degree of severity at worst)
- Aggravating or precipitating factors (activity or time relationships)
- Alleviating or soothing factors (positon, medication, etc.; if medicated, with what?)
- Association with other symptoms or bodily functions
- Radiation to other organs or locations (have patient point again to area of radiation)
- Course (is it getting better or worse?)
- Has this patient had this pain before; if so, was he seen, by whom and what was diagnosed?

VITAL SIGNS

Complete vital signs (including level of consciousness—LOC), allergies, and immunizations should be recorded on *all* patients as well as all regular medications. Note skin color and diaphoresis, if present, and chart "skin appears....." or "patient appears....." All patients with abdominal pain or significant trauma should have *time of last meal* and/or *fluid ingestion* documented along with other findings and observations.

THE CRITICALLY INJURED PATIENT

- What position was the patient in when injury occurred?
- Where does the patient hurt *now?*

- Has patient ever had, or does he or she have, any other illnesses?
- Is patient on any drugs or medication of any kind, especially insulin, digitalis, or anticoagulants?
- Does patient have a bleeding tendency? (All you have to ask is "Are you a bleeder?" The patient who *is* a bleeder knows it and will tell you.)
- Does patient have any allergies, especially to antibiotics, that are likely to be used before or during an operation?
- When was the last meal or fluid intake and how much?

MOTOR VEHICLE ACCIDENTS (MVAs)

Obtain accident information from the police *and* from the patient, if possible, to demonstrate the degree of response and recall pertinent to the level of consciousness.

- When recording VS, always include PERLA (pupils equal, react to light and accommodation) and LOC (level of consciousness)
- Where did the accident happen?
- How many cars were involved?
- What speed was vehicle traveling? (Aortic tears occur on deceleration.)
- What time did the accident happen and on what date?
- Was the patient driving *or* a passenger?
- Were the police at the scene?
- What are the injuries and locations? (Driver's head and sternum hit windshield, dash and impact steering column; passenger's knees hit dash with femoral fractures as well as head and facial injuries.)
- Was patient thrown from vehicle?

OTHER INJURIES (SPRAIN, STRAIN, PAIN OF UNKNOWN ORIGIN, POSSIBLE FRACTURE)

- Location of injury and pain
- Where did injury occur? (work, home, school)
- Time of injury
- Treatment since injury
- Location of injury
  Ribs: pain worse on coughing or deep breathing?
  Foot or leg: more pain on motion or weight-bearing?
  Arm or fingers: pain on extension or flexion?
  Range of motion (ROM) and sensory perception intact?

ILLNESS

All illnesses should be questioned as to any sudden, recent weight loss or gain, and this must be carefully documented.

Upper Respiratory Infection
(URI or URTI—upper respiratory tract infection)

- Any symptoms of sore throat, painful ears, cough, nasal drainage?
- Temperature? Has patient had any aspirin within the last 3-4 hours, and if so, how much?
- How long has the patient had symptoms?
- Has there been any previous treatment for the illness and if so, when and what?

Nausea, Vomiting and/or Diarrhea

- Get full VS and temperature
    How long (days and hours)?
    How many times in 24 hours?
    Any related pain or injury?
- Any treatment given, including ASA?
- Any blood (bright or dark) noted in vomitus or stools?
- Any changes in appetite or diet in past 2-3 days?
- Amount of liquid being retained? What kind?

Urinary Tract Infection (UTI)

- Requires full VS and temperature.
- Location of pain (low abdomen and/or flank pain?)
- Urinary frequency, urgency, burning? Scant urine?
- Any blood in urine?
- Any chills or fever?
- Duration of problem in days and hours?
- History of any similar episodes? Treatment?

Always obtain a clean catch urine specimen if UTI is suspected, unless a catheterized specimen is ordered.

LACERATIONS

- Document location on body, and if on hand, note unconsciousness at any time as well as present LOC.
- How, when, and where was person at the time (work, school home)?
- What caused laceration (glass, metal, knife, etc.)?
- How long ago?
- Note type of bleeding, i.e., oozing versus spurting (if indicated).
- Is the range of motion (ROM) or sensory perception affected?
- Date of last tetanus booster and known allergies?

BURNS

- Take B/P if possible and TPR.
- Note area of body burned.

- Note type of burn (water, grease, chemical, thermal, electrical, etc.).
- How, when, where did burn occur (work, school home)?
- How long ago?
- Date of last tetanus booster and known allergies?

POISONINGS AND OVERDOSES

- Take full VS and record LOC.
- Note type and amount of material ingested if known (dosage per tablet); if unknown, write unknown.
- Time of ingestion?
- Any known reason for ingestion?
- Any symptoms (coma, nausea and vomiting (N&V), burns in mouth, odor, coughing, shortness of breath, burns in throat).

VAGINAL BLEEDING

Always put a clean pad on the patient so that the amount of bleeding can be accurately established while you proceed to obtain the history and full VS.

- Date of last menstrual period (LMP)?
- Is patient pregnant? Gravida? Para? What was the date of last birth?
- Is patient using oral contraceptives or an IUD?
- Is there any pain? Note type, location, severity, and duration (steady, intermittent, radiating).
- Note and document the severity, duration, and nature of bleeding (dark clots, heavy bright flow, etc.).
- Note color of skin (pale, blanched, flushed, etc.).
- Note quality and rate of radial pulse.

LABORATORY DIAGNOSTIC PROCEDURES

After the EDN has gone through the overview of the patient and the initial general assessment, appropriate laboratory tests should be anticipated and/or requisitioned as soon as possible to expedite treatment, presuming that the hospital and ED policies allow the triage or charge nurse to intake laboratory requistions.

Table 3.1 provides a list of laboratory tests usually employed by physicians in the ED with an adjacent list of disease states correlating with each test. The list should be studied carefully for indications and correlations, in anticipation of what may be ordered.

Table 3.1 Some Specific Indications for Laboratory Evaluation and Appropriate Tests*

EMERGENCY LABORATORY TESTS USUALLY EMPLOYED	DISEASE CORRELATION TO LABORATORY TEST TO HELP ESTABLISH DIAGNOSIS
Blood values	Blood values
1. Hematocrit (PCV)	1. Acute: Hypovolemic shock
2. Hemoglobin	2. Chronic Anemia
Blood chemistry	Blood chemistry
1. Alcohol (for medical purposes)	1. Intoxication, mental change
2. Amylase	2. Pancreatitis
3. Barbiturate	3. Mentation change
4. Bromide	4. Mentation change
5. Calcium	5. Tetany
6. $CO_2(HCO_3^-)$	6. Electrolyte balance
7. Chloride (Cl^-)	7. Electrolyte balance
8. Creatinine phosphokinase (CPK)	8. Smooth muscle damage (heart)
9. Fibrinogen	9. Hemorrhagic state
10. Glucose (blood sugar)	10. Diabetes mellitus
11. Lactic acid (serum lactate)	11. Shock state
12. Magnesium	12. Mentation change, tetany
13. PCO_2 pH, arterial PO_2	13. Respiratory functional capabilities, mentation change
14. Partial thromboplastin time (PTT)	14. Hemorrhagic state
15. Potassium (K^+)	15. Electrolyte imbalance and cardiac arrhythmias
16. Prothrombin time (Pro time)	16. Hemorrhagic state
17. Salicylate	17. Mentation change
18. Sodium (Na^+)	18. Electrolyte balance
19. Urea nitrogen (BUN)	19. Renal dysfunction

*Adapted from A Training Program for Hospital Emergency Room Personnel, U.S. Department of Health, Education and Welfare, Rockville, Md., 1972.

REVIEW

1. List the information which is basic to a concise and meaningful nursing history.
2. Identify some practical guidelines in the general approach to a patient interview.
3. Define a focused interview.
4. List at least eight guidelines for conducting a patient interview.
5. List some specific questions appropriate to the following situations:
   - The critically injured patient
   - Motor vehicle accident victims

- Other injuries
- Upper respiratory infections
- Nausea, vomiting and/or diarrhea
- Urinary tract infection
- Lacerations
- Burns
- Poisonings and overdoses
- Vaginal bleeding

6. Identify the important questions that must be asked to trace the origin of pain.

7. Identify the laboratory tests indicated for at least ten pathologic states.

BIBLIOGRAPHY

Bello TA: The Latino patient in the emergency department. JEN Vol. 6, No. 4, pp 13-16, July/August 1980

Buckingham W, Sparberg M, Brandfonbrener M: A Primer of Clinical Diagnosis, 2nd ed. Harper & Row, New York, 1979

Budassi SA, Barber JM: Emergency Nursing: Principles and Practice. C.V. Mosby Co., St. Louis, Missouri, 1981

Cosgriff JH, Anderson DL: The Practice of Emergency Nursing. J.B. Lippincott Co., Philadelphia, Pennsylvania, 1975

DeGowin E, DeGowin R: Bedside Diagnostic Examination: A Comprehensive Pocket Textbook. The Macmillan Co., New York, 1981

Dorland's Illustrated Medical Dictionary, 26th ed. W.B. Saunders Co., 1982

Eggland ET.: How to take a meaningful nursing history. Nursing 77, pp 22-30, July 1977

Navarro MR, LaCourt G: Helpful hints for use with deaf patients. JEN Vol 6, No 6, pp 26-28, November/December 1980

Ravel R: Clinical Laboratory Medicine. Year Book Medical Publishers, Inc., Chicago, Illinois, 1974

Warner C: Emergency Care: Assessment and Intervention, 2nd ed. C.V. Mosby Co., St. Louis, Missouri, 1978

CHEST SOUNDS   *4*

KEY CONCEPTS

This chapter will deal with promoting an understanding of the importance of assessing the status of the chest as the patient exchanges air, and with techniques employed in the evaluation.*

After reading and studing this chapter, you should be able to:

- Identify the important preliminary step to evaluating the chest.
- Define tachypnea and bradypnea.
- Identify the four skills employed in the chest assessment.
- Identify the key points relating to each skills.
- List the five sounds heard when the chest is percussed and their characteristics.
- Describe the proper use of the stethoscope.
- Describe the proper positioning of the patient for auscultation and percussion.
- Identify the two elements of normal breath sounds.
- Identify the four components of each breath sound.
- Define an adventitious breath sound.
- Describe what differentiates a musical rale from other types.
- Identify some nonpulmonic adventitious breath sounds.

---

*Much of the material on breath sounds in this chapter was adapted from George Druger, *The Chest: Its Signs and Sounds* and reprinted with permission of Humetrics Corporation, Los Angeles, California.

The nursing assessment of the chest should begin with an evaluation of the rate and quality of respirations that are observed with the patient at rest and placed in a position of comfort before proceeding with the examination. The normal adult respiratory rate at rest is between 14 and 18 breaths per minute. Children have a slightly higher rate, and infants may have rates as high as 40 per minute, with neonates breathing as rapidly as 60 per minute.

Tachypnea, or excessive rapidity of respiration, occurs in many normal situations. During exercise, people breath more rapidly and therefore become *tachypneic.* Patients who are anxious, apprehensive, febrile, anemic, obese, or who have heart or lung disease are often tachypneic. Adult patients are considered to be tachypneic when their respiratory rate exceeds 20 per minute.

Bradypnea, on the other hand , is an abnormal slowness in breathing and is usually a sign of some abnormality such as brain disorder, drug or alcohol overdose, or some metabolic imbalance. Adult patients may be considered *bradypneic* when their respiratory rates are *less than* 10 breaths per minute.

COMPONENTS OF THE CHEST EXAMINATION

The chest examination should begin with the posterior chest, proceeding to the anterior chest, and comparing one side of the chest to the other as the examination proceeds, from top to bottom.

Four skills are necessary for examining the chest: 1) *Inspection;* 2) *Palpation;* 3) *Percussion;* and 4) *Auscultation.* Inspection and palpation, or examining by touch, are techniques commonly used by nurses, but percussion and auscultation (by means of a stethoscope) are newer to the nursing profession generally.

INSPECTION

Inspection of the chest and lungs begins with some questions to be answered by your observations.

1. What is the patient's attitude lying in bed? Is he calm and at ease or apprehensive and restless, lethargic, dyspneic?
2. What is the quality of his respiration?
3. What is his color?
4. Does the chest move symmetrically with respiration?
5. What muscles are used during respiration? (Diaphragm, accessory muscles, intercostals?)
6. Is the skin dry or moist?
7. Do the respirations appear labored?
8. Is the trachea midline?
9. Is an abnormal pattern of respiration present?

Recognition of abnormal breathing patterns is frequently very helpful in early awareness of underlying disease. Three of the more common abnormal breathing patterns seen are the Cheyne–Stokes respiration, Biot's respiration and Kussmaul respiration:

Cheyne–Stokes (Chān'–stōks) *respiration,* named for John Cheyne, a Scottish physician (1777-1838) and William Stokes, an Irish physician (1804-1878), is breathing characterized by rhythmic waxing and waning of the depth of respiration with regular recurring periods of *apnea* lasting up to 20 seconds and seen especially in coma resulting from damage to the nervous centers.

Biot's (Bē–ōz') *respiration,* named for Camille Biot, a French physician of the 19th century, is breathing characterized by *irregular* periods of *apnea* alternating with periods in which four or five breaths of identical depth are taken. This condition is usually associated with patients who have increased intracranial pressure.

Kussmaul respiration is also known as "air hunger" and is a distressing dyspnea occurring paroxysms at a rate usually greater than 20 per minute. This respiratory pattern usually indicates a metabolic abnormality and is seen frequently in diabetic acidosis as well as renal failure.

PALPATION

The chest and neck should be palpated for the position of the trachea and any evidence of tenderness in the muscles of the chest wall and the chondrocostal (the ribs and costal cartilage) areas. The vibrations caused by resonance of voice sounds, which can be felt by placing the hands on the chest wall, are called *fremitus.* This examination is conducted on both posterior chest walls while the patient (in a sitting position if at all possible) repeats "ninety-nine" in as low a voice as possible, because a large number of vibrations are generated and transmitted through the chest in this manner.

Sound is conducted best through *solid* matter, which acts as a *bridge,* then water, and least through air. If consolidation is present in the lungs because of pneumonia, accumulated secretions, masses, etc., you should feel fremitus over the affected area. Conversely, fremitus will be absent or barely noticeable in the presence of pneumothorax, emphysema, and pleural effusion.

PERCUSSION

Percussion is accomplished by laying the middle finger against the chest and tapping it with the middle finger of the other hand. There is no normal percussion note as such. It will vary from person to person and even from place to place on the same individual.

Five sounds can be heard when the chest is percussed. They are:

Tympany

Tympany is heard over air-filled areas and has a high-pitched musical or drumlike quality of long duration. It is typically heard over hollow air-filled organs like the bubble of the stomach.

Hyperresonance

This sound is percussed between the head of the humerus and the base of the neck and is an exaggerated *resonance* with a low pitch.

Resonance

The sound heard over areas of normal fremitus, it is the prolongation and intensification of sound produced by the transmission of its vibrations to a cavity, as elicited by percussion, with a moderately low pitch.

Dullness

This sound is heard at the diaphragm and over the heart with a muffled quality and a moderately high pitch.

Flatness

The sound heard over large bone areas with a high pitch and a soft thud.

AUSCULTATION

Auscultation is defined as the act of listening for sounds within the body, chiefly for ascertaining the condition of the lungs and other organs. *Direct* auscultation is performed without the stethoscope, but with the naked ear. More commonly, *mediate* auscultation is performed, with the aid of the stethoscope interposed between the ears and the part being examined.

The Stethoscope

Most stethoscopes in use today are *binaural* (both ears). The chest piece may be either the bell-type, the diaphragm, or a combination of both (Sprague type). The bell chest piece (Ford model) is a hollow cone and transmits all sounds but is of particular value when listening for low-pitched sounds. It is also valuable for listening to the apices of the lungs, between ribs on thin patients, or other less accessible areas. It is necessary to use the bell to hear mitral stenosis and fetal hearts. The diaphragmatic chest piece (Bowle's model) is a flat, shallow cup covered with a diaphragm made of Bakelite or celluloid. This diaphragm filters out low-pitched sounds so that high-pitched sounds can be heard more clearly. Since most chest sounds are high-pitched, the diaphragmatic chest piece is usually used in auscultating the chest for breath sounds as well as the heart, for such sounds as regurgitant aortic murmurs.

Damaged stethoscope diaphragms *must* be replaced with the proper material (*not* x-ray film) or the acoustic quality of the instrument will be impaired. The soft rubber or plastic tubing should be thick-walled and its outside diameter should not be smaller than the caliber of the connecting tubes. Optimally, the tubing should not exceed 30 cm (about 12 inches). Shorter tubing is inconvenient and long tubing is thought to compromise the quality of the sound transmitted. It is also important that the ear pieces fit the listener's ears comfortably without pressure and discomfort, forming an air-tight seal to promote transmission of sound without extraneous noises, which is the only function of the stethoscope since it does *not* amplify sound.

When the stethoscope is used, the bell-type should touch the surface of the skin lightly but firmly enough to form an air seal on the surface; the diaphragm type should be held firmly on the skin so that external sound is filtered out. Extraneous noises are a common distraction in the use of a stethoscope, for example, your breath on the tubing or rubbing hair with the chestpiece may produce sounds like rales, and movements of muscles or tendons may sound like friction rubs. Proper interpretation takes a good deal of practice.

It should be added that stethoscopes require examination and service periodically to be certain that tubing diaphragms are intact and that the pieces are clean and free of ear wax, lint, and even, as one writer suggests, *flies!*

Positioning the Patient

The proper positioning of the patient for auscultation is as follows:

1. Place the patient in a relaxed sitting position with shoulders drooping forward slightly to reduce the bulk of the back muscles.
2. Instruct the patient to turn his or her face to the side and breathe a little more deeply than normal to increase the intensity of sounds and to breathe through the mouth, not the nose.
3. Inhalation should be *active* and exhalation should be *passive*. Do not let the patient force expiration. Often it is easier to demonstrate than to explain, thereby avoiding induced hyperventilation.
4. Start at the apices of the lungs and work downward, comparing both sides as you move down the chest wall posteriorly and then anteriorly.

BREATH SOUNDS

All normal breath sounds consist of either the *vesicular* sound or the *bronchial* sound, or a combination of both. There are four components of each breath sound to be evaluated on both inspiration and expiration: pitch, amplitude, quality, and duration.

Vesicular

The vesicular element is the sound produced by air entering the alveoli directly under the stethoscope and is thought to result as the alveoli distend and separate on inspiration. Vesicular breath sounds are *breezy* sounds, resulting from the air passage directly under the stethoscope, and although the actual time consumed for expiration is slightly longer than that of inspiration (approximately a 6:5 ratio), the *audible* range reverses and the inspiratory phase becomes 3:1 over the expiratory phase with no pause heard between the phases (Fig. 4.1A). These vesicular breath sounds are harsher in children with thinner chest walls and more elastic lungs.

Bronchial

Bronchial breath sounds (also called *tubular*) are harsher sounding than vesicular sounds and are usually heard only over the *manubrium* (body) of the sternum in normal patients. They are loud and high-pitched, with a short pause between phases; the expiratory phase is 1½ times longer than the inspiratory phase (Fig. 4.1B).

Bronchovesicular

In the normal lung, you will hear bronchovesicular breath sounds where the trachea and bronchi are closest to the chest wall, above the sternum and between the scapulas. Characteristically, these bronchovesicular breath sounds have an almost equal inspiratory and expiratory phase with no pause heard between phases and a medium to high pitch with a muffled blowing sound (Fig. 4.1C)

Tracheal

Tracheal breath sounds are heard only over the trachea as very high-pitched, loud, harsh tubular sounds. This is the purest form of the *glottic hiss* (Fig. 4.1D) having a short phase between inspiratory and expiratory phases.

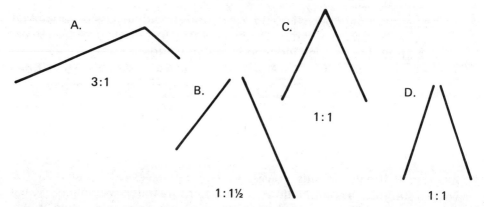

Figure 4.1. The four breath sounds that may be auscultated. A. Vesicular breath sound. B. Bronchial breath sound. C. Bronchovesicular breath sound. D. Tracheal breath sound (glottic hiss).

ADVENTITIOUS SOUNDS

Occasionally extra sounds, or *adventitious* sounds, are heard that are not normally heard in the chest and are superimposed on the breath sounds. Most commonly, these originate from the lungs or airways and are termed *rales* (rahls). Generally, there are considered to be five types of rales, the first of which is called musical and is composed of *continuous sounds,* as opposed to the four other types, which are essentially showers of discrete (or separate) individual sounds.

Musical Rales

Musical rales are both sibilant and sonorous. *Sibilant* rales are high-pitched hissing sounds similar to that produced by suddenly separating two oiled surfaces. They are produced by the presence of a viscid secretion in the bronchial tubes or by thickening of the walls of the tubes, as heard in asthma and bronchitis. (The second is also referred to as a *wheeze.*) *Sonorous* rales are fine moist sounds resembling the cooing of a dove and are produced by the passage of air through mucus in the capillary-bronchial tubes. They are heard in capillary bronchitis and asthma and are sometimes called a *snore.*

Crepitant Rales

Crepitant rales are very fine rales resembling the sound produced by rubbing a lock of hair between the fingers or by particles of salt thrown on a fire. This rale is heard at the end of inspiration and is also referred to as a *fine moist* rale.

Subcrepitant Rales

These sounds are heard in conditions associated with liquid in the small tubes and airways. They are also called *crackling* or *medium moist* rales, are not nearly as high-pitched, and are comprised of many discrete sounds that are usually present at the end of inspiration. Fluid from alveoli emptying into smaller airways can cause crepitant rales to become subcrepitant, as in pneumonia and pulmonary edema.

Bubbling Rales

Bubbling rales are moist and finer than a subcrepitant rale and are heard in bronchitis, the resolving state of exudative pneumonia, and over smaller cavities. They have a bubbling quality in sound and are produced when air passes through fluid.

Gurgling Rales

Very coarse rales resembling the sound of large bubbles bursting are called *gurgling rales.* In pulmonary edema, they are heard over large cavities that contain fluid and can be heard without a stethoscope. When present in the trachea, they are referred to as the *death rattle* and are very low-pitched, loud, wet-sounding, discrete rales.

NONPULMONIC ADVENTITIOUS BREATH SOUNDS

Other chest sounds to be considered on auscultation are the nonpulmonic adventitious sounds. These are extra sounds in the chest which are *not* pulmonic in origin. First among these would be the pleural friction rub.

Pleural Friction Rub

This sound is apt to be loud, grating, and intermittent and is produced by inflamed and roughened pleural surfaces rubbing together. Its pitch is similar to that of a crepitant rale but is more intense and of a different quality. Its *grating* or *scraping* quality is more commonly heard during inspiration and may disappear after the first few respiratory efforts when the pleural surfaces have become better lubricated. The sound produced when *hair* is moved under the diaphragm of the stethoscope can be confused with a pleural friction rub. To avoid this confusion, eliminate the possibility by wetting the chest hair and pressing the diaphragm firmly against the chest wall.

Subcutaneous Emphysema

Resembling crepitant rales or a pleural friction rub, the sounds of subcutaneous emphysema are not related to the respiratory cycle and should not be confused with any other sounds. Subcutaneous emphysema is produced by very small air pockets under the skin which are moved back and forth by the pressure of the diaphragm of the stethoscope on the skin. These air pockets under the skin may be the result of rupture of the trachea, bronchus, or esophagus, pneumothorax, mediastinal trauma, or elective neck surgery. Subcutaneous emphysema is a highly significant finding and is a harbinger of greater problems.

Bone Crepitus

This sound may be heard when the chest is auscultated following trauma. It is a grating sound related to the respiratory cycle and is produced when two ends of a fractured rib rub together. It may or may not be heard without a stethoscope.

In summary, remember to position your patient properly when preparing to evaluate chest sounds and to use a *binaural* stethoscope of good quality when auscultating the chest. A quality stethoscope is a most worthwhile investment for the EDN and should be carried at all times on duty. Experience is *still* the best teacher, and the most beneficial way to learn to recognize and evaluate chest sounds in your patients is to listen to every chest, if it is appropriate to the needs of the patient and time permits.

REVIEW

1. What is the first observation to be made before beginning with an assessment of the chest?
2. Define "tachypnea" and "bradypnea."
3. Name the four skills utilized in examining the chest.
4. List at least eight essential points of observation as inspection is carried out.
5. Define "Cheyne–Stokes respiration."
6. Define "Biot's respiraton."
7. Define "Kussmaul respiration."
8. Explain fremitus.
9. What provides the best "sound bridge?"
10. Describe the five types of sound heard during percussion.
11. Define the two types of auscultation.
12. What is a Sprague-type stethoscope?
13. Does a stethoscope amplify sound?
14. Describe the proper positioning of the patient for auscultation.
15. Identify the two main elements of a normal breath sound.
16. Each breath sound has four components or characteristics. Name them.
17. Describe the relative time components of each of the four breath sounds.
18. Define an "adventitious breath sound."
19. What differentiates musical rales from the other types?
20. Define "discrete."
21. List the four types of nonmusical rales.
22. What is the characteristic sound of a pleural friction rub?
23. What differentiates subcutaneous emphysema from crepitant rales or pleural friction rub when auscultated?

BIBLIOGRAPHY

Assessing vital functions accurately. Nursing 77 Books, Horsham, Pennsylvania, 1977

Bates B: A Guide to Physical Examination, 2nd ed. J.B. Lippincott Co., Philadelphia, Pennsylvania, 1980

Buckingham W, Sparberg M, Brandfonbrener M: A Primer of Clinical Diagnosis, 2nd ed. Harper & Row, New York, 1979

DeGowin E, DeGowin R: Bedside Diagnostic Examination: A Comprehensive Pocket Textbook. The Macmillan Co., New York, 1981

Delaney MT: Examining the chest, Part I: The lungs. Nursing 75, pp 12-14, August 1975

Druger G: The Chest: Its Signs and Sounds. The Humetrics Corp., Los Angeles, 1973

Jarvis CM: Perfecting physical assessment. 2. Nursing 77, pp 38-45, June 1977

Ruby EB, Gray VR: Handbook of Health Assessment. The Robert J. Brady Co., Bowie, Maryland, 1981

Timmons J: Breath Sounds. JEN Vol 6, No 6, pp 16-18, November/December 1980

CARDIAC STATUS AND HEART SOUNDS 5

This chapter is designed to promote an understanding of an initial recognition of the patient with an acute cardiac problem to be followed by further examination. The basic techniques in auscultation of heart sounds and their relative interpretations are explained, correlated with findings from visual observations and palpation of the chest wall and extremities.

After reading and studying this chapter, you should be able to:

- Identify cardinal signs of impending cardiac arrest.
- Describe the immediate nursing intervention necessary to avoid problems with possible impending cardiac arrests.
- Identify further indication of need for assessment of cardiac status.
- Describe the proper positioning for your patient preparatory to a cardiac assessment.
- Identify the areas to be checked on visual inspection.
- Describe the factors to be assessed in palpation of peripheral pulses.
- Describe the areas on the chest wall where the aortic valve, pulmonic valve, tricuspid valve, and point of maximum impulse (PMI) are best heard by auscultation.
- Describe the meaning of S_1 and S_2 heart sounds.
- Describe the gradation of heart murmurs.
- Explain the heart pathology that causes systolic murmurs and diastolic murmurs.

All patients with a potential for cardiac rhythm disturbances *must* be monitored for arrhythmia detection. Shock, hemorrhage, myocardial infarction, neurological trauma, septacemia, or any other process which results in hypoxemia or disturbances in ABG values/acid-base balance, or alteration in serum electrolyte levels, predisposes to the development of dysrhythmias and necessitates cardiac monitoring.

Initially, when a patient presents complaining of chest pain or *severe pressure, pain radiating from the chest,* shortness of breath, fainting spells, or any other signs of poor cardiac output, *assume the worst* and *move quickly* to initiate the necessary steps for intervention and management. Take the patient immediately to a bed in the area equipped to handle "codes," and after removing at least the top half of clothing to expose the chest and precordial area, proceed as follows:

1. Administer oxygen at a rate of at least 6 LPM (30-40%) oxygen delivery via nasal prongs *until further evaluation.*
2. Apply cardiac monitor leads in lead II configuration and assess for arrhythmia requiring immediate intervention.
3. Get an IV line in fast (antecubital vein is easiest and fastest in emergencies although it is bothersome later). If it is the ED's responsibility to draw blood for the lab, a 20 cc syringe of blood should be drawn at this time and injected into the appropriate Vacu-tubes. Run D5/W TKO (to keep open) with a pediatric microdrip set.
4. Position the patient comfortably (Fowler's or semi-Fowler's), call for a stat ECG, and continue *closely* monitoring vital signs and clinical status as they relate to the monitor tracing.

This information is outlined again and discussed further in Chapter 11 on ECGs and Arrhythmias but must be included here as an integral part of the initial assessment responsibility.

INDICATIONS FOR EXAMINATION OF THE CHEST

A nursing examination of the chest, including the lungs and the heart, should be conducted on patients who present with problems related to the cardiorespiratory system. Emergency nurses who have the opportunity should take the initiative and pursue development of their own skills in chest assessment; a valuable capability of this sort can only be acquired through practice. Patients generally appreciate the interest and attention shown during the initial assessment and whether or not a physician is apt to repeat the examination, a competent initial evaluation of the chest by the EDN is an appropriate procedure which can contribute important information toward effective nursing management.

Presenting problems which indicate the need for chest assessment would include:

1. History of angina
2. Palpitations
3. Intermittent claudications
4. Edema
5. Paroxysmal nocturnal dyspnea (PND)
6. Orthopnea
7. Other history of heart disease, *including* high blood pressure.

THE CARDIAC EXAMINATION

The assessment of cardiac status by examination of the chest wall includes *inspection, palpation, percussion,* and *auscultation,* combined with continued observation of blood pressure. The examination should be conducted with the patient properly and comfortably positioned in a semi-Fowler position, since the heart is assessed chiefly by examination through the anterior chest wall, with most of the anterior cardiac surface represented by the right ventricle. The left ventricle, lying to the left and behind the right ventricle, makes up only a small portion of the anterior cardiac surface; it forms the left border of the heart and produces the *apical* impulse, which is usually referred to as the *point of maximum impulse* (PMI). The PMI may not always be apical, however, depending on the existing pathology.

When assessing heart sounds, always stand to the patient's right and proceed with the examination using a quality stethoscope of the binaural type, employing both the bell and the diaphragm in the auscultation of the heart. Again, experience is the best teacher, and the nurse wishing to develop skills in this area must take advantage of every available opportunity to listen to heart sounds and develop an "ear."

INSPECTION AND PALPATION

The overall *inspection* of the patient begins with the head and goes all the way to the feet in order to check for visual evidence of effective circulation by the heart. Inspection is, in reality, carried out simultaneously with *palpation* which is defined in *Dorland's Medical Dictionary* as "the act of feeling with the hand; the application of the fingers with light pressure to the surface of the body for the purpose of determining the consistence of the parts beneath in physical diagnosis." In other words, it is necessary to *look* and to *feel.*

Head and Neck

Inspection begins with the *head* and *neck,* noting color of skin, lips, ears, nose, and mucous membranes and looking for distention of superficial vessels and/or cyanosis of any parts, the respiratory status, and the general appearance and behavior of the patient. With the bed in semi-Fowler position, the neck should be checked for distention of the jugular veins and any obvious pulsation. Visible distention of the jugular veins while the patient is lying at a 45° angle is an indication of an elevated central venous pressure (CVP). The carotid pulse should be lightly palpated for rate and quality, bilaterally, evaluating *one side at a time.*

Extremities

Extremities should be inspected for color and temperature. Cold skin, pallor, or cyanosis of an extremity may well be an indication of impaired circulation from cardiovascular disease or may be an indication of impending or incipient shock. Occluded arterial circulation will result in a reduction in pulses (or a decreased intensity) and possibly an entirely obliterated pulse so that no palpable pulse can be obtained. Super bruits may be heard; these are audible manifestations of turbulence in vessels from drastic changes in the caliber of the vessel wall. Atrophy of muscles from chronic occluded circulation is manifested by thin, shiny skin and thickened fingernails. Elevation of an occluded extremity will cause it to turn pale, placing it is a dependent position will precipitate rubor (redness or flushing).

Look for cold mottled extremities. Look at the color of skin on the legs; a brawny induration of the tibia and the malleolus develops from long-term congestion of venous return in the circulation. The presence of congestion in the venous circulation must *always* be evaluated and the EDN must always be observant for any signs of *dependent* peripheral edema of the ankles, sacrum, or scrotum.

Evaluating the Pulses

Pedal pulses should be checked. The *dorsalis pedis* pulse may be obtained on the dorsum of the foot, usually just lateral to the extensor tendon of the great toe, placing fingers lightly so as not to obliterate the comparatively fragile pulse (Fig. 5.1). The *posterior tibial pulse* may be obtained on palpation by curving the fingers posteriorly and slightly below the malleolus of the ankle on the soft tissue (Fig. 5.2). Both of these pedal pulses may be congenitally absent and, at best, may be difficult to palpate.

Peripheral pulses, whether radial or pedal, should be assessed bilaterally, noting the rate, quality, and bilateral equality. Pulses are rated on a scale of 0–4+ with 0 meaning *absent* pulse; 1+, *palpable;* 2+, *normal* or *average;* 3+, *full;* and 4+, *full* and *bounding* (may even occasionally be visible). Temporal, carotid, brachial, radial, femoral,and popliteal pulses should all test 2+ bilaterally. The posterior tibial and dorsalis pedis should test 1+ bilaterally.

Locating the Point of Maximum Impulse

Following inspection and the accompanying palpation of head, neck, and extremities, the anterior chest wall should be palpated over the precordial area for the *point of maximum impulse* (PMI), observing for precordial "lift," rocking motion, etc. The PMI is usually located in the *left fifth intercostal space,* within the *midclavicular line,* and will normally be felt as a single impulse (Fig.

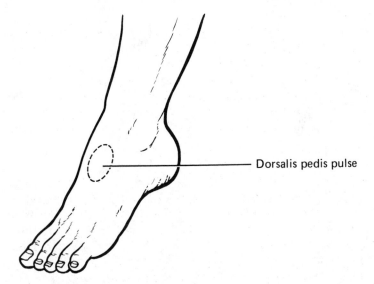

Figure 5.1. Dorsalis pedis pulse.

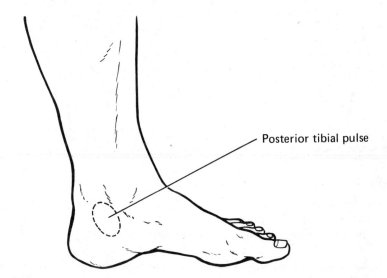

Figure 5.2. Posterior tibial pulse.

5.3). A double or paradoxical impulse that waxes and wanes with respirations may be indicative of myocardial disease, which could lead to congestive heart failure.

The PMI may be palpated by placing the right hand horizontally against the lower part of the sternum with the heel of the hand over the sternum and the fingers extending leftward to the region of the apex in the midclavicular line, feeling for:

1. Apical impulse (PMI), normal or exaggerated
2. Thrust against the chest wall

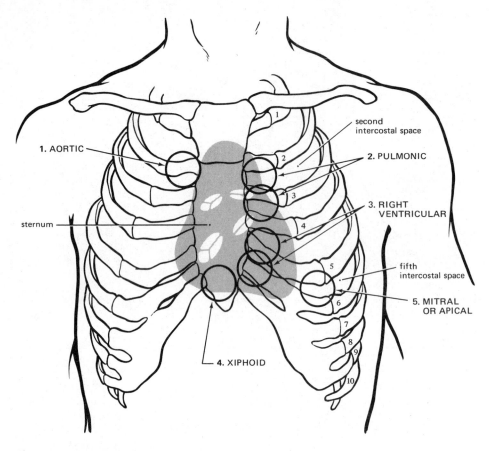

1. AORTIC

second intercostal space

2. PULMONIC

sternum

3. RIGHT VENTRICULAR

fifth intercostal space

5. MITRAL OR APICAL

4. XIPHOID

Figure 5.3. Suggested sequence for auscultating heart sounds.

3. Rocking motion within the chest wall
4. Systolic or diastolic thrills. (*Thrill* is defined in *Dorland's Medical Dictionary* as a "sensation of vibration felt by the examiner on palpation of the body, as over an incompetent heart valve.")

PERCUSSION

Percussion techniques are the same as those used in percussing the lungs and will help determine heart size. Normally, the left cardiac border (LCB) is near the PMI, usually at or within the midclavicular line (MCL). Place the patient recumbent in the semi-Fowler position and stand on the patient's right; begin percussing the left anterior axillary line at the fifth intercostal space, moving to the fourth intercostal space if necessary, percussing toward the sternum until you hear dullness. The point of dullness indicates the left border of cardiac dullness (LBCD). Normally, this is usually 10-12 cm from the midsternal line and most always within the midclavicular line. If the LBCD is greater than 12 cm from midsternum and is outside the MCL, the heart may be considered enlarged except in a highly trained athlete.

AUSCULTATION FOR HEART VALVE SOUNDS

When the stethoscope is used, one sound should be listened to at a time. Each heart valve sound is reflected to a specific area of the chest wall:

1. The *aortic* sound is best heard in the *second right intercostal* space (ICS).
2. The *pulmonic* sound is best heard in the *second left ICS.*
3. The *tricuspid* sound is loudest at the *fifth right ICS* near the sternum or at midline below it.
4. The *mitral* valve sound, or *apical* sound, will be heard in the *fifth left ICS* near the midclavicular line. This will approximate the PMI.

It should be noted that sound related to the movement of heart valves and the flow of blood across them are *not* heard best over the anatomic locations, but in the auscultatory areas bearing their names (Fig. 5.3).

The sounds of S_1, the first heart sound, and S_2, the second heart sound, differ according to location. S_1 is *louder at the apex* (if one pictures the heart as an upside-down pyramid), and S_2 is *louder at the base* (or actually at the top). Begin a systematic assessment by listening at the top of aortic and pulmonic valves, moving to the apex over the tricuspid and mitral valves. You may start the other way around but the important thing is to be consistent and systematic in order to train your ear. Listen for these four values:

1. Gross timing
2. Degree of intensity at the PMI
3. Pitch and quality
4. Fine timing

S_1 is thought to be the closure of both the mitral and tricuspid valves (atrioventricular) just before the ventricular systole. The closures occur almost simultaneously; however, the left-sided events in the heart occur slightly before the right-sided events. Thus, the mitral valve closes slightly before the tricuspid and because of the difference in timing, the first sound can actually be split into mitral (M_1) and tricuspid (T_1). The vibrations generated by the mitral valve closure are of higher intensity and frequency than those generated by tricuspid closure, and this mitral component is heard over much of the precordium and is the main component of the heart sound at the apex. The S_1 sound, then, is the *lub* of "lub-dub."

The second sound, S_2, is the closing of both semilunar valves (the aortic and pulmonic) just before diastole. Near the end of systole, the rate of ejection slows, as the ventricular and arterial pressure begin to diminish. Ventricular pressure drops rapidly at the onset of ventricular relaxation. Blood in the base of the aorta and in the base of the pulmonary artery rushes back toward the ventricular chambers, but this movement is abruptly stopped by the closure of the aortic and pulmonic valves. The momentum of the moving blood overstretches the valve cusps, and the recoil initiates oscillations in both the atrial and ventricular cavities. S_2 is the *dub* of "lub-dub."

For further definitive study of heart sounds, including S_3 and S_4, the student is referred to several excellent references, including Barbara Bates' *A Guide to Physical Assessment,* published by Lippincott in 1974; the American Heart Association's booklet on "Examination of the Heart, Part IV, Auscultation," published in 1967; and *Nursing 75,* September issue on "Assessing heart sounds, normal and abnormal."

PALPITATION

Palpitation is a frequently heard complaint, and though its cause may be trivial, it can seriously frighten the patient, requiring a determination of cause and a satisfactory explanation. The term is applied to the symptom in which the patient is conscious of his heart action, whether fast, slow, regular, or irregular. The sensation is often described as "pounding," "fluttering," "flopping," "skipping a beat," "jumping," and "turning over." The frequency, rate, and intensity depend on the underlying cause. Some causes of palpitations are exertion, high cardiac output at rest (anxiety, hypertension, thyrotoxicosis, flutter, or paroxysmal tachycardia), cor pulmonale, pressure on the heart (mediastinal tumor or tympanites), and stimulus of drugs (tobacco, tea, coffee, alcohol, epinephrine, etc.).

MURMURS

If you hear what you *think* are murmurs, try to evaluate and record their location, gross timing, intensity (PMI), pitch and quality, and the fine timing. Murmurs are graded 1 through 6, and *Dorland's Medical Dictionary* defines *murmur* as "an auscultatory sound, benign or pathologic, particularly a periodic sound of short duration of cardiac or vascular origin." The intensity grades for evaluating murmurs are:

Grade 1. Extremely faint, elusive, and diffcult to hear in all positions

Grade 2. Quiet but immediately obvious to the ear when the stethoscope is placed on the chest

Grade 3. Moderately loud with *no* associated *thrill*

Grade 4. Loud and *may* have an associated *thrill*

Grade 5. Very loud and may even be heard with the stethoscope partly off the chest and *may* have an associated *thrill*

Grade 6. Loud enough to be heard *without* the stethoscope and *has* an associated *thrill.*

The pitch of a heart murmur may be high, medium, or very low, and the quality may be that of "blowing," "rumbling," "harshness," or periodically harmonious sound. Remember that high-pitched sounds or relatively high-pitched sounds, such as the first two heart sounds and the murmurs of aortic and mitral regurgitation, can be heard with the diaphragm of the stethoscope. The bell is best used for hearing low-pitched sounds such as the S_3 and S_4 and the diastolic murmur of mitral stenosis. The bell of the stethoscope should *just* make contact with the skin, forming an air seal.

Murmurs are categorized either as *systolic* or *diastolic;* therefore, consider both. When the heart is in systole, noise may be created by:

- Aortic stenosis
- Pulmonary stenosis
- Mitral regurgitation
- Tricuspid regurgitation

Systolic Ejection Murmur

This murmur occurs predominantly in midsystole when ejection volume and velocity of blood flow are at their maximum. It is heard in aortic or pulmonary stenosis, is of a *medium pitch,* and can be heard when there is an increased stroke volume, as with anemia and pregnancy.

Diastolic Murmur

This murmur occurs during diastole—that is, after the second heart sound. Heard at the *apex,* it is a sign of *mitral obstruction;* heard at the *base* of the heart, it is due to *aortic regurgitation* or, more rarely, to pulmonary regurgitation with a back-flow into the ventricles. A murmur caused by *tricuspid* or *mitral stenosis* is best auscultated by using the bell of the stethoscope at the apex of the heart. *Regurgitation during diastole,* whether pulmonic or aortic, will cause a back-flow into the ventricles and a high-pitched murmur heard at the left sternal border. This murmur is best heard with the diaphragm of the stethoscope.

INDICATIONS FOR ASSESSMENT

A nursing examination of the chest, including the lungs and the heart, should be conducted on patients who present with problems related to the cardio-respiratory system. These would include:

- History of angina
- Palpitations
- Intermittent claudication
- Edema
- Paroxysmal nocturnal dyspnea (PND)
- Orthopnea
- Other history of heart disease, including high blood pressure

REVIEW

1. List the pathophysiological processes which can result in the need for cardiac monitoring.
2. Describe the protocol for immediate nursing intervention in cases of suspected impending cardiac collapse.
3. Describe the presentation of a patient with an impending cardiac arrest.
4. List at least six presenting complaints that indicate the need for a nursing examination of the chest.
5. Describe the proper positioning of the patient for an assessment of cardiac status.
6. Where should the examiner stand when conducting the examination, and what two components of the examination are carried out simultaneously?
7. Where does the inspection begin?
8. Distention of the jugular veins in the neck with the patient reclining at a 45° angle would be an indication of what?
9. List the observations that should be made of the extremities.
10. Where are the two pedal pulses found?
11. How should peripheral pulses be assessed?
12. Where is the PMI usually found?
13. Define *thrill*.
14. Describe the procedure for percussing the cardiac border.
15. Identify the two main heart sounds, what they represent, and where they are heard the loudest.
16. Describe the relationship of S_1 and S_2 to the "lub-dub" of the heartbeat.
17. Identify the grades and characteristics of heart murmurs.
18. Identify the heart pathology responsible for systolic and diastolic murmurs.

BIBLIOGRAPHY

Assessing Vital Functions Accurately. Nursing 77 Books, Horsham, Pennsylvania, 1977

Bates B: A Guide to Physical Examination, 2nd ed. J.B. Lippincott Co., Philadelphia, Pennsylvania, 1979

Buckingham W, Sparberg M, Brandfonbrener M: A Primer of Clinical Diagnosis, 2nd ed. Harper & Row, New York, 1971

DeGowin E, DeGowin R: Bedside Diagnostic Examination: A Comprehensive Pocket Textbook. The Macmillan Co., New York, 1981

DeLaney MT: Examining the chest. 2. The heart. Nursing 75, pp 41-46, September 1975

Dorland's Illustrated Medical Dictionary. W.B. Saunders, Philadelphia, Pennsylvania, 1982

Jarvis CM: Perfecting physical assessment. 2. Nursing 77, pp 38-45, June 1977

Lehman J: Auscultation of heart sounds. Am. J. Nursing, Vol 72, pp 1242-1246, 1972

Leonard J, Krootz F: Examination of the Heart, Part 4: Auscultation. American Heart Association, 1967

Ravin A: Auscultation of the Heart. Year Book Medical Publishers, Inc., Chicago, Illinois, 1967

Ravin A: Cardiac Auscultation: An Audio Presentation. Merck Sharp and Dohme, West Point, Pennsylvania, 1970

ACID-BASE BALANCE AND ARTERIAL BLOOD GAS ANALYSIS 6

KEY CONCEPTS

This chapter deals with the acid-base balance of the blood as it relates to oxygen transport and arterial blood gases. It should promote an understanding of the factors concerned in the regulation of the acid-base balance of the body, the mechanisms employed in that regulation, and the values and interpretations of arterial blood gases. The material is based largely on lecture content presented to EDNs in the Portland Metropolitan Area by Mona Motz, D.O., Tom Rich, ARRT, and Earl R. Showerman, M.D.

After reading and studying this chapter, you should be able to:

- Explain photosynthesis and the respiratory cycle.
- Explain the derivation of partial pressures of gases in the bloodstream.
- Explain the relationship between the partial pressure of arterial oxygen and oxyhemoglobin saturation.
- Identify the two factors that significantly affect the oxyhemoglobin dissociation curve.
- List the major cations and anions involved in maintenance of acid/base balance and their normal serum values.
- Describe the clinical signs of deficiencies and excesses of the major electrolytes.
- Identify the physicochemical and physiological factors that determine the acid-base balance of the body.
- Recognize the conditions under which fixed acids appear in the blood in significant amounts.
- Explain the role of the lungs and kidneys as they relate to the adjustment of pH in the body.
- Identify the criteria for easy accessibility of oxygen to the tissues.
- Define hypoxia and identify five manifestations.
- Define hypercapnia and identify five manifestations.
- Identify normal values in arterial blood gases and define base excess.

- List the equipment necessary to perform arterial puncture and obtain a sampling.
- Describe the technique of arterial puncture, identifying the hazards and listing the safeguards that must be employed.
- Explain the Allen test and its importance.
- Explain the formula for dosage determination when administering intravenous sodium bicarbonate.
- Identify the four steps in determining acid-base status of the patient.

OXYGEN, CARBON DIOXIDE, AND THE RESPIRATORY CYCLE

Oxygen is essential to life; the body can live for only a few minutes without it since *there are no body stores of oxygen.*

Oxygen in our atmosphere is produced by plant life as it utilizes carbon dioxide and sunlight to synthesize carbohydrates, giving off oxygen as a by-product. Algae in the oceans produce about 90% of the oxygen in our atmosphere, amounting to hundreds of billions of tons annually.

As the human body metabolizes fuel, oxygen is recombined with the carbohydrates yielding water and carbon dioxide which is carried back to the lungs to be exhaled into the atmosphere, where it is utilized again by the plant world in the process of *photosynthesis.* This is the respiratory cycle.

The oxygen content of *inspired* air is 21% at sea level while the carbon dioxide content is 4%. The proportion of water vapor in exhaled air is about ten times greater than that of the normal atmosphere, accounting for the insensitive water loss of approximately 500 ml per day which occurs in the normal individual.

PARTIAL PRESSURES OF GASES

We live at the bottom of what is literally an "ocean" of air which extends several miles above us. One half of the earth's atmosphere is below 20,000 feet, and most of the world lives in the first 5,000 feet where the air is denser and breathing is easier.

At sea level, atmospheric pressure measures 30 inches on a standing column of mercury which is the equivalent of about 15 pounds to the square inch. In order to apply this measurement to human physiology, the reading must be converted as follows:

Barometric pressure at sea level = 30 inches Hg
30 inches converted to centimeters = 30×2.54 cm (1 in.) = 76.20 cm Hg at sea level
76.20 cm Hg converted to millimeters Hg = $76.20 \times 10 = 760$ mm Hg (rounded off)
Thus, atmospheric pressure at sea level is represented as 760 mm Hg.

The *partial pressure* of a gas is the pressure exerted by each of the components of the gas mixture, the pressure of each component is proportional to the percent of the mixture occupied by that gas. The partial pressure of oxygen, then, would be 21% of the total atmospheric pressure of 760 mm Hg.

21% of 760 mm Hg = 159.60 mm Hg of oxygen in room air at sea level.
159.60 mm Hg − 47 mm Hg inhaled water vapor pressure = 112.60 mm Hg.
112.60 mm Hg − 15 mm Hg± from dilution of oxygenated blood by return flow of deoxygenated blood from the coronary and bronchial circulation = a PaO_2 (partial pressure of arterial oxygen) of 100 mm Hg.
P = partial pressure or tension exerted by a gas and is usually expressed in *mm Hg* or *torr*.

Normal Partial Pressures of Gases in Man (at Sea Level)

PaO_2 = 100 mm Hg on room air (90-100 mm Hg considered normal limits)
PCO_2 = 40 mm Hg (38-42 mm Hg considered normal limits)

OXYGEN TRANSPORT IN THE BLOOD

In the fetal stage, the lungs contain no air but nevertheless fill the thoracic cage. With the first inspiratory effort, the respiratory muscles contract powerfully to expand the chest wall creating an 80 cm H_2O negative pressure that forces air inward. During expiration, the lungs do not deflate completely; thus, from the first breath at birth to the last breath at death, the lungs are *never* airless.

Of the total amount of oxygen and carbon dioxide in the blood, less than 5% of the oxygen is in simple solution. Reversible chemical reactions are responsible for the transport of the remainder of the oxygen, and hemoglobin plays the major role in this process.

Oxyhemoglobin is oxygen-carrying hemoglobin, and the *oxyhemoglobin dissociation curve* expresses the relationship between blood oxygen tension and oxyhemoglobin saturation. The oxyhemoglobin dissociation curve should be utilized because oxygen tension and saturation frequently have different clinical implications (Fig. 6.1).

The PaO_2 (partial pressure of arterial blood oxygen) measures oxygen in solution in the blood, while the oxyhemoglobin saturation measures the amount of oxygen *attached to the hemoglobin*. The arterial blood oxygen tension is determined by the inspired oxygen tension, the adequacy of ventilation, and the efficiency of intrapulmonary gas exchange. Discrepancy between arterial blood and alveolar gas oxygen tensions indicate abnormalities of gas exchange even when blood oxygen tension has been relatively well maintained by oxygen therapy.

A tool that has gained recent attention in blood gas analysis is the alveolar (A) to arterial (a) pressure gradient (DO_2) written as A−a = DO_2. Minor ventilation-perfusion (V/Q) imbalances and diffusion defects lead to slightly lowered arterial oxygen tensions for given alveolar oxygen tensions; normal is around 15 mm Hg and increases with age and should not exceed 20-25

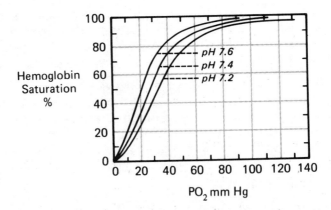

Figure 6.1. Oxyhemoglobin dissociation curve. A small increase in PO_2 in the 10-50 mm Hg range results in a large increase in the O_2 saturation of hemoglobin. Above a PO_2 of 60 mm Hg, a large increase in PO_2 results in very little increase in the O_2 saturation of hemoglobin. (Reprinted with permission of the American Lung Association)

mm Hg. An *elevation* of the A–a DO_2 is associated with the presence of an intrapulmonary process that interferes with gas exchange, such as V/Q imbalances, shunt, or diffusion disturbance.

In contrast, knowledge of oxyhemoglobin saturation is critical to appraise the adequacy of tissue oxygenation. A substantial reduction in oxygen tension is often accompanied by only modest lowering of saturation. A small increase in arterial blood oxygen tension, in the 10-50 mm Hg range, results in a *large* increase in the *oxygen saturation* of hemoglobin. An arterial blood oxygen tension of over 60 mm Hg, a large increase, results in *very little* increase in the oxygen saturation of hemoglobin.

Factors Affecting the Oxyhemoglobin Dissociation Curve

Two important conditions affect the oxyhemoglobin dissociation curve. They are the blood pH and temperature. A rise in temperature or a fall in the pH shifts the curve to the right. When the curve is shifted in this direction, hemoglobin binds less oxygen at a given arterial blood oxygen tension. The pH of blood falls as the PCO_2 increases, so that when the arterial blood oxygen tension rises, the curve shifts to the right and the oxygen-carrying capacity is decreased, making oxygen more available to the tissues.

During exercise, much more oxygen is removed from each unit of blood flowing through active tissues because the tissue arterial blood oxygen tension declines. At low arterial blood oxygen tension values, the oxyhemoglobin dissociation curve is steep, and large amounts of oxygen are liberated per unit drop in the arterial blood oxygen tension. The dissociation curve is also shifted more to the right than it is in resting tissues because the temperature rises in active tissues and carbon dioxide and metabolites accumulate, lowering the pH.

MAINTENANCE OF THE ACID-BASE BALANCE IN THE BODY—REACTION OF BLOOD

METABOLISM AND ELECTROLYTES

Maintenance of the acid-base balance of the blood is dependent upon normal metabolism and electrolyte balance *as well as* oxygen and carbon dioxide exchange with our environment. Electrolytes are chemical elements which, dissolved in water, carry an electrical charge; *cations* carry a positive charge and include sodium (Na^+), potassium (K^+), and calcium (Ca^{++}), while chloride (Cl^-) and bicarbonate (HCO_3^-) carry a negative charge and are called *anions*. With the exception of bicarbonate, which is constantly produced by the metabolic breakdown of carbohydrate, protein, and fat, all electrolytes are taken into the body as minerals in food and water. Intake of these ions should be equivalent to the output, under normal circumstances; deficiencies and surplus amounts of these electrolytes can present an interesting challenge in initial assessment and are frequently key to the underlying clinical problem.

The cells of the body require a liquid environment with a slightly alkaline reaction in order to perform their functions normally. The pH of the *blood* is 7.4 and this reaction, despite many widely fluctuating factors, is maintained at a constant level during the metabolic process.

Hydration

Water, which accounts for 60% of the total body weight (40% intracellular, 20% extracellular), is ingested, absorbed, and excreted by the kidneys, lungs, and skin in a balance that meets normal metabolic requirements. Initial patient assessment should include a rapid clinical appraisal of the patient's state of hydration; loss of skin turgor, wrinkling, and dark urine would indicate some degree of dehydration, while puffy tissues and/or edema would indicate fluid retention. Inquiry regarding food and fluid intake, vomiting, diarrhea, hyperventilation, polyuria or oliguria, will contribute to evaluation of recent fluid and electrolyte losses or gains, while observing the respiratory pattern closely for rate and depth may give clues to the pH of the blood.

Sodium

The cation sodium (Na^+), once absorbed from the intestinal tract, is maintained in the blood and extracellular fluid (ECF) in a normal concentration of 135-145 mEq/L which represents 40% of the total body sodium level; the balance is found inside the cells, bone, and connective tissue. Sodium is secreted in perspiration, pancreatic juices, bile and small intestines, and massive amounts may be lost in persistent vomiting or diarrhea, since normally much of the intestinal sodium content is reabsorbed and conserved. The kidney regulates sodium excretion according to body requirements, with reabsorption taking place in the distal tubule of Henle's Loop in exchange for hydrogen ion or potassium, again depending on body needs.

Hyponatremia	Hypernatremia
Decreased Na^+ intake	Decreased H_2O intake
Decreased absorption	Increased H_2O loss:
Heavy diaphoresis	• Skin
Increased loss from diuretics	• Lungs
Persistent nausea and vomiting	• Kidneys (e.g., diabetes in-sipidus)
Poor transport of H_2O to kidneys	Disorders of kidney regulation
H_2O retention out of proportion to salt	

Sodium retention seen in hypertension, renal failure, or congestive heart failure retains water with it so that low sodium concentration will probably be seen.

Potassium

Potassium (K^+) is the principal intracellular cation and is normally ingested in adequate amounts in the daily diet; fruits containing large amounts of potassium for additional needs include bananas, oranges, and prunes. The normal concentration in both blood and ECF is between 3.8 and 5 mEq/L, which represents only 2% of the total mEq within the body. Potassium has a profound effect on cellular activity and the acid-base balance, similarly, has a particular influence on the relationship between plasma and cellular potassium. Acidosis tends to shift potassium out of cells, while alkalosis favors movement of potassium from extracellular fluid into cells. It can be said, simply, that potassium goes where hydrogen ions go; therefore, when the pH is low, hydrogen ions in the serum are increased and so is potassium. When the pH is elevated, hydrogen ions are decreased and so is the *serum* potassium level. (Remember that a serum potassium level reflects only 2% of the whole body's potassium.)

Potassium is secreted in perspiration, gastric and pancreatic juices, and fluids of the small intestine, all of which represent a significant source of loss in GI diseases. Potassium is also released from the cells in great amounts with trauma or burns involving tissue destruction.

Hypokalemia	Hyperkalemia
Abnormal excretion	Tissue trauma
Decreased intake	• Burns
GI losses:	• Bruises
• Continual suction	• Lacerations
• Diarrhea	Acidosis of any kind
• Vomiting	Heavy IV administration
	Impaired kidney function

Under normal circumstances, the intracellular potassium level is about 110 mEq/L and extracellular potassium is about 4 mEq/L; specific clinical problems will result in potassium leaving the cells and passing into the interstitial/extravascular spaces. Code situations, both in trauma and cardiac arrest, which result in metabolic acidosis will require correction of the acidosis in order to drive potassium back into the cells and reduce the threshold of cellular excitability; more attention is being paid to replacing K^+ in cardiac emergencies now in order to reduce the greater incidence of ectopy. Recurrent ventricular fibrillation and ventricular tachycardia are known to be K^+ dependent arrhythmias and early recognition and correction of acidosis is essential to control.

Some important points to remember about administration of potassium are:*

1. *Never* inject directly into an IV line! A bolus is not only *extremely* dangerous but is extremely painful;
2. Always dilute in at least 500 cc of IV fluid and administer at a rate no greater than 20 mEq/hr for safety;
3. Be certain that urine output is established before potassium administration;
4. Monitor patient closely for: (see Chapter 11 on ECGs and Arrhythmias)
   A. Any change in heart rate, rhythm, or duration of QRS pattern
   B. Signs of toxicity such as:
      - Narrowed *peaked* T wave (potassium "tents" under T wave)
      - *Shortened* QT interval
      - *Prolonged* PR interval
      - *Diminished* P waves
      - Bizarre ECGs with *widened* QRS complex

An approach to treating hyperkalemia is to give both bicarbonate and insulin in order to 1) correct the acidosis and increase the pH (to drive the K^+ serum level down) and 2) to administer insulin and glucose in balance formula (to drive K^+ back into the cells *with* the glucose). Whatever the management strategy involved, close baseline monitoring of the patient is an essential nursing role and responsibility.

Calcium

Although calcium (Ca^{++}) is not generally considered a major serum electrolyte, essential to the acid-base balance, it is included here because of its implications in cardiac and trauma emergencies. Calcium enters the body through the alimentary track; half is absorbed and the rest is excreted in stool. It is transported in the blood in two forms, with half in a protein-bound form and the other half ionized with phosphate. The normal serum calcium level is 4.5 to 5.5 mEq/L.

---

*Meltzer LE, Pinneo R, Kitchell JR: Intensive Coronary Care, A Manual for Nurses. 3rd ed. The Robert J. Brady Co., Bowie, Maryland, 1977

Calcium is essential to the contractile apparatus of muscle cells, along with the Na^+-K^+ exchange across cell membranes; the *strength* of muscular contractions is dependent on the quantity of calcium which reaches the contractile sites; it is also essential to the normal clotting mechanisms of blood. Calcium is lost from the body by way of the GI tract, urine (kidney stones in hypercalcemia), and sweat, as well as serum loss in bone deposits.

Hypocalcemia	Hypercalcemia
Insufficient dietary intake	Abnormally high dietary intake
Malabsorptive disorders	Metabolic disorders
Blood loss	Iatrogenic causes
Hypothalamus malregulation	Kidney glomerular malfunction
Kidney glomerular malfunction	
Hyperphosphotemia	

Calcium deficiencies are observed clinically when manifested as neuromuscular irritability and Tetany syndrome with carpo-pedal spasms, anxiety, altered mental state, seizures, bronchospasm, laryngospasm (with classical crowing sound), and a lengthened Q-T interval. Treatment is administration of IV calcium.

Hypercalcemia, on the other hand, is demonstrated with anorexia, nausea and vomiting, constipation, some degree of hyponatremia, kidney stones, and frequently depression. Treatment includes Lasix to increase urinary excretion of calcium.

When administering calcium, some important points to remember are:

1. Never give in the presence of *ventricular fibrillation;*
2. Never give sub-Q or IM—it is extremely irritating to the tissues;
3. Calcium chloride is more potent than calcium gluconate and more irritating to the tissues—both can cause necrosis from IV infiltration;
4. Calcium gluconate acts like digitalis on the heart, increasing tone of muscle and force of contractions (positive inotropic effect);
5. When administering massive replacement of blood with *stored* units, coagulopathy may ensue unless calcium is replenished. (Binding of calcium by anticoagulants in banked blood is a problem with massive transfusions.) See Chapter 15 on Major Trauma.

The so-called calcium channel blocking agents are used to oppose calcium fluxes at the cellular membrane level, and since calcium is a critically important ion in cardiovascular function, this has important implications. The most widely used of these agents are verapamil, nifedipine, and diltiazem hydrochloride and have been found, by their calcium antagonism to 1) lower blood pressure, 2) raise cardiac output in heart failure, 3) effectively convert tachyarrhythmias to normal sinus rhythm and decrease heart rate, and 4) to give effective relief in angina.

Chloride

Chloride (Cl^-) is ingested, absorbed, transported and secreted along with sodium, potassium, and calcium and in the same manner. Chloride is excreted by the kidneys, and depending on the body's need for sodium bicarbonate, more or less chloride is excreted as ammonia to eliminate hydrogen ions in exchange for sodium. Regulation in the body, therefore, is passively related to sodium levels; when serum sodium increases, chloride usually increases but when more bicarbonate is needed, chloride will be sacrificed.

Hypochloremia	Hyperchloremia
Decreased intake with normal fluid intake	Dehydration
Malabsorption and diarrhea	Diamox diuretics
Increased secretion	Salicylate intoxication
• Profuse diaphoresis	Acute renal failure
• Vomiting	Diabetes insipidus
Increased excretion—diuretics	
Respiratory acidosis	
Adrenal insufficiency	
Diabetic acidosis	
Lactic acidosis	

ACID-BASE REGULATION FACTORS

Regulation of the acid-base balance is controlled by two groups of factors; these may be designated as physicochemical and physiologic.

Physicochemical Factors—Buffers

The ability of the body to neutralize acid or base in order to maintain a blood pH of 7.4 resides in buffers. A *buffer* is a substance which aids in preventing the change in reaction of a solution on the addition of acid and/or base. The blood is capable of combining with almost 300 times as much acid as an equal amount of distilled water before the reaction will change, and this is due to the buffers normally found in the blood such as carbonic acid (carbon dioxide), acid carbonate (HCO_3), diacid and dibastic phosphates, and proteinate (hemoglobin being the most important of the protein buffers). These buffer systems act within seconds.

Acid carbonate (HCO_3 or bicarbonate) is particularly important since it interacts immediately with any non-volatile acid which appears in the blood to form a neutral salt and carbonic acid (H_2CO_3) which then dissociates at once into water and carbon dioxide; the carbon dioxide is promptly eliminated by the lungs.

$$H^+ + \quad HCO^3 \longrightarrow H_2CO_3 \longrightarrow H_2O + \quad CO_2$$

acid   acid carbonate   carbonic acid   water   carbon dioxide
        (bicarbonate)

Fixed acids do not appear in the blood in significant amounts except under the following circumstances:

1. During violent exercise (lactic acid)
2. In severe anoxia (lactic acid)
3. In severe diabetes or starvation (beta-oxybutyric and aceto-acetic acids)
4. In advanced nephritis (phosphoric and sulphuric acids)

The alkaline reserve is base which is potentially available through hemoglobin and other blood proteins for the neutralization of acids; it will combine with bicarbonate but cannot be measured directly. The alkaline reserve is determined indirectly by the carbon dioxide combining power of the blood, which normally is between 55 and 65 volumes percent (ml CO_2 per 100 ml blood).

Physiologic Factors

Pulmonary ventilation and renal output of acid and base are the two physiologic factors concerned in the regulation of acid-base balance.

An increase in the carbon dioxide level in the blood stimulates breathing, the introduction of base into the blood decreases respirations and the balance is so regulated that the ratio of CO_2 to HCO_3 (bicarbonate) remains constant at 1:20.

If the numerator (CO_2) is increased, base will be made available in the blood to increase the denominator (HCO_3) proportionately.

The body continually produces CO_2 in metabolism, the amount being directly proportional to the rate of production and to the rate of elimination (ventilation). The CO_2 level can fluctuate in minutes and seconds through the lung activity; the kidneys take a longer time to compensate (several hours to days) with HCO_3 (bicarbonate). The kidneys also help maintain the acid-base balance by altering the relative amounts of acid and basic phosphates excreted. They also form ammonia; the amount of ammonia formed will be increased if fixed acids are present in large amounts as in diabetes mellitus or severe anoxia and decreased if sodium must be excreted. The acid-base balance must be disturbed for several days before the ammonia mechanism comes into play.

Acid-base adjustment is so effectively maintained by the lungs and kidneys that ordinarily the pH of the blood is kept at 7.4 and the CO_2 combining power at 60 volumes percent. Normally, changes associated with exercise and ingestion of acid or base are corrected by the physiologic factors, however, in some disease states the individual is unable to adjust normally to the change and *acidosis* or *alkalosis* results. If the pH remains unaltered in spite of symptoms of alkalosis or acidosis, the condition is said to be *compensated;* if the pH is altered, the acidosis or alkalosis is said to be *uncompensated.*

ARTERIAL BLOOD GASES

Arterial blood gases are a reflection of the normal and abnormal blood gas values in the body and should be considered a "look at the entire body." They should be the first laboratory test ordered and drawn in a number of acute conditions that enter the ED. The criteria for evaluating arterial blood gases are numerous but are often overlooked during the first inspection of the patient. Frequently, the result is a delay in treatment that is essential and relatively easy, once the need is recognized.

One indication for arterial blood gases (ABG) is *hypoxia,* the deficiency of oxygen at the *cellular* or *tissue* level. Hypoxia is present when there is an insufficient supply of oxygen to meet the metabolic requirements of the cell, as opposed to *hypoxemia,* which is a decreased amount of oxygen in the blood.

Hypercapnia, or *hypercarbia,* is an increased carbon dioxide concentration in the arterial blood. The condition occurs when alveolar ventilation cannot keep pace with body metabolism and carbon dioxide production. The degree of CO_2 retention is measured by the arterial PCO_2. Acute hypercapnia is CO_2 retention that occurs in a relatively short time, making the arterial blood more acid; chronic hypercapnia is CO_2 retention that occurs over several days, weeks, or months. The blood pH may be normal because of the kidney's ability to compensate by reabsorbing bicarbonate which usually takes 3-5 days.

Some cardinal signs of hypoxia and hypercapnia that would indicate the need for evaluation of arterial blood gases are presented in Table 6.1. When these clinical manifestations are present, it becomes obligatory to draw blood gases and to treat from these values as indicated.

Table 6.1 Cardinal Signs of Hypoxia and Hypercapnia

SIGNS OF HYPOXIA	SIGNS OF HYPERCAPNIA
Unconsciousness	Unconsciousness
Hypotension*	Hypertension
Combativeness (common)**	Dizziness
Confusion**	Confusion**
Dyspnea at rest	Cyanosis at rest
Restlessness	Headache
Tachycardia	Twitching
Central cyanosis	Diaphoresis
Warm extremities	Miosis (constricted pupils)

*Always a sign of the need for oxygen.
**Frequently a sign of the need for oxygen.

INTERPRETATION OF ARTERIAL BLOOD GAS STUDIES

pH

An indication of acidosis or alkalosis in the body. Normal pH is usually between 7.35 and 7.45, and the body functions normally in this state. A pH of lower than 7.35 is a determination of acidosis, and a pH of higher than 7.45 is a determination of alkalosis.

P_{CO_2}

An indication of partial pressure of CO_2 in the *arterial* blood. A normal value for CO_2 is 40 mm Hg $\pm$ 5mm. A high CO_2 pressure indicates hypoventilation of some type and is usually reflected by lowering of the pH. A low CO_2 pressure usually reflects hyperventilation with an accompanying rise in the pH. (CO_2 is 25 times more diffusable in the blood and tissues than O_2.)

Standard Bicarbonate

An indication of the buffering capacity of the blood with normal values of around 25 mEq/liter. (24 mEq/L $\pm$ 3 mEq/liter.)

Base Excess

An indicator of treatment with extraneous bicarbonate. Normal value is 0 ± 2 or 3. Treatment of a *minus* base excess ($-BE$) of significance should be based on the following formula for the amount of bicarbonate to be given:

$$(wt[kg] \times [-BE]/5) \times 0.5$$

PaO_2

An indicator of the pressure of arterial oxygen in the blood. Normal arterial oxygen pressure is from 90 to 100 mm Hg. Low PO_2 usually means hypoxia of some type. A high PO_2 is usually insignificant except when prolonged and the patient becomes oxygen-toxic.

Oxygen Saturation

An indicator of the oxygen saturation (SaO_2) of hemoglobin. Optimal oxygen saturation is 100%; the pH determines the availability of this oxygen to the tissues as shown on the oxyhemoglobin dissociation curve.

Respiratory Versus Metabolic

To effectively manage the patient it must be first determined whether the acidosis or alkalosis is of metabolic or respiratory nature. Some questions to ask in order to make this determination are:

1. Is the pH normal (7.40 ± 0.05), high (alkalosis), or low (acidosis)?
2. Is the main process respiratory (main abnormality is in PCO_2) or metabolic (main abnormality is in HCO_3)?
3. Is the process uncompensated, partially compensated, or completely compensated (indicated by a normal pH)?
4. If the main abnormality is respiratory, is the process acute (no compensatory change in HCO_3) or chronic (the kidneys have had hours to days to regulate HCO_3)?

Metabolic Acidosis

pH ↓, HCO_3 ↓ (primary), PCO_2 ↓. The acid-base status of the body shifts toward the acid side because of loss of base and excess production of organic acids or failure of the body to excrete accumulated acids. The body will try to compensate by hyperventilating in order to lower the CO_2 level in the blood. Some examples are: 1) lactic acidosis; 2) diabetic ketoacidosis; 3) salicylate intoxication; 4) chronic renal failure; 5) methanol poisoning.

Metabolic Alkalosis

pH ↑, HCO_3 ↑ (primary), PCO_2 ↑. The acid-base status of the body shifts toward the alkaline side because of retention of base, a deficit of H± ions in the blood caused by excessive intake of alkaline substances. The lungs will attempt to compensate by hypoventilating and thus raising the PCO_2. Examples: 1) vomiting; 2) nasogastric suction; 3) administration of long-term diuretics; 4) administration of steroids; 5) excessive HCO_3 therapy.

Respiratory Acidosis

pH ↓, PCO_2 ↑ (primary), HCO_3 ↑. This condition is due to excess retention of CO_2 in the body (also called hypercapnic acidosis). Occurring with alveolar underventilation with the lungs unable to eliminate CO_2 as rapidly as it is being produced by the body. Remember that whenever the PCO_2 rises, the PO_2 will fall when the patient is breathing room air. Examples: 1) acute airway obstruction (cafe coronary, for example); 2) pulmonary edema; 3) anaphylaxis; 4) cardiac arrest and acute respiratory failure.

Respiratory Alkalosis

pH ↑, PCO_2 ↓ (primary), HCO_3 ↓. Caused by excess loss of CO_2 from the body and may occur with overventilation of the alveoli when lungs eliminate CO_2 in excess of production. Examples: 1) hyperventilation; 2) respiratory maladjustments; 3) pulmonary embolus; 4) myocardial infarction; 5) mild to moderate asthma; 6) liver disease.

ARTERIAL PUNCTURE*

A sampling for blood gas analysis must be obtained by arterial puncture and an assembled or prepared kit should contain the following:

- 2-ml syringe with 25 gauge needle for infiltration if necessary
- 1% lidocaine (optional to have on hand)
- 10-ml syringe with 19 or 20 gauge needle (adult); or 22 or 25 gauge needle (child)
- Sodium heparin (1,000 units/ml mixed with normal saline)
- Rubber stopper or cap to seal air from needle
- Sterile sponges and skin germicide
- Small basin or bag for ice
- Tape for label

Selection of the puncture site will most likely depend on the clinical situation and the rapidity with which the sample must be obtained, as well as the circulatory status of the patient. The three readily available sites are the radial artery, brachial artery, and femoral artery; the latter is most frequently selected in trauma code situations when peripheral pulses are compromised and the femoral artery is not only accessible but frequently peripheral to the central areas of activity. When using the brachial or radial artery it is best to hyperextend the arm or wrist to facilitate palpation as the artery is located and puncture site is bracketed with your fingertips.

Precautions

1. The specimen placed in the basin of ice and properly labeled must be taken to the laboratory *immediately*. Blood gas determinations should be done immediately since gas tensions and the pH can change rapidly.

2. Following puncture, the site must be inspected frequently, along with other assessments of the patient. Hematoma, arterial thrombosis, arterial spasm, and ulnar nerve puncture are complications following this procedure.

3. If the radial artery is the site to be punctured, it is *essential* to first check the patency of the ulnar artery to assure circulation to the hand in case of radial artery spasm. This is done by means of the Allen test and the patient's record should reflect documentation of a patent ulnar artery. The Allen test is accomplished by elevating the patient's hand and arm while encircling the wrist, with thumb depressing the ulnar artery, and fingers depressing the radial artery. Instruct the patient to open and close the hand several times, which will cause the palm to blanch from the occluded blood supply. Release pressure over the ulnar artery and

---

*Excerpted from "Arterial Puncture" ROCOM Medical Skills Library. Annuals of Internal Medicine. American College of Physicians, with permission.

observe closely; a patent ulnar artery will allow the hand to flush with arterial blood and restore color.

Some important procedural points are:

1. Explain the procedure to the patient if the situation permits.
2. The patient's temperature, respiratory rate, and the amount of oxygen being received (i.e., room air, 10 LMP, etc.) must be noted on the laboratory slip since these measurements are taken into consideration when the sample is evaluated. (There is a 15-20 mm log time when O_2 is started or d.c.'d before blood reflects the change.)
3. The syringe must be heparinized by withdrawing a sufficient amount of heparin (1,000 USP units per ml) into the syringe to wet the plunger completely and prevent blood from clotting. The syringe must be held in an upright position and all excess heparin and air bubbles expelled.
4. Proper skin preparation with a germicide is essential. Using sterile technique, the fingertips of the free hand are used to bracket the area of maximum pulsation in the artery as the needle is inserted into the artery, bevel upward, at a right angle or slightly acute angle to the artery. As the needle enters the artery, the pulsating flow of blood will easily fill the syringe, after which the needle is withdrawn.
5. Firm pressure *must* be maintained on the puncture site for at least a *full five minutes* to prevent the formation of a hematoma, and if the patient is on an anticoagulant medication, direct pressure *must* be applied over the puncture site for 15 minutes and then a firm pressure dressing for 3-4 hours.
6. Again, immediately cap the needle by sticking the end into the rubber plug, thereby preventing room air from mixing with the specimen. Place it in the container of ice, labeled with the patient's name and the time drawn. Be certain that the accompanying laboratory requisition reflects the patient's temperature, respiratory rate, and the oxygen percentage being administered. If the patient is on room air, *indicate* room air.

REVIEW

1. Define photosynthesis and the respiratory cycle.
2. Explain the derivation of partial pressures of gases in the bloodstream.
3. Identify two significant factors that affect the oxyhemoglobin dissociation curve.
4. List the major cations and anions involved in the maintenance of acid-base balance, their normal serum values, and causes of deficiencies and excesses.

5. Describe the clinical findings with deficiencies and excesses of the major electrolytes.

6. Describe the most important points to remember in replacement and administration of potassium and calcium.

7. Describe the physicochemical and physiologic factors which determine the acid-base balance of the body.

8. List some examples of fixed acids appearing in the blood in significant amounts and under what circumstances.

9. Explain alkaline reserve and the method by which it is determined.

10. Describe the role of the lungs and kidneys as they relate to the adjustment of pH in the body.

11. Define hypoxia and identify five manifestations.

12. Define hypercapnia and identify five manifestations.

13. Identify the normal values in arterial blood gases.

14. Define base excess.

15. List the equipment necessary to perform arterial puncture.

16. Describe the proper technique to be employed in obtaining arterial blood samples.

17. Identify the hazards in sampling arterial blood.

18. Explain the Allen test and the rationale for using it.

19. Describe the formula for determining the correct dosage of sodium bicarbonate IV.

20. Identify the four steps in determining acid-base status of the patient.

21. Explain the pH and bicarbonate status in metabolic acidosis and give at least three clinical examples.

22. Explain the pH and bicarbonate status in metabolic alkalosis and give at least three clinical examples.

23. Explain the pH and carbon dioxide status in respiratory alkalosis and give at least three clinical examples.

24. Explain the pH and carbon dioxide status in respiratory acidosis and give at least three clinical examples.

BIBLIOGRAPHY

American College of Physicians: Arterial Puncture. American College of Physicians Medical Skills Library, ROCOM, Annals of Internal Medicine, Philadelphia, Pennsylvania, 1972

American Lung Association: Graphic Aids in Blood Gas Analysis. American Lung Association, New York

Barnes TA, et al: Brady's Programmed Instruction to Respiratory Therapy, 2nd ed. Robert J. Brady Co., Bowie, Maryland, 1980

Budassi SA: An emergency nurse's guide to drawing arterial blood gases. JEN, Vol 3, No 1, Emergency Department Nurses Association, Lansing, Michigan, 1977

Budassi SA, Barber JM: Emergency Nursing: Principles and Practice. C.V. Mosby Co., St. Louis, Missouri, 1981

Collins RD: Illustrated Manual of Fluid and Electrolyte Disorders. J.B. Lippincott Co., Philadelphia, Pennsylvania, 1976

Cosgriff JH: Atlas of Diagnostic and Therapeutic Procedures for Emergency Personnel. J.B. Lippincott Co., Philadelphia, Pennsylvania, 1978

Engberg S: Blood gases. JEN, Vol 2, No 6, Emergency Department Nurses Association, Lansing, Michigan, 1976

Filley G: Acid-Base and Blood Gas Regulation. Lea and Febiger, Philadelphia, Pennsylvania, 1967

Goldberger E: A Primer of Water, Electrolytes and Acid-Base Syndromes. Lea and Febiger, 6th ed. Philadelphia, Pennsylvania, 1980

Guyton AC: Medical Physiology. W.B. Saunders Co., Philadelphia, Pennsylvania, 1977

Hunsinger D, et al: Respiratory Technology, 2nd ed. A Procedure Manual. Reston Publishing Co., Reston, Virginia, 1980

Karlsberg RP: Calcium Channel Blockers for Cardiovascular Disorders. Arch Intern Med, Vol 142, March 1982

Meltzer LE, Pinneo R, Kitchell JR: Intensive Coronary Care, A Manual for Nurses. Robert J. Brady Co., Bowie, Maryland, 1977

Oakes A, Morrow H: Understanding blood gases. Assessing Vital Functions Accurately. Nursing 77 Books, Horsham, Pennsylvania, 1977

Shrake K: The ABCs of ABGs—or how to interpret a blood gas value. Nursing 79, Vol 9, No 9, pp 26-33, September 1979

Thorn GW, Adams RD, Brawnwald E, et al: Harrison's Principles of Internal Medicine, 8th ed. McGraw-Hill, New York, 1977

Wade AM, Wilson RF: Management of Trauma: Pitfalls and Practice. Lea and Febiger, Philadelphia, Pennsylvania, 1975

Wade J: Respiratory Nursing Care, 3rd ed. C.V. Mosby Co., St. Louis, Missouri, 1982

NEUROLOGICAL ASSESSMENT 7

KEY CONCEPTS

The aim of this chapter is to promote an understanding and a working approach to the components of a nursing neurological assessment. The material is based on lecture material presented to emergency nurses by Louise Queener, Neurological Nurse Specialist, and Susan Foster, Neurological Nurse Specialist, both of the Portland Metropolitan Area.

After reading and studying this chapter, you should be able to:

- Identify the first two priorities when receiving a patient with head injuries in ED.
- Identify the components of the neurological assessment.
- Name the most important parameter in observing a patient with head injuries.
- Describe the correct method of caring for contact lenses after removal.
- Identify some of the pupil patterns seen with various problems.
- Define direct reaction and consensual reaction.
- Identify the cranial nerves which control eye movements and their function.
- Describe the significance of a patient being unable to look laterally or medially.
- Explain the meaning of PERL–A.
- Explain the doll's-eye maneuver and its significance.
- Identify the areas tested in motor systems' assessment and the tests employed.
- List some of the methods employed in eliciting response from a partially or totally unresponsive patient.
- Describe the correct manner of eliciting a valid response to a Babinski test and define a positive Babinski finding.
- Describe decorticate posture and its implication.
- Describe decerebrate posture and its implication.
- Describe flaccid posture.
- Describe the Glasgow Coma Scale and explain its interpretation.

Probably for no other patient does the nurse rely so heavily on her senses to make a thorough assessment. A rapid, general assessment, insuring a patient airway and checking for possible cervical spine damage, is completed *prior* to moving an unresponsive or head-injured patient onto the ED cart. Vital signs are taken and recorded immediately and should be repeated at regular intervals, initially every 15 minutes during the patient's stay in the department until they are stabilized. The patient must be completely disrobed once the initial assessment has revealed that no cervical spine fracture is present and the patient is secure on the emergency cart.

COMPONENTS OF NEUROLOGICAL ASSESSMENT

The level of consciousness (LOC) is the single most important baseline observation required, but pupil reaction and eye movements, and motor system assessment (it is important to develop systematic approach) are also essential.

LEVEL OF CONSCIOUSNESS

Evaluate and document the appropriatness of responses as you observe them. Determine confusion, degree of orientation, lack of response, etc. Question the patient as to the day, year, name, and relevant information, making every effort to distinguish between speech impairment and confusion, as well as ability to respond to specific commands. Again, documentation is essential to establish a baseline for evaluation of changes which may or may not occur.

EYE SIGNS

The sclera should be searched for contact lenses, which may be used by patients of any age. Often the lenses may be displaced from the cornea and found beneath the eyelid; they should be removed with a small suction-cup device. The soft-type lens may have adhered to the cornea if the patient's eyes have been closed for any considerable length of time and should *not* be removed until normal saline irrigant has been used to soften the lens and "float" it free. Corneal damage can be sustained otherwise. If lenses are present, they should be removed and stored for safekeeping with identification of right and left lenses; soft lenses must be stored in normal saline. Any other solution containing buffers will permanently damage the very expensive lenses.

Pupil size and shape are an important sign. Under ordinary circumstances, the pupils should be round, regular and equal, and reactive to light. Inequality of pupils usually results from an intracranial lesion such as subdural hematoma. Constricted or pinpoint pupils may indicate narcotic addiction; dilated pupils accompany barbiturate intoxication or anoxia. In functional disorder, the pupils are characteristically dilated, equal, and reactive. Failure of the pupils to constrict when stimulated by light may indicate severe brain damage.

The nurse is cautioned to be alert for an ocular prosthesis (glass eye), which can be very misleading to the uninitiated. There is also an occasional person with a condition known as *anisocoria,* congential inequality of the pupils in diameter.

For pupil reaction and eye movement, check with a penlight with strong batteries as follows:

1. Observe if the pupils are round, normal sized, and moving together.

2. Check for light reaction, keeping one eye closed as you check the other. This is called *direct reaction.* If both eyes are left open, the light may be perceived on the opposite side by *consensual reaction.* This is because the third nerve nucleus on one eye can transmit to or innervate the nucleus of the opposite eye.

3. Check for extraocular eye movements (EOM). Eye movements are controlled by the third, fourth, and sixth cranial nerves. A third nerve lesion renders the eye unable to look *inward* or *medially.* A sixth nerve lesion renders the eye unable to look *laterally.* The affected eye stays midline. (Cranial nerve signs are usually *ipsilateral* or same sided.)

   It is important to have the patient hold his head in one position while asking him to follow your finger with his eyes. For instance, inability of the left eye to look laterally indicates a sixth nerve lesion on the left.

   The third and sixth cranial nerves have long courses through the intracranial vault, and very frequently, the *first* sign of increasing intracranial pressure will be the inability of the patient to look laterally or medially.

4. *Chart* if pupils are normal size and reactive to light: *PERL* means pupils equal, reactive to light. In the term *PERL–A,* the *A* is for *accommodation.* This means the patient is able to follow your finger as you hold it up, from a distance to a near point, and as you watch the eyes converge, the lenses thicken and the pupils constrict slightly.

5. The doll's-eye maneuver refers to the fact that normally, as the head is rapidly turned to one side, the eyes go to the opposite side. An absent or positive doll's-eye sign is produced when the head is turned to the side and the eyes stay midline. You *cannot* test for doll's-eye in an alert patient since voluntary control would be present. The lesion causing loss or absence of doll's-eye is at the point where the third, fourth, and sixth cranial nerves travel closely together in the brain stem. (*Caution:* Do not use doll's-eye maneuver unless the possibility of cervical spine fracture has been ruled out!)

6. Remember that the lesion (clot) is on the same side as affected eye, with the possible exception of contre coup injuries.

MOTOR SYSTEM ASSESSMENT

It is important to develop a *systematic* approach to assessment of movement by starting at the top and working down. The responses elicited depend on the patient's LOC, but it is often helpful to demonstrate what you are asking for as you test the patient.

Facial Weakness

Have the patient:

- Show teeth
- Wrinkle forehead
- Open eyes wide and close tightly
- Stick tongue way out (tests twelfth cranial nerve).

Arm and Hand Strength Compared Bilaterally

Test grip by having patient hold just two of your fingers and pull fingers out to test for strength.

Close eyes and extend arms. Watch for downward drift of one arm in 30-60 seconds (an indication of weakness).

Leg Strength Compared Bilaterally

Ask patient to lift one leg and then the other off the bed.

Place hand at the bottom of foot and ask patient to tap his foot against your hand. Any weakness will show.

Babinski Reflex

This is elicited by stroking the sole of the foot firmly upward starting at the lateral aspect of the heel and curving medially toward the big toe. A Babinski reflex should be elicited with the very least painful stimulus. A normal or negative Babinski reflex is demonstrated when the big toe flexes downward and the other toes flex down or stay in normal position. A positive Babinski, indicating a lesion anywhere along the corticospinal tract is demonstrated when the big toe flexes upward on stimulus.

TECHNIQUES OF ELICITING RESPONSE

In the partially or totally unresponsive patient, it may require everything in your power to determine whether or not that patient responds at all. The effort may include:

- Voice stimulus
- Shaking
- Vigorous shaking
- Painful stimuli, such as 1) pinching under arm or inner aspect of leg; 2) applying pressure on supraorbital nerve notch near the nasal margin; 3) applying pressure on the nail bed.

Responses To Be Documented

It is extremely important to document all findings and note any changed from the initial baseline information. In the unresponsive patient, several areas can be readily evaluated and documented. The most likely of these are:

- Facial grimaces and types of posturing in response to painful stimuli
- Withdrawal from painful stimulus without moving the extremity tested and grabbing or deflecting with the other extremity is a normal protective defense and demonstrates a good deal of thought process. Be certain to *chart* such an instance. This tells you the patient is not paralyzed in that extremity and that cognizance of pain exists.
- Posture and movement (Fig. 7.1)
  1. Decorticate posture indicates a lesion high near the brain cortex or high midbrain and is manifested with the arms rigidly flexed on the chest and hands rotated internally along with stiffened legs.
  2. Decerebrate posture indicates a descending lesion invading the brain stem and is a rigid extension of *all* extremities, abduction of the arms, arching of the back, and toes pointed inward. It usually indicates the elimination of cerebral function either transient or otherwise.
  3. Flaccid posture is weak and limp with no response or muscle tone.

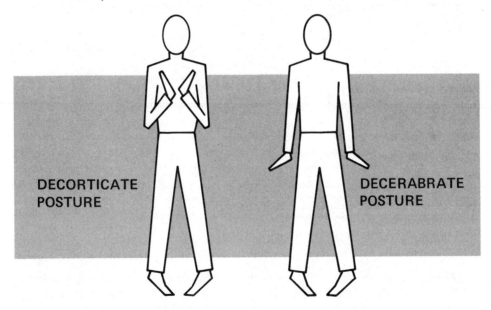

DECORTICATE POSTURE

DECERABRATE POSTURE

Figure 7.1. Inappropriate postures seen in the severely brain-damaged patient.

THE GLASGOW COMA SCALE

The Glasgow Coma Scale (GCS) is a neurological evaluation tool being used widely in the prehospital phase of care and is included here for the EDN's reference (see Table 7.1).

Table 7.1 Glasgow Coma Scale

EYES:	OPEN	Spontaneously	4
		To verbal command	3
		To pain	2
	NO RESPONSE		1
BEST MOTOR RESPONSE:	**TO VERBAL COMMAND**	Obeys	6
	TO PAINFUL STIMULUS*	Localizes pain	5
		Flexion—withdrawal	4
		Flexion—abnormal (decorticate rigidity)	3
		Extension (decerebrate rigidity)	2
	NO RESPONSE		1
BEST VERBAL RESPONSE**		Oriented and converses	5
		Disoriented and converses	4
		Inappropriate words	3
		Incomprehensible sounds	2
	NO RESPONSE		1
TOTAL			3-15

*Apply knuckles to sternum; observe arms.
**Arouse patient with painful stimulus if necessary.

The GCS is based upon eye opening, verbal, and motor responses and is a relatively practical way of monitoring changes in the level of consciousness. Various responses on the scale are given a number value; the responsiveness of the patient can then be expressed by summation of the figures, the lowest score being 3 and the highest 15.*

*Adapted from Upjohn, January 1980, based on Teasdale, G, and Jennett, B, Glasgow Coma Scale. *Lancet,* No. 7872, p 81

REVIEW

1. Name the two priorities when receiving a patient with head injury in the ED.
2. Identify the components of the neurological assessment.
3. Identify the single most important parameter when observing a patient with head injury.
4. Describe the proper removal and care of both soft and hard contact lenses.
5. Describe the meaning of unequal pupils.
6. Describe the meaning of constricted equal pupils.
7. Describe the most likely meaning of dilated pupils.
8. Describe the characteristic pupil status in functional disorders.
9. Explain the meaning of direct reaction and consensual reaction.
10. Identify the cranial nerves that control eye movements and their function.
11. Describe the significance of a patient's inability to look laterally with either eye without moving the head.
12. When charting PERL-A, what is the significance of A?
13. Describe the doll's-eye maneuver and its significance.
14. Describe the systematic tests employed in evaluating motor systems.
15. Describe the means by which response can be elicited from a partially responsive patient.
16. Describe decorticate posture and explain its meaning.
17. Describe decerebrate posture and explain its meaning.
18. Describe the Glasgow Coma Scale (GCS).
19. Explain the clinical areas of evaluation using the GCS.

BIBLIOGRAPHY

Buckingham WB, Sparberg M, Brandfonbrener M: A Primer of Clinical Diagnosis, 2nd ed. Harper & Row, New York, 1979
Cosgriff JH, Anderson DL: The Practice of Emergency Nursing, J.B. Lippincott Co., Philadelphia, Pennsylvania, 1975
Dagrosa T: Brainstem damage associated with cerebral injury. JEN, Vol 2, No 5, 1976
Glass SJ: Nursing care of the neurosurgical patient Head injuries. J Neurosurg Nursing, Vol 5, No 2, pp 49-55, 1973
Luckmann J, Sorenson K: Medical-Surgical Nursing. W.B. Saunders Co., Philadelphia, Pennsylvania, pp 430-431, 1974

Plum F, Posner JB: The Diagnosis of Stupor and Coma, 3rd ed. F.A. Davis Co., Philadel-
   phia, Pennsylvania, 1980
Teasdale G, Jennett B: Glasgow coma scale. Lancet 7872, p 81
Valencius J: Guidelines for neuroassessment, AORN J, Vol 20, No 442, 1974
Young MS: Understanding the Signs of Intracranial Pressure. Nursing 81, Vol 11, No 2,
   Intermed Communications, Horsham, Pennsylvania, February 1981

BASIC RADIOLOGY IN THE EMERGENCY DEPARTMENT

8

KEY CONCEPTS

This chapter represents the compilation of some very basic guidelines that will hopefully contribute to cooperative and constructive effort between emergency and radiology departments in the interest of quality patient care, as well as developing the abilities of EDNs to perform at certain levels of competency in assessing the need for specific X-ray procedures and the use of pertinent terminology. Much of this material represents the contributions of Raymond F. Friedman, M.D., Clinical Associate Professor of Diagnostic Radiology, and of J. Richard Raines, M.D., Clinical Professor of Diagnostic Radiology, both of the Oregon Health Sciences University.

After reading and studying this chapter, you should be able to:

- Describe the proper procedure for preparing a patient for X-ray examination.
- Identify the areas of important information that should be contained on the X-ray requisition.
- Explain the reasons for including all of the requested information in accurate fashion.
- Describe the correct nomenclature used for requisitioning fingers and toes on X-ray.
- Define radiology and roentgenology, radiopaque, and radiolucent.
- Identify the five basic roentgen densities in order of increasing density.
- List the routine views utilized when obtaining X-ray films.
- Identify the prime example of metal density *normally* found in the body.
- Describe the effect of water density in *anatomic* contact with another water density.
- Describe the views usually included in a skull series.
- Identify the situation which requires a Water's view.
- Explain the importance of visualizing the pineal gland in skull films.

- Describe the views taken normally of the cervical spine unless there are extenuating circumstances.
- Specify how many vertebrae *must* be visualized in each section of the spine.
- Identify the two most important abnormal findings in abdominal films.
- Describe at least four important normal baseline findings in the chest X-ray.

An understanding of some of the very basic concepts of radiology and departmentl procedures as they relate to the ED should be helpful to emergency personnel in understanding 1) why certain X-ray are requisitioned with specific views; 2) which X-rays the nurse should be able to requisition to expedite management of single-extremity trauma when the physician is tied up with more severe problems; 3) how the patient should be prepared and transported to the radiology department, as well as which patients should remain in ED and have portable films done; 4) why the requisition itself is extremely important, as it relates not only to the diagnostic interpretation but to the medical record as well; and 5) how to apply some very basic radiologic concepts and guidelines in a gross examination of an X-ray as it relates to the patient and the available history.

PREPARATION OF THE PATIENT

In many hospitals, the intramural relationship between the radiology department and ED is too often laced with misunderstandings, petty criticisms, loss of valuable time for patient care, and, too frequently, unnecessary films. A constructive working rapport between the two departments is essential if the patient is to receive the best possible care and if members of both departments are to work at their most effective levels.

Very frankly, the radiology technologist frequently has every reason to be upset when, at the busiest times, the procedure must be delayed while 1) someone finishes undressing the patient, 2) valuable time is lost checking back on incorrect spellings, and 3) having to clean and sweep down the entire examination room before receiving the next patient because the last one from ED was sent over as he had arrived—generously coated with roadside accumulations of mud, grass, broken glass, etc. It should go without saying that any patient being transported to X-ray for futher diagnostic evaluation must be disrobed to the extent that the area being filmed will be totally unencumbered by clothing or metal parts (including jewelry, safety pins in garments, bra snaps, etc.), and relatively clean. There is no reason to transport the dirt that accompanies the patient into the ED further into the X-ray department. Every trauma victim (usually the most heavily soiled) should be totally disrobed for a thorough examination in the ED before being sent on to X-ray dressed in a patient gown and covered with clean warm blankets.

Stretcher patients should go to X-ray on their stretchers, wheelchair patients go in wheelchairs, and the rare walking patient should also be accompanied.

Never allow a patient to wander off to X-ray and assume he will get there! Department policy should state that *all* patients are accompanied to the X-ray waiting area.

Patients with any significant head trauma should not be allowed to wait in the hall unattended, nor should any acutely ill or unstable patient. As a general rule, it is wise to request portable films in the ED with *any* seriously compromised patient (if portable equipment and a technician are available), since the X-ray room is rarely equipped or staffed to handle a real crisis situation.

One further consideration involves the patient's valuables. Purses and wallets containing credit cards and money should never be left behind unattended in the ED but should go with the patient or to a waiting family member. This will avoid *many* problems.

LOGICAL REQUISITIONING

Most X-ray requisition slips ask for a given amount of information, and there is a good reason for all of it; therefore, it is important to make a consistent effort to be thorough and accurate. Not only is the requisition necessary for the sake of complete medical and fiscal records but for the evaluation of the problem and the decision as to which examination should be employed so that the radiologist may render an accurate interpretation.

The patient's name (including middle initial) *must* be spelled correctly and written legibly, with hospital numbers and the patient's age included. Generally, it should be noted whether the patient has ever had previous films taken in that department. In the space usually provided for "reason" the film is being ordered, the problem may be stated as:

1. The chief medical complaint of the patient, i.e., swelling, unexplained pain, limited range of motion, hemoptysis, etc., or
2. Rule out (R/O) fracture, foreign body, renal stone, pneumothorax, dissecting aortic aneurysm, cervical spine fractures, etc.

The purpose is to provide the technician with a brief indication of the reason for films as given above and if, for instance, the chief complaint is pain in the abdomen, it should be noted for how long, which side, whether the patient is febrile, and if so, the temperature. Chronic pain without injury connotes quite a different sort of evaluation than pain following injury. If the film is to be a "recheck," the time interval should be noted and whether a procedure (such as thoracentesis, remanipulation of a fracture, passage of catheter, etc.) has been done since the last examination.

Emergency personnel should not be concerned with "views" but, rather, the area to be examined. They are, and should be, expected to use correct terminology in these requisitions to avoid confusion, error (costly to the patient), delay, and personal criticism. There is a strong economic consideration to be kept in mind, so specific areas must be defined and filmed only as needed diagnostically. Remember, too, that the patient should not be exposed to any more radiation than absolutely necessary.

Specific nomenclature should be used with hands and feet: thumb, index finger, middle finger, ring finger, fifth finger, great toe, second toe, fourth toe, and fifth toe, etc. The foot and ankle areas should be indicated specifically: ankle, tarsal area, toes, and os calcis (heel), etc. In other words, the actual area desired to be X-rayed should be specified with the correct anatomic terms as indicated by the physician, and this will then be interpreted by the X-ray technician into the most meaningful views of the indicated area, with the minimum radiation and expense to the patient.

BASIC UNDERSTANDING OF THE PRINCIPLES OF RADIOLOGY

Radiology is defined in *Dorland's* as the science of radiant energy and radiant substances, especially that branch of medical science dealing with the use of radiant energy in the diagnosis and treatment of disease. *Roentgenology* is defined as the branch of radiology which deals with the diagnostic and therapeutic use of roentgen rays, producing *roentgenograms,* or X-rays. The roentgen (pronounced rent'–gen) was named for Wilhelm Konrad Roentgen (a German physicist, 1845-1923), who discovered roentgen rays in 1895, and was awarded the Nobel prize in physics for 1901. The roentgen is the recognized international unit of *x* or *y* radiation. It is abbreviated as *R*. The principle of utilizing roentgenograms (X-rays) to visualize diagnostic evidence is based on the fact that dense materials such as bone are *radiopaque* and will not permit the passage of radiant energy (X-rays), with the representative areas appearing light or white on the exposed film, whereas other materials such as air are *radiolucent* and permit the passage of radiant energy while offering some resistance to it (depending on density) with representative areas appearing dark on the exposed film. The basic roentgen densities are shown in Table 8.1.

Table 8.1 Basic Roentgen Densities

ELEMENT OR AGENT	ROENTGEN DENSITY
Gas, air	Dark
Fat	Intermediate (dark)
Water, organs, blood	Intermediate (light)
Bone, contrast media	Whitish (lighter) or grey scale
(metal—barium, lead)	Solid white

The views that are typically taken are PA (posterior to anterior), AP (anterior to posterior), lateral (sagittal), and oblique (angled). *Decubitus films* are films taken while the patient is lying down with the X-ray beam horizontal and are designated as right lateral decubitus when the patient is lying on his or her right side and left lateral decubitus when lying on his or her left side.

It should be remembered that in X-ray films, the farther away the part, the larger it shows on film; therefore, angulations and displacements farther from the film will tend to be exaggerated.

In looking at a film, it is important to think about it three-dimensionally since the X-ray is a composite "shadowgram" and represents the added densities of many layers of tissue, requiring the viewer to think in layers when looking at any given X-ray film and remembering that 1) calcium is the prime example of metal density *normally* found in the body and 2) water density in *anatomic* contact with another water density obliterates the existing interface. An example of the latter is pneumonia (water density) in anatomic contact with a heart border (water density) *will obliterate* that border.

GENERAL GUIDELINES FOR FILMS OF SPECIFIC AREAS

Some generalities regarding the basics of radiology are included here, but it should be borne in mind that procedures and standard views for specific examinations may vary somewhat, as does terminology, from hospital to hospital and the EDN should be familiar with those used in the specific hospital of practice.

SKULL SERIES

The skull series, when ordered, usually includes:

1. PA (posterior to anterior)
2. Lateral (both sides)
3. Towne view (an oblique view from the anterior hairline caudally for visualization of basal skull area)

This makes four views in all, and a Water's view (for visualization of orbital structures) is sometimes indicated in addition to the skull series if an orbital fracture is suspected. However, if facial bone or orbital fracture is suspected, order the specific area, *i.e.,* orbitus or facial bones, and the technician will determine which views will be required.

Skull films are not an immediate priority if taken just to see fractures. Emergency requisitioning of a skull series is justified when it is unclear as to whether the patient is deteriorating, or when one who is apparently stable begins to develop lateralizing neurological signs. The rationale in ordering these films is to determine if the patient has a calcified *pineal gland*. The position of a normally calcified pineal gland on a skull film can confirm without a doubt the presence of an intracranial hematoma, if the pineal gland has been displaced from its normal midline position more than 1 cm. (The pineal gland calcifies in 75%-80% of people at about 15 years of age.)

Again, remember that the busy radiology department is unable to closely monitor a patient with head injury who is lying unattended in the waiting area.

If the EDN assigned to that patient does not stay close by and in attendance, a lethargic patient may rapidly become comatose before returning from X-ray without anyone being aware of the deterioration. *Never* leave a seriously ill patient unattended in X-ray.

FACIAL FRACTURES

Specific films are taken in most X-ray departments and generally do not include mandible and nasal bone views. Most facial fractures are diagnosed by observation and palpation (light ballottement) with follow-up confirmation by film.

1. Facial bones require multiple zygoma views.
2. Mandible examination requires an exaggerated Towne view, specifically for evaluation of the mandibular condyles. Right and left oblique views are taken of the mandible, and over 90% of fractures reveal medial displacement of the fractured superior segment of the condyle.
3. Films of the temporomandibular joint may require tomography (body section roentgenography, a special technique to show in detail images of structures lying in a predetermined plane of tissue while blurring or eliminating detail in images of structures in other planes).
4. Nasal bones are a specific examination and will not be adequately examined in routine facial bone or mandible examination.

EPIGLOTTITIS

When acute epiglottitis is suspected, a lateral examination using a soft tissue technique should be taken of the neck for confirmation of epiglottitis with the accompanying soft tissue swelling. Airway management equipment must be close at hand in case of sudden airway obstruction during procedure.

SPINAL FILMS

Patients requiring examination of the cervical spine should have the head immobilized in whatever fashion is required if they have been victims of severe trauma. If the patient is comatose, it is probably safe to use sandbags, with 3" tape across the forehead to sides of stretcher or backboard, but if the patient is conscious and either cooperative or not, it is essential for someone to assume the responsibility of applying and maintaining head traction until X-ray films have ruled out a fracture. This may entail portable X-rays in the ED before the patient is even moved off the ambulance stretcher, or it may mean accompanying the patient to the X-ray room and staying throughout the filming procedure. With the seriously injured patient or the real candidate for permanent damage, *never* assume someone else will do it. Be certain!. Again, when possible, order portable films in the ED. The patient who walks in complaining of a whiplash injury may be more comfortable in a cervical collar until evaluated but does not require the rigorous regimen that has just been described. Let common sense be the guide.

1. Three films are taken of the cervical spine (anterior, odontoid, and lateral). Lateral flexion and extension views may be indicated, but these should not be obtained unless a radiologist is in attendance.
2. Always be certain that *all* 7 cervical vetebrae are *fully* visualized.
3. The odontoid process may be congenitally absent or very small. Fracture of the odontoid is a high-risk injury and may not heal. The odontoid process is hooked to C_2 upon which C_1 swivels.
4. Films of the thoracic spine must visualize *all* 12 thoracic vertebrae.
5. Films of the lumbar spine must visualize *all* 5 lumbar vertebrae and usually will include T_{11} and T_{12}, where unsuspected fractures are often seen.
6. When a film of the spinal column is traced, there should be midline alignment of *all facets,* with clear interspaces.
7. Suspected hip fractures require special handling until ruled out. These may be subtle and impacted (at times difficult to diagnose) or grossly deformed.

CHEST

Anatomic structures are recognized on X-ray by their differences in density, as discussed earlier. The *normal* chest X-ray shows them as water density of the heart, muscles, and blood, the metal (calcium) density of the ribs; the gas (air) density of the lungs; and streaks of fat density around the muscles. The fifth density, that of heavy metal and contrast media, is not present in the normal chest film. The normal cardiac silhouette falls within the range of less than half the distance across the chest area.

Lateral films of the chest are routinely taken on the left because this does not enlarge the cardiac silhouette and provides a standardization for follow-up comparison. Normally the chest contains air, arteries and veins, the heart, and the ribs. There should be the following (which are but a few of the *many* things looked for in the normal chest film):

1. Sharp symmetrical angles at the diaphragm (fluid blunts the angle)
2. Symmetry of the diaphragm with a little more bulge on the left side
3. Midline trachea with clavicular heads in the center
4. Costophrenic gutter on the lateral view

Pneumothorax will show a blacker line around one lung, most prominent at the top, and density (more whiteness) within the lung area may indicate pneumonia, tumor, embolus, and other conditions.

The chest X-ray in trauma is an important part of diagnosis for injuries but is *not the most* essential step. After initial resuscitation and/or stabilization, the X-ray film assesses the status of the heart, lungs, and mediastinum.

ABDOMEN

To repeat, it is important to be certain all clothing has been removed, as well as jewelry which might clutter and obscure the film. This should be done in the ED, since the X-ray technician is *entitled to assume* it has been done. For abdominal films requiring contrast media, preparation (prep) is not always necessary, depending on what the physician wants to know.

1. An intravenous pyelogram (IVP) can be done without prep for stones and renal trauma.

2. Upper GI studies are not usually done on an ED basis, but plain films can be made for perforated ulcers. If there has been massive bleeding, an upper GI series will be helpful after the stomach has been cleared of blood by 8-12 hours of suction.

3. The colon needs adequate prep for visualization of polyps, diverticulitis, etc., but emergency films of intussusception, massive internal bleeding, or obstruction can be done without prep. A massive rectal bleed is frequently from the upper GI tract (stomach), and a barium enema is not the first examination needed. A massive rectal bleed often occurs from the right side of the colon and should be suspected unless the patient is also vomiting blood.

4. The old "flat plate" of the abdomen is obsolete.

5. Ordering a kidney, ureter, and bladder film (KUB) or abdominal film will net the same results.

6. Abdominal films for foreign bodies (IUD, bullets, etc.), kidney stones, pregnancy, gallstones, etc., all require *one* AP view.

7. Abdominal series and/or surgical abdominal series and/or surgical series all mean that three or four times will be taken: one supine (lying with face upward) abdomen AP, one upright abdomen AP, and one chest PA. A lateral decubitus view may also be taken, especially if the patient cannot be upright. This is a highly useful diagnostic series when, for instance, a right lower lobe (RLL) pneumonia can present as abdominal pain.

8. There are five densities to be aware of when looking at films: gas, fat, water, calcium (bone), metal (lead and barium).

9. Cartilage does not show on X-ray unless calcified.

10. On acute abdominal films there are two common conditions to consider:

    A. Perforation of the bowel with free air (this air shows between the diaphragm and liver)

    B. Obstruction, most often of small bowel. The small bowel loops will be dilated and there will be air-fluid levels on the upright and lateral decubitus views.

       Detection of free air and air-fluid levels requires horizontal X-ray beam films, either upright or lateral decubitus, or both. Free air in the abdomen and/or chest is a *bad* sign.

11. When sending a pregnant (or possibly pregnant) female to X-ray, specify on the requisition that the abdomen be shielded, unless of course the studies are to be abdominal in nature.

EXTREMITIES

1. Air splints or cardboard splints are suitable for immobilization of an injured extremity prior to X-ray examination.
2. Again, all clothing and jewelry *must* be removed to prepare for X-ray examination, so that snaps, pins, zippers, rings, etc., do not occlude findings.
3. It is generally considered good practice to film the joint nearest to a suspected fracture.
4. Foot and ankle films should always include PA, lateral and oblique views. In most departments, this is a routine practice, but if not, the oblique view should be requisitioned, requesting only the part involved.

SUMMARY

The basic concept presented here is that after evaluating the patient, the EDN should order specific examinations or examination by area as required, and X-ray personnel will obtain the specific views that will enable the radiologist to make the roentgenologic diagnosis.

If, due to unusual circumstances, additional information is thought to be necessary, consultation with the radiologist is indicated. Most radiologists and X-ray technicians will be more than willing to assist ED personnel in the best care for their patients.

REVIEW

1. Explain the proper procedure for preparing a patient for X-ray.
2. Describe the situations requiring that portable films be taken in the ED.
3. Explain the importance of each area of information which is required on the average X-ray requisition.
4. Describe the correct nomenclature to be employed when requisitioning films of specific fingers or toes.
5. Explain the reason for using correct anatomic terms when requisitioning films.
6. Identify the five basic roentgen densities in order of increasing density.
7. Explain the definitions of radiology and roentgenology.

8. Define radiopaque and radiolucent.

9. List the routine views most frequently utilized when obtaining X-ray films.

10. Identify the prime example of metal density *normally* found in the body.

11. Identify the most frequently utilized contrast media in roentgenology.

12. Identify the component views included in a skull series.

13. Explain when a Water's view is necessary in addition to skull series.

14. Describe the location of the normal pineal gland and explain the significance of deviation from its normal position.

15. Explain the technique known as tomography.

16. Identify the two cervical spine views that are not routine and should be eliminated in certain situations.

17. Identify the number of vertebrae that *must* be visualized in each section of the spine when X-ray films are requisitioned.

18. Explain the significance of the two most important abnormal findings in abdominal films.

19. Describe at least four important normal baseline findings in the chest X-ray.

20. Explain what would indicate an enlarged cardiac silhouette.

BIBLIOGRAPHY

Budassi SA, Barber JM: Emergency Nursing: Principles and Practice. C.V. Mosby Co., St. Louis, Missouri, 1981

Cosgriff H, Anderson DL: The Practice of Emergency Nursing. J.B. Lippincott Co., Philadelphia, Pennsylvania, 1975

Felson M, Weinstein A, Spitz H: Principles of Chest Radiology, A Programmed Text. W.B. Saunders Co., Philadelphia, Pennsylvania, 1965

Harris JH, Harris WH: The Radiology of Emergency Medicine, 2nd ed. Williams & Wilkins Co., Baltimore, Maryland, 1981

Squires F: Fundamentals of Roentgenology. Harvard University Press, Cambridge, Massachusetts, 1964

Warner C: Emergency Care: Assessment and Intervention, 2nd ed. C.V. Mosby Co., St. Louis, Missouri, 1978

SECTION II

EMERGENCY INTERVENTION AND CARE

AIRWAY MANAGEMENT 9

KEY CONCEPTS

This chapter reviews the respiratory system based on the concept that the human respiratory system is a living bellows. The absolute and essential need for early and effective airway management is stressed in discussion of the methods of airway management available to ED personnel. Much of the content is derived from lectures presented to EDNs by Guy Guffey, M.D., John Naron, American Registry of Respiratory Therapists (ARRT), and Bill Brown, ARRT, all of the Portland Metropolitan Area, and by Gerald E. Ferguson, CRNA (Certified Registered Nurse Anesthetist). The balance has been adapted from the supplement to JAMA, August 1980, on Standards for Cardiopulmonary Resuscitation, with permission of the American Heart Association.

After reading and studying this chapter, you should be able to:

- Define the terms "clinical death," "biological death," and "functional death."
- Identify the anatomy of the respiratory tract.
- Describe the physiology of external respiration.
- Explain spirometry and the measurements of lung volumes.
- List the steps to be taken in clearing an airway.
- Name two indications for the Heimlich maneuver abdominal thrust.
- Describe conditions contraindicating use of oropharyngeal airways.
- List the advantages and disadvantages of the S-tube.
- List four advantages of the pocket mask.
- Describe the principle applied with an esophageal obturator airway and list some of the advantages, disadvantages, and contraindications of its use.
- Identify the indications and advantages of endotracheal intubation.
- Identify the indications and advantages of the cricothyroid stab.
- Describe circumstances under which a tracheostomy should be done.
- Identify criteria for an adequate bag/mask unit.
- Identify four requirements to provide effective suction capability.
- Identify the guidelines for oxygen administration.
- List at least eight airway management guidelines for the EDN.

119

This chapter may well be the most important chapter in the book since it deals directly with providing oxygen, the essence of life, to the compromised patient. It is now universally recognized that when *clinical death* (the cessation of cardiac and respiratory function) occurs, there is an incredibly short period of *only four minutes* before *biological death* (death of the brain cells) occurs (Fig. 9.1). After this length of time, there will have been irreversible brain damage from *anoxia* to the brain cells, even though the cardiovascular function of the patient may have been effectively restored. This deprivation of oxygen can manifest itself all the way from a permanently dull mentality following an otherwise apparently successful resuscitation to a condition termed *functional death,* which is defined as the "total and permanent destruction of the central nervous system, with vital functions sustained by artificial means."

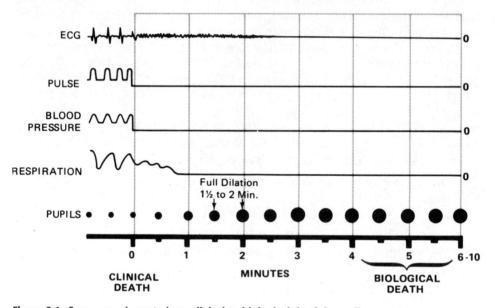

Figure 9.1. Sequence of events from clinical to biological death in cardiac arrest.

A frequently quoted reference to this sort of tragedy is attributed to John Scott Haldane (1860-1936), a physician and physiologist born and educated in Edinburgh, Scotland, who pioneered the field of anesthesia and respiratory studies. His major work, done from 1905 to 1911, involved the physiology of respiration, and he is chiefly noted for his elucidation of the gas exchange during respiration from which evolved his now classic remark: "Anoxia not only stops the machine, but wrecks the machinery."

Professional nursing personnel functioning in acute situations that often require rapid and effective intervention must be constantly alert and dedicated to the concept of preserving not just life but the quality of life as we know it. To suppose that anyone would wish to be responsible for another human being's continuing existence in a vegetative state is incomprehensible, but it not only can happen, it *does* happen!

It is basic and essential that every EDN possess the knowledge, skills, and common sense required to anticipate airway problems and to rapidly establish and maintain a patent airway for the compromised patient, realizing that integrity of the airway with adequate ventilation and perfusion is that patient's lifeline and must be the EDN's primary responsibility.

RESPIRATION

Respiration is the interchange of gases between an organism and the medium in which it lives. The main functions of the human respiratory system are the exchange of oxygen and carbon dioxide as air moves in and out of the lungs with diffusion or the passive movement of gas across the alveolar capillary membrane (external respiration) and the circulation of oxygen via the bloodstream to the cells, returning carbon dioxide to the alveoli (internal respiration).

External respiration begins and ends with the nose.* The nose has been compared to an air conditioning unit because it controls the temperature and humidity of the air entering the lungs and filters foreign particles from the air. The interior of the nose is divided by a wall of cartilage and bone called the septum. Near the middle of the nasal cavity, and on both sides of the septum, are a series of scroll-like bones called the conchae, or turbinates. The purpose of the turbinates is to increase the amount of tissue surface within the nose so that incoming air will have a greater opportunity to be "conditioned" before it continues on its way to the lungs. The surfaces of the turbinates, like the rest of the interior walls of the nose, are covered with mucous membranes. The membranes secrete a fluid called mucus. The film of mucus is produced continuously and drains slowly into the throat. The mucus gives up heat and moisture to incoming air and serves as a trap for bacteria and dust in the air. It also helps dilute any irritating substances. In addition to the mucus, the membrane is coated with cilia, or hairlike filaments, that wave back and forth a dozen times per second. The millions of cilia lining the nasal cavity help the mucus clean the incoming air. When we breathe through the mouth, we lose the protective benefits of the cilia and mucus.

The incoming air that has been filtered, warmed, and moistened in its trip through the nasal cavity next passes into the pharynx. The pharynx is one of the more complicated parts of the body since it serves as a passageway for both food and air. The incoming air travels through the nasal cavity, into the pharynx, and through the larynx, or voice box, by crossing over the path used by food on its way to the stomach.

Similarly, food crosses over the route of air on its way from the nose to the larynx. But, when food is swallowed, a flap of cartilage called the epiglottis folds over the opening of the larynx. The base of the tongue pushes down the epiglottis as the food is moved back into the throat during the swallowing

*Reprinted with permission of the American Medical Association from The Wonderful Human Machine, 1971

action. At the same time, the larynx moves up to help seal the opening. This action can be observed by watching a person's "Adam's apple" move up at the start of swallowing. The Adam's apple is part of the larynx. [The Adam's apple is actually the upper part of the thyroid cartilage, below which lies the cricoid cartilage; the cricothyroid membrane separating the two.]

On each side of the pharynx, behind the mouth cavity, are tonsils. Tonsil tissue is also located at the base of the tongue, and it may appear at the back and sides of the pharynx as adenoids. Tonsils usually are more prominent in children than adults. Their purpose is to guard the body against infections that may enter through the mouth or nose.

The larynx, also called the voice box, is at the top of the column that finally takes the air into the lungs, the trachea. Two folds of membrane, the vocal cords, are attached to the front of the larynx wall and held [posteriorly] by a pair of tiny cartilages [the aretynoids]. The cartilages are attached to muscles that contract and relax to move the vocal cords toward or away from the center of the larynx.

Below the larynx, the trachea, also called the windpipe, continues down the neck and into the chest. A series of C-shaped rings of cartilage hold open the trachea. Lack of rigidity of the trachea permits us to bend the neck. The path of the esophagus, which carries food to the stomach, runs immediately behind that of the trachea. At the point behind the middle of the breastbone, where the aorta arches away from the heart, the trachea divides into two branches— [the point at which the trachea divides, or bifurcates, is called the corina] the right and the left bronchi [also referred to as the right and left mainstem bronchi]. Each bronchus divides and subdivides many times into smaller cartilage-ringed branches that reach deep into the right and left lungs.

The tiniest bronchi, almost too small to be seen without a microscope, have cartilage rings in their walls. However, as the tubes become still smaller, they have little or no cartilage but have, instead, muscle cells in their walls. Bronchi of this size are called bronchioles. Finally, the bronchiole ends in a tiny air sac called an alveolus. The lungs contain nearly a billion of these microscopic, balloon-like alveoli. The alveoli, with their spaces air-filled, make the lungs appear somewhat like large sponges.

Each alveolus has a thin membrane wall, one cell thick. Networks of blood capillaries surround the alveoli. When air is breathed into the lungs, the molecules of oxygen gas pass through the thin membrane wall of the alveolus and through the capillary wall to become attached to the hemoglobin in the red blood cell. The blood turns a bright red after it picks up the oxygen.

Each lung is enclosed in a double-membrane sac called the pleural sac. The sac is air-tight and contains a lubricating fluid. The pleural layers keep the lung surface from rubbing against the chest wall. The pleural lining which covers the lungs is called visceral pleura, while that which lines the chest wall is called the parietal pleura. A negative pressure of -4 to -6 mm Hg exists between the pleura during expiration.

The right lung has three lobes: the upper, middle, and lower; the left lung has two lobes: the upper and lower. A small tongue-like structure projects from the lower portion of the upper lobe of the left lung called the lingula. All lobes of the lungs have separate bronchi.

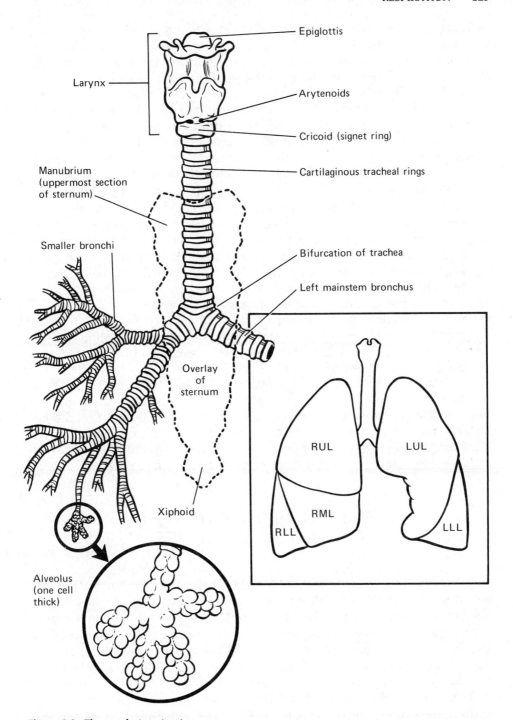

Figure 9.2. The respiratory tract.

Breathing is controlled by a series of respiratory centers in the nervous system. One center is in the medulla, the part of the brain at the top of the spinal cord. Breathing action can be triggered by the centers, when there is an increase in the amount of carbon dioxide in the blood or when there is a drop in the oxygen level of the blood. Forced breathing sometimes depletes the carbon dioxide in the blood. When there is not enough carbon dioxide to trigger the respiratory center, breathing will be interrupted for a moment.

[The lungs, living bellows, are formed by the rib cage, diaphragm, and intercostal muscles. There are 12 pairs of ribs, with the top 10 pairs attached by strips of cartilage to the sternum and the bottom 2 pairs attached only to the spinal column and called floating ribs. The first 7 pairs of ribs are attached directly to the sternum by cartilaginous joints and work like a bucket handle, moving up and down with the intercostal and diaphragmatic action.]

The primary moving force is the diaphragm, a dome-shaped sheet of muscle fibers and tendons separating the organs in the chest from the organs in the abdomen. The diaphragm is attached to the breastbone on the front, to the spinal column at the back, and to the lower ribs on the sides. When the muscle fibers of the diaphragm contract, the sheet of tissue is drawn downward, creating a partial vacuum in the chest cavity. This causes air to flow into the trachea, the bronchi, and the alveoli. Expiration occurs when the diaphragm muscles relax, closing the "bellows" and forcing the air out again.

[During expiration, the diaphragm rises up to the level of the fifth intercostal space at the mid-axillary line. The diaphragm receives its innervation from the phrenic nerve which originates at the level of C-4 and C-5 and runs down along the esophagus and near the heart.]

The intercostal muscles between the ribs also participate in the breathing action. In forced breathing, abdominal muscles assist in expiration and the neck muscles assist in inspiration by pulling upward and outward on the first rib and the breastbone. This has a chain-reaction effect on the other ribs, increasing the capacity of the chest. [This is referred to as the use of accessory muscles and is seen in varying degrees of respiratory distress.]

TIDAL VOLUMES AND VITAL CAPACITIES OF LUNGS

Spirometry is the measurement of breathing capacity of the lungs or the lung volume. The tidal volume (TV) is the amount of air exchanged in easy breathing and is approximately 500 cc per respiration in the normal adult at rest.

The vital capacity (VC) is the amount of air a person can exhale maximally after maximal inhalation. Normally, this vital capacity is 3000-6000 cc, with 5000 cc being the norm for a 70-kg man. Normal lungs should exhale 80% of the vital capacity in 1 second when being tested; this is referred to as the forced expiratory volume in 1 second (FEV_1).

The functional residual capacity (FRC) is the volume of air or gas that remains in the lungs at the end of normal expiration; the residual volume (RV) is the volume of air or gas remaining in the lungs after maximal expiration. Remember that once the lung is inflated at birth there will *always* be a reservoir of gas present.

ESTABLISHING A PATENT AIRWAY

Establishing and maintaining a patent airway is *always* of the highest priority. The best method depends on the cause and degree of obstruction, along with the patient's relative condition. The treatment must be related directly to the degree of the problem; this usually requires rapid evaluation and prompt intervention.

The goal is to accomplish improvement of exchange at the cellular level with a reversal of signs and symptoms resulting from inadequate pulmonary ventilation. It is necessary to be able to recognize *when* the exchange of air is adequate and when improvement is seen. Recognition of adequate exchange can be tricky, but if the symptoms of anoxia begin to reverse, exchange is then adequate.

PRECAUTIONS

The inappropriate use, meaning unnecessary use, of oropharyngeal airways can cause vomiting and laryngospasm, as may the use of endotracheal (ET) intubation at any time during resuscitation attempts. As the patient rises from unconscious to semiconscious with improvement, gagging and vomiting frequently occur, and aspiration of vomitus is all too common.

Prevention of aspiration, then, is the real key. If the patient is conscious, there should be no real problem since the patient will react and take care of it, as a rule. If the patient is semiconscious, have suction on standby, be ready for a Trendelenburg position, and turn the head to the side to mechanically remove vomitus with a rigid tonsil suction tip (Yankauer type), tongue blade, fingers, or whatever is available.

Remember it is best to *undertreat* when insertion of an airway is possibly indicated *until the real need* for the use of one is determined.

AIRWAY MANEUVERS

The Head Tilt

Initially, the mouth and pharynx must be cleared of all blood, mucus, vomitus, foreign bodies, and frequently dentures, by reaching with fingers, gauze wipes, or suction tip. *The tongue is the most common cause of airway obstruction,* and this can be managed easily and quickly by tilting the patient's head backward as far as possible. Sometimes this simple maneuver is all that is required for breathing to resume spontaneously.

To perform the head tilt the patient must be lying on his or her back. The rescuer places one hand beneath the patient's neck and the other hand on the forehead. The neck is lifted with one hand, and the head is tilted backward by pressure with the other hand on the forehead. The maneuver extends the neck and lifts the tongue away from the back of the throat. Anatomic obstruction of the airway caused by the tongue dropping against the back of the throat is thereby relieved. The head must be maintained in this position at all times with an unconscious patient* (Fig. 9.3).

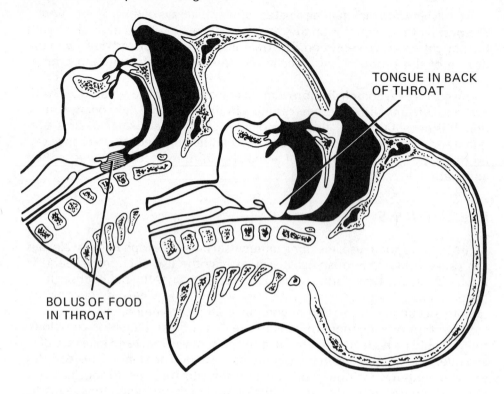

TONGUE IN BACK OF THROAT

BOLUS OF FOOD IN THROAT

Figure 9.3. Two major causes of airway obstruction.

Triple Airway Maneuver

The head tilt method is effective in most cases. If the head tilt is unsuccessful in opening the air passage adequately, additional forward displacement of the lower jaw (the jaw thrust) may be required. This can be accomplished by a *triple airway maneuver,* in which the rescuer's fingers are placed behind the angles of the victim's jaw and 1) the mandible is forcefully displaced forward while 2) the head is tilted backward; 3) the rescuer's thumbs then retract the lower lip to allow nasal *and* mouth breathing. Remember that the jaw thrust is best performed from a position at the top of the patient's head.** [If the respirations persist in sounding somewhat obstructed, sometimes turning the head to one side or the other can make an appreciable difference.] If both of these maneuvers fail to provide an open airway, one must assume there is an upper airway obstruction.

---

*Reprinted with permission of the American Medical Association from *The Wonderful Human Machine,* 1977, 1971

**Reprinted with permission from the American Heart Association from *Standards for CPR,* Supplement to JAMA, Vol 244, No 5, August 1980

The patient will probably be making strong inspiratory efforts, and a cursory look at the neck will reveal contraction of the cervical muscles with retraction at the suprasternal notch and the supraclavicular fossae, coincident with each inspiration. The intercostal spaces and epigastrium will also retract on inspiration. The patient's color may be cyanotic or ashen gray.*

The Heimlich Maneuver/Abdominal Thrust

A simple and relatively new first aid technique now being employed for airways obstructed by a bolus of food or by drowning is known as the "Hemlich maneuver," developed by an Ohio surgeon, Henry J. Heimlich, M.D., Director of Surgery and Physician-in-Chief of the Esophagus Center at the Jewish Hospital in Cincinnati. The rescuer stands behind the victim and wraps his or her arms around the victim's waist. Making a fist, the rescuer places it against the abdomen above the navel and below the xiphoid process. The fist is then grasped with the other hand and pressed forcefully into the patient's abdomen with a quick upward thrust. The *quick* thrust is important for if the movement is slow, it will be ineffective. If the victim is lying face up, the rescuer kneels astride him or her and, facing the head, places one hand on top of the other, then places the heel of the lower hand against the victim's abdomen slightly above the navel and below the xiphoid process. The rescuer then presses forcefully into the abdomen with the same *quick* upward thrust, repeating if necessary. This maneuver is not used on infants or pregnant women; the chest thrust is used placing the fist over the sternum on pregnant women, while infants are placed over the hand and forearm. See below on First Aid for Choking.

First Aid for Choking**

Subsequent to a report submitted by the National Academy of Sciences on Emergency Airway Management, the American Heart Association is currently advocating "First Aid for Choking," as follows, rather than the Heimlich Maneuver:

For the conscious victim:

1. If the victim *can* speak, cough, or breathe, do *not* interfere.
2. If the victim *cannot* speak, cough, or breathe, give 4 quick back blows.
3. If unsuccessful, give 4 upward abdominal thrusts or 4 backward chest thrusts.
4. Repeat above sequence. Be persistent. Continue uninterrupted until advanced life support is available.

---

*From Clinical Symposia, Vol 22, No 3, by Emil A. Naclerio, M.D. Copyright © 1970 CIBA-GEIGY Corporation, Reprinted with permission.

**Information excerpted from Report on Emergency Airway Management Committee on Emergency Medical Services. National Academy of Sciences, Washington, D.C. 1976

If the victim becomes unconscious:

1. Open the airway and try to ventilate, or
2. If unsuccessful, give 4 quick back blows.
3. If unsuccessful, give 4 abdominal *or* chest thrusts.
4. If unsuccessful, try finger probe.
5. Attempt to ventilate.
6. Repeat above sequence. Be persistent. Continue uninterrupted until advanced life support is available.

A revised interim statement from the Heart Association discusses abdominal and chest thrusts with the following comments: "Differences in the airway flow, pressure, and volume between abdominal and chest thrusts have been demonstrated not to be significant. The chest thrust is preferred for special circumstances, *i.e.*, advanced pregnancy, or marked obesity."

A significant consideration in either abdominal or chest thrust is the possibility of damage to internal organs such as rupture or laceration of abdominal or thoracic viscera. The rescuer's hands should never be placed on the xiphoid process of the sternum or on the lower margins of the rib cage. They should be below this area for abdominal thrust and above this area for chest thrust. Use of the abdominal thrust instead of the chest thrust in the older age might avoid the fracture of brittle ribs. Regurgitation may occur as a result of abdominal thrust.

Training and proper performance should minimize these problems.

When the rescuer is dealing with an unconscious supine victim, the preferred position for performing abdominal thrusts or chest thrusts is at the side of the unconscious victim. At his side, the rescuer has more maneuverability and is in the proper position to perform many procedures that may be required, including manual thrusts, back blows, turning the head if regurgitation occurs, finger probes, head tilt to open the airway and mouth-to-mouth ventilation. Of these, only the abdominal thrust (Heimlich maneuver) can be performed while astride the victim. Although a small rescuer astride a large victim can use body weight to assure an effective abdominal thrust in the proper direction toward the diaphragm, proper hand and body position by a rescuer at the side can also provide for an effective thrust.

The general public should be taught and encouraged to use the "distress signal of choking," which is clutching the neck between the thumb and index finger.

Following removal of a foreign body from an unconscious victim, artificial ventilation or cardiopulmonary resuscitation may be required. If so, this should be performed according to the *Standards for Cardiopulmonary Resuscitation (CPR) and Emergency Cardiac Care (ECC)* and the training programs of the American Heart Association, the American National Red Cross, and other agencies that provide basic life-support training.

Mouth-to-Mouth Resuscitation

If mouth-to-mouth resuscitation is necessary, supplemental oxygen should be used as soon as it becomes available. Rescue breathing (exhaled air ventilation) will deliver about 16% oxygen to the patient; ideally, this will produce an alveolar oxygen tension of about 80 mm Hg. However, because of the low cardiac output associated with external cardiac compression and the presence of intrapulmonary shunting and *ventilation-perfusion abnormalities,* marked discrepancies will occur between the alveolar and arterial oxygen tension, and *hypoxemia* may ensue. Hypoxemia leads to *anaerobic metabolism* and *metabolic acidosis,* which frequently impair the beneficial effects of chemical and electrical therapy in a "code" situation when resuscitation and advanced life support procedures are being carried out.

Because of this, the recommendation of the National Conference on CPR is that *supplemental oxygen always be used* when bag-valve-mask or bag-valve-tube systems are used. This will enhance myocardial and cerebral oxygenation, which is essential for successful resuscitation.

The Pocket Mask

An effective alternative to mouth-to-mouth resuscitation is the use of a "pocket mask," a clear-domed collapsible mask with an inflated cushion and an optional oxygen port. When held in place and properly seated over the patient's mouth and nose, it is possible to deliver an inspired oxygen content of upwards of 50% with oxygen attached at a flow rate of 10 L/min. The pocket mask allows both hands to position the patient's head and maintain an open airway, it protects the operator from direct contact and contamination from the patient's nose and mouth, and provides a clear dome to observe for regurgitation during resuscitation. Personnel with less expertise in airway management are able to achieve better lung ventilation with the pocket mask.

In pediatric resuscitation efforts, the mask may be used, even on infants, if applied to the face upside down with the narrower nose portion covering the patient's chin and the wider section covering the child's mouth and nasal area.

Airways

Oropharyngeal airways should be used whenever a bag-valve-mask system or automatic breathing device with a mask is used, but only if done by a person properly trained in their use. *Airways should be used only on deeply unconscious persons!* If introduced into a conscious or stuporous person, an airway may promote vomiting or laryngospasm. Care is required in the placement of the airway because incorrect insertion can displace the tongue back into the pharynx and itself produce airway obstruction. Oropharyngeal airways should be available in infant, child, and adult sizes in every ED.

An oropharyngeal airway should be held between the thumb and first and second fingers, inserted into the patient's mouth with the tip of the airway curving and pointing toward the roof of the mouth. As the airway is carefully advanced, it should be rotated 180° and dropped into place at the base of the tongue (Fig. 9.5). *Nasopharyngeal airways* also may be used for adults; however, as with all adjunctive equipment, explicit training and practice must

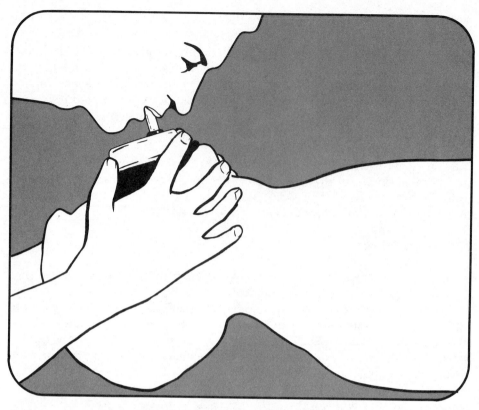

Figure 9.4. The Pocket Mask. Mask is applied to the face and held firmly by placement of the thumbs on sides of mask. The index, middle, and ring fingers grasp the lower jaw just in front of the ear lobes and jaw is pulled forcefully upward. The victim's mouth should remain open under the mask; the operator then blows in through the opening of the mask.

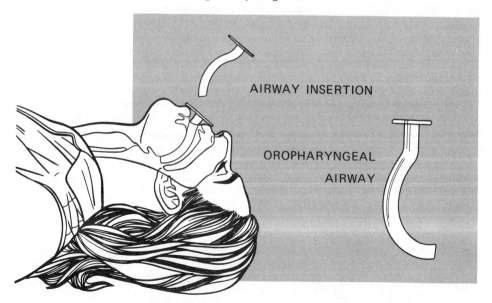

Figure 9.5. Placement of oropharyngeal airway with 180° rotation.

be required for their use. A nasal tube is first lubricated with a water-soluble lubricant, the nares are lifted, and the tube is inserted along the *floor* of the nose with gentle steady pressure. The left nostril is most generally employed because it is thought to be of a larger size in most people.

S-tubes are an extension of the oropharyngeal airway, and they are available in numerous styles. S-tubes range from simple tubes with mouth pieces and bite blocks to more elaborate devices with valves. Despite many different designs they share certain limitations:

1. They do not provide as effective an airway seal as mouth-to-mouth or mouth-to-mask ventilation.
2. They do not reduce potential transmission of infection.
3. They require training for safe and effective use.
4. They induce vomiting if used improperly.
5. They require the single rescuer to move to the victim's head and reposition the S-tube to inflate the lungs between chest compressions and CPR.

S-tubes do offer useful features, such as 1) overcoming esthetic problems of direct mouth-to-mouth contact; 2) assisting and maintaining a patent airway; and 3) keeping the mouth open. *However, it is generally found that direct mouth-to-mouth or mouth-to-mask ventilation provides more effective artificial ventilation.*

The Esophageal Obturator Airway

The esophageal obturator airway is a fairly recent innovation in the management of cardiac arrest and victims of extensive facial trauma. It appears to be a useful airway adjunct, but its future role remains to be determined.

The airway consists of a 15″ cuffed tube (similar to an endotracheal tube) mounted through a face mask and modified with a soft plastic obturator blocking the distal orifice, with multiple openings in the upper one-third of the tube at the level of the pharynx *with the mask in place on the tube, the tube is passed down the back of the throat into the esophagus.* The mask is then tightly seated on the face and the 30-cc cuff of the tube is inflated, utilizing a one-way valve system. When mouth-to-tube or bag-valve-tube ventilation is performed, the air is discharged through the pharyngeal openings in the tube and passes down the trachea since the esophagus is blocked. Theoretically, this will prevent gastric distention and regurgitation during resuscitation. *The esophageal obturator airway should be inserted only in patients who are not breathing or who are deeply unconscious (Fig. 9.6).*

The potential advantages of the esophageal obturator airway are that no visualization is required for introduction, and that it can be placed more easily and quickly than an endotracheal tube without hyperextension of the head and neck. In a large series of cardiac arrest cases, successful use of the airway was documented without injury to the esophagus when used by professional allied health personnel who had been trained in its use on intubation manikins

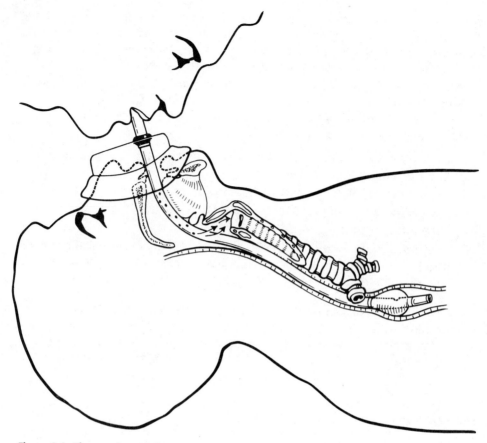

Figure 9.6. The esophageal airway.

and unconscious patients. However, the potential for damage to the esophagus is *always* present unless use of the airway is restricted to adequately trained individuals.

Removal of the esophageal airway, like an endotracheal tube, frequently is followed by immediate regurgitation. To cope with this, the airway should *not* be removed until the patient is becoming conscious and is breathing *or* has a return of reflexes. When it is to be removed, the patient should be turned onto his or her side and *adequate suction* should be *available and ready*. A standard cuffed endotracheal tube should be introduced into the trachea *prior* to removal of the esophageal airway if necessary.

Remember that a patient coming into the emergency department with a YELLOW, WHITE or RED, tipped intubation tube in place probably has an esophageal obturator airway. *The 30-cc balloon cuff must be deflated fully before any attempts at extubation are made in order to avoid trauma to the soft tissue of the esophagus.*

Cricothyroid Stab

In desperate situations of complete or near complete upper airway obstruction secondary to injuries of the face, mandible, throat, or entrapped foreign bodies in the larynx, any measure short of an emergency cricothyroid stab may prove fatal. In these situations (if none of the previously described measures can be used), the cricothyroid membrane must be opened at once using any relatively sharp instrument, a penknife, scissors, or even a nail file.

The cricothyroid membrane can be identified by feeling for the transverse indentation which is located about 1/2 inch (1.5 cm) below the Adam's apple. This area is relatively avascular and serious bleeding does not occur. The instrument should be inserted transversely to obtain a sufficient opening. Once the trachea has been entered, a piece of rubber tubing, if available, should be inserted into the airway to keep the edges of the aperture apart. [A small tracheostomy tube or infant airway will work very well.]

The insertion of intravenous needles in the cricothyroid membrane has been recommended, but even those of large bore will improve the airway very little* unless two #14 ga. or one #10 ga. X 3" angiocath are placed. The needle is directed at a 45° angle caudally, aspirating as it is advanced; aspiration of air signifies entry into the tracheal lumen.

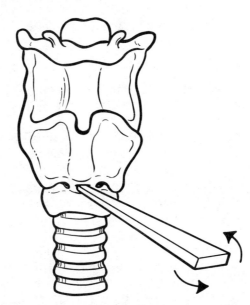

Figure 9.7. The cricothyroid stab.

Percutaneous Translaryngeal Oxygen Jet Insufflation

Percutaneous translaryngeal O_2 insufflation (TLOJI) consists of intermittent high pressure oxygen insufflation into the larynx via a small bore (e.g., 14- or 16-gauge) catheter-outside-needle inserted percutaneously. This is a technique for oxygen and ventilation, increasingly employed for selected cases in intrahospital resuscitation and anesthesia. *It is not recommended for use at*

---

*From Clinical Symposia Vol. 22, No. 3, by Emil A. Naclerio, M.D. Copyright © 1970 CIBA-GEIGY Corporation. Reprinted with permission.

this time in prehospital care. In contrast to cricothyrotomy, TLOJI requires compressed oxygen and special equipment, consisting of tubings, connectors, stopcocks, and flexible cannulas.

TLOJI can be an alternative when tracheal intubation is not possible, if the necessary equipment is immediately available. Cricothyrotomy can be accomplished with pocket-size equipment only and permits an adequate airway through the cannula for exhalation of air. In addition to requiring special equipment, TLOJI also depends upon the victim's upper airway, above the point of its insertion in the larynx, for exhalation. Therefore, in using TLOJI, inability to exhale must be watched, and if the lungs do not deflate, cricothyreotomy should be performed.

The National Academy of Sciences, in a 1974 report on emergency airway management, identified cricothyrotomy as a technique meriting further exploration for *intractable acute asphyxia with total upper airway obstruction,* including food choking. Now, both the 1980 ACLS Standards and the 1981 ATLS Standards include cricothyrotomy as part of the optional adjunct capability for such emergencies; the August 1981 AHA Standards specify that EDs have the necessary equipment readily available for use.

Endotracheal Intubation

American Heart Association Standards for Advanced Life Support (Part III) recognize endotracheal intubation as one of the quickest and easiest ways to insure a protected airway, when simpler airway adjuncts have been ineffective. Endotracheal intubation will isolate the airway, keep it patent, prevent aspiration, and assure delivery of a high concentration of oxygen to the lungs.

The 1979 AHA Conference recommended that all emergency department training programs and equivalent programs give satisfactory training to all professional personnel in the safe and effective introduction of endotracheal tubes.*

Because of the difficulties, delays, and complications in properly placing an endotracheal tube, its use should be restricted to medical personnel and professional allied health personnel who are highly trained and either use endotracheal intubation frequently or are retrained frequently in this technique.

The indications for endotracheal intubation include:

1. Cardiac arrest
2. Respiratory arrest
3. Inability of rescuer to ventilate the unconscious patient with conventional methods
4. Inability of the patient to protect his own airway (coma, areflexia)
5. Prolonged artificial ventilation

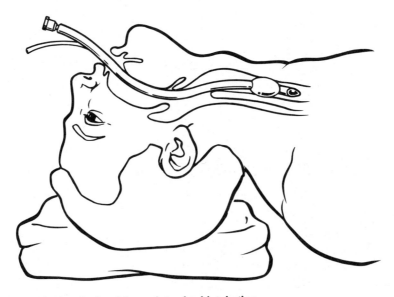

Figure 9.8. Positioning the head for endotracheal intubation.

Blind Intubation

Nasal route without hyperextension of the neck. There is a procedure available for use on the patient who has sustained a neck injury and cannot have the neck hyperextended. This is the so-called "blind intubation" procedure in which the patient is effectively intubated without direct visualization of the vocal cords. An endotracheal tube is inserted into the nostril for a distance equivalent to that from the tip of the nose to the tragus of the ear. Insertion of the tube for that distance places the tip of the tube right above the epiglottis; *when the patient breathes,* you can slide it into place and by listening to the end of the tube, you can quickly tell whether or not you've entered the trachea. It is said that most of the time it is relatively simple to do because of the curve of the tube. This can be done in most patients with neck injuries, but remember that it *cannot be accomplished in a patient who is not breathing!* Figure 9.9 presents another method of blind intubation.

Oral route. Place bite block to prevent being bitten, hyperextend the head, locate larynx with index finger of non-dominant hand, and pull epiglottis forward (Fig. 9.9).

Pass E/T tube, using placed index finger as a guide with the curvature of tube pointing the tip anteriorly.

Tracheostomy*

"A tracheostomy procedure may be life-saving in chest-injured patients. However, in an acute emergency, tracheostomy is far inferior to endotracheal

---

*Excerpted from Clinical Symposia, Vol 22, No 3, by Emil A. Naclerio, M.D. © Copyright 1970. CIBA GEIGY Corporation. Reprinted with permission.

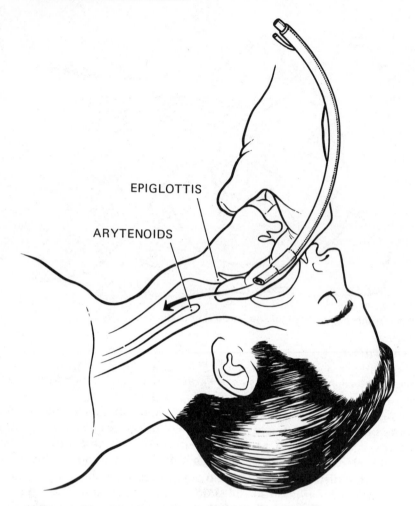

EPIGLOTTIS

ARYTENOIDS

Figure 9.9. Blind intubation. Hyperextend the neck and pull the epiglottis toward you with the index finger. Insert the tracheal catheter, using the top surface of the inserted finger as a guide, and slowly advance the tube past the arytenoids into the trachea.

intubation. In the first place it will take 10-15 minutes, as compared to the few seconds required to insert an endotracheal tube. Furthermore, a hastily done tracheostomy with inadequate assistance, poor lighting, and improper instruments in a patient who is rapidly expiring often leads to troublesome bleeding which may significantly increase the airway difficulty.

Tracheostomy, therefore, should be deferred until it can be carried out carefully under suitable conditions, preferably in the operating room, and as an *elective* procedure. The endotracheal tube should not be withdrawn until the tracheostomy has been completed."

OXYGEN ADMINISTRATION

Oxygen is listed as a drug in the national formulary and requires a doctor's order for administration. Oxygen-enriched air must be given continuously to a compromised patient, regardless of the cause, because there are *no body stores of oxygen available*. However, some patients with chronic obstructive pulmonary disease and chronic respiratory failure depend on *hypoxemia* to stimulate the respiratory drive. When they present with acute-on-chronic respiratory failure they need oxygen, but *only* enough to restore their small PaO_2 to what is normal for *them* which is probably a PaO_2 of about 50 mm Hg. In other words, they need continuous *controlled* oxygen therapy.

In emergency situations, the vast majority of patients with any form (or suspicion) of respiratory failure should be given continuous high concentrations of oxygen; when administration is prolonged, the concentration is adjusted to give a normal PaO_2. Oxygen toxicity does not occur with low-flow methods of delivery (nasal prongs) or with concentrations below 50% even after prolonged administration.

The effect of oxygen therapy in a chronic lung patient should be monitored with arterial blood gases (ABGs). Oxygen administered by nasal cannula or mask for a short term of 30 min to an hour should not require humidification unless the patient is asthmatic or emphysemic, or unless the relative humidity of the air itself is very, very low and the patient is stressed. When humidifier bottles are used for oxygen administration, they must be changed after each patient usage. Disposable humidifier bottles should be removed from the flow meter when they are no longer in use and *disposed of*. Reusable humidifier bottles should be removed from the flow meter, emptied, cleansed, and replaced in dry condition. Water-filled bottles hanging at room temperature for any considerable length of time have been found to be prolific sources of *Pseudomonas* growth and represent a severe health hazard to the next patient receiving humidified oxygen from that source.

Oxygen may be administered in the emergency setting by nasal catheter, nasal cannula, face mask without reservoir bag, and face mask with reservoir or rebreathing bag.

A comparison of oxygen concentrations available to the patient with various delivery systems is presented in Table 9.1; it is interesting to note that both the nasal catheter and the nasal cannula produce relatively high percentages of oxygen at a low flow, while the face mask with the reservoir or rebreathing bag produces the highest percentage of oxygen at a high flow rate.

HAZARDS OF AIRWAY MANAGEMENT

The three major hazards of airway management are airway trauma, the introduction of infection, and aspiration of gastric contents. Of the three, *aspiration* is by far the greatest hazard encountered in attempts to adequately manage the patient's airway.

Aspiration is defined as the act of inhaling. Several types of aspiration syndromes may be seen in the ED and are probably due either to a diminished gag reflex or to poor dentition and could be classified as follows:

1. Toxic or chemical fluid (aspiration of acids, hydrocarbons, alcohol, or mineral oil)

Table 9.1 Oxygen Delivery Percentages by Different Delivery Systems*

OXYGEN FLOW (LITER/MIN)	OXYGEN DELIVERY (%)			
			FACE MASK	
	NASAL CATHETER	NASAL CANNULA	WITHOUT RESERVOIR BAG	WITH RESERVOIR BAG
2	24	24	–	–
4	35-44	32-37	28-48	–
6	48-60	38-48	34-50	40-50
8	70	45	36-50	50-60
10	77	53	38-54	90-95

*Smith R, Petruscak BJ, Solosko D: Am J Nurs Vol 73, No 1, p 72, 1973

2. Bacterial pathogens, both aerobic *and* anaerobic (poor dentition)
3. Inert substances (steak, etc., also known as "cafe coronary").

The aspiration of gastric contents during emergency resuscitation procedures is associated with a very high mortality of approximately 30-70% and possibly a good deal higher than that. The symptoms of aspiration should be included in the caution index and are as follows:

1. Dyspnea within several hours of aspiration
2. Bronchospasms with wheezing
3. X-rays showing white fluffy changes in the lung fields
4. Frothy sputum without purulence
5. Frequent hypotension
6. Lungs filling with fluid and demonstrating reduced compliance in the volume/pressure relationship.

It may be well to mention something here regarding the problem of the full stomach in emergencies. Gastric emptying time after an ordinary meal is probably 3.5-4 hours; gastric emptying slows greatly or *may cease altogether* with the onset of pain, trauma, emotional crisis, or the onset of labor in the pregnant woman. Furthermore, administration of analgesic drugs following injury or the use of amnesic drugs during labor will also prolong gastric emptying time. Accordingly, accident victims and women in labor, when brought to the hospital as emergencies, are most likely to have delayed gastric emptying and, therefore, are predisposed to vomiting and aspiration. A good rule of thumb is to assume that if the patient has eaten within 4 hours of injury, the stomach will not be empty for up to *10 hours* following injury and possibly longer.

Emergency personnel should always be ready to immediately position and suction a patient who is a candidate for vomiting/aspiration and *should be able to anticipate* the problem.

ESSENTIAL SUPPORTIVE EQUIPMENT AND ITS USE

When bag-valve-mask units are used, they usually provide less ventilatory volume than mouth-to-mouth or mouth-to-mask ventilation because of the difficulty in providing a leakproof seal to the face while maintaining an open airway. *Extensive* specialized training and demonstrated *continuing proficiency* is required with the bag-valve-mask device (Fig. 9.10).

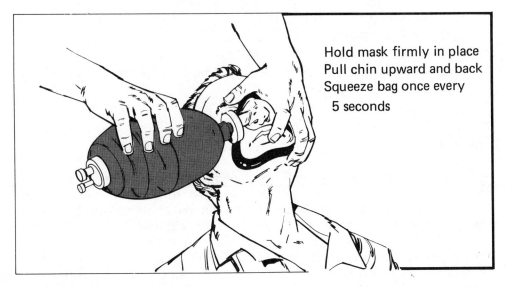

Hold mask firmly in place
Pull chin upward and back
Squeeze bag once every
5 seconds

Figure 9.10. Bag/mask resuscitation.

The rescuer must assume a position at the top of the patient's head and must then maintain the head and extension, keep the lower jaw elevated, and secure an optimum mask fit with one hand while using the other hand to squeeze the bag. Attempts have been made to achieve effective ventilation with these devices by using two rescuers, one to hold the mask and one to squeeze the bag, but this is an awkward procedure. However, some bag mask units have an extension tubing from the bag to the mask which allows the bag to be placed between the arm and the chest wall while holding the mask in place with both hands and forming the seal as the bag is squeezed between the arm and the body. When an endotracheal tube or esophageal obturator airway is used, the rescuer may assume a position at the patient's side. When a mask is used, the rescuer should *always* be positioned at the top of the patient's head and *not* at the side, maintaining a leakproof seal between the mask and the face to achieve maximum ventilation. This is a technique which requires a great deal of skill.

An adequate bag-valve-mask unit should fulfill these criteria:

1. Self-refilling, but without sponge rubber inside because of the difficulty in cleaning, disinfecting, eliminating ethylene oxide, and fragmentation

2. Non-jam valve system at 15 liters/min oxygen inlet flow
3. Transparent, plastic face mask with an air-filled or contoured resilient cuff
4. No pop-off valve, except on pediatric models
5. Standard 15 mm/22 mm fittings
6. System for delivery of high concentrations of oxygen through an ancillary oxygen inlet at the back of the bag or via an oxygen reservoir
7. A true nonbreathing valve
8. Oropharyngeal airway
9. Satisfactory for practice on manikins
10. Satisfactory performance under all common environmental conditions and extremes of temperature
11. Available in adult and pediatric sizes

Suction

It is *essential* that portable and/or installed suction equipment be available for airway management emergencies. The portable unit should provide vacuum and flow adequate for pharyngeal suction. It should be fitted with large-bore, non-kinking suction tubing and semirigid pharyngeal suction tips (Yankauer or "tonsil" type). There should be multiple sterile suction catheters of various sizes for suctioning via endotracheal or tracheostomy tubes, a non-breakable collection bottle, and a supply of water for rinsing tubes and catheters.

The installed suction unit should be powerful enough to provide an airflow of over 30 liters/min (LPM) at the end of the delivery tube and a vacuum of over 300 mm Hg when the tube is clamped. The amount of suction should be controllable for use on children and intubated patients.

There should be an additional set of rigid pharyngeal suction tips (tonsil suction tips) and sterile, curved, tracheal suction catheters of various sizes. For tracheal sucton, a Y- or T-piece or a lateral opening should be between the suction tube and the suction source for on/off control. The suction yoke, collection bottle, water for rinsing, and suction tubes should be readily accessible to the attendant at the head of the litter. The tube should reach the airway of the patient, regardless of his position. Suction apparatus must be designed for easy cleaning and decontamination.*

An excellent fail-safe procedure to utilize when anticipating the arrival of a patient who may suddenly require immediate vigorous suctioning is to have the suction equipment assembled, turned on, and clamped off with an instrument or by wedging a fold of tubing into an IV pole receptacle on the stretcher.

---

*Adapted from the American Heart Association Standards on Advanced Life Support. Reprinted in JAMA, August 1, 1980, Vol 244, No 5, (III). With permission from the American Heart Association.

This seemingly small item of preparedness can save precious seconds of time when a desperately compromised patient vomits and is in danger of aspiration.

If the patient requires suctioning beyond the oropharyngeal area or through an ET tube, sterile suction catheters must be used with sterile gloves if possible. The one-hand sterile technique is generally most workable, handling the catheter tip with a sterile glove as it is advanced down the airway. Catheters used for suctioning bronchial secretions should be soft plastic or rubber with a whistle tip and should be *discarded* after each use.

The diameter of the catheter is important since this displaces the passage of air or oxygen in the airway. Usually a #14 French catheter is adequate for adults and a # 10 French is adequate for children.

The catheter should have a "Y" connection or a thumb port so that the tube can be passed into the bronchus without sucking out the oxygen supply and then slowly withdrawn as the suction is applied and as the catheter is gently rotated.

The same rule applies for endotracheal intubation: never occlude the patient's airway with a tube any longer than you can hold your own breath and never suction a patient for more than 10 sec at a time, maximum, allowing several minutes between suctioning efforts so that the patient does not become even more hypoxic.

Endotracheal Intubation Tray

1. Straight blade (Miller) or curved blade (MacIntosh), laryngoscope with *bright* light and *fresh* batteries (adult sizes numbers 2, 3, and 4 as well as pediatric size blades should be on hand)
2. Rubber or plastic endotracheal tubes with *intact* cuffs; average adult French-gauge sizes are 32, 34, 36, 38; average adult millimeter sizes are 7, 7.5, 8, 8.5, 9. Pediatric sizes should be on hand. (Many experienced anesthesia people say that one can "guestimate" the adequate size of an endotracheal tube according to the size of the patient's little finger.)
3. Wire guides should be available *with* clamps but should *never* be used *except* by a physician or anesthesia personnel.
4. One 10- to 20-cc syringe with large blunt needle for cuff inflation
5. One shod hemostat to clamp pilot tube and maintain cuff inflation
6. A selection of adaptors for connection of tube to respirator or bag unit
7. Contoured forceps (Magill and/or Rovenstein)
8. Spray for topical anesthetics (for the conscious, alert patient)
9. *Water-soluble* lubricant (for use with cuffed tubes)
10. Suction capability
11. One-half inch adhesive tape, tincture of benzoin, applicators
12. Oxygen and resuscitation equipment, including manual resuscitation bag
13. Pillow, folded towel, sand bag, or other under-shoulders support.

N. B.

A primary responsibility of *all* ED personnel is to check the status of the intubation tray at the beginning of each *and* every shift. Rechargeable handles should be plugged into wall outlets for charge, and batteries should be replaced in other handles if the light is dimming. The full supply of tubes should be checked as well as the presence or absence of the filling syringe, "shod" clamp, McGill forceps, and *water-soluble* lubricant. Any nurse who has been in the miserable situation of having a dead battery or light on the laryngoscope during a code procedure well knows the importance of checking at the beginning of each shift to be *certain* that there is a dependable light source on the laryngoscope should the equipment be needed.

Guidelines for endotracheal intubation are presented in Table 9.2.

Table 9.2 Guidelines for Endotracheal Intubation*

Indications for Intubation

Inadequate ventilation
Prior to gastric lavage in drug-overdosed patients to prevent aspiration
Maintenance of airway during tracheostomy
Assisting ventilation during resuscitation
Acute severe pulmonary edema

Contraindications to Intubation

ANY question of cervical spine fracture
Presence of foreign bodies in upper airway
Previous long-term or repeated tracheal intubations
Laryngeal edema, usually accompanied by acute laryngitis
Mandibular fractures
Open pulmonary tuberculosis

Common Errors of Intubation

Intubating inappropriately in emergency situations when an oropharyngeal airway and bag/mask unit are adequate
Wasting time excessively
Failing to see tracheal opening
Passing tube too far into right mainstem bronchus with resulting collapse of left lung
Choosing too small an E/T tube

Helpful Hints During Procedure

Remember to reassure even an apparently comatose patient
Assemble *all* equipment in advance and check the cuff of the tube for leaks
Check working condition of laryngoscope light
Position the patient's head carefully
Protect patient's teeth
Never persist in intubation attempt *any longer than you can your own breath,* without reoxygenating the patient
Always listen to breath sounds and the apexes of both lungs after intubation
Secure the tube in proper position with 0.5-inch adhesive or an elastic holding device, being careful to avoid any pressure on the nares
Recognize excessive coughing as a possible sign of irritation to tracheal carina (the point at which the trachea bifurcates into right mainstem bronchus, approximately 2 inches below suprasternal notch.

*Excerpted from the Medical Skills Library, American College of Physicians with Permission of the American College of Physicians.

SUMMARY

Airway distress in a patient is usually quite obvious, but the EDN should evaluate every patient closely by *looking* and *listening*. Evaluate the respiratory *pattern* (rapid or slow), *quality* of respiration (shallow or deep), the *sound* (quiet, raspy, crowing, gurgling), *skin color* (pale, cyanotic, ashen), *facial expression* (relaxed, anxious, frantic), and check for *use of accessory muscles*.

Some guidelines to remember for competent and effective airway management are:

1. The airway is always the first concern.
2. Proper positioning of the head will be the major factor in clearing most airways, remembering the *tongue* is the commonest form of airway obstruction.
3. *Never* use an airway on a responsive patient if a gag reflex is present.
4. Be careful to avoid soft-tissue damage when inserting and removing oropharyngeal and/or nasopharyngeal airways.
5. Have the suction *on* and *ready* for *all* extubations.
6. Have rigid tonsil suction tips and large-bore tubing available at all times on the suction apparatus.
7. Always check the laryngoscope at the beginning of every shift. *Never* assume that the last shift has done this.
8. Keep only water-soluble lubrication on the endotracheal tray.
9. *Always* auscultate the apexes of both lungs after intubation to be certain breath sounds are present bilaterally.
10. Never persist in the intubation attempt any longer than you can hold your own breath without reoxygenating the patient.

REVIEW

1. Explain the difference between clinical death and biological death.
2. Define functional death.
3. What purpose does the film of mucus serve that is constantly secreted by the membranes lining the upper airways?
4. What does the larynx house?
5. Describe the structure of the trachea.
6. What is an alveolus? Describe its structure.
7. What is the pressure gradient between the visceral pleura and parietal pleura?
8. How do the lungs operate?

9. Define the respiratory cycle.

10. Define external respiration.

11. What is the average tidal volume in the normal adult?

12. What would be the normal vital capacity for a 70-kg man?

13. Identify the most essential steps in establishing an airway.

14. Describe the Heimlich maneuver and the indications for its use.

15. When is the placement of an oropharyngeal airway contraindicated?

16. List the criteria for an adequate bag/mask unit.

17. List five indications for placement of an endotracheal tube.

18. What is the most essential adjunct to airway management?

19. List the important guidelines in airway management.

BIBLIOGRAPHY

American College of Physicians Medical Skills Library, ROCOM: Endotracheal Intubation. Ann Intern Med, American College of Physicians, Philadelphia, Pennsylvania, 1972

American College of Surgeons: Advanced Trauma Life Support (ATLS) Course Manual. ACS, Chicago, Illinois, 1981

American Medical Association: The Wonderful Human Machine, Part V. The American Medical Association, Chicago, Illinois, 1971

Boyce B: Nursing Practice: Respiratory Care Terminology. American Lung Association, New York, 1976

Budassi SA, Barber JM: Emergency Nursing: Principles and Practice. C.V. Mosby Co., St. Louis, Missouri, 1981

Bushnell S: Respiratory Intensive Care Nursing. Little, Brown & Co., Boston, Massachusetts, 1973

Fuchs P: Getting the best out of oxygen delivery systems. Nursing 80, Vol 10, No 12, pp 34-43, December 1980

Grigsby J, Rottman S: Prehospital airway management: Esophageal obturator airway or endotracheal intubation? Controversies in Emergency Medicine, TEM, Vol 3, No 2, pp 25-29, July 1981

Jacquette G: To reduce hazards of tracheal suctioning. Nurs, Vol 71, pp 2362-64, 1971

Kirilloff L, Maszkiewicz R: Guide to respiratory care in critically ill adults. AJN, Vol 79, No. 10, pp 2005-2012, 1979

Moody A: Oxygen therapy. JEN, Vol 5, No 4, pp 15-20, July-August 1979

Naclerio A: Chest Trauma. The Ciba Pharmaceutical Co., Summit, Pennsylvania. 1970

Perro K, Goetze C, Monaghan J: Making every minute count with an esophageal gastric tube airway. Nursing 80, Vol 10, No 8, pp 61-65, August 1980

Promisloff RA: When, why, and how to administer oxygen safely. Nursing 80, Vol 10, No 10, pp 54-56, October 1980

Standards for cardiopulmonary resuscitation (CPR) and emergency cardiac care (ECC). JAMA, Vol 244, No 5, August 1980

Stringer LW: Emergency Treatment of Acute Respiratory Diseases, 3rd ed. The Robert J. Brady Co., Bowie, Maryland, 1982

Sweetwood H: Nursing in the Intensive Respiratory Care Unit, 2nd ed. Springer Publishing Co., Inc., New York, 1979

RESPIRATORY FAILURE STATES *10*

KEY CONCEPTS

This chapter provides an overview of the disease states that lead to and culminate in respiratory failure. Some management concepts for each state are outlined. Much of this material is based on lecture content presented to Emergency Nurses by Guy Guffey, M.C., Tom Rich, ARRT, John Naron, ARRT, Keith Ironside, M.D., and Gideon Bosker, M.D., all of the Portland Metropolitan Area.

After reading and studying this chapter, you should be able to:

- Categorize the disease states leading to respiratory failure.
- Recognize the signs of acute airway obstruction.
- Describe the protocol that should be followed with acute airway obstruction.
- Identify the disease states that are included as chronic airway obstructions.
- Describe the protocol to be followed with chronic obstructive airway problems.
- Recognize the signs of acute hypercapnia.
- Identify some of the disease states that are considered restrictive defects.
- Describe the implications of A-a gradients substantially larger than normal.
- Describe the emergency management of pulmonary edema.
- Describe the emergency management of near-drownings.
- Explain the difference in the pathophysiology of salt water versus fresh water near-drownings.
- Identify some of the drug hazards encountered in the management of respiratory failure.
- Identify some of the symptoms of aminophylline toxicity.

Basically, respiratory failure is due to hypoxemia or hypercapnia or a combination of both. The normal PaO_2 for a given patient depends on his or her age, the altitude of the environment, and the fraction of oxygen in the inspired air. Generally 80-90 mm Hg is considered normal breathing room air. Clinically, *respiratory failure is a fact when the PaO_2 is less than 50 mm Hg and the PCO_2 is greater than 50 mm Hg.* Since the lungs are a simple symmetrical unit dealing with the exchange of blood and gases and the airway is the means of conducting atmospheric gases into those lungs, respiratory failure, then, is a disease state caused by either 1) impaired ventilation (transport of atmospheric gases to the alveoli), or 2) impaired diffusion and gas exchange at the alveolar or cellular level.

The degree of alveolar ventilation for clinical purposes is reflected by the level of a $PaCO_2$, and some basic significant factors to remember are:

- A normal $PaCO_2$ indicates *effectiveness* of alveolar ventilation.
- An increased $PaCO_2$ means *hypoventilation* is occurring.
- A decreased $PaCO_2$ means *hyperventilation* is occurring.

There are other factors that affect tissue oxygenation which must be taken into consideration including cardiac output, the hemoglobin concentration of the blood, pH, and temperature.

IMPAIRED VENTILATION

The causes of impaired ventilation can be categorized as 1) acute airway obstruction, 2) chronic airway obstruction, and 3) restrictive defects.

ACUTE AIRWAY OBSTRUCTION

Acute obstruction of the airway (by the tongue, decreased swallowing reflexes, epiglottitis, croup, laryngeal edema, or foreign bodies) is a commonly seen occurrence in children, and assessment for respiratory embarrassment must be done early and carefully.

The acutely ill child in a toxic state from severe respiratory infection, such as croup or epiglottitis, may progressively and quietly hypoventilate from the degree of soft tissue obstruction as well as fatigue, and be in serious and too often irreversible straits unless carefully and continually monitored for rate and quality of respirations. An infant exhibiting grunting respirations and flaring nostrils with the use of accessory muscles of respiration and a bulging abdomen on expiration is in serious respiratory trouble.

The healthy child suffering an airway obstruction from the aspiration of a common foreign body such as beans, toys, peanuts, or any other item small enough to find its way into the trachea or bronchi, will probably have noisy respirations (although not necessarily) and will be anxious and probably coughing, depending on where the foreign body lodges. Sometimes these children can be all but asymptomatic and the diagnosis is confirmed by auscultation and x-ray.

A foreign body lodged deeply and causing serious obstruction may result in heavy coughing, retching, struggling, laryngospasm and even bronchospasm. The patient by this time will be extremely cyanotic; foreign bodies can be a serious management problem and rarely allow for wasted time or movement! Treatment will vary with the definite diagnosis. Frequently the Heimlich maneuver is considered an effective means of dealing with upper airway obstruction. In children, however, the maneuver requires modification by holding the small child over either the arm or hand and delivering a sharp blow between the shoulder blades in order to "pop" the object out of position by the forceful expulsion of a sudden gust of air from the lungs. Bronchoscopy in the operating room is sometimes necessary and on rare occasions pneumonostomy is required.

Croup

Croup (laryngotracheobronchitis) is an upper airway infection usually seen in small children under age 6, more frequently between ages 4 and 6 (see Chapter 23 Pediatric Emergencies). Croup is a viral infection which causes inflammation and edema in the subglottic area with a characteristic "seal bark" type of cough which can frequently be recognized over the telephone.

These children can present serious management problems and should be seen in the ED for intervention and treatment with cold mist and administration of corticosteroids if necessary in severe cases. Constant assessment of the airway must be maintained and the endotracheal tray should be close at hand.

Epiglottitis

Epiglottitis occurs less frequently than does croup but it fulminates *rapidly* and must always be considered an eventuality in children, *and* with high temperatures and respiratory difficulty. The evaluation and emergency management of epiglottitis is discussed in the chapters on Pediatric and EENT emergencies.

CHRONIC AIRWAY OBSTRUCTION

Emphysema, chronic bronchitis, and chronic asthma all produce chronic airway obstruction. Although the etiologies differ, the essential clinical approach to relief for these patients is very similar as it relates to airway management and the administration of oxygen.

Emphysema

Emphysema is frequently referred to as *chronic obstructive pulmonary disease* (COPD) or *chronic obstructive lung disease* (COLD) and is a generalized obstructive condition of the lungs which producess varying degrees of dyspnea and disability due to hyperinflation of the lungs with a loss of elasticity in the alveoli. The alveoli remain overdistended with air which cannot be expelled, and this can produce acute respiratory embarrassment on exertion; the patient will be apprehensive, short of breath, and may exhibit tachycardia and even cyanosis. It is important to remember that a patient with chronic respiratory obstruction may be severely hypoxemic without necessarily being cyanotic and will require humidified *low flow* oxygen at 2-3 liters per min (LPM) as discussed in the previous chapter.

Breathing for these patients is generally characterized by the use of the accessory muscles of respiration, by a characteristic forward-leaning position, and by a prolonged expiratory phase through pursed lips, with occasional audible wheezes and rales. ABGs generally show a lowered pH with hypoxemia and hypercapnia.

Chronic Bronchitis

Chronic bronchitis is another disease which is referred to as COPD and is a long-standing disease of the tracheobronchial tree, frequently associated with emphysema, and characterized by chronic inflammation and atrophic changes in the mucous membranes and deeper bronchial structures. It is also frequently associated with pulmonary fibrosis and other chronic pulmonary disease and is not a reversible airway obstruction since there have been degenerative changes taking place. The resulting bronchial rigidity often restricts normal ventilation and becomes a factor in the patient's ventilatory insufficiency and a prominent cause of dyspnea. There is usually a chronic cough with expectoration, becoming more troublesome during the winter months. Chronic bronchitis is characteristically afebrile, and the physical signs are few, other than those of chronic pulmonary disease. When the need for oxygen is indicated, it should be administered at a *low flow* rate of 2-3 LPM.

Asthma

A *reversible* obstructive airway disease, asthma is a disease of unknown etiology until proved otherwise and is characterized by spasm and increased secretion of the bronchial tree. Some of the factors responsible for precipitating asthmatic attacks are cold air, strong odors, infections (especially viral), and emotional factors (after asthma is an established entity).

The acute asthmatic attack exhibits characteristic signs of labored respiration, particularly in the expiratory phase, frequently associated with audible wheezing. On auscultation, the expiratory phase, and occasionally the inspiratory phase, is accompanied by rales and wheezes, with the typically prolonged expiratory phase. Unless there is an upper respiratory infection present as well, the vital signs, white blood count, and chest x-ray will all be within normal limits. If the asthma is of the allergic type, there may be an eosinophilia present in the differential count. The patient may be severely dyspneic, apprehensive, and even diaphoretic without exhibiting central cyanosis initially but will develop cyanosis shortly unless the obstruction is eased and finally reversed.

Most recognized asthmatic patients have their own medication regimen and know what works best for *them*; they rarely present to the ED unless their problem is complicated by an upper respiratory infection, or they have not responded effectively to their medications. When this occurs, alveolar collapse may develop secondary to dehydration following prolonged labored respiration, with formation of mucus plugs in the small airways, unless the patient is managed properly and without delay.

Epinephrine (Adrenalin) is the drug of choice, given subcutaneously in doses of 0.3-0.5 ml of 1:1000 solution in adults and 0.01 ml/kg in children. Many physicians feel it is wise to avoid giving SusPhrine (epinephrine, aqueous suspension) on the initial administration until the action of the aqueous epinephrine can be evaluated. If no relief is obtained, the dose may be repeated in 15-20 minutes. During this time, it is essential to observe and document the vital signs, since epinephrine may cause tachycardia or hypertension.

The theophylline group of drugs (Xanthine derivatives), which includes aminophylline, is well established in the treatment of asthma. Aminophylline or theophylline is given to relax bronchial musculature, to stimulate respiration, and as a diuretic with the dose computed per kilogram of body weight. The average dose of aminophylline is generally 5-7 mg/kg body weight diluted in 250 ml of D5/W and given IV over a period of 20-30 min. If aminophylline is given too rapidly, vomiting and dizziness will occur; there may be stimulation of vagal response with severe bradycardia and cardiac arrest. In adults, the safe administration rate is 0.9-1 mg/kg/hour IV drip after the initial dose. Rectal administration of aminophylline or theophylline is generally ill-advised because of the variable absorption and mucosal toxicity. Many patients use aminophylline suppositories at home, however, and it is essential to know how much medication they have on board before giving more in the ED.

Humidified oxygen should be administered at 4-5 LPM. Mucus plugging is a common factor, and a number of investigators feel that mucus plugging with attendant shunting accounts for the severe arterial hypoxemia of these states. Although humidification is thought by most to be essential, there are some who have demonstrated that aerosolized mist has no effect whatsoever on humidification below the glottis.

Further general management includes systemic hydration with 1000 ml D5/NS (normal saline) or 1/2 NS solution IV, correction of hypercapnea and acidosis (according to ABG results if done) with appropriate sodium bicarbonate IV, ultrasonic nebulized oxygen if indicated and avoidance of sedatives which could result in respiratory depression. Steroids are sometimes administered IV as a last measure in controlling the asthmatic attack.

If the acute episode does not reverse with marked improvement in the patient's condition within an hour, arterial blood gases should be drawn and further evaluation done. This patient may well be approaching respiratory failure with an increasing hypoxemia, even though cyanosis has not developed. Cyanosis may not manifest itself until the PaO_2 falls to around 55 mm Hg.

Status Asthmaticus

Status asthmaticus is defined in a variety of ways but generally is considered to be a state of bronchial asthma which is refractory to bronchodilating drugs, particularly epinephrine, and which persists for more than

24 hours. This is a life-threatening episode, and many physicians feel that the time to treat status asthmaticus is *three days before it happens*. Status is considered, by physicians who specialize in the treatment of asthma, to be a "crisis of neglect," and a patient who is still refractory to treatment of the initial problem within 24 hours should not be treated again and sent home but admitted to the hospital for "pre-status" evaluation (as it were) and management *before* the status becomes an established clinical fact.*

RESTRICTIVE DEFECTS

Defects resulting in decreased lung expansion and oxygenation include the following:

1. Limited thorax expansion from kyphoscoliosis, multiple rib fractures, thoracic surgery, and spinal arthritis
2. Decreased diaphragmatic movement from abdominal surgery, ascites, peritonitis, and severe obesity
3. Neuromuscular defects such as Guillain-Barré syndrome, multiple sclerosis, myasthenia gravis, brain or spinal injuries, and drugs or toxic agents such as curare and acetylcholinesterase inhibitors
4. Respiratory center damage or depression from narcotics, barbiturates, tranquilizers, anesthetics, cerebral infarction, or trauma and *uncontrolled high-flow oxygen* therapy
5. Tumors.

IMPAIRED DIFFUSION AND GAS EXCHANGE

Knowledge of alveolar oxygen tension is fundamental to adequate clinical appraisal of ventilatory status and the recognition of impaired diffusion and gas exchange. For any given alveolar oxygen tension (PAO_2), there is a corresponding expected arterial blood oxygen tension (PaO_2) which is only slightly lower than the alveolar level in normals. The difference between the PAO_2 and the PaO_2 is called the *A–a gradient* and is normally about 30 mm Hg at high PO_2 and 10 mm Hg at low PO_2. If A–a gradients are substantially larger, the presence of an *intrapulmonary* process is indicated which interferes with gas exchange such as shunt, diffusion disturbance, or ventilation-perfusion imbalance.

By way of contrast, failure to find an increased A–a gradient in the presence of hypercapnia indicates hypoventilation caused by extrapulmonary factors, such as narcosis, muscle weakness, or paralysis. The patient will be hypoxemic while breathing air, but this results only from the hypoventilation.**

---

*Excerpted from Asthma, the State of the Art, by R. Farr. Oregon Thoracic Society Spring Conference, Salishan, 1977.

**Excerpted from Graphic Aids in Blood Gas Analysis with permission of the American Lung Association.

Pulmonary Edema

Pulmonary edema is usually of cardiac origin with acute left ventricular failure but it may be of noncardiogenic origin with damage to pulmonary capillary tensions from chemical irritation of fumes, smoke, radiation, nitrogen oxides, particulate matter, or heroin overdose. Whatever the cause, there is an increased permeability of the alveolocapillary membrane with seepage of plasma from the capillaries of the lung bed into the alveoli. This directly results in a compromised gas exchange with varying degrees of *hypoxemia;* later *hypercapnia* develops with dyspnea, tachycardia, apprehension, hemoptysis (there may be copious frothy blood-tinged sputum), distended neck veins, tender liver, cool sweaty extremities, cyanosis, orthopnea, paroxysmal nocturnal dyspnea (PND), and loud gurgling rales.

Nursing intervention guidelines for the patient with pulmonary edema are geared to reducing venous return to the heart and to increase left ventricular output.

The patient must immediately be placed in an upright position to facilitate breathing, the legs and feet should be dependent to reduce return venous flow.

1. Give oxygen at high liter flow by mask or intermittent positive-pressure breathing (IPPB).

2. Give morphine sulfate IV in increments of 2-4 mg to allay anxiety and slow the respiratory rate. Morphine should not be given if respiratory depression might result and naloxone (Narcan) should be on hand just in case.

3. Furosemide (Lasix) is generally the diuretic of choice, and it should be given IV for rapid diuresis.

4. Insert a Foley catheter to monitor output.

5. Aminophylline may be given to relax the bronchospasm caused by irritation of the pulmonary edema. (See page 155 on drug hazards at end of chapter.)

6. Digoxin (Lanoxin) may be given to strengthen the cardiac contractility as well as to enhance the action of the diuretic.

The patient with pulmonary edema will be extremely apprehensive and anxious, and the EDN should stay close by with a confident, reinforcing attitude to help alleviate the anxiety as much as possible, helping to calm respirations, and letting the medications do their work.

Arterial blood gases are essential, and a CBC and electrolytes should be done. Chest films should be requisitioned *stat* and a large bore IV line (heparin lock) initiated for administration of medications, as well as for possible use in carrying out phlebotomy to reduce the patient's circulating blood volume. Rotating tourniquets may also be indicated.

Near-Drowning*

With both fresh and sea water inhalation, the lungs are "messed up" and resemble a combination of pulmonary edema and status asthmaticus. Experiments on animals have shown that the damage is worse with sea water, although fresh water stopped the heart faster. With massive fresh water inhalation, the water passes as quickly into the circulation, overloads the circulating blood volume and may even double it in two minutes. Hemodilution, ballooning and destruction of red cells, and ventricular fibrillation may result. Kidney shutdown is not uncommon.

Sea water, on the other hand, is hypertonic compared to blood since it contains 3.5% mixed salts. Sea water in the lungs in large amounts pulls fluid out of the circulating blood volume into the lungs with a resulting pulmonary edema, a low circulating blood volume, and shriveled, crenated red blood cells. The patient may die of hypovolemia as well as hypoxia from the severely impaired diffusion and gas exchange of pulmonary edema.

These changes depend, of course, on whether fluid is actually aspirated and, if so, in what quantities. Severe laryngospasm may result from aspiration of the first small amount of water, causing the victim to die of actual suffocation rather than drowning, in the true sense of the word, with the lungs full of water.

Although the effects of salt water versus fresh water in the lungs differs, the resulting severe hypoxia is the same and immediate resuscitative efforts are directed to correcting the hypoxia and existing acidosis.

Information is appearing now in the literature about the so-called "diving reflex"** which is nature's way of inducing profound bradycardia to conserve oxygen in man and animals, elicited by placing the face in a pan of cold water. This is said to cause a reduction in heart rate between 15-30% in normal subjects, according to a Dallas, Texas, team of investigators and is thought to account for some of the prolonged survival times in children who were submerged in cold water and presumed drowned, but who responded to prolonged resuscitation efforts.

Patients suffering severe prolonged periods of hypoxia will sustain significant brain damage if global brain ischemia (GBI) occurs. Reducing or preventing brain damage secondary to GBI is being achieved with *barbiturate coma* through administration of thiopental or pentobarbital, IV bolus, followed by maintenance infusion for a minimum of 48 to 72 hours or until normal intracranial pressure and blood pressure are obtained. Demonstrations in both laboratory animals and groups of patients including such ischemic-anoxic states as stroke, severe hypotension/shock, asphyxiation/drowning, cerebral edema, head trauma, and cardiac arrest showed that 1) cerebral metabolic oxygen requirements were reduced, 2) glucose resaturation was enhanced, 3) direct reduction of intracellular edema occurred, 4) direct change of cerebral metab-

---

*Excerpts taken from Simkins T., Drowning: Physicians discuss respiratory complications in victims who survive. Respiratory Therapy, May/June 1972, p 22

**For PAT: go soak, (Author not given): Emergency Medicine, August 1975, p 64

olism improved cellular viability, 5) convulsions and lactic acidosis were suppressed, and 6) intracranial pressure was reduced. Although still controversial, with many questions still to be answered, the barbiturate coma is receiving more interest; emergency personnel are encouraged to learn more about its application and potential.*

Nursing Guidelines

It should be remembered that *all* drowning or near-drowning victims exhibit some degree of hypoxia, hypercarbia, and acidosis. The nursing management guidelines for immediate intervention include the following steps:

1. Maintain airway, breathing and circulation, defibrillating, and suctioning as necessary.
2. Administer 100% oxygen by bag/mask unit or bag/tube if intubated. Positive and expiratory pressure (PEEP) of 5-10 cm water is frequently used to improve exchange at the alveolar level and allow a lower concentration of oxygen administration. Occasionally, ethyl alcohol is nebulized with the oxygen because of its mucolytic properties.
3. Place patient on cardiac monitor.
4. Draw serial arterial blood gases (ABGs) before administering bicarbonate.
5. Give sodium bicarbonate as indicated by ABGs with the dosage computed.**
6. Initiate IV line and give lactated Ringer's solution (10 ml/kg body weight) for the first hour except in fresh-water drowning. Then establish IV line and run to keep open (TKO) or use a Heparin lock.
7. Insert Foley catheter into bladder and connect to metered output container.
8. Order laboratory studies: arterial blood gases, serum electrolytes, hemoglobin, and hematocrit.
9. Place a nasogastric tube and empty stomach contents.
10. Have suction on hand, connected and ready to use.
11. Order portable chest x-ray films.
12. Monitor vital signs closely.
13. Transfer as soon as possible to an intensive care facility.

---

*Thomas RG, Brenneise K: High-Dose Barbiturates After Cardiac Arrest. Pediatric Emergencies. Rockville, Maryland, TEM, Vol 3, No 1, April 1981

**Formula for computing sodium bicarbonate dosage is as follows:

Body wt. in kg $\times$ minus base excess (−BE) $\div$ 5 $\times$ 1/2 = mEq of bicarbonate or

$$\frac{\text{Body wt. in kg} \times -BE}{5} \times 1/2 = \text{mEq of bicarbonate}$$

Initially, one half the dose is given until the effect has been reevaluated, in order to avoid overcorrection and alkalosis.

Caution: *Do not* a) inflate the stomach during resuscitation; b) hesitate to administer the bicarbonate and oxygen before getting any lab studies. Time may be the essence!

Pulmonary Embolus

Pulmonary embolus (obliterative pulmonary vascular disease) can be caused by thromboembolism of blood, fat, bone marrow, or amniotic fluid obstructing the pulmonary artery.

Patients who have acute pulmonary edema due to pulmonary thromboemboli will usually have some predisposing causes that can be identified. Thrombosis of the leg veins, use of oral contraceptives, long bone fractures, and prolonged immobilization (frequently following trauma) are most often the cause. The patient presenting with respiratory distress, pleuritic pain, and blood-tinged sputum of sudden onset should be regarded with a high degree of suspicion and treated as a possible pulmonary embolus until proven otherwise. The patient will probably, additionally, be extremely apprehensive with a sense of impending doom and may exhibit pallor, cyanosis, and engorged neck veins.

Nursing Guidelines

Immediate nursing intervention should include the following:

1. Administration of oxygen by mask at high liter flow
2. Cardiotonic drugs or diuretics are indicated
3. Electrocardiogram (ECG)
4. Portable chest X-ray
5. Arterial blood gases (ABGs) and partial prothrombin time (PIT)
6. Heparin administration as indicated
7. Large bore IV line with heparin lock
8. Foley bladder catheter with metered output container
9. Continuous monitoring of vital signs and close observation.

Carbon Monoxide Poisoning*

Inhalation of the products of incomplete hydrocarbon combustion will result in carbon monoxide poisoning. The causative agent can be automobile exhaust, smoke inhalation, use of burning charcoal in a closed space for cooking or even, to a minor degree, cigarette smoking. The onset can be insidious, since carbon monoxide has no color, odor, or taste; early symptoms can be confused with an upper respiratory infection.

Carbon monoxide binds with hemoglobin to produce carboxyhemoglobin (COHB) and has 200 times the affinity of oxygen for hemoglobin, producing a profound anemia. The symptoms will usually, but not always, correlate with the COHB level and a level above 25% *can* be irreversible and fatal.

---

*Koenig S: Utilization of the Hyperbaric Unit, Providence Hospital, Portland, Oregon, 1977

Nursing Management

The most important thing to understand is that COHB has displaced oxygen in the blood stream, and this profound anemia must be reversed as rapidly as possible.

1. Administer 100% oxygen.
2. Notify the laboratory to activate the co-oximeter and draw specimens for CO (carbon monoxide) level and ABGs.
3. If there is a Hyperbaric Unit in the area, check the availability.
4. Stat ECG.
5. Intubate if necessary (particularly with smoke inhalation).

A patient who has inhaled carbon monoxide eliminates half of his absorbed CO while breathing room air in 5 hours and 20 minutes. If he is given 100% oxygen to breathe, the time for eliminating half of the absorbed CO is now reduced to 1 hour and 20 minutes. If he receives hyperbaric oxygen (HBO) at 3 atmospheres of pressure (ATA), the time for elimination is reduced to 23 minutes. HBO is indicated for carboxyhemoglobin percentages of 25 or greater, CNS signs other than headache (especially confusion progressing to coma), and ECG changes showing evidence of increasing hypoxia (especially with evidence of a prior normal cardiogram).

It is important to note that heavy cigarette smokers will have increased levels of CO already in their blood, and if they are exposed to heavy air pollution, daily levels of 6-7% may be present normally. Obviously, these people are already at increased risk when exposed to carbon monoxide in heavier concentrations.

DRUG HAZARDS

Sympathomimetic drugs (those which mimic the sympathetic nervous system) include epinephrine (Adrenalin) and isoproterenol (Isuprel). These drugs, when given in respiratory crisis, may produce restlessness, anxiety, headache, palpitation, tachycardia, nausea, hypertension, and cardiac arrhythmias. The latter possibility *increases* with respiratory acidosis. Since these drugs may also reduce arterial oxygen saturation, they should be given together *with oxygen* to any patient who is already hypoxemic.

The hazards of giving aminophylline too rapidly have been discussed earlier in this chapter, but remember that very large doses given rapidly may cause dizziness, light-headedness, anxiety, confusion, tachycardia, *or* bradycardia, coupled with a drop of blood pressure and precordial pain which may progress into stupor, convulsions, and coma.

Even when giving safe doses of aminophylline IV, *too rapid* an injection may stimulate the vagus nerve causing bradycardia and possibly cardiac arrest. The effects of aminophylline on arterial oxygen have not been clearly established, so it would be advisable to administer oxygen along with the drug, and *extreme* caution should be taken when administering aminophylline in cases of severe hypoxia.

Again, before giving *any* aminophylline, attempt to find out if the patient has taken it earlier by another prescribed route, and if so, how much.

REVIEW

1. State the clinical definition of respiratory failure.
2. Identify the two causative factors of respiratory failure.
3. Give three significant factors in the determination of alveolar ventilation reflected by the Pa_{CO_2} level.
4. Describe the appearance of a child brought to the ED with a foreign-body obstruction of the upper airway.
5. Describe the appearance of a child with a probable lower airway obstruction and the clinical findings.
6. Explain the rationale employed with the Heimlich maneuver.
7. Describe the protocol to be followed generally with chronic obstructive airway problems.
8. Identify the cardinal signs of severe hypercapnia (CO_2 narcosis).
9. Explain the significance of an A–a gradient substantially higher than normal and the absence of a high A–a gradient in the presence of hypercapnia.
10. Describe the emergency management protocol of the asthmatic patient.
11. Define status asthmaticus.
12. Describe the emergency management protocol of pulmonary edema.
13. Describe the pathophysiology and emergency management protocol of pulmonary embolus.
14. Explain the difference in pathophysiology of fresh and salt water near-drownings and outline the steps in emergency management.
15. Explain the mode and rate of administration of aminophylline in the ED, and identify some of the symptoms of aminophylline toxicity.
16. Identify some of the sympathomimetic drugs employed in treating respiratory problems, and describe some of the undesirable side effects frequently seen.
17. Describe the immediate management of the patient with carbon monoxide poisoning.

BIBLIOGRAPHY

Abramson NS, Safar P: Barbiturate therapy following cardiac arrest, Controversies in Emergency Medicine. TEM Vol 3, No 2, Rockville, Maryland, July 1981

American College of Surgeons: Advanced Trauma Life Support (ATLS) Course Manual. ACS, Chicago, Illinois, 1981

Bennett RM: Drowning and and near drowning; Etiology and pathophysiology. AM J Nurs 76, pp 209-221, 1976

Bishop CM: Pulmonary emboli management. JEN, Vol 4, No 3, pp 35-39, May-June 1978

Budassi SA, Barber JM: Emergency Nursing: Principles and Practice. C.V. Mosby Co., St. Louis, Missouri, 1981

Cahill SB: The asthmatic patient: A practical perspective. JEN, Vol 6, No 5, pp 14-16, September-October 1980

Caudle J: Emergency nursing of near-drowning victims. Am J Nurs 76, pp 922-923, 1976

Cosgriff JH, Anderson DL: The Practice of Emergency Nursing. J.B. Lippincott Co., Philadelphia, Pennsylvania, 1975

Doti R: Emergency management of bronchial asthma. JEN, Vol 4, No 2, pp 11-17, March-April 1978

Emergency Nurse Drug Reference, Aminophylline. JEN, Vol 3, No 4, 1977

Guyton A: Textbook of Medical Physiology. W.B. Saunders Co., Philadelphia, Pennsylvania, 1977

Jodice J: Management of acute pulmonary edema. JEN, Vol 4, No 2, pp 19-22, March-April 1978

Petty T, Nett L: For Those Who Live and Breathe with Emphysema and Chronic Bronchitis, 2nd ed. Charles C. Thomas, Springfield, Illinois, 1972

Ravin MB, Modell JH: Introduction to Life Support. Little, Brown & Co., Boston, Massachusetts, 1973

Rivers JP: Near drowning. Nursing Mirror, Vol 139, pp 50-51, 1974

Rothstein R (ed): Respiratory Emergencies—Part I. TEM, Vol 2, No 1, Rockville, Maryland, April 1980

Rothstein R (ed): Respiratory Emergencies—Part II. TEM, Vol 2, No 2, Rockville, Maryland, July 1980

Seaman-Bates VJ: Emergency Management of Status Asthmaticus. JEN, Vol 6, No 5, pp 9-12, September-October 1980

Shrake K: The ABC's of ABG's—or how to interpret a blood gas value. Nursing 79, Vol 9, No 9, pp 26-33, September 1979

Stewart RD: Drowning and Near Drowning. Environmental Medical Emergencies. TEM, Vol 2, No 3, Rockville, Maryland, October 1980

Stringer JW: Emergency Treatment of Acute Respiratory Diseases, 3rd ed. Robert J. Brady Co., Bowie, Maryland, 1982

Wade J: Respiratory Nursing Care, 3rd ed. C.V. Mosby Co., St. Louis, Missouri, 1982

Young S: Preventing the adult respiratory distress syndrome. JEN, Vol 5, No 1, pp 17-22, January-February 1979

ELECTROCARDIOGRAMS AND ARRHYTHMIAS *11*

KEY CONCEPTS

The aim of this chapter is to provide an understanding of the electrical conduction system of the heart, the factors controlling it, the recording and interpreting of the heart's electrical activity, and the recognition and management of lethal arrhythmias. The concept presented here, of assigning top priority attention to the clinical status of the patient vis a vis the ECG tracings and the critical importance of early control of arrhythmias, has been prepared by Marilyn Marcy, RN, BSN, Portland, Oregon, an emergency nurse who teaches extensively in the cardiac care field. Much of the material has been excerpted from *Emergency Cardiac Care* by Robert J. Huszar, MD, with permission of The Robert J. Brady Co., Publisher, and from the "Standards for Cardiopulmonary Resuscitation and Emergency Cardiac Care," *JAMA* Supplement 244:5, August 1980, with permission of the American Heart Association. It is *strongly* suggested that the reader do further study of the interpretation of dysrhythmias and the current standards.

After reading and studying this chapter, you should be able to:

- Describe the electrical conduction system of the heart.
- Describe the factors that control the heart and the relationship between the sympathetic and parasympathetic nervous systems.
- Explain the electrical principle involved in electrocardiography and describe correct electrode placement for Leads I, II, III and MCL_1.
- Discuss the electrical basis of the ECG, explaining the P-QRS-T pattern, and the relationship to depolarization and repolarization.
- Describe the normal time intervals for ECG tracings and their lengths, with the steps to be followed in examining a rhythm strip systematically.
- Identify characteristics of dysrhythmias and those which are considered lethal.
- Identify the arrhythmias which all emergency personnel should be able to recognize, and the management protocols for each of them.
- Describe recognition and management of pacemaker problems and their initial insertion when indicated.

- Describe rationale and procedure for use of defibrillator and/or synchronized cardioversion.
- Describe protocols to be followed for all patients whose cardiac problems may otherwise go unrecognized and some guidelines to avoid these problems.
- List the suggested Code Cart inventory for essential airway management equipment, circulatory management essential drugs, and useful drugs as found in the American Heart Association Standards.
- Outline the most recent criteria for termination of resuscitative efforts in cardiac arrest.

In order to more fully understand ECG's and arrhythmia's interpretation and treatment, this chapter will include a brief overview of the anatomy and electrophysiology of the cardiac conduction system.

THE CONDUCTION SYSTEM

The cardiac conduction system is comprised of thick, interwoven networks of specialized pacemaker and conductive tissues which perform the functions of spontaneous electrical impulse formation and transmission of these impulses to the myocardial muscle cells in order to induce cardiac contraction.

The cells of the myocardial conduction system are distinctive from myocardial muscle cells in that they display certain unique characteristics:

1. *Automaticity.* The cells of the myocardial conduction system (and especially those of the Nodes) are capable of spontaneously generating their own electrical impulses, without stimulation from another source. This is called *impulse formation.*

2. *Rhythmicity.* This is the ability of conduction system tissues to form impulses repeatedly, at specific intervals, in a reliable, rhythmic fashion. This rhythmic repetition of impulse formation is responsible for the creation of *inherent rates* in all parts of the conduction system.

3. *Conductivity.* This is the ability of conductive tissues to spread electrical impulses beyond themselves to other cells.

Conduction system tissues also share the property of *excitability* (ability of cells to respond to an electrical stimulus/electrical potential) with myocardial muscle cells, but are *non-contractile,* in contrast to muscle tissues.

These are the specific characteristics of conductive tissues which provide for the spontaneous initiation of an electrical impulse and its conduction through specialized channels which deliver that impulse to the myocardial muscle.

Conduction tissues are prioritized in order of their dominance in determining the capture and rate of the cardiac cycle. The specific components of the conduction system are as follows (See Fig. 11.1):

1. *Sino-Atrial Node* (SA Node) is a highly specialized bundle of pacemaker tissue which is located high in the right atrium, near the junction of the

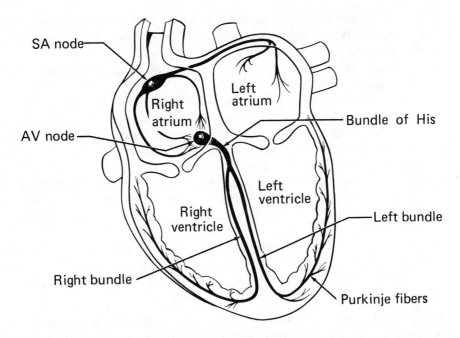

Figure 11.1. Cardiac electrical conduction system. (From Huszar RJ: Emergency Cardiac Care, 2nd ed. Robert J. Brady Co., Bowie, Maryland, 1982)

superior vena cava. This tissue is the dominant pacemaker of the heart, due to its rapid rate of impulse formation and high degree of rhythmicity, which produces an inherent rate of 60-100 impulses per minute. The SA node fires and recovers most rapidly to "capture" the cardiac rhythm.

2. *Atrial Internodal Tracts* (also called Atrial Preferential Pathways or Internodal Bundles). Although it is controversial as to the exact type of tissue which these tracts represent, research shows that the right atrium contains several bundles of specialized tissues which seem to be a part of the conduction system. It is thought that these atrial preferential pathways serve to triage sinus impulses to the atrioventricular junction in order to aid in achieving an effective heart rate and organized atrial excitation. These tracts are designated as:
   A. Anterior internodal
      • Bachman's bundle
      • Descending bundle
   B. Middle internodal
   C. Posterior internodal

3. *Atrioventricular Junction* (AV Junction). The atrioventricular junction consists of the *Atrioventricular node* (AV Node), which is located on the junction of the atria and the ventricles on the fibrous cardiac skeleton, and the *Bundle of His,* which penetrates the fibrous cardiac skeleton and gives rise to the ventricular bundle branches. The combined function of the AV Junction is to slow sinus impulses to the ventricles so that the maximal atrial emptying ("atrial kick") and ventricular filling can occur, enhancing the cardiac output to meet metabolic demands. The inherent

rate of these "junctional" tissues is 40-60/min, and there is a high degree of rhythmicity in these tissues, so that when cardiac capture is achieved the resulting junctional rhythm is *very* regular.

4. *Ventricular Bundle Branches.* The bundle branches arise from the *Bundle of His* and branch to both ventricles to spread the sinus impulses to the ventricular myocardium. The *Left Bundle Branch* is the larger of the two main bundle branches; it divides into the *anterior left bundle branch,* which stimulates the majority of the left ventricle and a portion of the ventricular septum, and the *posterior left bundle branch,* which conducts impulses to the posterior portion of the left ventricle. The *Right Bundle Branch* is somewhat smaller and is responsible for the stimulation of the right ventricle and the upper one-third of the ventricular septum. The bundle branches are very rhythmic and are capable of an inherent rate of 20-40/min.

5. *Purkinje System.* The Purkinje system is a fine network of conductive fibers which surround the ventricular myocardium and spread the impulse to the myocardial muscle cells. This system has an inherent rate of approximately 20/min.

The formation of a sinus impulse and its spread through the conductive tissues to the myocardial muscle cells is known as one *cardiac cycle.* It is helpful to remember that *the farther from the SA node that an impulse arises, the slower its inherent rate.* The Purkinje system, for example, has a much slower inherent rate than the AV Junction; this assists one in determining the origin of an arrhythmia and evaluating its clinical significance.

Myocardial contraction is both an electrical and a mechanical phenomena. This chapter deals specifically with the electrical functioning of the heart. Refer to Chapter 12 for discussion of the heart's mechanical activity.

CELLULAR PHYSIOLOGY OF THE MYOCARDIUM

Depolarization and repolarization, the electrical activity of the heart, can best be understood by examining a single myocardial cell.

The myocardial cell may be defined as a series of contractile protein filaments surrounded by a semipermeable cell membrane which allows for the flow of sodium, potassium, calcium, and chloride ions. This ion flow produces electrical activity and precipitates a series of chemical reactions which causes a shortening of the myocardial cell (myofibril). Myocardial contraction results (Fig. 11.2).

DEPOLARIZATION

The surface of each myofibril in the resting state has a positive charge on the outside, due to the higher sodium concentration, while the inside of the cell has a relative negative charge. This is called *resting potential.* When an electrical stimulus is applied to one end of the cell (from the conduction system), there is a disruption of the electrical balance of the myofibril. Cell membrane permeability is increased, allowing sodium ions to rush *into* the interior of the

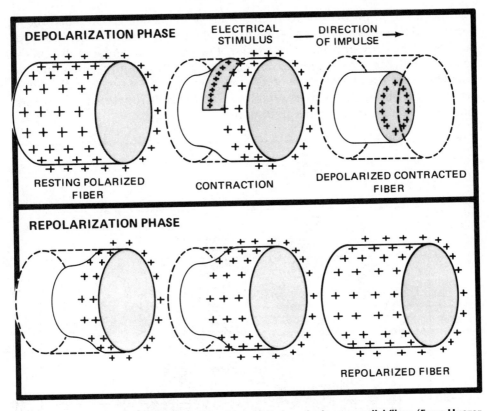

Figure 11.2. Depolarization and repolarization activity in a single myocardial fiber. (From Huszar RJ: Emergency Cardiac Care, 2nd ed. Robert J. Brady Co., Bowie, Maryland, 1982)

cell, and as a result, the electrical charges are reversed across the cell membrane to become + on the inside and − on the outside. Once this occurs, the wave of + charges sweeps through the interior of the cell; this is *depolarization*.

When the depolarization wave has passed through the interior of the myofibril, a chemical reaction is triggered which causes the formation of calcium bonds between the protein filaments inside the cell. These calcium bonds pull the protein filaments closer together and myofibril contraction results. The *concerted* contraction of the myofibrils results in the coordinated myocardial contraction.

REPOLARIZATION

Following myofibril contraction, a physiological pump mechanism called the *sodium pump, actively* pumps sodium out of the cell, restoring the electrical charges across the cell membrane to the resting potential state. In effect, the cell interior recovers its relative negative charge again in a wave-like manner as the sodium ions are actively pumped to the cell exterior. This wave of recovery to the resting potential state is called *repolarization*.

Repolarization occurs in two stages: that of the absolute refractory phase, (about the first one-half of the repolarization process), when the myofibril has only partially recovered and is incapable of responding to any stimuli; and the *relative refractory phase* (vulnerable phase period), when the myofibril has recovered more and is capable of responding to some stimuli. Ectopic stimuli which occur during the relative refractory phase may disrupt the repolarization process and capture the cardiac rhythm.

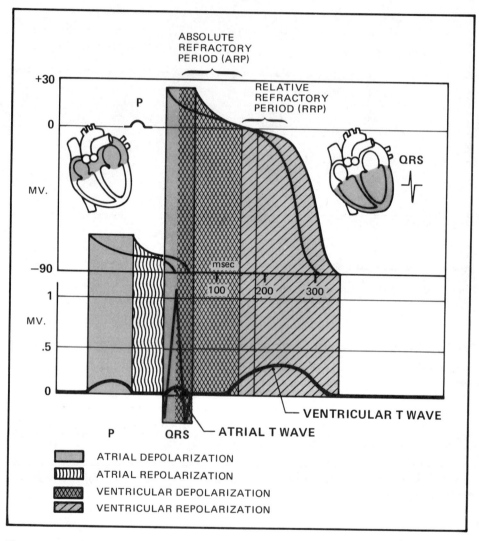

Figure 11.3. Relationship of depolarization and repolarization of the heart to the ECG. (From Huszar RJ: Emergency Cardiac Care, 2nd ed. Robert J. Brady Co., Bowie, Maryland, 1982)

The processes of depolarization and repolarization (Fig. 11.3) are influenced by catecholamines, serum electrolyte levels, drug therapy, hypoxia and acidemia, as well as central nervous system autonomic controls. These factors influence cell membrane permeability or ion flow, which in turn affects the electrical activity of the myocardium.

Although the heart is automatic and originates its own contractions, the frequency and strength with which it beats *are* partly under the control of the central nervous system. If this control is abolished by cutting the nerves to the heart, its rate will be more than 100 per minute and will be relatively constant. The nerves exercising this control are *motor* to the heart. Sensory nerves that carry messages from the heart to the central nervous system (CNS) are also present. Sensations arising in the heart may reach consciousness, as does pain; or they may belong to that class of sensory impulses of which we are unconscious, some of which aid in the regulation of heart rate and blood pressure.

AUTONOMIC NERVOUS SYSTEM

The CNS controls voluntary muscle activities, such as walking and talking, while the *autonomic* nervous system, which is composed of several control centers in addition to its own network of nerves, regulates *involuntary* body activities such as digestion, respiration, and cardiac function. The autonomic system is further divided into the *sympathetic* (adrenergic) and parasympathetic (cholinergic or vagal) components, each producing opposite effects when they are stimulated (Table 11.1). These two systems work together to bring about changes in cardiac output by regulating blood pressure, heart rate, and respiration.

Table 11.1 Autonomic Nervous System

SYMPATHETIC NERVES (CARDIO-ACCELERATOR)	PARASYMPATHETIC NERVES (CARDIO-INHIBITOR)
Increase: Heart rate AV conduction rate Strength of contractions	Decrease: Heart rate AV conduction rate Force of contractions

Nervous control of the heart emanates from a section of the brain called the *medulla,* where the two separate nerve centers are located. One is the *cardio-inhibitor,* which is part of the parasympathetic nervous system; the other is the *cardio-accelerator* center, which is part of the sympathetic nervous system (Fig. 11.4).*

Stimulation of the sympathetic (adrenergic) system will cause an *increase* in the firing rate of the SA node, will enhance the electrical conductivity through the AV node, and will strengthen atrial and ventricular contractions. Thus stimulation of this network produces a more rapid heart rate, increased cardiac output and an elevation of blood pressure.**

---

*Reprinted from Huszar, R: Emergency Cardiac Care, copyright © 1974, the Robert J. Brady Co., p. 20. With permission.
**Ibid, p. 21.

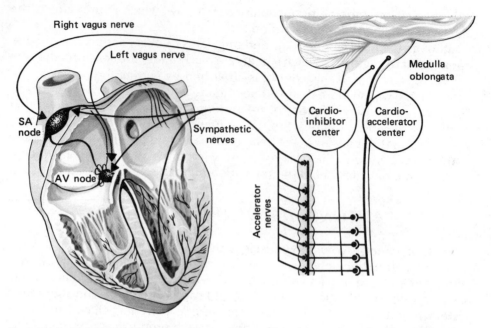

Figure 11.4. Sympathetic and parasympathetic innervation of the heart. (From Huszar RJ: Emergency Cardiac Care, 2nd ed. Robert J. Brady Co., Bowie, Maryland, 1982)

Stimulation of the parasympathetic (cholinergic or vagal) system will cause just the opposite effects. It will result in a *slower* heart rate, decreased cardiac output, and a drop in blood pressure. Nausea, vomiting, bronchial spasm, sweating, faintness, and hypersalivation are effects of excessive parasympathetic activity.

Again, the SA node is normally the dominant pacemaker of the heart, although any component of the conduction system can act as a secondary pacemaker, should the SA node fail to function. There is a direct relationship between the secondary pacemaker's location in the conduction system and the firing rate. As the secondary pacemaker becomes further removed from the SA node, the heart rate becomes slower. The SA node normally fires 60-100 times a minute, the AV junction in the region of the AV node fires 45-55 times a minute and the ventricular Purkinje system fires 30-40 times a minute. Spontaneous firing of either the dominant or secondary pacemaker does not depend entirely on stimulation from the autonomic nervous system, but will occur even if all nerve connections are severed or if the electrical conduction system is blocked. The heart will continue to beat *automatically;* only the rate will be affected. This distinctive characteristic is known as *automaticity.*

As the blood requirements of the body change, impulses are relayed from multiple regions of the body to the cardio-inhibitor and cardio-accelerator centers in the medulla. The impulses are then transmitted through the sympathetic and parasympathetic nerves, which terminate in the electrical conduction system and in the atrial and ventricular myocardium. A nerve center is located at the point of branching of the common carotid artery, and at this point there is a slightly dilated section called a *carotid sinus,* which contains sensory nerve endings important in the regulation of blood pressure and heart rate. Another important cardio-inhibitor (parasympathetic) center affecting the electrical conduction system is located in the lower posterior wall of the *interatrial septum* of the heart.

MONITORING ELECTRICAL ACTIVITY OF THE HEART

The rhythmic ebb and flow of electrical activity in the myocardium can be sensed via skin electrodes (galvanometers) which are placed on the surface of the body. The electrodes pick up the impulses and conduct them through the patient cable to the monitor, where transducers translate the electrical impulses into waveforms and amplify them to be displayed as the configurations that we see on the oscilloscope.

The monitor measures impulses in amplitude (height) and duration or interval (time). Thus, the myocardium's electrical activity is translated into waves, complexes, and intervals which coincide with each cardiac cycle and may be seen and measured against a normal standard. It must be remembered that the use of cardiac monitoring equipment gives information regarding only the *electrical* functioning of the heart, without assessment of the mechanical/pumping activity of the myocardium. Refer to Chapter 12 for discussion of cardiac pump disturbances.

Although cardiac monitors come in many different styles and models, all operate on the same principles of sensing the impulse within the myocardium and translating and amplifying that impulse for display and comparison. The EDN must be familiar with points of operation of monitoring equipment which is in use in individual departments.

GUIDELINES FOR THE USE OF MONITORING EQUIPMENT

All patients with a potential for cardiac rhythm disturbances must be monitored for arrhythmia detection. Shock, hemmorhage, myocardial infarction, neurological trauma, septicemia, or any other process which results in hypoxemia or disturbances in arterial blood gas values/acid-base balance, or alteration in serum electrolyte levels predisposes to the development of dysrhythmias, and necessitates cardiac monitoring.

Lead Placement for Cardiac Monitoring

The initial step in treating any patient complaining of sudden chest pain is to place him on a cardiac monitor via electrodes and observe for any cardiac arrhythmias; when placing electrodes of *any* variety on the body surface for monitoring, it is essential that the best possible contact be made between the skin surface and the electrode, regardless of the type being used. The skin must be cleansed thoroughly of dirt, oil, and hair. A slight abrasive rubbing with an alcohol pledget is beneficial; then the electrode with conductive jelly or paste is applied to the skin.

Standard Limb Leads

Basic electrode placement for the standard limb leads (lead I, II, III) is done according to Einthoven's trangle (Fig. 11.5), placing the right arm lead (RA-white) just below the clavicle at the right midclavicular line, the left arm lead (LA-black) just below the clavicle at the left midclavicular line, the left leg lead (LL-red) just below the costal margin in the left midclavicular line, and the right leg lead (RL-green) opposite, below the costal margin in the right midclavicular line for *ground*. The RL lead will *always* be ground when using the standard limb leads.

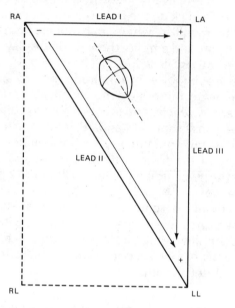

Figure 11.5. Einthoven's triangle. The sum of electrical impulses of lead I and lead III is equal to lead II.

For monitoring purposes in the ED, lead II is preferred by many because it conforms more closely to the long axis of the heart (sinus node to ventricular apex), giving a clear picture of myocardial activity in all phases. In addition, the majority of pre-hospital care personnel monitor in lead II, lending uniformity to monitoring the patient in the field and in the ED. Finally, although lead II may not be ideal for more sophisticated or extended cardiac monitoring, an advantage to its use in the ED is that the central chest and left lateral rib cage remain relativly free of wires and electrodes, in the event that defibrillation or other chest procedures becomes urgently necessary.

Modified Chest Leads

Alternative monitoring leads are increasing in popularity in many units. The most preferred of the anterior chest leads is Modified Chest Lead 1 (MCL_1), where the heart is monitored across the chest from the left shoulder to an electrode which is placed in the fourth intercostal space, along the right sternal border. This "view" of the heart's electrical activity provides a more detailed and adequate assessment of the conduction system within the ventricles. Such information is vital when there is a disturbance of impulse conduction through the ventricles (i.e. Bundle Branch Block), when it is necessary to pinpoint the conduction disturbance and evaluate its significance.

When a lead is chosen for cardiac monitoring purposes, that "channel" must be selected on the oscilloscope so that the monitor is sensing through the appropriate electrodes. This is accomplished by turning the lead selection knob to the appropriate setting. MCL_1 is sensed when the lead selector is set on the "V" channel; in pre-hospital and ED situations utilizing monitors and patient cables without chest lead capability, an interim MCL_1 is most easily obtained by selecting lead III and placing electrodes in standard chest lead configuration, *except* that the positive LL electrode is placed across the chest at the fourth intercostal space, right sternal border. This "exploring" LL electrode can easily be moved back to the left anterior axillary costal margin for lead II placement, again with reselection of the appropriate channel (Fig. 11.6).

THE TWELVE-LEAD SYSTEM

The 12-lead electrocardiogram (ECG) is a multi-dimensional picture of the electrical activity within the heart. The ECG utilizes the standard limb leads (I, II, & III), which are *bipolar,* meaning that the impulse is sensed between the two poles (electrodes), and the *augmented limb leads,* so called because these leads are designed to increase the amplitude of the standard limb leads by 50%. Because they record activity from the *right* and *left* shoulders and *left* leg, they are identified as AVR (augmented vector *right*), AVL (augmented vector *left*), and AVF (augmented vector *foot*). Studying all six leads will provide more information than the three standard leads alone.

The remaining six leads of the 12-lead system are the *unipolar* precordial leads, or chest leads. They are designated by the letter V and a number that represents the position of the electrodes on the chest wall, or precordium. These positions are:

- V_1 Fourth intercostal space, right sternal border (utilized in MCL_1)
- V_2 Fourth intercostal space, left sternal border
- V_3 Midway between V_2 and V_4 on a "line" joining these two locations
- V_4 Fifth interspace in midclavicular line
- V_5 Fifth interspace in anterior axillary line
- V_6 Fifth interspace in midaxillary line

The placement of the precordial leads in relation to the ventricles gives a good picture of the electrical activity within the ventricles themselves. Leads V_1 and V_2 represent the right ventricle (and also the right atrium), while leads V_3 through V_6 represent the larger left ventricle. Therefore, these six leads will increase the amplitude of the R wave and decrease the amplitude of the S wave. If you keep in mind that each lead gives a picture of a different

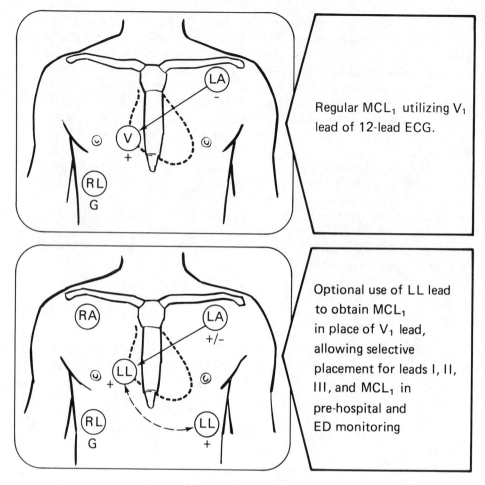

Regular MCL$_1$ utilizing V$_1$ lead of 12-lead ECG.

Optional use of LL lead to obtain MCL$_1$ in place of V$_1$ lead, allowing selective placement for leads I, II, III, and MCL$_1$ in pre-hospital and ED monitoring

Figure 11.6. Modified chest lead I (MCL$_1$).

anatomic part of the heart, it will be easier to pinpoint areas of damage or problems in interpreting ECGs.

A 12-lead ECG is required in order to diagnose specific areas of the myocardium which are injured or ischemic. A rhythm strip, on the other hand, is a single-dimensional view of the cardiac cycle in order to determine rate and rhythm and to compare the waves, complexes, and intervals against the norm.

THE P-QRS-T PATTERN

The ebb and flow of depolarization and repolarization within the myocardium is sensed by the cardiac monitor and translated into waveforms, complexes and intervals which correspond to the cardiac cycle (See Fig. 11.7).

The *excitation impulse* begins in the SA node (the normal pacemaker site), initiates depolarization of the atria, and rapidly proceeds through three atrial conduction pathways to the only entrance to the ventricles—the atrioventricular (AV) node located in the atrioventricular junction. The impulse travels slowly during its passage through the AV node before it enters the bundle of His. From this point, the transmission of the impulse proceeds more rapidly through the right and left bundle branches to the endocardial and intramyocardial Purkinje fibers. Depolarization of the ventricles begins in the endocardium while the excitation impulse is still passing through the Purkinje fibers.

When a sinus impulse initiates the depolarization of the atria, the resultant waveform which this electrical activity produces on the monitor is designated as the *P wave*. The *PR interval* represents that period of time from the beginning of the sinus impulse until the depolarization of the ventricles. Thus, the SA node has fired, the impulse has spread through the atria and been slowed slightly through the AV junction during the PR interval.

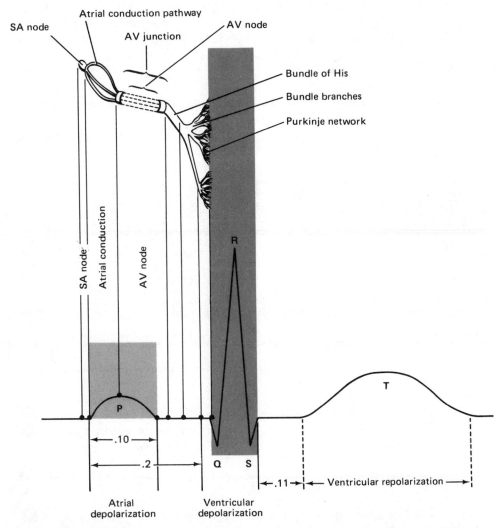

Figure 11.7. The P-QRS-T. (From Huszar RJ: Emergency Cardiac Care, 2nd ed. Robert J. Brady Co., Bowie, Maryland, 1982)

The following rapid depolarization of the ventricles produces the QRS complex. The *ST segment* is isoelectric (neutral) normally, and represents the brief delay between ventricular depolarization and recovery. Repolarization of the ventricles appears as the *T wave* on the ECG. The *QT interval* is the period between the onset of the QRS complex and the end of the T wave. It represents the full cycle of depolarization and repolarization.

Thus, the normal P-QRS-T complex in the ECG directly represents the following sequence of electrical events occurring in the heart during one complete cycle: P, depolarization of the atria; QRS, depolarization of the ventricles; and T, repolarization of the ventricles.

The R-to-R interval is the period of time between one QRS complex (measured at the peak of the R wave) and the next (See Fig. 11.7).

All complexes and waveforms in lead II are normally positive (upright) deflections. This is because the impulse, when "viewed" in lead II, is traveling toward the positive (LL) electrode. When the impulse is moving away from the positive/exploring electrode, it is displayed as negative or inverted. When we look at the cardiac cycle as viewed from MCL$_1$, the P wave is upright, because the depolarization wave is traveling toward the exploring electrode in the right 4th intercostal space; The QRS is inverted in MCL$_1$ because as the depolarization wave continues along the long axis of the heart, it travels away from the electrode and is thus seen as negative.

The normal, rhythmic cardiac cycle is reflected on the monitor as normal sinus rhythm (NSR), which becomes the standard against which all rhythm strips are compared (See Fig. 11.8).

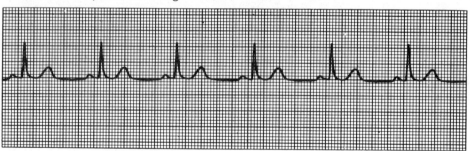

Figure 11.8. Normal Sinus Rhythm (NSR) strip. (From Huszar RJ: Emergency Cardiac Care, 2nd ed. Robert J. Brady Co., Bowie, Maryland, 1982)

Ectopic Focus

When the excitation impulse arises in a site other than in the SA node, the abnormal or secondary pacemaker site is known as an *ectopic focus*. An ectopic focus can be present in the atria, AV junction, or ventricles.

ELECTROCARDIOGRAPHIC PAPER

Electrocardiographic tracings are recorded on rolls of specially marked graph paper, which is divided into small 1 × 1 mm squares by light lines and into larger 5 × 5 mm squares by heavier lines. Thus, a grid is formed. Every small square (1 mm) represents 0.04 sec in time, every large square (5 mm) represents 0.2 sec, and five large squares (25 mm) represent 1 sec. These units of measure are applicable only to electrocardiograms recorded at a speed of 25 mm/sec.

The grid is used to measure the amplitude and duration of the waves, complexes, and intervals of the ECG complex. The amplitude is measured vertically in millimeters, and the duration of the waves, complexes, and intervals are measured horizontally in seconds. An interval is determined by counting the number of small squares between two points and multiplying that number by 0.04.*

THE ECG TRACING

The configuration of ECG complexes in lead II is as follows:

P wave

Normal—upright, smooth, rounded

Abnormal

1. Peaked, biphasic, notched—indicative of atrial hypertrophy; delayed conduction through atria
2. None definable—erratic or undulating baseline—indicative of atrial fibrillation
3. Sawtooth pattern—indicative of atrial flutter
4. Absence of P wave—absence of atrial activity; may be indicative of atrial fibrillation
5. Inverted—retrograde conduction from AV node

QRS Complex

Normal—upright, narrow (0.04-0.10 sec), shallow Q wave, if present

Abnormal

1. Deep, widened Q wave—indicative of myocardial death
2. Notched or primed R wave—indicative of bundle branch block (BBB)
3. Broadened QRS (usually greater than 0.12 sec)—interventricular conduction defect
4. Shallow R wave—indicative of lead placement away from long axis of heart; obesity
5. Electrical alternans—SICK HEART—inability of the heart to depolarize efficiently

---

*Reprinted from Huszar R: Emergency Cardiac Care, p. 106. With permission from the Robert J. Brady Co.

S-T Segment

Normal—isoelectric (flat—no deflection)

Abnormal

1. Elevated—indicative of myocardial injury
2. Depressed—indicative of myocardial ischemia; digitalis effect (spooning of segment)

T Wave

Normal—upright, smooth, rounded (larger than P wave)

Abnormal

1. Inverted—indicative of myocardial ischemia
2. Flattened or inverted—hypokalemic
3. Tall, peaked—hyperkalemic
4. Notched—may be indicative of pericarditis

U Wave

Rarely seen, but when present usually follows configuration of T wave.

ELECTROGRAPHIC INTERVALS

R-R Interval (refers to ventricular response only)

Normal—regular, recurring 60-100 times per minute

Abnormal

1. Irregular—indicative of a whole gamut of arrhythmias
2. Recurring over 100/min—tachycardia
3. Recurring less than 60/min—bradycardia

P-P Interval (refers to atrial response only)

Normal, as in RR

Abnormal, as in RR

P-R Interval

Normal—0.12-0.20 sec. isoelectric

Abnormal

1. Prolonged—indicative of delayed conduction through the AV node, if P wave large and wide and the isoelectric portion of the P-R is short, delay may be due to delayed conduction through the atria rather than through the AV node (measure of P wave to R segment)

2. Shortened—indicates aberrant conduction pathway as in nodal (P usually inverted) or WPW syndrome

QRS Interval

Normal—0 04-0.10 sec

Abnormal: Prolonged—indicative of aberrant conduction through the ventricles as in BBB

Q-T Interval

Normal—0.35-0.40 sec

Abnormal

1. Prolonged—in myocardial disease especially severe, *i.e.*, CHF; with use of certain drugs (quinidine and procainamide); hypocalcemia; indicative of weak heart
2. Shortened—digitalis; hyperkalemia; indicative of increased speed of depolarization and repolarization (See Fig. 11.7 on page 171.)

FORMAT FOR RHYTHM INTERPRETATION

It is important to develop the habit of examining the rhythm strip in a uniform and systematic way. In emergency care, it is also very important to determine *quickly* whether the rhythm is life-sustaining or lethal in terms of rate and point of origin:

1. *Identify the QRS complexes and ascertain the ventricular rate.* Heart rate is calculated from the ECG strip utilizing the number of QRS complexes that are recorded in one minute. Two relatively simple ways to do this are 1) run a 6-sec strip, count the number of R waves and multiply by 10, or 2) count the number of 0.2-sec boxes between R waves and determine: 2 boxes = 150/min; 3 boxes = 100/min; 4 boxes = 75/min; 5 boxes = 60/min; 6 boxes = 50/min.
   Is it fast?
   Is it slow?
   Is it normal?
2. *Is the rhythm regular?*
   R to R – QRS to QRS?
3. *Is there a P wave present before every QRS?* Calculate the atrial rate and determine whether the atrial and ventricular rates differ. Are the P waves regular in rhythm?
4. *Look at the PR interval* and determine whether it is normal or abnormal in duration (0.12-0.20 sec.).
5. *Does the QRS appear normal in configuration and duration,* or is it abnormally shaped or prolonged in duration?

6. *Are ectopic/premature beats present?* If so:
   Does each have a P wave preceding the QRS?
   Is the P wave absent, buried, or retrograde?
   Is the QRS normal in configuration, or is it bizarre and wide/prolonged?
   Are the ectopic beats frequent (more than 5 per minute)?

If the QRS rhythm is irregular, is there a noticeable pattern, or is it haphazard?

If the P waves are absent, are they hidden/buried, or retrograde to the QRS complexes?

Have the P waves been replaced by the sawtooth "F" waves of atrial flutter, or by the fine, chaotic "f" waves of atrial fibrillation?

DYSRHYTHMIA OR ARRHYTHMIA

Arrhythmias are identified according to:

1. Point of origin (i.e. AV junction)
2. Rate (tachycardia, bradycardia)
3. Mechanism, where applicable (i.e. heart blocks)

Dysrhythmias/arrhythmias or abnormal rhythms are generated from several factors, including myocardial ischemia, acid-base imbalance, digitalis intoxication, mechanical interference with cardiac tissue, or, in general, a disturbance in the impulse conduction system. Arrhythmias may be classified as tachycardias, bradycardias, or *irregular rhythms.* The term *tachycardia* means that the heart rate exceeds 100/min. The term *bradycardia* identifies a heart rate which is less than 60/min. *Accelerated* is a term used to describe a heart rate which is faster than the normal inherent rate for that portion of the conduction, but is still less than 100/min (thus accelerated junctional rhythm describes an arrhythmia which arises from the AV junction and exceeds the inherent junctional rate of 40-60 but is not tachycardic).

Dysrhythmias disrupt the mechanical function of the heart because they alter the formula for cardiac output (CO = HR × SV).

Tachycardias interfere with normal cardiac output because they decrease ventricular filling time and, therefore, *stroke volume.* The arrhythmias included in this classification are as follows:

1. *Sinus tachycardia* arises from the SA node
2. *Supraventricular tachycardias* arise from some part of the conduction system which is "above" the ventricles. Paroxysmal atrial tachycardia, atrial flutter, and junctional tachycardia are included under this term. Atrial fibrillation with uncontrolled ventricular rate may also be included as a tachycardia.
3. *Ventricular tachycardia* arises from a point somewhere in the ventricles.

Bradycardias interfere with normal cardiac output because they decrease the *rate* of ventricular ejection. The arrhythmias included in this classification are as follows:

1. *Sinus bradycardia*—a slowing which occurs in the SA node
2. *Heart blocks*—a blockage, partial or complete, in the AV junction causes a decrease in the sinus impulses which conduct on to depolarize the ventricles
3. *Junctional rhythm*—arises in the AV junction; has inherent rate of 40-60/min
4. *Ventricular rhythm* (idioventricular or accelerated ventricular)—arises in ventricles; inherent rate 20-40/min.

Irregular rhythms compromise the cardiac output because they create *both* a variable heart rate and an erratic stroke volume due to irregular ventricular filling times. Irregular rhythms include:

1. *Atrial fibrillation* arises somewhere in the atria and causes a disorganized "quivering" of the atria, rather than the concerted contraction of the atrial kick.
2. *Ectopic premature beats* may arise from anywhere within the conduction system. These "early" beats give rise to an impulse which comes before the sinus impulse is due and capture the cardiac cycle. May be rare or frequent in appearance.
3. *Ventricle fibrillation* is only disorganized, chaotic activity in the ventricles, with cessation of cardiac output.

RECOGNITION OF ARRHYTHMIAS

Basically, all rhythm strips are compared with the standard normal "picture" of the conduction functioning in normal sinus rhythm (NSR). Deviations from NSR are checked by this comparison and are identified, as previously mentioned, according to site of origin, rate, and/or mechanism of action.

MANAGEMENT OF ARRHYTHMIAS

There are many dysrhythmias but we will not consider all of them in this text; this portion is directed at lethal or potentially lethal arrhythmias (refer to cardiology text for detailed arrhythmia descriptions and treatments). Emergency department personnel must be proficient in recognizing and treating the following *lethal* and *serious* arrhythmias:

1. Cardiac standstill (ventricular asystole)
2. Idioventricular rhythm
3. Ventricular fibrillation
4. Ventricular tachycardia
5. Premature ventricular contractions (PVCs)

6. Bradycardias
7. Atrioventricular blocks of all degrees
8. Supraventricular tachycardias
9. Malfunctioning pacemakers
10. Electromechanical dissociation

Arrhythmia management is largely based upon the hemodynamic effect and clinical picture which result from the rhythm disturbance. It is, therefore, mandatory that the patient be *rapidly* clinically assessed to determine the affect of the dysrhythmia:

1. Is he conscious?
2. Has he become confused, disoriented since the onset of the dysrhythmia?
3. Is the blood pressure normal, or hypotensive?
4. Is the skin warm/dry or cool/clammy since the onset of the dysrhythmia?

Any or all of these signs indicate that the rhythm disturbance has compromised cardiac output sufficiently to demand *immediate* treatment. Remember: *treat the patient, not the monitor!*
Some intervention protocols are as follows:

CARDIAC STANDSTILL/ VENTRICULAR ASYSTOLE (Fig. 11.9)

This disturbance represents the total or near-total cessation of ventricular activity and the collapse of all cardiac activity/output. The patient appears clinically dead, with absent blood pressure, pulse, and respirations, and widely dilated pupils. The monitor shows a "straight line," no ventricular activity.
It is imperative that cardiopulmonary resuscitation (CPR) be started at once, in order to perfuse cerebral tissues and preserve brain function, following the

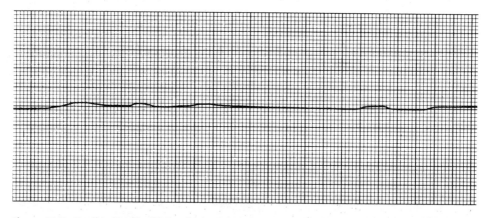

Figure 11.9. Cardiac Standstill/Ventricular Asystole. (From Huszar RJ: Emergency Cardiac Care, 2nd ed. Robert J. Brady Co., Bowie, Maryland, 1982)

guidelines in the American Heart Association Standards for CPR and ECC, JAMA 244:5, August 1980:

- Call (yell) for help.
- Place patient on flat surface (backboard, tray, removable bed headboard or floor).
- Clear airway (leaving dentures in place unless they are ill-fitting).
- Ventilate with 4 breaths.
- Compress sternum (1.5-2 inches for adult).
- One operator—rate of 80 compressions per minute; ratio of 15 compressions to 2 ventilations.
- Two operators—rate of 60 compressions per minute; ratio of 5 compressions to 1 ventilation (synchronized).
- Resuscitation efforts must be maintained between attempts at defibrillation and intubation, allowing no more than 15 sec of interruption.

Administer immediately epinephrine 0.5-1.0 mg (5-10 ml of a 1:10,000 solution) either IV push or per endotracheal tube. Follow this by pushing sodium bicarbonate 1 mg/Kg body weight IV. Continue CPR and administer epinephrine every 5 minutes as required. ABGs should determine following doses of sodium bicarbonate. If these measures are unsuccessful, calcium chloride may be administered in an attempt to enhance the electrophysiologic functioning of the myocardium. Give 5 ml of a 10% calcium chloride solution IV slow push. Repeat at 10-minute intervals as indicated. Isuprel infusion or pacemaker insertion may be attempted if all other treatments are unsuccessful.

Prognosis is poor for victims of ventricular asystole. Still, good basic life support which provides perfusion of the vital organs may give this patient a chance for survival.

IDIOVENTRICULAR RHYTHM (Fig. 11.10)

This dysrhythmia occurs when, for some reason, the "higher pacemakers" of the heart fail, and the cardiac rhythm is captured and supported by the ventricles. The rate is extremely bradycardic, between 20-40/minute; the rhythm is

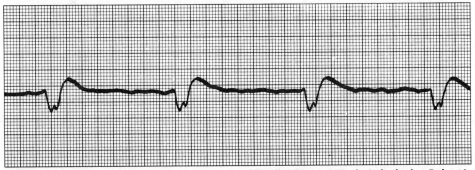

Figure 11.10. Idioventricular rhythm—dying heart. (From Walraven G: Basic Arrhythmias. Robert J. Brady Co., Bowie, Maryland, 1980)

regular. Since this rhythm arises in the ventricles, there is no P wave or PR interval, and the QRS complex is wide and bizarre in appearance. When the rate falls very low (down to below 10/min in some cases), we call this rhythm "dying heart rhythm."

Because of the extreme compromise to cardiac output, idioventricular rhythm (IVR) has a similar clinical appearance to that of cardiac standstill: cardiopulmonary arrest. Treatment is similar:

1. Start CPR.

2. Give sodium bicarbonate IV 1 mg/Kg, then titrate according to ABG results.

3. Start an IV of 1 mg isoproterenol (Isuprel) in 500 cc D5/W at 2-20 g/min and titrate to effect.

4. If IVR continues, epinephrine 0.5-1.0 mg (5-10 ml of a 1:10,000 solution) may be administered IV push or per endotracheal tube. Be prepared to defibrillate, if necessary.

VENTRICULAR FIBRILLATION

Ventricular fibrillation (V Fib) is disorganized, chaotic ventricular activity, with no cardiac output. No P waves, PR intervals, or QRS complexes are seen, only an erratic configuration of fibrillation. Clinical death occurs immediately with onset of V Fib, presenting the classic picture of cardiopulmonary arrest as previously described. Ventricular fibrillation is characterized in two different ways and treated somewhat differently:

Coarse ventricular fibrillation. (Fig. 11.11) Administer a precordial blow if the patient is monitored. Defibrillate at 200 watt seconds.

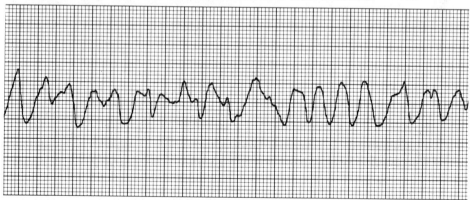

Figure 11.11. Ventricular fibrillation—coarse. (From Huszar RJ: Emergency Cardiac Care, 2nd ed. Robert J. Brady Co., Bowie, Maryland, 1982)

Fine ventricular fibrillation. (Fig. 11.12) Administer a precordial chest thump, if monitored. Since this rhythm is virtual cardiac standstill, with little electrical activity apparent, it is treated as asystole. Hopefully, the fibrillation will become coarse, indicating increased electrical potential, and the patient may then be defibrillated to convert the rhythm.

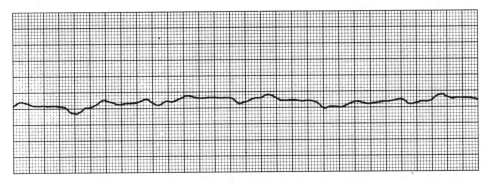

Figure 11.12. Ventricular fibrillation—fine. (From Walraven G: Basic Arrhythmias. Robert J. Brady Co., Bowie, Maryland, 1980)

Attempt to convert at 200 w/s × 2, then increase to 360 w/s. If unsuccessful, start CPR and treat as cardiac standstill until defibrillation can be attempted again, after five minutes. (See Page 189 on use of a defibrillator.)

When V Fib is *converted* to a normal rhythm, administer lidocaine, 1 mg/Kg IV bolus stat. Start a lidocaine drip of 2 Gms. lidocaine in 500 cc D5/W, and infuse at 1-4 mg/min.

Repeated V Fib which is refractory to lidocaine may be treated with procainamide HCl (pronestyl), bretylium tosylate (bretylol), or propranolol HCl (Inderol). Refer to ACLS Standards, 1980, for protocols in use of these drugs.

VENTRICULAR TACHYCARDIA (Fig. 11-13)

Ventricular tachycardia (V Tach) arises from the ventricles and, thus, presents as a wide, bizarre QRS, with T waves sloping away in the opposite direction from the main QRS (Fig. 11-13). P waves are absent or buried; therefore there is no PR interval. The rhythm is regular, and the rate is 100+.

V Tach is treated according to the clinical appearance of the patient:

1. If the patient is *unconscious* in the presence of V Tach: *cardiovert* immediately on *synchronized* countershock at 100-200 w/s. (See section

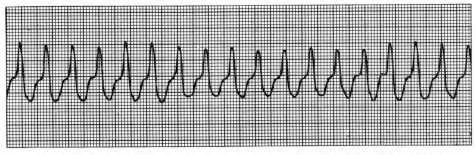

Figure 11.13. Ventricular tachycardia. (From Walraven G: Basic Arrhythmias. Robert J. Brady Co., Bowie, Maryland, 1980)

on synchronized countershock) Attempt × 2, then proceed to use 200-360 w/s as indicated. Give lidocaine *after* sinus rhythm has returned.

2. If the patient is *conscious* in the presence of V Tach: administer lidocaine 1 mg/Kg in an IV bolus, and start a lidocaine infusion at 1-4 mg per minute. Since V Tach may deteriorate at any time into ventricular fibrillation, be prepared to treat this appropriately, as described above. Procainamide, bretylium, or propranolol may be used to treat refractory V Tach.

PREMATURE VENTRICULAR CONTRACTIONS
(frequent, multifocal, coupled, R-on-T pattern) (Fig. 11.14 and 11.15)

PVCs are ectopic premature beats which arise from the ventricles and disrupt the regular cardiac cycle. QRS complexes are wide and bizarre in configuration, with T waves sloping away in the opposite direction as the main QRS. P waves are absent or buried, and there is no PR interval.

Treat PVCs with lidocaine, as discussed above in the treatment of V Tach. The same medications may be used to treat persistent PVCs if lidocaine is ineffective: procainamide, bretylium, or propranolol.

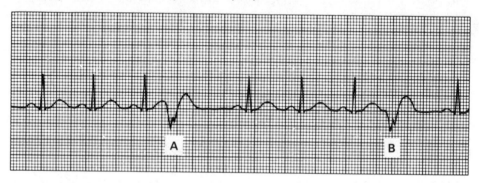

Figure 11.14. Premature Ventricular Contractions—R-on-T. (From Walraven G: Basic Arrhythmias. Robert J. Brady Co., Bowie, Maryland, 1980)

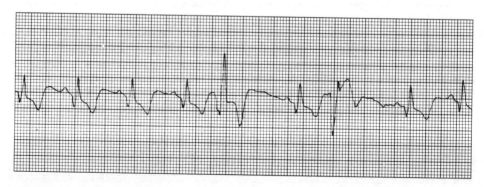

Figure 11.15. Multifocal PVCs. (From Walraven G: Basic Arrhythmias. Robert J. Brady Co., Bowie, Maryland, 1980)

BRADYCARDIAS

The bradycardias (sinus, junctional rhythm, idioventricular rhythm, or atrioventricular blocks) present varying clinical pictures, depending upon the rate and cardiac output (Fig. 11.16). The focus of treatment is to administer medication which will increase impulse formation and enhance conduction and contraction:

1. Administer atropine 0.5-1.0 mg IV bolus every 5 min to a limit of 2.0 mg.
2. If unsuccessful, start an infusion of dopamine HCl (Intropin) 400 mg in 500 cc D5/W at 1-10 μg/Kg/mkn, and titrate to effect,

OR

3. Start an infusion of isoproterenol (Isuprel) 1 mg in 500 cc D5/W at 2-20 μg/min.

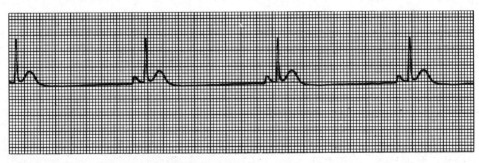

Figure 11.16. Sinus Bradycardia. (From Huszar RJ: Emergency Cardiac Care, 2nd ed. Robert J. Brady Co., Bowie, Maryland, 1982)

If unsuccesful, and the patient is unconscious, CPR may be utilized to maintain cerebral perfusion until effective drug therapy can be implemented, or until a temporary pacemaker can be placed.

ATRIOVENTRICULAR BLOCKS

The atrioventricular blocks vary greatly as to clinical picture and concern. Here we will discuss 3rd degree heart block (complete heart block) (Fig. 11.17). With this arrhythmia, the AV junction prevents any of the sinus impulses from being conducted on to the ventricles. Thus, we will see the atrial rate (regular P waves), that is completely unrelated to the ventricular rate, which is from another origin in the conduction system. There is no relationship between the Ps and the QRS complexes; the P waves are said to "march through" the strip. Therefore, we can measure no PR intervals, because they do not exist. The atrial and ventricular rhythms are each regular. The appearance of the QRS in complete heart block (CHB) is dependent upon where in the conduction system that it arises:

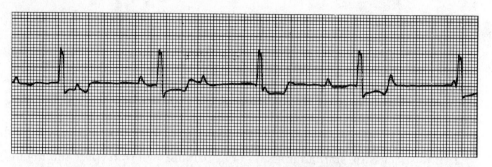

Figure 11.17. Complete Heart Block/Atrioventricular Block/3° Block. (From Huszar RJ: Emergency Cardiac Care, 2nd ed. Robert J. Brady Co., Bowie, Maryland, 1982)

1. If the AV junction has become the cardiac pacemaker, the QRS may appear normal or near-normal.
2. If the rhythm arises from the bundle branches or the Purkinje system, the resultant ventricular rhythm will have the typical wide, bizarre QRS appearance.

Treatment is based upon the clinical picture: if the patient has a reasonable junctional pacemaker at a rate of 55, he may not need urgent treatment because he has a life-sustaining ventricular rate. If, however, the patient has been hemodynamically compromised (decreased mentation, lowered BP, cool/clammy skin), immediate treatment is required. This is usually the case in the presence of CHB with an idioventricular pacemaker, and a rate of less than 40, where cardiac output has fallen so low that the patient may even have lost consciousness. Therefore, treat as follows:

1. If the patient is conscious, administer atropine 0.5-1.0 mg every 5 min until total dose of 2.0 mg has been given. If unsuccessful, start an iso-proterenol infusion of 1 mg Isuprel in 500 cc D5/W at 2-20 μg/min, and titrate to effect.
2. If the patient is unconscious, start CPR and give atropine as above. Start an Isuprel infusion as above if atropine is unsuccessful. Continue CPR until the patient responds to drug therapy, or until a temporary pacemaker can be placed. (See page 185 for information regarding emergency pacemakers). If complete cardiac asystole or V Fib occur, treat accordingly.

SUPRAVENTRICULAR TACHYCARDIAS (SVT) (Fig. 11.18)

SVTs may arise from anywhere above the ventricles and may have ventricular rates between 150 and 300 (i.e. 2:1 atrial flutter) (Fig. 11.18). Again, treatment is largely determined by the patient's clinical presentation:

1. If *unconscious*, use *synchronized* countershock at 50-200 w/s to convert to NSR. Once converted, the patient may be digitalized with Digoxin 0.5 mg slow IV and follow-up doses orally or IV to total 1.0 mg within 24

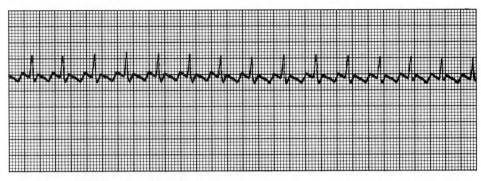

Figure 11.18. Supraventricular Tachycardia—2:1 Atrial Flutter. (From Walraven G: Basic Arrhythmias. Robert J. Brady Co., Bowie, Maryland, 1980)

hours, the digitalizing dose. Oral propranolol (Inderal) may be employed, if appropriate, for long-term therapy.

2. If the patient is *conscious* and symptomatic, several drugs may be tried, depending upon the origin of the arrhythmia:

- Digoxin 0.5 mg IV slowly or the more rapid-acting Ouabain 0.5 mg IV or Cedilanid 0.6 mg IV slowly.
- Verapamil (Calan) 5-10 mg slow IV push. This new calcium-channel blocker shows great promise in treating SVT.
- Phenylephrine HCl (Neo-synephrine) 1.0 mg diluted in 10 cc NSS and given slow IV push to a dose of 0.5-1.0 mg. This drug causes an increase in BP, with reflex slowing/conversion of the heart rate.
- Propranolol (Inderol) may be given 1.0-2.0 mg *slow* IV push. Start on oral long-term therapy when converted.

It may be necessary to digitalize a patient or to start long-term propranolol therapy after just one episode of SVT, but frequently, further treatment is not necessary unless the arrhythmias is recurrent.

MALFUNCTIONING PACEMAKERS

Occasionally, patients with permanent pacemakers will present to the ED with malfunction of the pacemaker:

1. With *loss of capture* (Fig. 11.19) the pacer will fire, and a pacer spike will be seen, without being followed by a QRS response. This is caused frequently when the pacing catheter has either dislodged from its position in the apex of the right ventricle, or when scar tissue (which is a poor conducter) has hypertrophied around the pacing tip, "smothering" the pacing impulse.

   If this occurs, turn the patient to his left side in an effort to lay the pacing catheter against the ventricular septum and achieve capture, or adjust the patient's position as indicated. Increase the voltage of the pacemaker impulse if possible. If necessary, administer atropine or Insuprel infusion as previously discussed to achieve an effective heart rate, or do CPR.

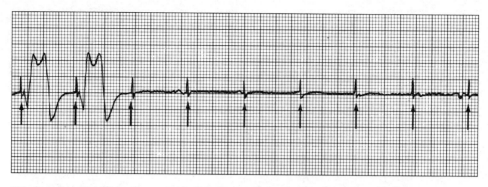

Figure 11.19. Pacemaker loss of capture. (From Phillips RE, Feeney MK: The Cardiac Rhythms. W.B. Saunders Co., Philadelphia, Pennsylvania, 1973)

2. When *loss of sensing* occurs (Fig. 11.20), it is usually for the same reasons. Try positioning the patient as above. If ineffective, use a magnet to turn the pacemaker *off!* When the pacer isn't sensing, the pacer spike falls indiscriminately throughout the cardiac rhythm and acts as an ectopic focus—it may even cause ventricular fibrillation. Support with drug therapy, if necessary, until the patient can have the pacemaker catheter surgically replaced or reimplanted.

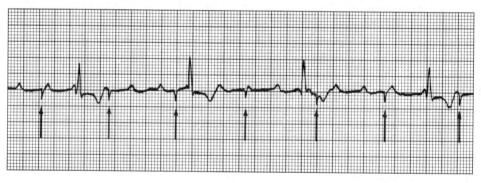

Figure 11.20. Pacemaker loss of sensing. (From Phillips RE, Feeney MK: The Cardiac Rhythms. W.B. Saunders Co., Philadelphia, Pennsylvania, 1973)

ELECTROMECHANICAL DISSOCIATION (EMD)

This phenomenon occurs when the electrical activity of the heart somehow fails to produce a myocardial contraction. A number of mechanisms may be involved, but since there is little or no cardiac output produced, the clinical picture is one of *cardiopulmonary arrest.*

1. Start CPR.
2. Administer epinephrine 0.5-1.0 mg IV push or per E/T tube. Give sodium bicarbonate 1 mg/Kg initially and then titrate to blood gas values.
3. May start isoproterenol infusion as previously discussed.

4. Calcium chloride may be administered in a 5 ml (of 10% solution) bolus in order to enhance the myofibril formation of calcium bonds and provoke contraction.

5. Continue advanced life support until the drugs have had sufficient time to become effective, or until it is determined that the code must be terminated.

PACEMAKER INSERTION

Pacemaker equipment varies according to each ED. The EDN *must* be familiar with the pacemaker equipment and know how to use it *immediately and correctly!* The patient's life may depend upon the prompt insertion and proper function of a pacer.

The EDN should open and manipulate the pacemaker equipment in order to become comfortable and familiar with it and should review at intervals the procedure for insertion. The equipment can be easily repackaged, sealed, and gas sterilized after being handled.

Basically, the procedure for transvenous pacemaker insertion is as follows:

1. The skin is prepped with Betadine.

2. The physician inserts the pacing catheter percutaneously into either subclavian vein or brachial vein and threads it into the right ventricle.

3. The exterior tip of the pacemaker catheter is attached via an adapter or alligator clips to the chest lead of the ECG machine. A continuous ECG strip is run from the chest lead.

4. The pacer is then advanced until the "injury pattern" (ST elevation) is seen on the ECG.

5. The pacing catheter is then taken from the ECG machine attachment and connected to the patient cable, with the pacer battery box (Fig. 11.21) connected at the other end.

6. The pacemaker battery is turned on at the designated voltage (milliamperes) and at the designated demand rate (which is slightly higher than the patient's own rate).

7. The pacing wire is secured to the chest, and battery settings secured.

DEFIBRILLATION

It is essential to thoroughly understand the rationale involved with defibrillation of a life-threatening arrhythmia and to have a working knowledge of the defibrillator machine used in the department, both for the defibrillation mode and the cardioversion mode of operation. (See Standards for CPR and ECC JAMA 244:5, August 1980, p 490 for additional definitive information.)

Defibrillation produces a simultaneous depolarization of all muscle fascicles of the heart, after which a spontaneous beat *may* resume if the myocardium is oxygenated and not acidotic. Direct current (dc) defibrillator shocks should be

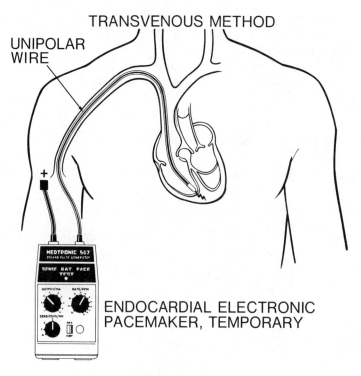

Figure 11.21. Diagram of Pacemaker; Battery Box/Controls.

delivered *as soon as possible* when the heart is known to be in ventricular fibrillation. Countershocks are also indicated on an emergency basis in the presence of ventricular tachycardia without a peripheral pulse. It has not been demonstrated that defibrillation is useful in cases of ventricular asystole, although it is sometimes used when it is impossible to be sure whether the heart is in a fine ventricular fibrillation or true ventricular standstill.

For defibrillation, the standard electrode position (lead II), always should be used; one electrode just to the right of the upper sternum below the clavicle and the other electrode paddle just to the left of the cardiac apex or left nipple. Standard electrode paste may be used but saline-soaked 4×4 gauze sponges are also excellent conductors with care taken to avoid soupy wet sponges "arcing" with the electrical discharges. These sponges may be applied rapidly, and external cardiac compression may be resumed after defibrillation without the problem of hand slippage on the chest that occurs when electrode paste is used.

A single defibrillator shock does not produce serious functional damage to the myocardium; there is no reason to withhold it in the unconscious, pulseless, adult patient when a direct current defibrillator is available, even though the patient is unmonitored. In these circumstances, unmonitored defibrillation with a single shock may be performed by medical or properly trained, authorized allied medical personnel. It must be emphasized that this single shock must not delay the prompt application of basic cardiac life support

(BCLS) measures in any way. *Unmonitored defibrillation is not recommended for children.*

In instances of apparent cardiac arrest secondary to hypoxemia (e.g., drug overdose), CPR for a period of 2 min is recommended, with reevaluation prior to the delivery of an unmonitored defibrillator shock.

The optimum amount of electrical energy has not been established, and there are no conclusive data concerning the ideal defibrillator output waveform. In emergency situations, it has been customary in the past to deliver a maximum shock of 400 w/s for cases of ventricular fibrillation. However, lower settings have been observed to be frequently effective in converting ventricular fibrillation and ventricular tachycardia and produce less myocardial damage. The damage resulting from defibrillator shocks is directly proportional to the energy used, and maximal setting, when not required, may further impair an already damaged myocardium.

The new standards direct that the initial attempt at defibrillation should be made using 200 to 300 w/s of *delivered* energy (this amount is less than the charge load indicator on most defibrillators). If a second defibrillation is necessary, it should be done immediately using, again, 200 to 300 w/s of delivered energy. A third attempt at defibrillation should not be made until BCLS has been resumed long enough to administer CPR with supplemental oxygen, epinephrine, and sodium bicarbonate if metabolic acidosis is documented by ABG determinations; the third defibrillation charge should be made at a setting not to exceed 360 w/s of delivered energy. For recurrent refractory V Fib, it is not necessary to increase the defibrillation energy on each successive shock, and, in fact, it is frequently possible to *reduce* the energy of the shock as the patient's condition improves with good BCLS and ACLS, minimizing the chances of electrical injury to the heart. (Again, see the new Standards on page 187 for complete guidelines and rationale.)

USE OF DEFIBRILLATOR

Rationale

- Stoppage of chaotic lethal rhythms
- Stoppage of automaticity of sinus node to resume control

Procedure

1. Plug in and set for *defibrillation* (synchronizer switch *off*).
2. Turn to appropriate setting for w/s *delivered* (initially 200-300).
3. Lubricate paddles with conduction paste or place saline pads on chest.
4. Apply to lead II configuration with firm presure (20-25 lb) to prevent "bridging" of the charge with skin burns.
5. Do *not* place over monitor electrodes on chest.
6. Caution others to stand back.

7. Be certain *you* are not in contact with the patient, bed, or any other equipment.

8. Fire paddles.

9. Repeat as indicated, rapidly if necessary, until effective, but *continue* CPR *between firings* with no longer than a 15-sec pause between breaths!

10. Transfer to CCU as soon as effective heart rate is restored. Be sure to have someone *notify CCU* that a code is underway and to prepare a bed for the patient, since frequently this involves moving one patient out before another can be admitted.

SYNCHRONIZED CARDIOVERSION

Rationale

- To treat any ectopic rhythm with definite R waves which causes unconsciousness or profound hypotension.
- To prevent shock from being delivered on the T wave (vulnerable phase).

Procedure

1. Prepare the patient with IV diazepam (Valium) if possible
2. Plug machine in; turn on.
3. Set for *cardioversion, synchronized*.
4. Attach synchronizing wire to monitor if necessary. (Some models are "all in one" and no additional wires are necessary.)
5. Test synchronization by button which will cause a "spike" to fire on the monitor screen with R wave of the patient's complex. If no synchronization test can be done, test by firing the paddles, faces together, using no more than 10 w/s to see if the machine delays the shock until an R wave is detected.
6. Set voltage to 50 w/s.
7. Proceed as with defibrillation; no CPR is needed, unless asystole is produced.

TERMINATION OF BASIC OR
ADVANCED LIFE SUPPORT

The American Heart Association Standards for CPR and ECC teach the following:

> The decision to terminate resuscitative efforts is a medical one (also see *Medicolegal Considerations*) and depends on an assessment by a physician of the cerebral and cardiovascular status of

the patient. Clinical criteria of the adequacy to cerebral circulation include the reactivity of the pupils, level of consciousness, and the presence of movement and spontaneous respiration. Deep unconsciousness, absence of spontaneous respiration and brainstem reflexes, and pupils that remain fixed and dilated for 15 to 30 minutes are usually ominous prognostic signs, but they are not foolproof indications of cerebral death.

To avoid curtailment of ACLS on an arbitrary basis, the end point of cardiovascular unresponsiveness is suggested as the most reliable and certain basis for this decision, both medically and legally, and is discussed in more detail in the medicolegal section.

In children, or in unusual circumstances, e.g., when the arrest is associated with hypothermia, *resuscitative efforts should be continued for longer periods,* since recovery has been seen even after prolonged unconsciousness.

AVOIDING PROBLEMS

As soon as a patient presents complaining of chest pain, shortness of breath, fainting spells, or any other signs of poor cardiac output, *assume the worst* and move quickly to initiate the necessary steps for intervention and management. Take the patient immediately to a bed in the area equipped to handle "codes," and after removing at least the top half of clothing to expose the chest and precordial area, proceed as follows:

1. Administer oxygen at a rate of at least 6 LPM (38-40% oxygen delivery) via nasal prongs *until further evaluation.*
2. Apply cardiac monitor leads in lead II configuration.
3. Get an IV line in fast (antecubital vein is easiest and fastest in emergencies although it is bothersome later). If it is the ED's responsibility to draw blood for the lab, a 20 cc syringe of blood should be drawn at this time and injected into the appropriate Vacu-tubes. Run D5/W TKO (to keep open) with a pediatric microdrip set.
4. Fowler's or semi-Fowler's position, as the patient's comfort dictates.
5. Call for ECG stat and possibly a portable chest X-ray.
6. Monitor VS and heart rhythm *closely.*
7. Assess any changes in LOC, peripheral perfusion, and skin temperature frequently.
8. Have emergency equipment (intubation tray, suction apparatus) and drugs at hand and ready to use.
9. If the patient is to be admitted, transfer as soon as possible to the coronary care unit (CCU).
10. When transporting a patient to CCU, always accompany the transport

with the patient monitored, portable oxygen running, and a bolus of lidocaine and bag/mask unit with oropharyngeal airway on the stretcher.

If the patient arrives in serious condition, the physician will probably also want arterial blood gases (ABGs) drawn; any administration of O_2 *must* be noted on the lab slip with the liter flow, method of administration, and patient's temperature, if possible.

GUIDELINES FOR MINIMUM LIFE SUPPORT EQUIPMENT AND DRUGS: CODE CART INVENTORY*

RESPIRATORY MANAGEMENT

Oxygen supply with reserve of two cylinders (or wall oxygen)
Oropharyngeal airways/nasopharyngeal airways
Pocket masks (Optional)
Laryngoscope with blades (curved and straight, for adult, child, and infant) and extra batteries and bulbs
Assorted adult-size (cuffed) and child-size (uncuffed) endotracheal tubes with malleable stylet and 15mm/22 mm adapters
Syringe with clamp or plastic two-way or three-way valve for E/T tube cuffs
Acceptable bag-valve-mask unit, with provisions for 100% oxygen ventilation (see specifications in Standards on page 139)
Suction (preferably portable), with catheters (sizes 6 to 16) and Yankauer-type (rigid) suction tips
Esophageal obturator airway
Cricothyrotomy set or #10 over-the-needle catheter.

CIRCULATORY MANAGEMENT

Portable monitor/defibrillator with ECG electrode-defibrillator paddles or portable DC defibrillator and portable ECG monitor
Portable ECG machine, direct writing, with connection to monitor
Venous infusion sets (microdrip and regular)
Indwelling venous catheters:
- Catheter outside needle (sizes 14 to 22)
- Catheter inside needle (sizes 14 to 22)
- Central venous pressure (CVP) catheters and manometer
Intravenous solutions (D5/W and lactated Ringer's)

*Adapted from Standards for CPR and ECC, JAMA, Vol 244, No 5, August 1980

Cutdown set
Thoracotomy tray
Transvenous and transthoracic pacers (wires, cables, and battery pack)
Assorted syringes, needles, stopcocks, venous extension tubes
Tourniquets, adhesive, disposable razors
Sterile gloves
Anti-shock trousers (optional)

ESSENTIAL DRUGS—ALL LIFE SUPPORT UNITS MUST HAVE THESE DRUGS AVAILABLE

Sodium bicarbonate (prefilled syringes, 50 ml ampules, or 500 ml 5% bottles)
Epinephrine (Adrenalin) in prefilled syringes
Atropine sulfate in prefilled syringes
Lidocaine (Xylocaine) in prefilled syringes and in 2 Gm vials for infusions
Isoproterenol HCl (Isuprel)
Dopamine HCl (Intropin)
Morphine sulfate
Calcium chloride in prefilled syringes

USEFUL DRUGS—THESE DRUGS ARE RECOMMENDED FOR HOSPITAL AND PREHOSPITAL LIFE SUPPORT UNITS:

Aminophylline
Bretylium tosylate (Bretylol)
Dexamethasone (Decadron)
Dextrose 50% (Ion-O-trate Dextrose 50%)
Digoxin (Lanoxin)
Diphenhydramine HCl (Benadryl)
Dobutamine HCl (Dobutrex)
Diphenyhydantoin (Dilantin)
Furosemide (Lasix)
Lanatoside C (Cedilanid)
Levarterenol bitartrate/norepinephrine (Levophed)
Methylprednisolone sodium succinate (Solu-Medrol)
Naloxone HCl (Narcan)
Nitroglycerine Tabs (sublingual)
Nitroglycerine creme (Nitrolpaste)
Phenylephrine HCl (Neo-synephrine)
Potassium chloride
Procainamide HCl (Pronestyl)
Propranolol HCl (Inderal)
Succinylcholine Chloride (Anectine, Sucostrin for muscle paralysis)
Tubocurarine Chloride (muscle paralysis)
Verapamil HCl (Isoptin)
Sodium nitroprusside (Nipride), the potent, rapidly acting direct peripheral

vasodilator, is recommended to have available but because of its profound action, *hemodynamic monitoring is mandatory.*

REVIEW

1. Describe the electrical conduction system of the heart.
2. Describe the chemical factors that control the heart.
3. Explain depolarization and repolarization of the myocardium.
4. Describe the sympathetic and parasympathetic control of the heart.
5. Explain the electrical principle involved in electrocardiography.
6. Identify guidelines for use of monitoring equipment and clinical situations which necessitate cardiac monitoring.
7. Explain Einthoven's triangle and describe the electrode placement for cardiac monitoring in leads I, II, III & MCL_1.
8. Describe the purpose of and lead system for the 12-lead ECG.
9. Identify the wave forms on a normal ECG tracing.
10. Identify the electrocardiographic intervals and their lengths.
11. Explain at least one method of ascertaining the heart rate from a rhythm strip in normal sinus rhythm.
12. List the steps to be followed in examining a rhythm strip systematically.
13. Describe the important characteristics which identify dysrhythmias.
14. Describe the essential signs of decreased cardiac output which require immediate intervention and preparation for life support.
15. Identify the arrhythmias which require immediate intervention to prevent rapid death.
16. Identify the arrhythmias which all emergency personnel should be able to recognize.
17. Describe the management protocols for each of the life-threatening arrhythmias.
18. Describe the management options with a non-functioning pacemaker.
19. Describe the procedure for insertion and activation of a pacemaker.
20. Describe the procedure for use of the defibrillator.
21. Identify a potential hazard when using wet saline gauze pads for defibrillating.
22. Describe the correct positioning of defibrillator paddles on the chest wall.
23. Describe the rationale and procedure for use of synchronized cardioversion.

24. Explain the criteria for termination of resuscitative efforts in cardiac arrest.

25. Describe the protocol to be followed when receiving a patient with chest pain, shortness of breath, or any signs of poor cardiac output and identify management guidelines which will help avoid problems.

26. Describe the suggested inventory for code cart equipment.

27. Identify key items of airway management equipment and their specifications.

28. Identify the essential and useful drugs which are recommended for availability on Code Carts by the American Heart Association.

BIBLIOGRAPHY

Alspach J: Electrical axis: How to recognize deviations on the ECG and interpret them. AJN, Vol 79, No 10, pp 1971-83

American Heart Association: Standards for Cardiopulmonary Resuscitation (CPR) and Emergency Cardiac Care (ECC). JAMA Suppl, Vol 244, No 3, pp 453-509, 1980

Atcheson R: Cardiac Arrest, Comprehensive Review of Emergency Care (to be published). Aspen Systems Publications, Rockville, Maryland

Braun HA, Diettert GA, Willis VE: Coronary Care Unit Nursing: Part II, A Workbook in Clinical Aspects. Mountain Press, Missoula, Montana, 1969

Brunner LS, Suddarth DS: The Lippincott Manual of Nursing Practice, 2nd ed. J.B. Lippincott Co., Philadelphia, Pennsylvania, 1982

Corday E, Irving EW: Disturbances of Heart Rate, Rhythm and Conduction. W.B. Saunders Co., Philadelphia, Pennsylvania, 1968

Guyton A: Basic Human Physiology, 2nd ed. W.B. Saunders Co., Philadelphia, Pennsylvania, 1977

Hudak C, Gallo B, Lohr T: Critical Care Nursing, 3rd ed. J.B. Lippincott Co., Philadelphia, Pennsylvania, 1982

Huszar RJ: Emergency Cardiac Care, 2nd ed. Robert J. Brady Co., Bowie, Maryland, 1982

Introduction to Arrhythmia Recognition. California Heart Association, San Francisco, California, 1968

Meltzer LE, Pinneo R: Intensive Coronary Care, 3rd ed. Robert J. Brady Co., Bowie, Maryland, 1977

Phibbs B: The Cardiac Arrhythmias. C.V. Mosby Co., St. Louis, Missouri, 1973

Vinsant M, Spence M, Chapell D: A Commonsense Approach to Coronary Care: A Program, 3rd ed. C.V. Mosby Co., St. Louis, Missouri, 1981

Walraven G: Basic Arrhythmias. Robert J. Brady Co., Bowie, Maryland, 1980

Whipple GH, Peterson MA, et al: Acute Coronary Care. Little, Brown & Co., Boston, Massachusetts, 1972

CARDIOVASCULAR EMERGENCIES *12*

KEY CONCEPTS

This chapter presents a general review of the heart and circulatory system, followed by material discussing the etiology, pathophysiology, and emergency management of heart disease, including the progressions of coronary artery disease (CAD) and the acute myocardial infarction (AMI). Heart/pump failure is addressed with the governing factors relating to events in decompensation, left ventricular decompensation (LVD), right heart failure, and cardiogenic shock. Guidelines for treatment, drug protocols, and key points of clinical assessment are included.

Information based on lectures prepared for EDNs by Sharon Saty, R.N., CCRN and Barbara Coombs, R.N., PA, have been augmented with additional materials by Marilyn Marcy, R.N., BSN, an emergency nurse who teaches extensively in the cardiac care field. All are actively involved in acute patient care in the Portland area.

After reading and studying this chapter, you should be able to:

- Describe the major components of the cardiovascular system and trace the flow of blood through the heart.
- Describe the supportive circulatory role of the lymph vascular system.
- Describe the location and function of the coronary arteries.
- Identify the major and minor risk factors involved in Coronary Artery Disease (CAD).
- Discuss CAD, its pathophysiology and stages of development with accompanying clinical manifestations.
- Describe the general variable pictures of a myocardial infarction with the diagnostic steps employed and the immediate nursing action that should be taken.
- Discuss Starling's law of the heart and identify some of the factors that contribute to an increased cardiac output as well as the manifestations of a decreased cardiac output.
- Discuss the profound ramifications of left ventricular decompensation (LVD).
- Describe the stages of pulmonary edema and the goals of management.

197

- Discuss the classic findings in right heart failure and the current treatment modalities employed.
- Describe the clinical manifestations of cardiogenic shock, the specific areas of clinical assessment involved, the essential goals of treatment, and the standard drugs employed.

CIRCULATORY SYSTEM

To provide an opportunity to refresh memories on the anatomy and physiology of the cardiovascular system, this portion of the chapter will cover a relatively simple review of the structures and functions of the heart and the circulatory system.

CARDIOVASCULAR SYSTEM

The blood vascular system is responsible for uninterrupted delivery of oxygenated blood and its nutrients to all tissue cells, their exchange for waste products of metabolism, and transportation of wastes to points of elimination. No body system has graver responsibility than the circulatory system, for without a supply of oxygenated blood, tissues and cells quickly die.

At the center of the cardiovascular system is its "pump," the heart. This powerful muscular organ has four inner chambers or cavities which fill with blood and collect it to be pumped through the body's vascular system. The heart's chambers are divided into two basic categories, depending upon function:

1. The *right heart* consisting of the right atrium or auricle (upper chamber) and the right ventricle (lower chamber). The right heart is a lower pressure system which is primarily responsible for pumping blood to the lungs for oxygenation and metabolic waste elimination.

2. The *left heart,* consisting of the left atrium and the left ventricle. It is the left heart which carries the bulk of the circulatory load in pumping oxygenated blood through the systemic circulation under much higher pressures.

The *aorta* arises from the left ventricle of the heart and is the largest artery in the body. *Arteries* are elastic, smooth-muscled vessels through which oxygenated blood is pumped in pulsatile waves to all parts of the body. Arteries branch off the aorta and into increasingly smaller units, eventually becoming *arterioles,* which connect with *capillaries.*

Capillaries are the smallest of the vascular units and are the link between arterioles and venules, the smallest veins. Everywhere in the body, capillaries form networks of tiny vessels, called capillary beds, which deliver oxygenated blood and retrieve metabolic waste products at the cellular level. Thus, it is in the capillary bed that the true function of the cardiovascular system is evident.

Venules are small vessels which pick up deoxygenated blood and metabolic waste products from the capillary bed and transport them for elimination. Venules/veins are much less elastic than arteries and must depend upon their many valves and the muscular support and massaging action of surrounding skeletal muscles to overcome gravity in returning blood to the heart. This network of vessels carrying waste products gradually increased in size from venules in *veins,* eventually flowing back into the largest veins in the body, the inferior and superior venae cavae. The *superior vena cava* empties blood from the head, neck, and upper extremities into the right atrium of the heart, and the *inferior vena cava* drains blood from the rest of the body into the right atrium.

The heart and the arteries, capillaries, and veins form the network of circulation in the body and are often called the *cardiovascular tree* (Fig. 12.1).

ROUTE OF BLOOD FLOW THROUGH THE CARDIOVASCULAR SYSTEM*

Trace the route of blood flow by following the diagram in Figure 12.2.

Start at *1,* the right lower chamber called the *right ventricle.* Venous blood with a heavy concentration of carbon dioxide is pumped out of the right ventricle through the *pulmonary valve 2,* into the *pulmonary artery 3,* which carries it to both lungs. The pulmonary artery is the *only* artery in the body that carries non-oxygenated venous blood. In the air sacs of the lung (*alveoli*), carbon dioxide is exchanged for oxygen and the oxygenated blood flows back to the left upper heart chamber called the *atrium 4* via the *pulmonary veins 5.* The four pulmonary veins are the *only* veins in the body which normally carry oxygenated blood.

From the left atrium, blood flows through the *mitral* or *bicuspid valve 6* into the lower left chamber or *ventricle 7.* The valves of the heart open and close to prevent backflow of blood. The left ventricle contracts and forces the oxygenated blood out through the *aortic valve 8* into the *aorta 9* to start its systemic journey. Because the left ventricle must pump blood in large volume into the largest artery, the aorta, this heart chamber is normally the largest and most powerful.

At the *aortic arch 10,* where the aorta bends to turn downward, the *innominate 11, left common carotid 12,* and *left subclavian 13* arteries branch off to carry oxygenated blood to the head and upper extremities. As the downward course of the aorta continues, other large arteries branch off to carry blood to the kidneys and other organs. At a point called the *bifurcation* (see Fig. 12.1), the aorta divides into two major common iliac arteries, which supply blood to each leg. The common iliac arteries, in turn, branch off into smaller units and eventually become arterioles.

Blood reaches the capillary bed through the arterioles, and there oxygen flows through the *semipermeable capillary membrane, which is one cell thick,* into the body tissues. Carbon dioxide passes through the capillary membranes

---

*Reprinted from *The Human Body* with permission of Ethicon, Inc.

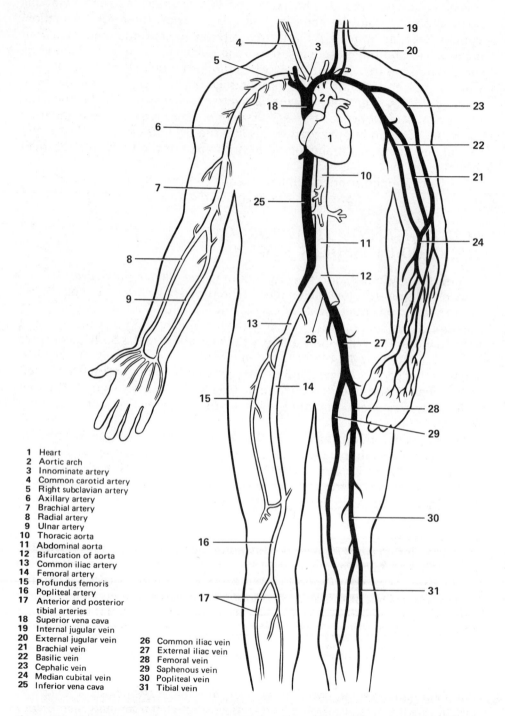

1   Heart
2   Aortic arch
3   Innominate artery
4   Common carotid artery
5   Right subclavian artery
6   Axillary artery
7   Brachial artery
8   Radial artery
9   Ulnar artery
10 Thoracic aorta
11 Abdominal aorta
12 Bifurcation of aorta
13 Common iliac artery
14 Femoral artery
15 Profundus femoris
16 Popliteal artery
17 Anterior and posterior
    tibial arteries
18 Superior vena cava
19 Internal jugular vein
20 External jugular vein
21 Brachial vein
22 Basilic vein
23 Cephalic vein
24 Median cubital vein
25 Inferior vena cava

26 Common iliac vein
27 External iliac vein
28 Femoral vein
29 Saphenous vein
30 Popliteal vein
31 Tibial vein

Figure 12.1. The blood vascular systems (cardiovascular tree). The venous system is illustrated by dark vessels. However, both arteries and veins are present all over the body to assure uninterrupted delivery of oxygenated blood and nutrients to cells and their exchange for wastes. (Reprinted through courtesy of Ethicon, Inc., Somerville, New Jersey)

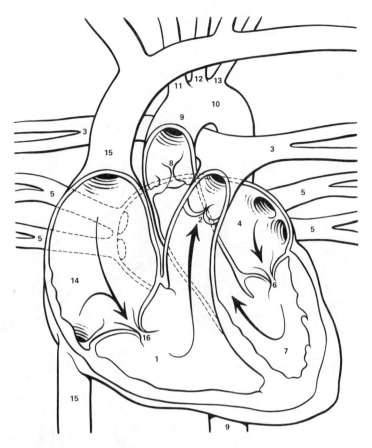

Figure 12.2. The route of blood flow through the heart. (Reprinted through courtesy of Ethicon, Inc., Somerville, New Jersey)

1 Right ventricle	**9** Aorta
2 Pulmonary valve	**10** Aortic arch
3 Pulmonary artery, right and left	**11** Innominate artery
4 Left atrium	**12** Common carotid artery
5 Pulmonary veins, right and left	**13** Subclavian artery
6 Mitral (bicuspid) valve	**14** Right atrium
7 Left ventricle	**15** Venae cavae, inferior and superior
8 Aortic valve	**16** Tricuspid valve

in the opposite direction, back into the bloodstream. As a result of this cellular blood gas exchange, blood becomes *deoxygenated* venous blood, carrying metabolic waste products away from the body tissues.

Venous blood flows back toward the heart in venules which become veins. It is emptied into the right upper heart chamber or *atrium 14* through the inferior and superior *venae cavae 15,* then passes through the *tricuspid valve 16* into the right ventricle 1. Another round trip begins at this point.

In summary, then, the primary function of the cardiovascular system is to carry oxygen and nutrients to cells, exchange them for wastes, and carry the wastes to points of elimination. This system is equipped to adjust flow rate, blood volume, and composition to meet varying body needs. The major organs of the circulatory system are: the heart, aorta, arteries, arterioles, capillaries, venules, and veins.

THE LYMPH VASCULAR SYSTEM*

The lymph system (see Fig. 12.3) functions as a mechanism of drainage, supplementing the work of the veins and capillaries. Tissue fluid is returned to the

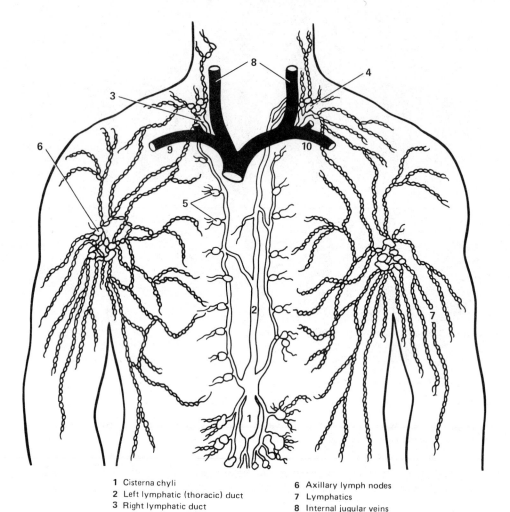

1 Cisterna chyli	**6** Axillary lymph nodes
2 Left lymphatic (thoracic) duct	**7** Lymphatics
3 Right lymphatic duct	**8** Internal jugular veins
4 Jugular lymph nodes	**9** Right subclavian vein
5 Intercostal lymph nodes	**10** Left subclavian vein

Figure 12.3. The lymph vascular system. Tissue fluids gathered all over the body by the lymph system are emptied into the bloodstream at the junction of the internal jugular and subclavian veins, right and left. (Reprinted through courtesy of Ethicon, Inc., Somerville, New Jersey)

---

*Adapted from *The Human Body* with permission from Ethicon, Inc.

bloodstream to prevent the accumulation in tissue spaces. The fluid is gathered all along the network of lymph channels to be emptied into the venous blood circulation via the lymphatic ducts at the junction of the internal jugular and subclavian veins bilaterally.

In contrast to the complete circle made by blood flow, lymph travels in one direction only—always *toward* the heart. The lymph vascular system has no pumping force and no pulsating vesels comparable to arteries; its functioning more nearly resembles only the venous portion of the blood circulatory system. From tiny lymph capillaries between cells to larger lymphatics, the channels are usually found in close proximity to and parallel with veins carrying blood back to the heart. Lymph itself is a substance continuously filtered from tissue fluids, ordinarily containing fluid plasma, some white blood cells, and carbon dioxide. Other chemical components of lymph vary, depending on body location of particular lymph vessels, e.g., the fat content of lymph usually is high in the intestine during digestion.

In summary then, the major components of the lymph vascular system include the channels (capillaries, lymphatics, and ducts) and lymph fluid itself, which is thought to play a defensive role in the spread of infection with filtering action of its nodes and distribution of antibodies, as well as the supplemental action in helping the return of tissue fluids to the blood stream.

CORONARY ARTERY DISEASE

THE CORONARY ARTERIES

The coronary artery system consists of two major branches, the *right* and the *left coronary arteries,* which arise from the base of the ascending aorta in the sinus of Valsalva, near the leaflets of the aortic valve. The *left coronary artery* immediately divides into the *left anterior descending* (LAD) branch, which supplies oxygenated blood to most of the muscle of the left ventricle, and the *left circumflex* branch, which supplies the posterior left ventricle and goes on to anastomose with the right coronary artery. *The right coronary artery,* via the *posterior descending branch,* which runs in a groove between the right atrium and right ventricle around behind the heart to join with the left circumflex, supplies approximately 60% of the oxygenated blood to the sino-atrial (SA) node and approximately 90% to the atrioventricular (AV) node. The *coronary venous system* empties into the posterior wall of the right atrium close to the superior vena cava (Fig. 12.4).

The coronary arteries supply oxygenated blood to the myocardium during the diastolic phase of the cardiac cycle, when the aortic valve leaflets are closed to prevent backflow of blood into the left ventricle. *Systole* is that portion of the cardiac cycle in which the ventricles are contracting to eject blood into the circulation; *diastole* is conversely the "resting phase" of the ventricular activity, during which coronary blood flow oxygenates the muscular myocardium.

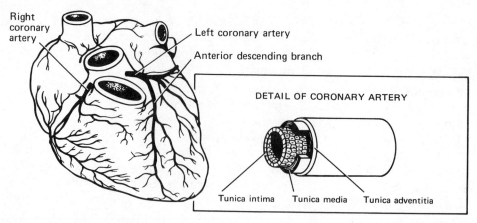

Figure 12.4. Coronary arteries.

ATHEROSCLEROSIS

Any artery of the body, regardless of its location or size, can be affected by *arteriosclerosis* (hardening of the arteries), which is a common term for several kinds of degenerative arterial disease. The associated signs, symptoms, and mortality vary, depending on which vessels are involved, and to what extent.

A common type of arteriosclerosis, *intimal atherosclerosis,* is of special concern, since it involves the aorta and its main branches as well as the coronary and cerebral arteries. Turbulent blood flow and the numerous bends and befurcations make the coronary system especially prone to this degenerative process. Constant bending or torsion of the coronary vessels as they comply with the muscular pumping action of the heart makes them subject to mechanical damage as well. Intimal atherosclerosis causes thickening, hardening, and loss of elasticity of the walls of the blood vessels. The result is narrowing of the internal lumen of the arteries and reduced blood flow. Diffuse deposits of cholesterol and other fatty products accumulate to form plaques, which further narrow the arterial lumen, and may embolize to totally obstruct the lumen distally (see Fig. 12.5).

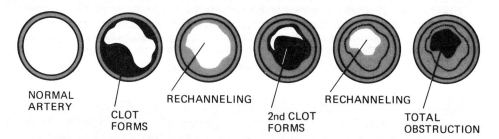

Figure 12.5. Atherosclerosis. (From Huszar RJ: Emergency Cardiac Care, 2nd ed. Robert J. Brady Co., Bowie, Maryland, 1928)

RISK FACTORS IN DEVELOPMENT OF CORONARY ARTERY DISEASE

The degree and rapidity of the formation of the atherosclerotic lesion leading to coronary artery disease (CAD) vary among individuals and depend upon a variety of risk factors, some of which can be remedied and some of which cannot. These risk factors are noted in Table 12.1 below.

Table 12.1 Risk Factors in Coronary Artery Disease

NONMODIFIABLE	MODIFIABLE
Age Sex Familial history of premature CAD	**Major:** Elevated serum lipids Diet rich in cholesterol and other lipids Hypertension Cigarette smoking Carbohydrate intolerance **Minor:** Obesity Sedentary living Personality type Psychosocial tensions Others

*Adapted from Hurst JN (Ed), Logue RB, Schlant RC, Wenger NK. *The Heart,* 3rd Ed. New York, McGraw Hill, 1974.

In certain societies, studies have isolated several incriminating factors that provide logical hypotheses for the causes and high incidence of CAD. Included among these factors are stressful living, high cholesterol diets, and high carbohydrate diets. Metabolic disorders such as diabetes, gout, and hypothyroidism also predispose to CAD.

Since cholesterol (a lipid found in eggs, dairy products, and animal fat) is almost always found in atherosclerotic lesions, some researchers feel that the dietary intake of cholesterol and saturated fats is the basic cause of atherosclerosis and is largely responsible for the high incidence of CAD in affluent, civilized countries. Primitive and poor societies with different dietary habits have been found to have a low incidence of CAD. Other researchers have suggested that high sugar intake is the prime cause of atherosclerosis. Recently, there have been demonstrations that excessive blood platelet adhesiveness, due to a high level of adrenalin (resulting from stress) and perhaps cigarette smoking, can cause clot formation within the coronary arteries. These demonstrations have lead to speculations that excessive platelet adhesiveness may be one of the basic causes of atherosclerosis. However, although many studies have been made and many theories have been proposed, the exact causes of CAD are not yet known.

Once the vital coronary arteries have become obstructed by the gradual laying down of the atherosclerotic plaques, they can no longer carry enough blood to the area that they have previously supplied. At this point, small interconnecting (collateral) arteries may dilate to provide an alternate route for blood to reach otherwise blood-starved areas of the myocardium.

STAGES OF CORONARY ARTERY DISEASE

The various stages of coronary artery disease are 1) *asymptomatic,* 2) *angina pectoris* (stable), 3) *unstable angina* (preinfarction angina), and 4) *myocardial infarction.*

Asymptomatic

The early stages of atherosclerosis are usually asymptomatic and can remain so for many years. If only minimal or moderate obstruction of the coronary arteries exists, or if an efficient collateral circulation is established, the myocardium will continue to receive a sufficient amount of blood flow, even during exertion. Chest pain and associated symptoms will not be present.

Stable Angina

When atherosclerosis of the coronary arteries has progressed to the point where blood flow can no longer meet myocardial demands, an acute discrepancy exists between oxygen requirements and the available supply. Pain of angina pectoris results. At this point, symptomatic coronary artery disease exists. *Angina pectoris* literally means *pain* or *choking* in the chest. Episodes of angina are caused by a temporary lack of oxygen (ischemia) in the myocardial tissue and the accumulation of carbon dioxide and lactic acid. Decreased blood flow through partially obstructed coronary arteries is responsible for the pain. Angina pectoris has two forms, *stable* and *unstable.* Stable angina is the less ominous of the two and its manifestations are predictable and follow an established pattern. For the individual with stable angina, equal amounts of physical exertion (such as climbing two flights of stairs or walking four blocks on a cold day), and/or situations with similar degrees of emotional impact will usually precipitate anginal pain of the same intensity, duration, and location.

Unstable Angina

Unstable angina is more serious and indicates further obstruction of the coronary arteries, with myocardial ischemia or coronary insufficiency. It is differentiated from stable angina by noticeable changes in frequency, intensity, or duration of anginal pain. Since unstable angina often precedes an acute myocardial infarction by a few hours or weeks, it is also called *preinfarction angina.*

It is questionable whether adequate oxygenation ever returns to the blood-starved areas of the myocardium once CAD advances to such a degree or if the myocardial cells in these areas can simply survive prolonged ischemic episodes.

Myocardial Infarction

An acute myocardial infarction (AMI) occurs when a portion of the heart muscle is deprived of an adequate supply of arterial blood long enough so that the tissue in that area dies (necrosis). The length of time that the heart muscle can withstand a lack of oxygen (anoxia) without dying depends upon the work load of the myocardium at the time of deprivation of oxygenated blood and on the amount of blood that can be supplied to the stricken area by collateral circulation.

The precipitating causes of AMI are 1) occlusion of an atherosclerotic coronary artery by a blood clot (thrombus); 2) hemorrhage into an existing diseased arterial wall; 3) reduced blood flow following shock from any cause; 4) arrhythmias; 5) spasm of a coronary artery; 6) pulmonary embolism; 7) unaccustomed effort; 8) emotional stress; or 9) unrelieved fatigue. All of these result in an inadequate oxygenated blood supply to the myocardium. If the myocardium remains ischemic for a long enough period of time, tissue death and necrosis results and myocardial infarction *has occurred*.

TREATMENT OF CORONARY ARTERY DISEASE

Asymptomatic CAD does not require treatment, since it proposed no compromise to the patient's lifestyle or, necessarily, survival. Rather, present research is directed at finding methods of preventing this degenerative process instead of merely dealing with its aftermath.

Stable angina is treated primarily by having the patient rest and use nitrates to abort the attack. Such patients may benefit by the use of longer-lasting nitrate therapy, as with Isosorbide dinitrate or nitrol ointments, while others may improve with beta-blockade agents such as Inderal (propranolol) or Corgard (nadolol). Supervised cardiopulmonary exercise programs may bring relief to the angina sufferer by promoting the development of collateral circulation to help assume some of the myocardial work load and oxygenation.

Unstable angina, because it indicates a precarious condition of the myocardium, is treated aggressively to drastically reduce the myocardial work load while improving oxygenation as much as possible. This patient must be placed on bed rest and administered supplementary oxygen. In addition, vigorous use of nitrates (including possibly Nitroprusside, the IV nitrate preparation) and beta-blocking agents is advocated to bring the myocardial ischemia under rapid control. It is at this time when evaluation of the benefits of coronary artery bypass surgery is appropriate, *before* myocardial infarction has occurred. Current studies are exploring the use of calcium channel-blocking drugs in the treatment of angina in selected patients.

ACUTE MYOCARDIAL INFARCTION

Myocardial infarction occurs when a portion of the myocardium has been deprived of oxygen (ischemic) for a long enough period of time to cause cellular death and necrosis. The overwhelming symptom of myocardial ischemia is *chest pain,* and it is for this reason that the majority of AMI patients seek medical attention.

The pain of acute MI is usually quite distinctive, being described most frequently as crushing (like an elephant standing on the chest), *squeezing* (like a band around the chest), or *pressure-like* in character. Typically, the pain is located *substernally,* but frequently it will radiate across the chest, to the shoulders, or down the arms, with a preference for the left arm and shoulder. The pain may radiate up into the throat, neck, or jaw, with an occasional patient complaining of pain in the teeth.

Pain of MI is more intense than the pain of angina and may be unlike any sensation that the patient has ever experienced before. Though infarction pain occurs suddenly, it is not necessarily associated with exertion, as is angina, but in fact frequently has onset during sleep. Its frequent appearance after eating (when blood is shunted toward the gut to aid digestion) explains why many patients interpret the pain as indigestion.

Myocardial infarction pain is steady, continuous, and is refractory to nitroglycerin, oxygen, changes in position, rest, or home remedies for indigestion such as bicarbonate of soda.

Shortly after the onset of *substernal pain, drenching perspiration* usually begins, and *nausea* or *vomiting* may occur at this time. *Dyspnea* and a feeling of *sudden weakness* may be manifested, along with *pallor* and *cool/clammy skin. Fear* and *apprehension* are generally present and most patients sense that a catastrophe has happened or is about to happen; this sense of catastrophic occurrence is often called *fear of impending doom* and is a hallmark of acute MI. In many instances, the patient will present with his fist clenched to the sternum in an unconscious gesture known as *Levine's sign,* which many consider to be virtually diagnostic of AMI.

This is the picture of the typical acute myocardial infarction. Not all patients present such typical histories, and there may be an absence of pain with sudden collapse and no prior warning. If an AMI is sustained without chest pain or other symptoms and the ECG shows evidence of an old infarction, it is termed a *silent infarction.* The diabetic patient seems to be more prone to suffer a silent MI, probably because widespread neuropathy causes disturbances in pain sensing and interpretation.

The left anterior descending (LAD) branch of the *left* coronary artery (Fig. 12.4) is the most commonly affected (and is frequently called "the widowmaker"), but frequently the posterior descending branch of the *right* coronary is involved. The lesion is less often in the posterior descending branch of the left coronary and still more rarely in the *left circumflex.* Generally, occlusion of the left anterior descending branch causes the "anterior" type of infarct in which the apex of the heart, the anterior wall of the left ventricle, and the adjacent portion of the interventricular septum are the chief regions involved. The "posterior" type of infarct usually is associated with thrombosis of one of the large posterior descending branches and involves mainly the posterior portion of the *interventricular septum* and the *diaphragmatic* and *posterior* portions of the *right* and *left* ventricles. Occlusion of any of these branches may take place gradually, or even suddenly, without causing myocardial infarction. This is not infrequent in patients who have an efficient collateral coronary circulation.

Because of the many variants involved, e.g., location, extent of infarct, degree of collateral circulation, etc., several possible clinical pictures may occur with the AMI, and ED personnel should be alert enough to recognize any and all as they present.

The extent of myocardial damage determines the patient's *hemodynamic stability,* and is responsible for the *clinical picture* which is observed. The patient may be asymptomatic, as with a silent MI, or he may be in one of various stages of heart/pump failure. When the myocardium has been extensively damaged, the cardiac output may fall severely enough to precipitate cardiogenic shock, which progresses rapidly into a lethal spiral ending in death to more than 80% of all patients who develop this serious complication.

Sudden deaths are almost always the result of *lethal arrhythmias,* which develop because of temporary, though extraordinary, electrical instability of the damaged myocardium. *Most of these arrhythmias are transient and treatable.* Studies have shown that up to 60% of all deaths from acute MI occur *within the first hour of onset of pain,* and almost all of these deaths are attributable to these transient, though lethal, arrhythmias. (Refer to Chapter 11 for management of arrhythmias.)

DIAGNOSIS OF ACUTE MI

The diagnosis of AMI is made essentially in three steps:

1. The clinical picture—the complex of information obtained through observation, physical examination, and history

2. The electrocardiogram (ECG)

3. Enzyme studies of blood

A definite diagnosis is usually made by electrocardiographic means. When injury and local death (infarction) of myocardial tissue occurs, characteristic findings reflecting these changes are found in the ECG tracings. Elevation of the ST segment is generally said to indicate myocardial injury ("injury pattern") or death, while ST segmental depression demonstrates myocardial ischemia.

In some instances the patient may give an impressive history suggesting an acute episode but the ECG shows equivocal (rather than definite) changes; this requires other studies to verify the diagnosis, the most important of which are the laboratory determinations of certain enzyme blood levels. Several enzymes normally reside within muscle and organ cells, and those of the myocardium are released into the bloodstream upon injury, causing a characteristic elevation in the serum, permitting detection and evaluation.

The three most useful enzyme studies employed to confirm the diagnosis of AMI are the following:

1. *Creatine Phosphokinase (CPK).* This enzyme is the *first* to rise after infarction, and elevated levels can be detected within 6 hours. After 2-3 days, the CPK levels usually return to normal. For this reason, the determination should be made at the *time of admission* to provide baseline information and repeated in 24 and 48 hours (serial enzymes). It should also be borne in mind that this enzyme is released from other muscle structures in the body as well and that *intramuscular injections* given prior to the CPK can reflect in the laboratory results. This is another reason emergency cardiac medications are best administered IV. Some hospital laboratories are able to give levels for *isoenzymes,* separating enzymes that are specifically myocardial in origin by a process of fractionating each group of enzymes and determining accurate indications of myocardial damage.

CPK normals for males and females are 5-50 mU/ml and 5-30 mU/ml respectively, using the Oliver-Rosalki method.

2. *Serum Glutamic Oxaloacetic Transaminase (SGOT).* Levels of SGOT rise less rapidly than CPK after infarction. Typical increases are usually noted after 24 hours and persist for 3-4 days. Therefore, the concentrations of this enzyme should be measured at 24, 48, and 72 hours after the attack. While SGOT levels are generally reliable in confirming myocardial damage, it should be recognized that this particular enzyme can also be elevated from other sources, especially the liver. Normal levels of SGOT are generally regarded as between 5 and 40 mU/ml according to most methods employed.

3. *Lactic Dehydrogenase (LDH).* The serum levels of LDH increase at a slower rate than CPK or SGOT following infarction. Significant elevations do not usually occur until the second or third day, and they last for 5-6 days. Accordingly, this determination should be performed on days 3, 4, and 5 after the attack if the other enzyme levels have not solved the problem. Normal levels of LDH vary greatly according to the method employed in the laboratory of each hospital.

It should be fully appreciated that the diagnosis of acute myocardial infarction must never be solely on the basis of these enzyme studies; the value of these tests is only supplemental. Conversely, negative results of these studies should not be grounds to abandon the diagnosis of AMI in the presence of a typical history and characteristic ECG findings.

MAJOR COMPLICATIONS OF THE AMI

There are five major complications that threaten life after an acute myocardial infarction, and the EDN must be aware of them and prepared to meet the worst:

1. Arrhythmias that reduce the pumping efficiency of the myocardium, leading to acute pump failure. Probably 80% of AMIs have some distur-

bance of rate and rhythm during the acute phase of the disease. Such arrhythmias may produce sudden death.

2. Acute heart failure is observed in about 60% of patients with the degree of pump deficit varying considerably.

3. Cardiogenic shock is by far the most serious complication of AMI, with a mortality of at least 80%, even with current method of therapy.

4. Thromboembolism from the left ventricle (or more likely from leg vein) can produce sudden death but is uncommon and accounts for a small percentage of all deaths.

5. Rupture of the left ventricle into the pericardium with tamponade and rapidly ensuing death develops most oftern 7-10 days after the original infarction but is uncommon and accounts for only a small percentage of deaths after an AMI.

NURSING MANAGEMENT GUIDELINES FOR THE AMI

Nursing intervention with the AMI patient begins with a *rapid* visual assessment of the ABCs and then should follow these guidelines:

1. Give humidified oxygen via nasal prongs or mask with rebreathing bag to increase the blood oxygen tension and thereby deliver more oxygen to the hypoxic heart muscle. An oxygen flow rate of 2-3 liters per minute (1pm) is appropriate for patients with reactive airway disease, while high flow (minimum of 4-6 1pm) may be used with the majority of patients.

2. Attach ECG monitoring electrodes and begin continuous monitoring for arrhythmia detection.

3. Start an intravenous line of D5/W running TKO or cap the IV injection site with a heparinized lock to ensure access to the venous circulation in event of a sudden complication (i.e. arrhythmia).(Use micro-drop set and large bore needle.)

Vital Signs

Measure and record the vital signs. Baseline information is essential to determine the presence of impending complications and to begin to develop an assessment of the patient's clinical status, which is based upon evaluating *trends* in the vital signs.

1. Assess both radial and apical pulses for rate and quality. Not the presence of pulse deficits.

2. Count the respiratory rate and note the quality of respirations. Tachypnea may indicate congestive failure or pulmonary embolus.

3. Evaluate the blood pressure. Low arterial pressure may be a sign of shock, which is a dangerous complication of AMI. A low BP *in itself* does not signal shock, but a *fall in systolic BP of 30 mm Hg or more* is worrisome regardless of the actual reading; a *narrowing pulse pressure* is an early and

ominous sign of impending shock. *Hypertension,* on the other hand, strains the myocardium by greatly increasing the cardiac work load and adding to ischemia which is already evident.

4. Note the appearance of the ECG (12-lead). A myocardial infarction produces distinctive changes such as ST segment elevation and pathological Q waves. Abnormalities in R wave potential may also be noted; *decreased R wave potential may be indicative of impending shock.*

5. Check the temperature. Both elevations and decreases in body temperature can predispose to the development of arrhythmias due to their separate effects on myocardial oxygenation.

6. Auscultate the chest for heart and lung sounds, and note the presence of cardiac murmurs, rubs, and gallops, and of pulmonary rales, ronchi, or wheezes.

7. Note the mental status and/or level of consciousness of the patient; impaired cardiac output will gradually manifest itself with cerebral hypoxia, among other things.

Relief of Pain and Anxiety

Anxiety raises the heart rate and the blood pressure, and causes the adrenal glands to release epinephrine, which may in turn produce arrhythmias. According to the new ACLS Standards*, nitroglycerine sublingual may be tried first to relieve pain if the patient is normotensive or hypertensive. Titrated doses (2 to 5 mg) IV morphine sulfate should be utilized for pain relief if required; these doses may be repeated at five-minute intervals for several doses as necessary. Experience has indicated that the titration of small doses at frequent intervals provides the desired therapeutic effect without significant respiratory depression.

Reassurance and psychological support should preface every interaction with the patient and should certainly precede, along with simple explanations, every procedure the patient undergoes. The EDN must be particularly sensitive to the intelligent reassurance which the AMI victim and his family need. Continue to monitor the vital signs and clinical status, and reinforce both patient and family with frequent progress reports.

Electrocardiograms

Order a stat ECG.

Laboratory Studies

Order stat serum enzymes (CPK with isoenzymes, SGOT, LDH), CBC, sedimentation rate, and serum electrolytes. Note particularly the serum

---

*Standards and Guidelines for CPR and ECC, JAMA Supplement, Vol 244, No 5, p 488, August 1980

sodium and potassium levels, since these electrolytes are intimately associated with the electrophysiologic functioning of the myocardium; imbalances may rapidly precipitate arrhythmias. In the presence of AMI, serum potassium levels between 4.0 and 5.0 mEq/L is a most acceptable balance, and serum sodium levels should hover near 140 mEq/L.

Lidocaine Prophylaxis

Many units prefer at this time to administer lidocaine prophylactically in the presence of AMI due to the high potential for ventricular arrhythmias from myocardial ischemia. Refer to Chapter 11 on management of arrhythmias for lidocaine dosage and administration.

Complications of Acute MI

Management of the AMI patient demands that the EDN be alert for developing complications, and be prepared to rapidly and efficiently treat such complications should they occur.

Since arrhythmia is by far the most frequent and lethal complication of the AMI, and because it is the most treatable, information regarding arrhythmia detection, recognition, and treatment is presented in the preceding chapter (Chapter 11). Following is a discussion of pump failure as a complication of acute MI.

HEART/PUMP FAILURE

DEFINITION OF TERMS

Let us begin by defining a few terms that will occur repeatedly in the discussion of the hemodynamic mechanisms and treatment of cardiac failure.

Stroke volume: The quantity of blood ejected during each ventricular contraction

Cardiac output: The volume of blood ejected by the heart per minute, this may be stated by the formula: Cardiac Output (CO) = Stroke Volume (SV) × Heart Rate (HR) (Fig. 12.6).

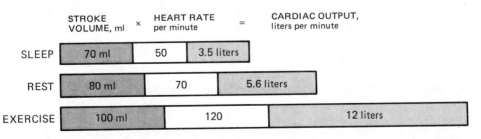

	STROKE VOLUME, ml	×	HEART RATE per minute	=	CARDIAC OUTPUT, liters per minute
SLEEP	70 ml		50		3.5 liters
REST	80 ml		70		5.6 liters
EXERCISE	100 ml		120		12 liters

Figure 12.6. Stroke volume and cardiac output.

End-diastolic volume: The volume of blood contained in the ventricle at the end of diastole just before contraction begins

Inotropic: Having the effect of increasing the contractile state of the ventricle; thus, a drug may be said to have a positive inotropic effect if it increases the force of contraction

Chronotropic: Affecting heart rate; thus, a drug with a positive chronotropic action would increase the heart rate

Heart failure: A state in which cardiac output is insufficient to meet the metabolic demands of the body. This state may occur when cardiac output is increased, decreased, or normal.

Heart failure, in the presence of a higher than normal cardiac output, occurs infrequently, but as a phenomenon in keeping with the foregoing definitions, it may be important to keep in mind. This phenomenon occurs when peripheral demands exceed even the capacity of a normally functioning heart to perfuse the tissues and may be seen in patients with severe anemia, thyrotoxicosis, and in those who have arteriovenous fistulas.

Low-output cardiac failure is much more common and occurs when there is failure of the heart as a pump to supply tissues whose demands are otherwise normal. A number of underlying heart disorders may be responsible for inadequate performance:

Myocardial infarct: May injure a sufficient number of muscle fibers as to compromise the pumping ability.

Valvular dysfunction: Resulting in either stenosis of an outflow tract or in regurgitation through an incompetent valve, severely increasing the cardiac work load and lowering cardiac output sufficiently to precipitate failure.

Constrictive pericarditis and *pericardial effusion:* May act similarly to mechanically restrict the heart's ability to fill and empty.

Arrhythmias: May compromise the cardiac output by altering either the heart rate, stroke volume, or both to the point where there is mechanical pump failure due to a disturbance in the electrical "drive" system of the heart (refer to Starling's Law on page 215).

FACTORS IN THE HEART'S ABILITY TO FUNCTION

The basic defect in heart failure is a decrease in the contractile state of the heart, expressed in the literature as V_{max}; that is, the velocity with which cardiac muscle fibers shorten during ventricular systole. Recently, methods have been described for measuring V_{max} in the intact heart of conscious patients from high fidelity recordings of isovolumic ventricular pressure and its rate of rise.* These concepts were applied to the study of patients with cardiac hypertrophy and/or failure, and it was found that left ventricular hypertrophy alone

---

*Mason DT, Spann JF, Zelis R: Myocardial contractile state in hypertrophy and congestive failure in conscious man: Determination by the maximum velocity of contractile state shortening. (abst) Circulation 40 (Suppl III):111-141, 1969

was associated with a depression of left ventricular contractility in the absence of less sensitive indicators of cardiac performance, such as stroke volume, cardiac output, ventricular end-diastolic volume, and arteriovenous oxygen difference. Thus, overt heart failure is viewed as a *late* manifestation of the severely depressed heart, occurring rather far down the road from the original problem of decreased cardiac contractility.

As the heart begins to fail, the body responds wih certain cardiac and circulatory compensatory mechanisms in an effort to maintain cardiac output. Although these are in many cases the same mechanisms used by healthy individuals to respond to an increased demand for cardiac work (as in strenuous exercise or a response to fright), it is helpful clinically to think of the relationship between symptoms manifested by a person in congestive heart failure and the compensatory mechanisms which have been called into play. Symptoms of failure may be viewed as the side effects of these compensatory mechanisms.

One of the first mechanisms to be called into play is the reflex increase autonomic sympathetic excitation of most cardiac muscle and the vascular system, complemented by inhibition of cardiac parasympathetic activity. Augmentation of sympathetic impulses to the heart improves the contractile state, increasing the velocity and force of contraction. Sympathetic discharges and an increase in circulating catecholamines affect peripheral circulation with peripheral vasoconstriction, thus working with the mechanisms in the heart to maintain arterial pressure in spite of a decrease in stroke volume. The *cool skin, increased sweating,* and *tachycardia,* common clinical findings in the congestive heart failure state, are all side effects of the utilization of the sympathetic nervous system as a compensatoy mechanism.

Another very important aspect of increased sympathetic activity is that it yields an increase in central and peripheral venous tone. This increases venous pressure, and helps to improve venous return to the heart, which augments ventricular filling during diastole and increases ventricular end-diastolic volume. This process leads to a direct increase in stroke volume, using the mechanism of Starling's law.

STARLING'S LAW

Starling's law of the heart states that there is a direct proportion between the end-diastolic volume of the heart (that is, the length of cardiac muscle fibers during diastole) and the force of contraction of the following systole. It is helpful to use the analogy of a rubber band with this concept. We know that the farther we stretch a rubber band, the greater will be the strength with which it snaps back. Within certain critical limits, the same may be said for heart muscle. The farther it is stretched by venous filling during diastole, the stronger will be the following systolic contraction and the greater will be the stroke volume.

Cardiac compensation by sympathetic stimulation also serves to increase heart rate. This alone, without an increase in stroke volume, can increase cardiac output by threefold (remember that $CO = SV \times HR$), but above a certain rate, cardiac output may actually begin to decrease. This rate varies from person to person but is usually around 170-180 for normal individuals. The rate of continued efficiency may climb as high as 200-220 in trained athletes or be as low as 120-140 in older, untrained individuals. Decrease in cardiac output above a certain rate is due to shortening of the diastolic phase of the cardiac cycle, which eventually allows insufficient time for filling of the ventricles. Shortening of diastole also inhibits coronary artery blood flow, since it is *during relaxation of the ventricles that these arteries are filled;* this helps explain why exercise, or tachycardia associated with anxiety, may elicit the pain of ischemia.

ROLE OF THE KIDNEYS

Another early homeostatic (tendency to stability) mechanism that occurs when cardiac output falls is that the kidneys are stimulated to retain sodium and water. The process involved may be related to sympathetic stimulation causing vasoconstriction and resultant decreased renal blood flow. This activates the renin-angiotensin system, which triggers antidiuretic hormone (ADH) and aldosterone release, with sodium retention. An expansion of the intravascular blood volume follows with a resultant increase in venous return and end-diastolic volume, again utilizing the Starling law to increase cardiac output. The cost, however, of maintaining ventricular pressure at an elevated level is an elevated systemic and pulmonary capillary pressure, which may ultimately result in the transudation of fluid from the vascular bed with edema formation.

FORMATION OF EDEMA

Transudation of fluid may be seen as a fairly reliable indicator of elevated venous pressure, with an elevation equivalent to approximately 5 mm Hg above normal at the capillary bed, resulting in edema. This is evident since the fluid exchange is modulated by the forces of hydrostatic pressure, which varies from 30 mm Hg at the arterial end of the capillary bed to 20 mm Hg at the venous end. The counteracting force is osmotic pressure, which remains at a constant 25 mm Hg throughout the capillary bed. As soon as the hydrostatic pressure is raised above 25 mm Hg at the venous end, edema will result.

Expansion of plasma volume through the sodium retention process has another significant drawback: the increase in end-diastolic fiber length serves as a compensatory mechanism *only* until optimal length is reached. Beyond this critical length, further stretching may actually *decrease* the strength of the following contraction. Thus, a greatly increased plasma volume may so decrease contractility as to produce a rapidly progressing downhill course. As with heart rate, again, each compensatory mechanism has limitations that may not be exceeded without deleterious side effects. As these limits are approached, their side effects become the signs and symptoms of compensated heart failure. Signs of cough, rales, peripheral edema, or hepatomegaly may give clues that the critical limits of compensation are being approached.

VENTRICULAR HYPERTROPHY

Ventricular hypertrophy is considered to be the major chronic hemo-dynamic adjustment of the failing heart, but it is interesting to learn how rapidly this mechanism may take place. Two experimental models of conges-tive heart failure have been studied to a considerable extent: right ventricular hypertrophy, with and without overt failure, was produced in a cat by constric-tion of the pulmonary artery, and left ventricular hypertrophy, with failure, was produced in the second instance by constriction of the ascending aorta of a guinea pig.* Only two days after constriction of the pulmonary artery, the right ventricular weight had doubled, and within a month, it had tripled in associa-tion with an increase in protein synthesis. After constriction of the aorta, left ventricular hypertrophy also promptly followed.

Hypertrophied myocardium is inherently less efficient than normal heart muscle in several ways. First, its contractility is less than normal per unit of mus-cle. Second, it demonstrates an imbalance between energy production and energy utilization, which may be due in part to an inability to use fatty acids at the mitochondrial level. Even so, the total mass of myocardium may be so increased by this mechanism as to maintain a compensated cardiac output. This compensation may be so complete that the other chronic adjustments of tachycardia and edema may disappear.

EVENTS IN DECOMPENSATION

When the various compensatory mechanisms of the heart can no longer per-form adequately to overcome the depressed myocardium and pump suffi-ciently to meet the metabolic demands of the body tissues, *decompensation* occurs. Cardiac decompensation may be of a subtle, gradual nature, or it may occur suddenly and dramatically, as in acute pulmonary edema. Occasionally, the oversimplified terms *forward failure* and *backward failure* are used. For-ward failure related to the symptoms primarily due to low cardiac output, such as fatigue, weakness and cachexia, while backward failure indicates the symptoms of elevated venous pressure from a failing ventricle, such as edema, organomegaly, and pulmonary congestion.

It is helpful again to think of the heart as being composed of two separate pumps, the right and left ventricles, which are in series with one another. Remembering that the right heart pumps primarily to the lungs, while the left heart is the systemic circulatory pump, it is possible to conceptualize impair-ment of one side and then the other as separate physiological events. Although both sides of the heart work in tandem and are never completely separate in functioning, some events may alter performance on one side without initially

*Spann JF, Buccino RA, Sonnenblick EH, et al: Contractile state of cardiac muscle obtained from cats with experimentally produced ventricular hypertrophy and heart failure. Circ Res, Vol 21, pp 341-354, 1967 from "Modern Concepts of Cardiovascular Disease, Vol XXXIX, No 1, January 1970

impairing function of the other side. Myocardial infarction, for example, often inflicts the majority of injury on the left ventricle, but cor pulmonale is a condition of the right heart, secondary to chronic lung disease.

LEFT HEART FAILURE

In left heart failure, the ability of the left ventricle is compromised; it is unable to move blood adequately, while the right heart continues to pump blood into the lungs with normal vigor. This results is an accumulation of blood in the lungs and an increase in the pulmonary capillary pressure. Consequently, the following symptoms are often exhibited by the patient:

Dyspnea. Increased pressure in the lung leads to loss of elasticity in the lung parenchyma. The resulting sensation of shortness of breath may be exacerbated by exercise (in early LV failure), when the cardiac work load is increased and the barely compensated heart is unable to meet the tissues' demands for oxygenation, or dyspnea may occur suddenly when there is an acute cardiac decompensation at critical pulmonary pressure levels.

Orthopnea. Dyspnea which occurs when the patient lies down is called orthopnea. Lying down increases venous return to the heart, thus increasing the output of the right heart and rapidly increasing pulmonary capillary pressure. Sitting up potentiates the use of accessory muscles of respiration and relieves abdominal pressure of the diaphragm.

Paroxysmal Nocturnal Dyspnea. Often abbreviated PND, this is a classic picture of a patient awakening at night suddenly breathless and either sitting at the bedside to obtain relief or rushing to open a window for "fresh air." This phenomenon represents a form of acute pulmonary edema, the cause probably being the mobilization of fluid while in the recumbent position. The fluid, which has been stored in dependent areas, increases circulating volume which exceeds the capacity of a failing heart. Also, excessive fluid may simply become redistributed to the lungs because of their now relatively dependent position.

On physical examination the patient in left heart failure will also demonstrate certain common findings.

Rales

Rales are often regarded as one of the first physical signs of left ventricular failure, although pulmonary capillary pressure is already quite high before they occur. They are a moist, crackling sound heard toward the end of the inspiratory phase, first at the bases if the patient has been upright or sitting, and especially on the right. Their presence represents the transudation of fluid from the pulmonary vasculature into the alveolar spaces and are theoretically the sound of the alveolar walls overcoming the "sticky" quality of this fluid as they pop open.

Gallop Rhythms

These include the third heart sound (S_3) (ventricular gallop), and the fourth heart sound (S_4) (atrial gallop). An S_3 is a low-pitched sound, occurring shortly after S_2, and is thought to represent the vibrations caused when rapid ventricular filling (rapid because pulmonary venous pressure is high) meets the abrupt limitation of ventricular distensibility. An S_3 is normal in children but is an early sign of congestive heart failure in any adult. An S_4 occurs just prior to the first heart sound and is thought to be the sound of the atrium contracting against the increased resistance of an already overburdened ventricle. It, too, is considered to be a relatively early sign of congestive heart failure.

Acute Pulmonary Edema

During left ventricular decompensation, when pulmonary capillary pressure becomes high enough to leak significant amounts of fluid into the lung parenchyma and alveoli, acute pulmonary edema occurs. The situation may be defined in terms of several stages. In the *first stage* the patient becomes restless and orthopneic. There may also be rales and some wheezing if bronchospasm is occurring or fluid is blocking a bronchial passage. In the *second stage*, the sympathetic nervous system begins to increase its discharge, with resultant tachycardia, pupil dilation pallor, sweating, and elevation of systemic arterial blood pressure. With worsening of the condition, copious amounts of frothy, blood-tinged sputum is expectorated, and rales become coarser and bubbling, indicating the progression of fluid into larger airways. Gas exchange is impaired and this results in a lowered PaO_2 and central cyanosis. With the *third stage*, this hypoxia makes the patient's anxiety more acute before the mental state deteriorates to confusion and then stupor. Respirations are noisy, and gurgling rales can be heard without the aid of a stethoscope. Blood-tinged fluid is now present in the bronchi and trachea, and the patient is literally drowning in his secretions. It is obvious that acute pulmonary edema represents a medical emergency and requires immediate and specific action.

Management of pulmonary edema is directed toward five goals:

1. Open airways. Clear fluids with suctioning and positive pressure ventilation to provide for reopening of the alveolar spaces and relief of hypoxia.
2. Support breathing and respiratory drive in the presence of altered arterial blood gas (ABG) levels.
3. Improve cardiovascular functioning.
4. Retard venous return.
5. Provide mental and physical relaxation.

TREATMENT OF LEFT VENTRICULAR DECOMPENSATION

With these goals in mind the following treatment measures are quickly implemented when left ventricular decompensation (LVD) is recognized:

1. Institute IPPB, delivering 100% oxygen via a well-fitting, non-rebreathing mask, using an airway pressure of 4-9 cm H_2O. Positive pressure ventilation serves both to force fluids from the airways and provide for expansion of the alveolar spaces with resultant relief of hypoxia and to help retard venous return by replacing normally negative intrathoracic pressure with a positive pressure.

2. Help the patient assume a sitting position (high Fowler's) and support with pillows. This position provides the upright chest positioning which allows the patient to more easily utilize accessory respiratory musculature for improved respiratory effort. In addition, it causes decreased venous return because of the relative dependent position of the legs and trunk.

3. Draw arterial blood gases immediately and correct acidosis with incremental doses of Sodium bicarbonate, 1 mg/Kg body weight. It may be necessary to intubate the patient and control ventilation mechanically if the arterial pCO_2 is rising; this indicates that the patient is fatigued and losing ground in his fight to maintain arterial oxygenation.

4. Administer morphine sulfate 8-15 mg in incremental doses IV to sedate and decrease catecholamine discharge. This will decrease myocardial irritability, decrease venous return to the heart, and possibly depress the nervous system pathways that participate in the formulation of pulmonary edema, as well as provide sedation and relief of anxiety.

5. Treat arrhythmias with appropriate medications and convert, if possible, to normal sinus rhythm (NSR). Digitalis, administered IV in a rapid-acting form, is used both to slow the heart rate and to improve cardiac output through better LV filling and stroke volume (see Starling's Law of the Heart on page 000) and for its positive inotropic effect on the myocardium. Specific anti-arrhythmics or electrocardioversion should be utilized in the presence of other arrhythmias which compromise cardiovascular functioning.

6. Aminophylline, in an IV drip infusion, is sometimes administered to relieve bronchospasm, increase cardiac output, and decrease venous tone.

7. Diuretics, usually rapidly-acting furosemide (Lasix) or ethacrynic acid (Edecrin), help eliminate excess fluid and reduce circulating blood volume.

8. Vasodilator therapy, such as the use of Isosorbide Dinitrate or Nitrol ointment, may be utilized to decrease venous return by the vasodilation actions.

The use of *rotating tourniquets* has been advocated in the past as a treatment for acute pulmonary edema, but this is now under vigorous controversy. Advocates feel that application of rotating tourniquets is an instantaneous method of reducing venous return and supporting cardiovascular function until drug therapy can take effect. Disclaimers argue that rotating tourniquets may trap blood centrally and cause an actual increase in intrathoracic pressure. In addition, there is a buildup of lactic acid in the blood which rotating tourniquets pool in the legs; each time a tourniquet is released, a bolus of acidotic blood rushes into the general circulation.

Phlebotomy is no longer recommended as a treatment for LVD. Modern medications and treatments leave little need for such a drastic measure.

The patient who develops acute left ventricular decompensation (ALVD) may benefit from advanced hemodynamic monitoring and specific treatment of cardiovascular dysfunction. In settings where early central monitoring is utilized, the EDN *must* become familiar with the equipment, insertion procedures, and use of the hemodynamic monitoring parameters.

RIGHT HEART FAILURE

It is often said that the most frequent cause of right heart failure is left heart failure, meaning that in the usual course of events, the left heart suffers injury and as a result exhibits acute or chronic compensated congestive heart failure. The right heart then must chronically pump against the increased resistance of elevated pulmonary pressures. In response, the right ventricle hypertrophies and dilates but soon passes the increased fluid load and venous pressure upstream to the systemic venous circulation. Organs and tissues that are normally drained by veins become congested, yielding certain signs and symptoms:

1. *Neck veins* become distended and stay distended even when the patient is sitting up. Usually, these veins flatten when a person raises his head 30-45°, but when the neck veins remain full at that elevation, they reflect an elevated pressure in the right atrium.
2. *Edema* develops in the body, most classically in these specific areas: *Skin,* where it is evident in any dependent area. Ask the patient if his shoes are tight at night and press a thumb firmly over the pretibial areas noting any indentation. The *liver* becomes enlarged when increased hepatic venous pressure forces fluid into interstitial areas. Hepatomegaly and liver tenderness are elicited on physical examination. Venous pressure can force fluid into the pleural cavity and cause a *pleural effusion.* In much the same way, fluid in the pericardium yields a *pericardial effusion.*
3. *Nocturia* can be a symptom of right heart failure when the recumbent position mobilizes fluid which is excreted during the night.

TREATMENT OF RIGHT HEART FAILURE

The treatment of right heart failure does not usually involve emergency measures and often includes the following:

1. Treat arrhythmias with specific medications as indicated to improve cardiovascular function.

2. Bedrest to reduce the work load of the heart and to mobilize intracellular tissue fluid.

3. A low-sodium diet to counteract the sodium-retaining tendency of the kidneys. Sometimes fluids are also restricted.

4. Digitalis to increase the force of myocardial contraction.

5. Diuretics, usually the thiazides, furosemide (Lasix), or aldosterone antagonists (spironalactone or triamterene).

6. Monitored intake, output, and body weight to determine response to treatment.

CARDIOGENIC SHOCK

If we look at heart failure in degrees upon a scale of severity, with compensated pump failure the least severe, cardiogenic shock falls into the area of *severe, overwhelming pump failure*. A current term for cardiogenic shock is "power failure," and in many ways this is quite descriptive of the state in which the heart simply lacks the power to propel blood forward and deliver oxygen and other nutrients to the cells of the body. Recent years have produced intensive research attempting to characterize this circulatory disturbance, but agreement as to the pathophysiologic disturbances involved, or the most efficacious treatment, is yet to be reached. Survival rates have not been appreciably altered despite all modes of therapy studied, with mortality remaining near 80-85%. Ten to fifteen percent of all patients who suffer MI develop this catastrophic complication.

Shock is a descriptive term, denoting a clinical picture that develops in the presence of *inadequate tissue perfusion*. Characteristics are:

1. A systolic blood pressure of less than 80 mm Hg, or 30 mm below the previous normal level. This variable alone, however, does not define shock but a narrowing pulse pressure *is* highly significant.

2. Pallor—cool clammy skin—denoting decreased peripheral perfusion and increased vasoconstriction.

3. Peripheral cyanosis indicative of the increased AV oxygen difference. This results because of increased tissue extraction of oxygen during the passage of blood from arterial to venous circulation; the tissues need to extract more from each passage of the blood, since the total number of "passages" (cardiac output) is reduced.

4. Mental confusion or marked dullness, resulting from diminished cerebral circulation and hypoxia and frequently beginning as anxiety and restlessness.

5. Urine output of less than 30 cc per hour. This reflects decreased renal artery flow.

TREATMENT OF CARDIOGENIC SHOCK

Since there is no clear-cut, effective treatment for cardiogenic shock once it develops, vigilant *hemodynamic/clinical monitoring* and aggressive treatment of pump failure in early stages is vital. Intelligent decisions in the treatment of shock depend upon watching for *trends* in the cardiovascular functioning of the patient, and so there is a need for as much current, frequent hemodynamic information as possible.

To this end, many care units routinely insert *intra-arterial catheters* to follow minute changes in mean arterial blood pressure, arterial oxygen saturation, blood pH and pCO_2, arterial-venous O_2 difference, and calculated peripheral resistance. Pulmonary artery catheters are most frequently used now to more accurately monitor cardiac output, and LV pressures and function; some units may continue to utilize the CVP as a *reflection* to LV function.

Respiratory support is vital to relieve hypoxemia, and the patient should rest in a supine position to improve cerebral circulation. A *Foley catheter* is always inserted to monitor urinary output. In addition to these measures, *relieve the patient's pain and anxiety* as much as possible, working within the confines of maintaining cardiovascular function, and *reassuring and supporting the patient and family. Essential goals are as follows:*

1. *Maintain the airway* and *provide ventilatory assistance* to relieve hypoxemia. If the patient is unable to maintain PaO_2 levels at 70-75% on nasal 02, intubation with positive pressure or volume assistance must be considered.*

2. *Correct arrhythmias* and establish an effective heart rate. Specific anti-arrhythmics, cardioversion, or electrical pacing may be required to abolish arrhythmias and improve cardiac function.*

3. *Correct hypovolemia.* Patients with a low cardiac output syndrome not associated with an elevated CVP or severe pulmonary congestion should be given a trial of fluid loading. Initiate IV line with D5/W. (Occasionally low-viscosity dextran is used for this purpose.)*

4. *Correct acidosis.* Metaolic acidosis develops when tissue perfusion is impaired, largely because of the lactic acid produced by anaerobic metabolism and released into the vascular system. This is corrected with administration of sodium bicarbonate, calculating the dosage, and taking care not to precipitate a sodium overload or overcorrect the acidosis.*

5. *Replace systemic catecholamines* (which may be decreased due to prolonged sympathetic discharge in the onset of shock) and improve renal blood flow along with enhanced myocardial contractility, cardiac output, and blood pressure by administering a titrated dopamine (Intropin) IV drip.*

6. *Improve circulation.* To make intelligent decisions regarding this goal, an estimation or calculation of peripheral vascular resistance must be made. Clinical estimates may be made on the basis of amount of increased venous pressure, amount of decrease in pulse pressure, state of cutaneous blood flow (temperature and color), character of peripheral pulses as compared with central pulsations, and the *clinical appearance of the patient.* The degree of this estimated vasoconstriction dictates the

*Andreoli KC, et al: Comprehensive Cardiac Care. C.V. Mosby Co., St. Louis, pp 45-47, 1971

choice of drug as to its alpha and beta adrenergic effects. Other techniques, such as the intraaortic balloon pump (which enhances coronary blood flow and myocardial oxygenation as well as decreasing peripheral vascular resistance) or heart-lung piggyback or bypass machines, may also be attempted. *Antishock garments/MAST pants* may be applied to the patient in cardiogenic shock as a reversible fluid challenge. If the patient improves, the garment should be left in place until appropriate volume/fluid load can be infused.**

7. *Maintain kidney function.* Normally 25% of the total cardiac output flows to the kidneys. In cardiogenic shock the renal arterial blood flow is drastically reduced and renal ischemia is a serious consequence. If urine output falls significantly, mannitol is sometimes given as an "obligatory" diuretic which works osmotically and increases renal blood flow.*

8. *Search for potentially correctable causes of shock,* such as pericardial tamponade, papillary muscle rupture, septal rupture, or ventricular aneurysm. Aggressive surgical management may save a certain number of patients.*

DRUGS EMPLOYED IN MANAGEMENT OF CARDIOGENIC SHOCK

Drug therapy employed for cardiogenic shock involves the use of the sympathomimetics, which are drugs that mimic the sympathetic nervous system. They have a few basic mechanisms by which they operate called *alpha* and *beta* effects (see Table 12.2).

Alpha effect means the drug is a *vasoconstrictor,* which increases the venous return to the heart by decreasing the area within which the blood circulates.

Beta effect means the drug affects the *contractility* of the heart muscle itself.

In the same manner, drugs that affect the contractility and the rate of the heart are classified as *inotropic* and *chronotropic.*

Inotropic means the drug affects the contractility of the heart. A *positive* inotropic drug *increases* the contractility; digitalis, for example, is a *positive* inotropic drug.

Chronotropic refers to the rate at which the heart contracts. A *positive* chronotropic drug *increases* the heart rate; digitalis, for example, is a *negative* chronotropic drug because it *slows* the heart rate.

The commonly employed sympathomimetic drugs found in most EDs and Code Carts and recommended in the 1980 ACLS Standards** are:

1. Dopamine HCl (Intropin) is used for its alpha and beta effects, which result in general vasoconstriction, increased cardiac output from its inotropic action, and improved renal and mesenteric blood flow due to its

---

*Andreoli KC, et al: Comprehensive Cardiac Care. C.V. Mosby Co., St. Louis, pp 45-47, 1971

**Standards for CPR and ECC. JAMA, Vol 244, No 5, p 483, August 1, 1980

Table 12.2 Sympathomimetic (Adrenergic) Drugs

Sympathomimetic (Adrenergic) drugs affect the sympathetic nervous system by acting on its alpha (α) and beta (β) receptor sites found in the heart, lungs, and blood vessels. Whenever one of these receptor sites is activated by an appropriate drug or hormone, a predictable sequence of responses will occur. Lungs and arteries have both alpha and beta receptors while the heart has only beta receptors; any beta agent given will have the same effect on the heart.

	α	β
HEART	No Action	Heart Rate Force of Contractions Contractility
ARTERIES	Constriction	Dilation
LUNGS	None or Mild Bronchoconstriction	Bronchodilation

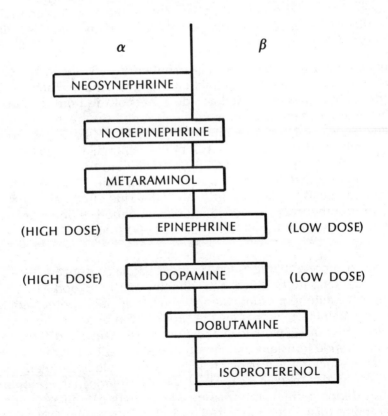

*Adapted from Atcheson R: Pharmacology Update on Sun River ACEP Conference, 1980

vasodilation of those areas specifically. Mix dopamine 400-800 mg in 500cc D5/W. Dose is based upon μg/Kg/min and usually start at 2-5 μg/Kg/min. Doses greater than 20 μg/Kg/min may result in reversed alpha effect and declining perfusion of renal and mesenteric vessels.

2. Dobutamine HCl (Dobutrex), a synthetic catecholamine, is a direct B-adrenergic receptor stimulating agent and produces little systemic arterial constriction at *low* dose levels. Usual dosage range is 2.5 to 10 μg/Kg/min. Doses in excess of 20 μg/Kg/min may cause tachycardia or other dysrhythmias.

3. Norepinephrine (Levophed). Should be diluted 4-8 mg in 500cc D5/W for a dilution rate of 8-16 μg/cc. The usual dose is up to 8 μg/min. If more than 8 μg/min are given, the inotropic effect is lost. Precaution: Best given through a central IV rather than peripheral and must be watched carefully for infiltration of drug into the tissues which will cause severe vasoconstriction, necrosis, and sloughing!

4. Isoproterenol (Isuprel). Should be diluted 1-2 mg in 500cc D5/W and given 2-20 μg/min, titrated to effect. It increases the myocardial oxygen consumption, extends the size of an MI when given to someone in cardiogenic shock, (because of an MI), causes tachycardia and premature ventricular contractions (PVCs) almost consistently, and it is falling into disfavor for these reasons.

5. Epinephrine (Adrenalin) is an alpha/beta drug, a vasoconstrictor which also produces an inotropic effect on the myocardium. Tachycardia and other arrhythmias may result as side effects of this potent natural catecholamine. Dosage for continuous infusion in the treatment of cardiogenic shock is 1 mg Epinephrine diluted in 250cc D5/W, started at 1 μg/min. In treating cardiac arrest or fine ventricular fibrillation, administer 0.5 to 1.0 mg (5-10cc of a 1:10,000 solution) IV or per endotracheal tube; intracardiac administration of epinephrine is no longer recommended due to the disproportionate lethal side effects and is used *only* when no other route is possible. Recommended endotracheal administration dosage is 1 mg (10 ml) of 1:10,000 solution.

An additional important drug used to improve cardiac output and BP is sodium nitroprusside (Nipride), which acts directly on the blood vessels, independent of the autonomic innervation. Even though it is a *potent vasodilator,* Nipride may be helpful in treating the shock victim because there is a redistribution of the cardiac work load and a decrease in myocardial oxygen consumption. Nipride infusions may be titrated along with volume infusions to maintain the exact left ventricular filling pressure, volume, and end-diastolic pressures desired for maximal cardiac efficiency. *Hemodynamic monitoring is mandatory* during sodium nitroprusside administration. Prepare Nipride infusions by adding the contents of the 50 mg vial to 250-1000cc D5/W; wrap the solution promptly in foil to protect it from light. Nipride solutions should be discarded after 4 hours, due to deterioration.

POINTS OF CLINICAL ASSESSMENT

A review of some of the points of initial evaluation and clinical assessment useful to the EDN in evaluating cardiovascular emergencies is summarized as follows:

Symptoms (subjective) and recent history

Signs (objective) and observations with examination

1. Position with breathing; quality of respirations
2. Facies (anxious, gasping, apprehensive, pale, florid)
3. Skin (temperature, moisture, perfusion, cyanosis, degree of perfusion to knees and ears)
4. State of mentation
5. Peripheral pulse quality and rate (regular or irregular)
6. Carotid pulse quality and rate
7. Jugular venous pressure (Normally, when someone is at a 45° angle, the internal jugular vein is not distended. A patient in heart failure will have a distended jugular vein at that angle. Distension 2-3 cm above the manubrial notch indicates higher than normal cardiovascular pressure and distension as high as the chin is equivalent to a CVP of about 25 cm H_2O.
8. Blood pressure (Pay particular attention to the pulse pressure.)
9. Cardiac rate and rhythm, auscultating the apex and the PMI
10. Auscultation of the chest for rales and listening both anteriorly and posteriorly for quality of respirations.
11. Measure urinary output every 30 to 60 minutes.
12. Assess any available data from advanced hemodynamic monitoring systems and note *trends* in pressures, cardiac output readings.

REVIEW

1. Trace the flow of blood through the heart starting at the right ventricle.
2. List the major components of the blood circulatory system.
3. Describe the major functions of the blood circulatory system.
4. Define the major functions of the lymph vascular system.
5. Describe the directional flow and pathways of lymph.
6. Describe the tricuspid valve, where it is found, and what it does.
7. Describe the mitral valve, where it is found, and what it does.
8. Identify the form of arteriosclerosis that affects the aorta, cerebral arteries, and coronary arteries.
9. Identify the noncontrollable factors among the major predisposing factors which contribute to the development of CAD.

10. Identify the controllable factors among the major predisposing factors which contribute to the development of CAD.

11. Describe the pathophysiology of CAD and identify its four stges.

12. List three factors that differentiate stable angina from unstable angina.

13. List some major causes of occlusion of an atherosclerotic coronary artery.

14. Define an acute myocardial infarction and explain its probable evolution.

15. Describe the symptom complex that is considered the typical history of an AMI.

16. Identify the artery that is most often affected in CAD.

17. Identify the cause of an "anterior" type of infarct and the cardiac area affected.

18. Identify the cause of a "posterior" type of infarct and the cardiac area affected.

19. List the three diagnostic steps necessary to confirm an AMI.

20. Name the three serum enzymes and their normal range values, which are employed in the diagnosis of AMI.

21. Identify the five major complications that threaten life after an AMI.

22. Outline the three immediate steps to be taken by the EDN if a patient presents with complaint of chest pain of a steady constrictive nature, which is unrelieved by rest or nitrites and which radiates widely.

23. Identify the essential vital signs which must be monitored and documented for baseline information with the AMI.

24. Describe guidelines for management of pain with the AMI.

25. Define stroke volume, cardiac output, and end-diastolic volume.

26. Identify four underlying heart disorders which can be responsible for inadequate performance.

27. Identify three compensatory mechanisms that contribute to an increased cardiac output.

28. Explain Starling's Law of the heart.

29. Define left heart failure and identify the accompanying clinical findings.

30. Describe the signs and symptoms characteristic of acute pulmonary edema.

31. Identify five immediate goals in the management of acute pulmonary edema.

32. Outline the treatment measures to be implemented in achieving the five goals.

33. Explain the current controversy over the use of rotating tourniquets.

34. Identify the specific signs and symptoms which accompany right heart failure and outline the treatment measures employed.

35. Describe the early and late signs and symptoms of cardiogenic shock, the essential goals of treatment, and the groups of drugs employed in treatment.

36. Identify the most frequently used sympathomimetic drugs and explain the alpha/beta mechanisms by which they operate.

37. Identify the mechanism by which sodium nitroprusside operates and describe the safeguards which are mandatory with its administration.

38. List at least 10 key points of initial evaluation and clinical assessment in cardiovascular emergencies.

BIBLIOGRAPHY

American Heart Association: Examination of the Heart, Part Two, Inspection and Palpation of Venous and Arterial Pulses. AHA, 1967

American Heart Association: Examination of the Heart, Part Four, Auscultation. AHA, 1967

Andreoli K, Hunn VK, et al: Comprehensive Cardiac Care, 3rd ed. C.V. Mosby Co., St. Louis, Missouri, 1979

Atcheson R: Cardiac Arrest, Comprehensive Review of Emergency Care (to be published). Aspen Systems Publications, Rockville, Maryland

Braun HA, Diettert A, Wills VE: Coronary Care Unit Nursing: Part II. A Workbook in Clinical Aspects, 2nd ed. Reston Publishing Co., Reston, Virginia, 1980

Brunner S, Suddarth S: The Lippincott Manual of Nursing Practice, 2nd ed. J.B. Lippincott Co., Philadelphia, Pennsylvania, 1982

Crumlish CN: Cardiogenic Shock, Catch It Early. Nursing 81, Vol 11, No 8, p 46, August 1981

Friedberg K: Disease of the Heart, 3rd ed. W.B. Saunders Co., Philadelphia, 1966

Giving Cardiovascular Drugs Safely, Nursing Skillbook. Horsham, Nursing Books, Intermed Communications, Inc., 1978

Guyton A: Textbook of Medical Physiology, 2nd ed. W.B. Saunders Co., Philadelphia, Pennsylvania, 1977

Hurst JW (ed), Logue RB, Schlant RC, Wenger NK: The Heart, 3rd ed. McGraw Hill (A Blankiston Publisher), New York, 1974

Mason DT, Spann JF, Zelis R: Myocardian contractile state in hypertrophy and congestive failure in conscious man. Circulation 40: Suppl. III, Vol III, p 141, 1969

Meltzer LE, Penneo R, et al: Intensive Coronary Care. The Robert J. Brady Co., Bowie, Maryland, 1977

Phibbs B, Craddock L, et al: The Human Heart—A Guide to Heart Disease. C.V. Mosby Co., 4th ed. St. Louis, Missouri, 1979

Standards and Guidelines for Cardiopulmonary Resuscitation (CPR) and Emergency Cardiac Care (ECC). JAMA, Vol 244, No 5, pp 453-509, 1980

Symposium on Emergency Nursing. Nurs Clin North Am, Vol 8, No 3, September 1973

Van Meter M, Lavine PG: Reading EKGs correctly. Nursing Books, Intermed Communications, Jenkinstown, Pennsylvania, 1977

Vinsant M, Spence M, Chapell D: A Commonsense Approach to Coronary Care: A Program, 3rd ed. C.V. Mosby Co., St. Louis, Missouri, 1981

Walraven G: Handbook of Emergency Drugs. The Robert J. Brady Co., Bowie, Maryland, 1978

Washington University School of Medicine: Manual of Medical Therapeutics, 23rd ed. Little, Brown & Co., Boston, Massachusetts, 1980

Whipple GH, Peterson M, et al: Acute Coronary Care. Little, Brown & Co., Boston, Massachusetts, 1972

NEUROLOGICAL INJURIES 13

KEY CONCEPTS

This chapter was prepared from lecture content presented to Emergency Department nurses by Louise Queener, R.N., Neurological Nurse Specialist; Susan Foster, R.N., Neurological Nurse Specialist; and Paul Blaylock, M.D., all of the Portland Metropolitan Area, and is designed to provide an understanding of the pathophysiology of head and spinal cord injuries and the ED intervention which is essential in dealing with these patients.

After reading and studying this chapter, you should be able to:

- Explain the rationale for rapid action with a patient with head injuries.
- Describe the categorization of head injuries.
- Outline the steps of immediate evaluation of a patient with head injuries and describe the signs of increased intracranial pressure which might be seen.
- Explain the types, clinical findings, and management of skull fractures.
- Identify the three types of intracranial hemorrhage, their origins and pathophysiology, and the cardinal signs of each.
- Discuss the drugs employed therapeutically in patients with head injuries.
- Outline the initial management of the patient with spinal cord injuries.
- Discuss the complications commonly seen with spinal cord injuries and identify the nursing management considerations.
- Describe the manifestations of spinal cord shock and their pathophysiology.
- Discuss some observations that may be definitive in the unconscious patient who may have cord injuries.

THE HEAD-INJURED PATIENT

The human brain is an extremely delicate and highly complicated organ which is enclosed in a rigid cranial vault formed by the bones of the skull. After trauma, the approach to the neurologically damaged patient requires acting rapidly since maximal brain swelling can occur in 24-36 hours. *Speed is of the essence!* If an unconscious patient is brought to the ED with a simple concussion, he will go on to recovery no matter what is done for him or against him. However, if he has an intracranial hemorrhage, death will certainly occur unless the hemorrhage is properly diagnosed and treatment carried out. Unfortunately, most patients with more serious head injuries develop cerebral edema, and whether they live or die may easily depend on how they are managed initially. The important aspect of a mass lesion such as an intracranial hemorrhage or cerebral edema is brain displacement. The brain can be displaced through the tentorium or through the foramen magnum, and this must be prevented at all costs.

In instances of trauma, especially in vehicular accidents, when there is significant injury to the body, the head is frequently injured as well—in fact, up to 70% of the time. Therefore, when an unconscious patient is brought to the ED, carry out triage first and then a mini-neurologic examination, bearing in mind that cervical spine injury should *always* be suspected in the patient with head injury.

Within the head and neck is a complex variety of structures involving many different organ systems, all closely related anatomically. Injury to the head or neck may damage portions of the central and peripheral nervous systems, upper gastrointestinal tract, lungs and pleura, and musculoskeletal structures. Because of the close proximity of the structures, multiple organ injury is quite common.

Head injuries may be categorized as follows:

Minimal: Fifty percent are from motor vehicle accidents (MVAs), etc., and are seen in the ED for routine check. They are alert, talkative, and probably have mild contusion.

Moderate: Thirty to 40% are closed-head injuries with borderline levels of consciousness, and confusion, and complaining of the head "hurting a little."

Severe: These patients are generally comatose, probably stage 5 coma, are not arousable, and may be decerebrate, decorticate or flaccid.

Cardinal points of *immediate* management for ED personnel receiving a head-injured patient should include:

- The ABCs
  A. Airway
  B. Breathing, being certain the patient is breathing easily and perfusing well. Administer oxygen as the condition indicates. (If patient is hypoxic, ventilation is poor; ischemic hypoxia indicates poor circulation to the brain from poor perfusion.)

C. Cervical spine injury. The cervical spine must be kept immobilized until X-ray films have ruled out damage that could result in serious paralysis for the rest of that patient's life.

- Provision of adequate suction at hand to clear secretions and vomitus
- Observation of the patient for baseline data
- Maintenance of a neurological flow sheet with documentation of vital signs, the LOC (speech, what the patient will awaken to, nonverbal reaction to pain), pupil status, and ability to move extremities (Fig. 13.1)

  A CHANGE IN THE LEVEL OF CONSCIOUSNESS IS THE SINGLE MOST IMPORTANT FACTOR IN THE OBSERVATION OF A PATIENT WITH A HEAD INJURY.

- Cervical spine and skull X-rays.

The *neurological flow sheet* is a valuable tool for documenting changes in status of the head-injured patient but particularly so when monitoring the patient with an *epidural hematoma,* which is a surgically treatable lesion. Usually the patient is unconscious for a short time, then wakens to a *lucid* period during which he starts to complain of headache, and then begins to develop a progressive deepening of conscious level. The patient's blood pressure will go up, a bradycardia may develop, and respirations will become more rapid. Then the ipsilateral (same sided) pupil dilates, because the temporal lobe is now being pushed through the tentorium. It is causing pressure on the third nerve which normally causes constriction of the pupil. As the pressure hits the nerve, the pupil dilates. Right next to the third nerve is the cerebral peduncle which later crosses to the other side so the patient develops a contralateral (opposite side) weakness. As this process continues, the brain stem is pushed across to the other side of the tentorium and the same processes occur; the patient ends up with bilateral fixed pupils and decerebration. Finally, the extremities become flaccid, the brain stem fails, and the patient dies. This deterioration can happen in a matter of minutes to a matter of hours, but the life can be saved if effective intervention occurs *before* brain-stem failure.

As pressure from hemorrhage or edema formation is exerted within the rigid cranial vault, a number of clinical signs are elicited that reflect the body's ability to cope with the increased pressure (compensation) (Table 13.1).

Four major steps can be taken in the ED to reduce intracranial pressure. They are as follows:

Hyperventilation

- Intubate if necessary
- Use bag or ventilator with high oxygen concentration

In a breakdown of brain water compartments, about 1% of the brain is blood (130 cc), about 1% spinal fluid; the rest is fluid within the brain cells. At the normal CO_2 (40 mm Hg), intracranial pressure is below 180 mm. If the PCO_2 is increased to 50 mm Hg, the pressure increases because the blood flow and

Evaluate

airway

first!

OBTAIN BLOOD GASES

NEUROLOGICAL EXAMINATION RECORD

INSTRUCTIONS: Record vital signs in Unit I. If the patient can talk, check (√) one subdivision in Units II, III, and IV. An orientated patient should know his name, age, etc. A moan can be checked as "garbled" speech. If unable to talk, check "none" in Unit III and one block in Unit V. In an "inappropriate" response, the patient is not effective in removing the painful stimulus; when "decerebrate", the extremities reflexly extend and/or hyperpronate. In Unit VI, draw the size and shape of each pupil and (√) for a reaction to light. Under Unit VII, normal strength (4); slight weakness (3); a 50 percent reduction in strength (2); marked weakness and without spontaneous movement (1); total paralysis (0).

(From *J. Trauma*, 8:29, 1968)

UNIT		Time:						
I Vital signs	Blood pressure							
	Pulse							
	Respiration							
	Temperature							
II Conscience and	Oriented							
	Disoriented							
	Restless							
	Combative							
III Speech	Clear							
	Rambling							
	Garbled							
	None							
IV Will awaken to	Name							
	Shaking							
	Light pain							
	Strong pain							
V Non-verbal reaction to pain	Appropriate							
	Inappropriate							
	"Decerebrate"							
	None							
VI Pupils	Size on right							
	Size on left							
	Reacts on right							
	Reacts on left							
VII Ability to move	Right arm							
	Left arm							
	Right leg							
	Left leg							

Figure 13.1. Flow sheet.

blood volume increase since CO_2 is a most potent vasodilator. Carbon dioxide retention will "blow the brain," but if the patient can be well ventilated, the

Table 13.1 Signs and Symptoms of Increased Intracranial Pressure

SIGNS	CHARACTERISTICS, ETC.
1. Headache	Though not uncommon in patients with head trauma, it forewarns nurse to watch closely for other neurologic signs
2. Vomiting	Protracted in nature and often projectile in character
3. *Any* change in the level of consciousness	LOC I: Alert, wakeful, oriented LOC II: Drowsy, apathetic, agitated, confused LOC III: Dulled but responsive to stimuli with appropriate movement, like a drunk person LOC IV: Stuporous (arouses with persistent stimuli) LOC V: Comatose
4. Cushing's triad (makes accurate baseline data essential)	A. Increased respiration (first to rise) B. Increased BP (next to rise—systolic elevates, diastolic drops, pulse pressure widens) C. Decreased pulse (last to alter) becomes full and bounding
5. Pupil changes	Persistent fixation and/or dilatation or unequal pupils means progressive brain damage (papilledema *may* take 24 hr to develop and is not necessarily associated with increased intracranial pressure)
NB (note well)	Lumbar puncture is discouraged in presence of head injury with increased intracranial pressure! An LP can cause brain to descend with swelling and depress medulla into foramen magnum, causing herniation of brain stem. *If* LP is done, nothing larger than a 25-gauge needle should be used to minimize CSF leakage.

CO_2 level will drop, and the blood volume and intracranial pressure will decrease.*

Administration of Steroids

- To stabilize lysosome membrane of cells
- Slow metabolism of brain cells and reduce oxygen requirements
- Reduce swelling

Dexamethasone (Decadron), 10 mg IV and 6 mg q6h or 4 mg q4h, may be given, or methylprednisolone (Solu-Medrol), 30 mg/kg body weight in IV bolus, and then maintenance drip IV, may be given.

---

*Adapted from Bouzarth WF: Trauma at the top. Emergency Medicine, p 74, September 1975

Temperature Control

Maintain normothermic status. Oxygen metabolism increases rapidly if the temperature exceeds 99°. The brain itself utilizes 20% of the total oxygen uptake of the body, and oxygen consumption by the brain is increased 10-15% by elevations in temperature. It is *essential* to control temperature in all serious head injuries.

CNS Level Affected	Respiratory Pattern	LOC	Pupils	Posture	Doll's Eye
Thalamus 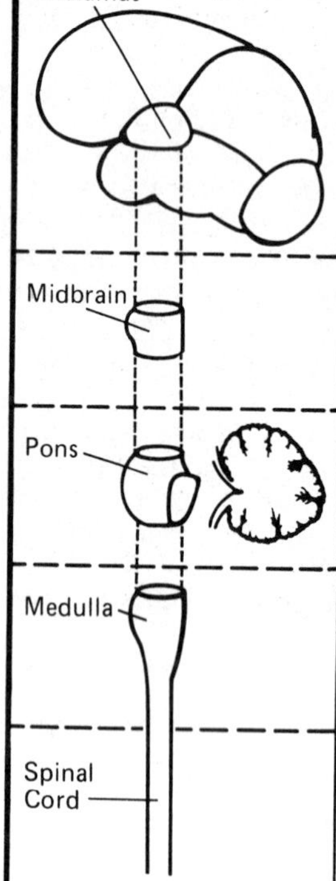	① 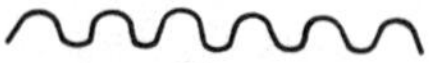 ～～～～～ or ② 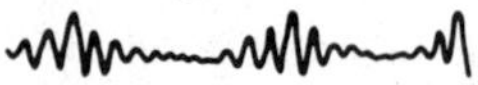 ～v\\\Mw～～\\Mw～～\\	Stupor / Semi-Coma	Small Reactive	Decorticate	—
Midbrain	③ 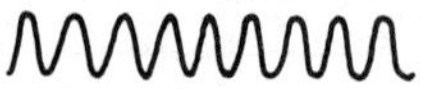 MMMMMM or	Coma	Mid-position Nonreact	Decerebrate	+
Pons	④ 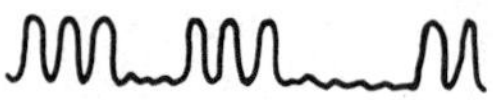 MwMw～M or	Coma	"	Flaccid	+
Medulla	⑤ 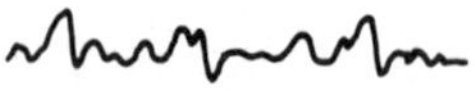 ～w～v～～	Coma	"	Flaccid	+
Spinal Cord	① Normal respiration ② Cheyne-Stokes with decreased response to pain and decreased corneal reflexes				
	③ Neurogenic Hyper-ventilation Not responsive to O_2 and "patterned"				
	④ Biot's respiration with regular periods of hyperventilation and irregular periods of apnea				
	⑤ "Apneustic" respiration with ataxic, gasping, shallow pattern				

Figure 13.2. Clinical signs in the neurologically damaged patient.

Administration of Mannitol (and/or Urea)

This should be given only if a neurosurgeon or neurologist is on the scene. A dosage of 20% mannitol in 500 cc D5/W IV in 30-45 min is administered when it is anticipated that the patient will be taken to the OR in 2 hours or less; mannitol may shrink the brain enough to permit additional bleeding if used too early.

Some practitioners support the theory that massive doses of barbiturates contribute to reduction of ICP; the ED nurse should be familiar with protocols involved in administration and management of the "barbiturate coma;" more specific reference will be found on page 152, Respiratory Failure States.

SUDDEN LOSS OF CONSCIOUSNESS

Sudden loss of consciousness in a neurologically compromised patient is a medical emergency; speed in starting treatment is of utmost importance. The steps to be taken and points of evaluation are as follows (Fig. 13.2):

1. Maintain airway and keep oxygenated.
2. Evaluate respirations:
   - Slow and shallow (barbiturates? alcohol?)
   - Deep and labored (diabetic? Kussmaul?)
   - Cheyne–Stokes (usually CNS structural damage with swelling around mid-brain)
   - Puffing cheek on one side (stroke?)
3. Evaluate level of consciousness.
4. Get all vital signs and temperature. Check every 10 min and *record*. *Constant* status check is essential.
5. Evaluate pupils and eye signs.
6. Evaluate posture and pain responses.
7. *Get history* from whoever accompanies the unconscious patient.
   - Establish LOC baseline prior to loss of consciousness.
   - Determine situation surrounding the accident. This is important but often missed.

     Example: The Emergency Room record says, "Patient fell." It should also state how far the patient fell; what were the circumstances? A fall down steps indicates a bad lesion. A fall on the ice would indicate a bad lesion. If the patient is intoxicated and fell on the floor, it may not necessarily be a bad lesion unless the patient is alcoholic. It should be noted that chronic alcoholics frequently sustain head injuries and may have *chronic* subdural hematomas. Certainly there should be a high index of suspicion with the alcoholic patient.

- Obtain past history of medical problems including allergies and drugs currently being taken on a routine basis, most especially, large doses of aspirin or anticoagulants of any sort.
- Pay particular attention to injured children under the age of 7 or 8 since battered children in that age category have been found to have a very high incidence of chronic subdural hemorrhage.

8. *Use senses of sight, smell, and touch:*

Sight—look *everywhere*

- Battle's sign (blush discoloration behind the ears in the mastoid area) is a strong indication of possible basal skull fracture. It is the extravasation of blood into the mastoid area and usually requires several hours to become evident.
- Needle marks in veins may be a sign of recent drug administration.
- Scarred tongue and lips may indicate seizure disorder.
- Constricted pupils may indicate narcotic use or severe pontine damage.

Smell

- Alcohol ingestion?
- Characteristic heavy sweetish odor of uremia, diabetes, ketoacidosis, kidney failure?
- Fetid odor indicative of bowel obstruction?

Touch

- Is skin hot or cold to touch? Damp?
- Increased temperature with dry skin in an unresponsive patient may be indicative of heat stroke.

9. Keep detailed records of intake and output, placing a Foley catheter.
10. Initiate gastric lavage if ingestion is suspected or if the patient is vomiting (the left nostril is said by some to be larger than the right nostril in approximately 85% of the people).

Repeat: Prevention of complications is accomplished by constant observation and adequate ventilation of the patient while keeping fluid intake and temperature down.

SKULL FRACTURE

The recognition and management of a *basal skull fracture* follows some very definite guidelines. Simple skull fracture by itself may not be a terribly serious injury. Linear fractures of the skull usually require no treatment unless they cross one of the meningeal arteries or one of the venous sinuses, whereas depressed fractures usually require elevation if pressure is being exerted on the dura and brain tissue. Open skull fractures, of course, require extensive cleansing, debriding, and surgical repair, as well as close neurological nursing follow-up and care.

When a severe scalp laceration presents with or without underlying skull fracture, the wound must be carefully evaluated to be certain that the galea is restored to an intact state. The galea is a freely movable "skull cap" of dense, fibrous tissue covering the skull, which helps to absorb the force of external trauma. The movement of the galea helps deflect blows to the skull, frequently causing them to slip off with no more damage than possibly extensive lacerations. Some laboratory studies have shown that without the protection given by the galea, the human skull can be fractured by as little as 40 lb/sq in (psi) of energy, while an intact head with scalp and galea attached requires 425-900 psi to fracture the underlying skull. For this reason, as well as others, every scalp laceration should be carefully evaluated to be certain the galea remains intact.*

X-ray evidence of a basal skull fracture may be positive only 5-10% of the time. (If the patient is a child, films should be taken of the chest and body as well.) The observant EDN should be alert for:

1. Battle's sign (bluish discoloration behind ear in mastoid area)
2. Rhinorrhea or otorrhea (indication of leakage of CSF)
3. Periorbital ecchymosis
4. Blood from external ear canal

Nursing management of the basal skull fracture after assuring a patent airway and adequate ventilation involves close observation and the following steps:

1. Talk straight and firm to the head-injured patient.
2. Avoid disruptions.
3. Restrict fluids. Give only enough IV for medications and maintenance.
4. Antibiotics are indicated whenever there is a break in the dura and should be given as ordered.
5. A head-injured patient in shock has another injury causing the shock. Look further.
6. Listen to the heart, chest, and bowels. Watch for pulmonary edema and paralytic ileus, which are common.
7. Look for movement:
   A. In light coma the normal limb will sink gradually if lifted from the bed.
   B. Symmetrical reflexes are important. Unilateral signs are indications for considering surgical intervention and must be reported immediately.
8. Record plus and/or minus on both sides for movements and reflexes.
9. *Never* leave an unconscious patient alone; X-ray studies should be done in the ED, and if the patient must be taken to X-ray, a nurse should accompany.

---

*Adapted from Jackson FE: The Pathophysiology of Head Injuries. CIBA Clinical Symposia, Vol 18, No 3, CIBA Corporation, 1966

10. Position the patient with the head to the side and slightly elevated. Never use the Trendelenburg position in a head-injured patient even if shock develops. Elevate legs for shock.

11. A conscious, head-injured patient with leaking CSF should be warned *not* to blow nose. (In rhinorrhea, dextro-stix may confirm presence of CSF.)

12. If suctioning is required, great caution must be exercised.

INTRACRANIAL HEMORRHAGE

Intracranial hemorrhage is a serious complication of head injury and may terminate fatally. Since the cranium is a closed rigid vault containing the brain, blood, and spinal fluid, bleeding within this rigid bony skull will result in increased intracranial pressure, which may cause local or generalized pressure on the brain itself. Varying types of neurologic deficit will be seen and progressive loss of consciousness is common to all.

Epidural Hematoma

This extradural blood tumor is:

- Most commonly caused by a tear in the middle meningeal *artery*.
- Usually happens *fast* with arterial bleed.
- Carries a mortality variously estimated at between 50% and 85%.
- Typical history is a severe blow to side of head, causing momentary unconsciousness, followed by a so-called "lucid interval" and then a progressively stuporous state with deterioration of vital signs.

Subdural Hematoma

Characteristics of the hemorrhage into subdural space, between dura and arachnoid are:

- *Venous* bleed which develops *slower* than an epidural.
- A mortality of between 65% and 70%.
- Usually loss of consciousness at time of injury, with a subsequent return to consciousness.

Subarachnoid Hemorrhage

This is the most common type of intracranial hemorrhage due to trauma. It is:

- Most commonly caused by cerebral artery aneurysm, trauma, and arteriovenous fistula and is frequently seen in the 30- to 40-year age group with hypertension.

- Managed without an operation unless a specific lesion is identified.
- Likely to manifest such cardinal signs and symptoms as headache or sudden onset and nuchal rigidity from bleeding into the subarachnoid space; resultant irritation of the meninges reflexly causes stiffness of the neck. Lumbar puncture will reveal grossly bloody fluid.

Rapid surgical intervention is indicated in cases of intracranial hemorrhage with increased intracranial pressure depressing the vital centers of the brain. Patients with major head injuries may survive with minimal aftereffects if there is early recognition and intervention. Too often, however, seemingly minor head trauma is treated lightly and as a result, not infrequently, leads to permanent damage that could have been prevented.

NURSING MANAGEMENT GUIDELINES AFTER ESTABLISHMENT OF AIRWAY

1. Any deterioration in the level of consciousness is a neurosurgical emergency.
2. Decerebrate posturing should alert the EDN to watch for respiratory distress, since it indicates secondary brain-stem damage.
3. Flaccid posture has a 20% association with neck injury. *Protect* the patient's position and order lateral cervical spine films (C_1 to C_7) *before* skull films are taken. C_5 to C_6 and C_6 to C_7 are usually involved in whiplash deceleration trauma.
4. The unconscious patient can be expected to have retrograde amnesia (RGA) or memory loss from the time of injury forward, to a degree. However, loss of memories established prior to trauma is an indication of more serious damage to the memory areas of the cerebrum and the brain in general. Loss or return of memory should be carefully documented.
5. A patient who has lost consciousness *should* be admitted for 24-hour observation.
6. Arterial Blood Gases (ABGs) and WBC should always be done on a head-injured patient with serious damage. The higher the white count, the greater the magnitude of the injury. PaO_2 and PCO_2 values are essential in the management of the patient.
7. Patients with concussion not serious enough to warrant admission must be turned over to family members who are carefully instructed in simple terms for danger signs to observe. A printed instruction sheet should be sent home with the family, outlining the following points as danger signs requiring further medical attention:
   A. Check the LOC and arousability: wake every 2-3 hours and ask questions for appropriate response
   B. *Persistent* or projectile vomiting
   C. Lateralizing weakness or hemiparesis (one-sided weakness)

  D. Respiratory difficulty
  E. Seizure activity
  F. Change in pupil size or inequality of pupils
8. Postconcussion syndrome must be explained carefully and again in simple terms to patients and their families.
  A. There will probably be a headache.
  B. There may be some difficulty in concentration.
  C. There may be some transient personality changes, *i.e.,* irritability, lack of motivation, withdrawal, aggressive behavior.
  D. There may be blurred vision which should resolve in several days.
9. Remember to talk back calmly and firmly to the loud, abusive patient and realize that this behavior is the effect of the injury.
10. Remember that the ideal person to provide reliable baselines of information on a head-injured child is the child's mother, who is more capable of identifying the norms for *her* child.
11. Seizures may occur following a head injury. If a patient has seizures, it is important to note the beginning area (such as the right arm), the duration of the seizure, and whether other areas of the body are involved. While the patient is convulsing, it is essential to maintain the airway and protect from further injury.

Drugs used in head injuries should be employed only for control of symptoms and never used indiscriminately. Some of the frequent usages and comparatively large pharmacologic dosages are as follows:

1. Cerebral edema
  A. Dexamethasone (Decadron) to prevent and reduce cerebral edema; 10 mg IV initial dose and 6 mg q6h or 4 mg q4h
  B. Methylprednisolone (Solu-Medrol) to prevent and reduce cerebral edema; 30 mg/kg body weight, IV bolus, followed by maintenance IV drip
  C. Mannitol, 20% given as an osmotic diuretic in 500 cc of D5/W in 35-45 min
2. Seizures
  A. Diazepam (Valium), 5-10 mg IV every 5-10 min if necessary for a total dose of 0.5 mg/kg (watch for depressed respirations and be ready for respiratory arrest)
  B. Phenobarbitol, 1.5-2 grains IM q4-6h
  C. Phenobarbitol for children, 5 mg/kg every 20 min $\times$ 2
3. Infection
  A. Ampicillin, used in most basal skull fractures and open wounds since most organisms (staph, strep, etc.) are gram positive
  B. Keflin, given when penicillin allergy exists
  C. Chloromycetin, most effective in crossing brain-blood barrier.
4. Tetanus—Diphtheria/Tetanus Booster; 0.5 cc IM

5. Analgesia (NB: use of analgesia is seldom appropriate in the ED)
    A. Codeine, 30 mg, is drug of choice for pain because it does not increase intracranial pressure or depress respirations
    B. Acetominophen (Tylenol) in lieu of acetylsalicylic acid (aspirin)
    C. Propoxyphene with Acetominophen (Darvocet N) which contains no aspirin
6. 2.5% glucose in 0.45 normal saline solution for IV administration, because of its isotonicity,* running TKO unless shock develops.

SPINAL CORD INJURY

Spinal cord injury is always suspect in the traumatized patient and especially one who has suffered head injury, regardless of the level of consciousness on arrival in the ED. Spinal cord injuries occur in motor vehicle accidents (MVAs), gunshot and knifing wounds, diving accidents, falls, and deceleration. It is interesting to note that the average age of the quadriplegic is 26 years. In quadriplegia the damage is to C_5 and C_6, while in the paraplegic the damage is to T_{11} and T_{12}. There are between 5,000 and 10,000 new occurrences of cord injury per year with approximately 125,000 persons so injured in the United States at the present time.

As with cardiopulmonary resuscitation, there are ABCs of management in patients who have head injuries or are heavily traumatized.

A. Airway. If the patient suspected of having a neck injury must be placed in a semiprone position, *turn the patient as a unit,* keeping the head in its original position.

   The laryngoscope is *contraindicated* for any patient who has been in an MVA or who has fallen any distance because there is a 10% chance that patient has a broken neck. The use of a laryngoscope will probably inflict a neurologic deficit that was not there to begin with. The flexible fiberoptic bronchoscope can be used by slipping the endotracheal tube over it and down into place; blind nasal intubation can be done; or the esophageal airway can be used.

B. Bleeding. Generally controlled by direct pressure.

C. Spinal Cord Injury. Again, any unconscious patient who has suffered a fall or been involved in a vehicular accident must be considered to have a spinal fracture until proved otherwise, and *all* precautions must be taken to prevent irreparable damage.

---

*Roberts JR: Pathophysiology, Diagnosis and Treatment of Head Trauma. Priorities in Multiple Trauma, TEM Vol 1, No 1, Rockville, Maryland, May 1979

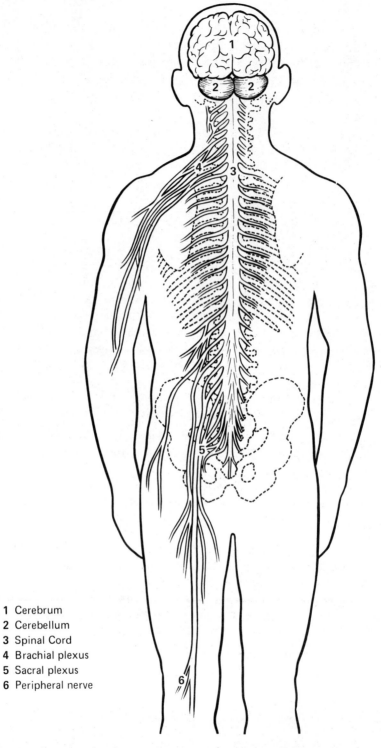

1 Cerebrum
2 Cerebellum
3 Spinal Cord
4 Brachial plexus
5 Sacral plexus
6 Peripheral nerve

Figure 13.3. The central nervous system. Messages to and from the brain travel along spinal cord and nerves seen branching off cord. (Reprinted from The Human Body with permission of Ethicon, Inc., Somerville, New Jersey)

THE SPINAL CORD

The spinal cord is composed of CNS tissue having both gray and white matter, just as the brain does, and lies within a body casing, just as the brain does. The cord is the pathway by which everything goes to and from the brain. All reflexes, all the integration for the autonomic nervous system, and all motor and sensory effectors pass through the cord (Figs. 13.3 and 13.4). Remember also that the neurons of the CNS do not regenerate.

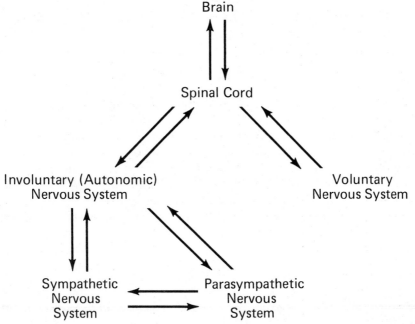

Figure 13.4. Flow of nerve impulses. (Reprinted from The Human Body with permission of Ethicon, Inc., Somerville, New Jersey)

The subarachnoid space surrounds the spinal cord and bathes it in cerebrospinal fluid. The space itself ends at the second sacral vertebra and the cord ends at L_2. Lumbar puncture is done at L_4 or L_5 below the termination of the spinal cord. Segments of the cord itself are usually about two positions higher than the vertebrae.

The main tracts in the spinal cord (Fig. 13.5) are:

1. Dorsal spinothalamic tract (through the spine to the thalamus) mediates:
   - Position
   - Deep pressure or touch
   - Vibration
2. Lateral spinothalamic tract mediates:
   - Pain
   - Temperature
3. Ventral spinothalamic tract mediates:
   - Light touch (stroke skin)

4. Lateral corticospinal track (80% of all motor fibers run through this tract)
5. Ventral corticospinal tract (Other 20% of motor fibers run through this tract)

THE SPINAL COLUMN

The spine is divided into five sections:

1. Cervical spine (neck), 7 vertebrae
2. Thoracic spine (upper back), 12 vertebrae (articulate with ribs)
3. Lumbar spine (lower back), 5 vertebrae
4. Sacral spine (part of the pelvis), 5 vertebrae (fused to form sacrum)
5. Coccygeal spine (coccyx, or tail bone), 4 vertebrae

The front part of each vertebra is a round solid bone. The back part of each vertebra is an arch open toward the inside. This series of arches forms a tunnel that runs the length of the spine and is called the spinal canal, which encloses the spinal cord. The vertebrae are separated from one another by cartilaginous disks, which act as cushions between the bones. The disks allow some motion, such as turning the head, bending the trunk forward or backward, and leaning it to either side, but they also limit motion of the vertebrae so that the spinal cord will not be injured. Where a fracture of the spine exists, full protection of the spinal cord is lost (Fig. 13.5).

SPINAL CORD DAMAGE

When spinal trauma is sustained, several systemic changes may occur, depending on the extent of damage. The first signs and symptoms may include such sensory changes as tingling and numbness followed by weakness or total paralysis distal to the level of injury. Since the greatest area of flexion and extension ability is found between $C_4 - C_5$ and $C_5 - C_6$, these are the areas where most cervical injuries are seen (Fig. 13.6).

Respiration may be seriously affected by damage to the phrenic nerve, which arises from C_3, C_4 (at shoulder level), and C_5. If there is an ascending cervical lesion (local edema secondary to the trauma), the respirations must be carefully watched for increasing involvement. The vital capacity of an individual can be reduced by as much as *one-fourth* to *one-half of normal*. The quality of respiration rate and pattern, therefore, must be carefully monitored.

Circulation may be seriously compromised without innervation of the autonomic nervous system secondary to the cord trauma, and hypotension may develop rapidly. The patient's legs should be elevated and atropine may have to be given for ensuing bradycardia.

Normal capillary pressure is 30 mm on the arterial side, decreasing to 15 mm on the venous side. When pooling occurs in capillary beds with vasodilation, the capillary pressure drops; decubitus ulcers begin to form when surface pressure exceeds capillary pressure. Therefore, careful management at the

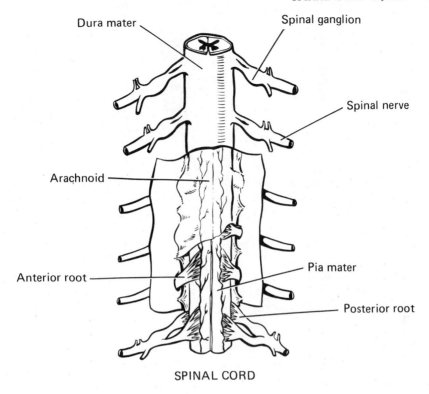

SPINAL CORD

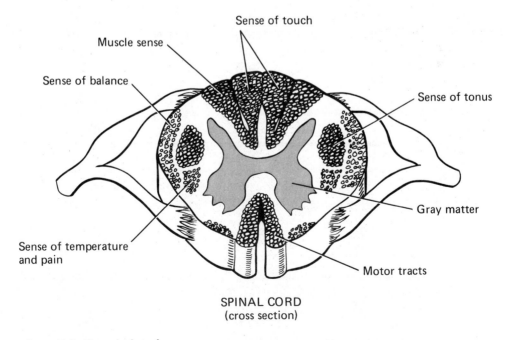

SPINAL CORD
(cross section)

Figure 13.5. The spinal cord.

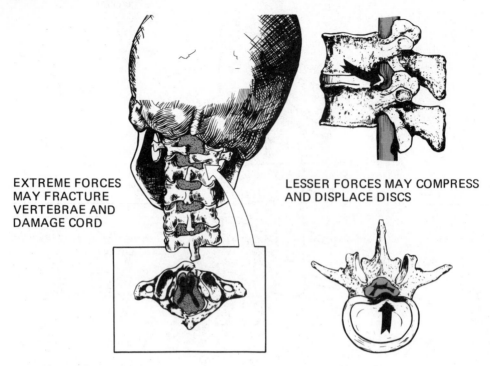

EXTREME FORCES MAY FRACTURE VERTEBRAE AND DAMAGE CORD

LESSER FORCES MAY COMPRESS AND DISPLACE DISCS

Figure 13.6. Spinal cord injury.

outset with spinal cord injury is an essential nursing responsibility, avoiding pressure points, keeping the patient turned frequently, and administering careful and thorough skin care.

Since the autonomic nervous system innervates smooth muscle and all the viscera, a problem with gastric dilatation and paralytic ileus must be anticipated. A nasogastric tube should be placed as soon as possible to decompress stomach distention and eliminate the hazard of vomiting and aspiration. A Foley bladder catheter should also be inserted and attached to a closed drainage and irrigation system. Scrupulous records must be kept on intake and output.

MANAGEMENT OF SPINAL CORD INJURY

1. Cardinal goal is to minimize movement and immobilize spinal column to prevent further damage to cord or nerve roots.
2. Stabilize vital processes—ABCs (airway, breathing, cervical spine).
3. Do *not* move patient off backboard until the physician is present and has done an initial evaluation.
4. Portable X-ray films are indicated with visualization of all 7 cervical vertebrae unless the physician insists films be done in the X-ray department. *Always* accompany and stay with the patient, and *never* assume anyone else will be responsible for keeping that patient immobilized!
5. Stabilize and support the head and neck at all times if cervical spine frac-

tures are suspected. Sandbags serve only to stabilize *unconscious* patients. The forehead must be kept down, and head traction is indicated, holding traction on the chin and occipital area of the head. *Hold* the traction. This could prevent paralysis for the rest of that patient's life. If necessary, use wide adhesive across the patient's forehead and tape him flat to the stretcher or use a short backboard in order to log-roll if necessary. Cervical collars are of little value in immobilizing the head unless they are the rigid, padded metal type or the rigid bi-valved foam collars of the "Philadelphia collar" variety.

6. Gardner-Wells or Crutchfield-type tongs are the *only* dependable skeletal traction for actually providing the necessary degree of traction and immobilization and are inserted into the outer table of the skull under local anesthesia. This can and should be performed in the ED before any further movement is attempted.

7. Initiate IV line.

8. Perform nasogastric intubation and connect to low intermittent suction.

9. Place Foley catheter with calibrated closed drainage unit.

SPINAL CORD SHOCK

Spinal cord shock is the result of sudden loss of continuity between the spinal cord and the higher nerve centers, with complete motor, sensory, and sphincter paralysis, as well as absence of reflexes and all autonomic nervous system function below the lesion. This can set in from the first few hours after trauma to three weeks post trauma, and the management involves maintenance of the body defenses and vital functions until the shock state subsides and the system has recovered.

Spinal cord shock can result in early respiratory arrest, cardiac arrest, and pulmonary embolus, and may later terminate in renal failure, septicemia, and dysreflexia (inappropriate response of the autonomic nervous system affecting the bladder).

All spinal cord injuries carry some degree of spinal cord shock (neurogenic shock) which may develop and last from hours to several weeks, and ED personnel must be prepared to support vital functions involved in the shock process and to understand the support system's rationale. Scrupulous technique must be used to prevent introducing infection into the patient, who will be a potential paralysis victim.

If a patient is admitted to the ED in an *unconscious state* following possible spinal cord damage, there are some valuable observations to be made that would tend to confirm a diagnosis of cord injury. They are included here for nursing alerts as follows:*

1. The lower extremities may be flaccid and areflexive, including the rectal sphincter, which *must* be examined.

---

*Adapted from Bouzarth WF: Trauma at the top. Emergency Medicine, p 82, September 1975

2. Respirations may be diaphragmatic in character.
3. The forearms may be flexed over the chest. This is one of the characteristic positions of a C_6 cord localization. The hands are half closed and are over the chest; straighten them out, and they'll come right back up. This is often overlooked.
4. Pain above the nipple line (but not below) will elicit a grimace from the patient if the injury is at the C_6 level.
5. Hypotension without other signs of shock may be seen initially, with an average systolic BP of about 70-80 mm. The pulse rate is usually slow since head-injured and cord-injured patients tend to bradycardia rather than tachycardia.
6. Priapism may be present, quite obviously in children but less so in adults.

Preparation for surgical intervention should be anticipated if any of the following are found:

- A progressive neurological deficit
- Bony fragments present in the spinal cord on X-ray film
- The presence of CSF block
- Locked facets, preventing reduction of the fracture

REVIEW

1. List the three categories of head injuries and their characteristic findings.
2. List the general guidelines for management of the head-injured patient.
3. Identify five cardinal signs of increased intracranial pressure.
4. List four major steps which can be taken in the ED to reduce intracranial pressure in the severely head-injured patient.
5. List the essential points of evaluation in the initial assessment of the unconscious patient.
6. Identify two laboratory studies indicated in the seriously head-injured patient and explain the rationale for each.
7. What instructions should be given to a patient being sent home following head trauma?
8. What is the neurosurgical fluid of choice for IV administration?
9. What is the analgesia of choice in the head-injured patient with significant pain?
10. Describe the pathophysiology of epidural, subdural, and subarachnoid hemorrhages.
11. List six circumstances of injury that would give a high index of suspicion for spinal cord damage.
12. Describe the functions of the spinal cord.

13. Identify the five main tracts of the spinal cord and the areas they account for.

14. List three options for airway management in the unconscious patient with a probable C-spine fracture.

15. Where does the spinal cord end?

16. Where is a lumber puncture done?

17. List three functions of the autonomic nervous system and how it relates to hypotension in the neurologically traumatized patient.

18. List at least six major points to be remembered in the management of spinal cord injuries.

19. Define spinal cord shock and the management of the patient.

20. What tube placements are indicated in a patient with spinal cord injury or shock and why?

21. Identify six findings that could be indicative of a cord injury in an unconscious patient who is unable to communicate verbally.

BIBLIOGRAPHY

Abramson N, Safar P: Barbiturate therapy following cardiac arrest. Controversies in Emergency Medicine. TEM, Vol 3, No 2, pp 45-55, July 1981

Advanced Trauma Life Support (ATLS) Course Manual. ACS, Chicago, 1981

Barber JM, Dillman PA: Emergency Patient Care. Reston Publishing Co., Reston, Virginia, 1981

Buckingham WB, Sparberg M, Brandfonbrener M: A Primer of Clinical Diagnosis, 2nd ed. Harper & Row, New York, 1979

Budassi SA, Barber JM: Emergency Nursing: Principles and Practice. C.V. Mosby Co., St. Louis, Missouri, 1981

Cain HD: Flint's Manual on Emergency Treatment and Management. C.V. Mosby Co., St. Louis, Missouri, 1980

Colohan DP: Emergency Management of Cervical-Spine Injuries (Emergency Physician Series). Abbott Laboratories, Chicago, 1977

Committee on Injuries, American Academy of Orthopaedic Surgeons: Emergency Care and Transportation of the Sick and Injured, 3rd ed. George Banta Co., Menasha, Wisconsin, 1981

Coping with neurologic problems proficiently: Nursing Skillbook. Intermed Communications, Inc., Horsham, Pennsylvania, Nursing 79 Books

Cosgriff JH, Anderson DL: The Practice of Emergency Nursing. J.B. Lippincott Co., Philadelphia, Pennsylvania, 1975

DeGowin E., DeGowin R: Bedside Diagnostic Examination: A Comprehensive Pocket Textbook. Macmillan Co., New York, 1981

Grant H, Murray R: Emergency Care, 3rd ed. Robert J. Brady Co., Bowie, Maryland, 1982

Haywood R: Management of Acute Head Injuries. C.V. Mosby Co., St. Louis, Missouri, 1980

Jackson FE: The Pathophysiology of Head Injuries. Clin Symp, Vol 18, No 3, 1966

Jackson FE: The Treatment of Head Injuries. Clin Symp, Vol 19, No 1, 1967

Kunkel J, Wiley J: Acute head injury: What to do when . . . and why. Nursing 79, Vol 9, No 3, pp 22-33, March 1979

Lamphier TA, Von Mizell, Mayer R: Manual of Routine Orders for Medical and Surgical Emergencies. Warren H. Green, St. Louis, Missouri, 1974

Millikan CH: Coma—Evaluating Depth of Consciousness. Patient Care, pp 127-144, September 1981

Nelson JR: The Comatose Patient. *In* The Management of Medical Emergencies, McGraw-Hill, New York, 1969

Start With A Good Coma Scale. Emergency Medicine, pp 199-200, March 1978

Todd M, Shapiro H: Barbiturate therapy following cardiac arrest: A call for caution. Controversies in Emergency Medicine, TEM, Vol 3, No 2, pp 57-67, July 1981

US Public Health Service, DHEW: Physicians in Hospital Emergency Departments. Bethesda: Health Services and Mental Health Administration, Division of Emergency Health Services, 1971

Warner C: Emergency Care: Assessment and Intervention. 2nd ed. C.V. Mosby Co., St. Louis, Missouri, 1978

SHOCK   14

KEY CONCEPTS

The aim of this chapter is to promote an understanding of the factors governing shock and the pathophysiology involved, with guidelines for intervention and management, based on lecture material presented to emergency nurses by John Schriver, M.D., Portland, Ore., and on material excerpted from "Shock, Its Definition, Classification, Diagnosis, Pathophysiology, Monitoring and Treatment," by Robert F. Wilson, M.D., and used with permission of Dr. Wilson and the Upjohn Company, as well as lecture content presented by Dr. Wilson at the 1977 Colorado ACEP Keystone Conference.

After reading and studying this chapter, you should be able to:

- Recognize the patient who is a candidate for developing shock and anticipate subsequent problems
- Understand the manifestations of inadequate tissue perfusion.
- Classify the types of shock and discuss the management concepts as well as the monitoring parameters.
- Describe the fluid challenge and the procedure to be followed.
- Outline the guidelines of nursing management to be acknowledged in caring for the shock victim.
- Discuss autotransfusion and MAST trousers as adjuncts in early shock management.

Definition

Shock may be defined in simple, straightforward terms as the inadequate perfusion of body tissues, or *perfusion failure*.

FACTORS GOVERNING SHOCK

The maintenance of an adequate circulating blood volume that provides adequate tissue perfusion is governed by three factors (Fig. 14.1).

- Cardiac output
- Plasma volume
- Peripheral vascular resistance

It follows, then, that any condition which significantly alters any one of these three factors can precipitate inadequate tissue perfusion and incipient shock unless the deficit is corrected. For this reason, emergency personnel should evaluate patients for potential problems, identifying shock *candidates,* and anticipating their needs before the shock state becomes an accomplished fact.

It is logical to anticipate at least altered perfusion in:

1. Hypoxia or anoxia
2. Massive trauma with hemorrhage and extensive tissue damage.
3. Cardiac decompensation with decreased cardiac output
4. Anaphylaxis
5. Severe infections

Manifestations of Inadequate Tissue Perfusion

Inadequate tissue perfusion, for whatever reason, will manifest itself with:

1. Altered mental status
2. Arterial hypotension (the degree varying with the patient)
3. Decreased urinary output
4. Metabolic acidosis

Metabolic Acidosis in Shock

When the tissues are deprived of adequate oxygen, anaerobic metabolism results, with a rise in the serum lactate from a normal level of 1.5 to 2 mEq/liter to a lactacidemia of up to 7-12 mEq/liter at the higher levels, causing a metabolic acidosis. Increased blood lactate is seen under other circumstances such as:

- Spontaneous lactic acidosis following violent exercise and in the postictal state
- Hyperventilation
- Excessive ethanol ingestion
- Glycogen storage disease
- Leukemia

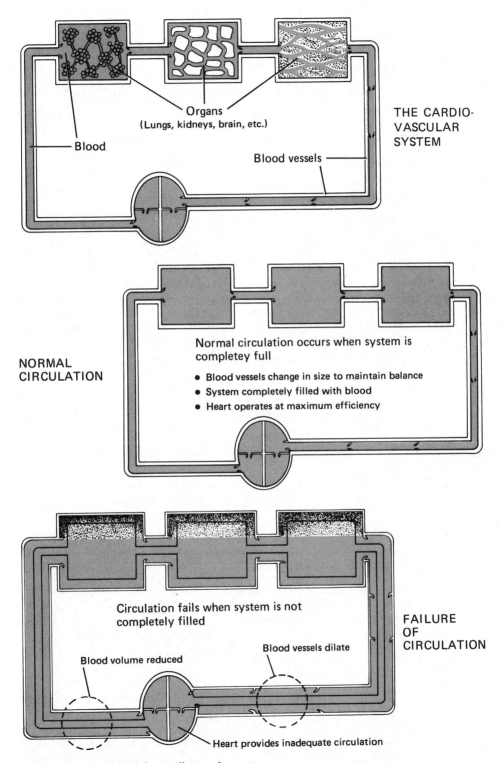

Figure 14.1. Shock and the cardiovascular system.

Criteria for Incipient Shock

A diagnosis of *incipient* shock, then, can safely be made if any *two* of these parameters are observed:

1. Altered mental status (frequently the first indication of poor perfusion and hypoxia, manifested usually with confusion and irritability)
2. Systolic blood pressure of less than 80 mm Hg with narrowing pulse pressure
3. Urinary output of less than 25 ml/hr
4. Metabolic acidosis (lactacidemia)

The blood pressure may be considered to consist of three parts: diastolic pressure, which correlates with the amount of vasoconstriction present; pulse pressure (the difference between the systolic and diastolic pressures), which is primarily related to stroke volume and to the rigidity of the aorta and its larger branches; and systolic pressure, which is determined by a combination of these factors.

Pulse pressure is the most important because it provides some indication of whether the stroke volume is increasing or decreasing. Changes in pulse pressure often correlate quite well with changes in stroke volume. For example, if a patient's blood pressure changes from 120/80 to 120/100, it is likely that the stroke volume has decreased by 40% to 60%.*

CLASSIFICATIONS OF SHOCK

Shock has been classified and reclassified variously by many knowledgeable physiologists, clinicians, and scientists. For these purposes, shock is classified as simply as possible:

1. Hypovolemic (the most common type, seen in 60-70% of shock victims not having enough circulating blood volume) shock results from hemorrhage, burns, and electrolyte imbalances.
2. Cardiogenic shock results from acute myocardial infarctions, cardiac failure, and arrhythmias.
3. Distributive shock results from sepsis with marked vasodilation, vasoconstriction, barbiturate intoxication with vasodilatation, CNS injury with vasodilatation secondary to autonomic nervous system damage, and anaphylaxis.
4. Obstructive shock seen with cardiac tamponade, pulmonary thromboembolus, and dissecting aneurysm.

---

*Wilson R: Shock, Its Definition, Classification, Diagnosis, Pathophysiology, Monitoring and Treatment. *From* a Manual of Practices and Techniques in Critical Care Medicine, The Upjohn Co., p 9, 1976

SHOCK MANAGEMENT

The basic concepts of management apply to *all* types of shock and involve bedside monitoring of as many of the following parameters as possible:

1. Arterial blood pressure
   A. Arterial catheter with pressure transducer or
   B. Sphygmomanometer and Doppler flow meter
2. Urinary output. (Foley catheter with closed one-way drainage and calibrated collection bag.)
3. Central venous pressure
4. Pulmonary artery pressure (Swan-Ganz catheter) and pulmonary wedge pressure (PWP)
5. Laboratory evaluations (serial)
   A. Arterial blood gases
   B. Arterial blood lactate
   C. Hematocrit, electrolytes, BUN, glucose
   D. Plasma osmolarity and colloid osmotic pressure
   E. Coagulation panel

The basic management options available for support (except in anaphylaxis and pulmonary thromboembolus) include:

1. Oxygen with mechanical ventilation if necessary
2. Supine position with legs elevated
3. Pneumatic anti-shock garment
4. Volume replacement (with fluid challenge if indicated)
5. Steroids given early and in massive doses
6. Catecholamines (epinephrine, dopamine, norepinephrine, etc.)
7. Surgical procedures
8. Antibiotics
9. Intensive nursing care with all

THE FLUID CHALLENGE*

The fluid challenge, or the technique of volume loading, has been described by Starchuk, Weil, and Shubin at the University of Southern California Shock Research Unit and involves monitoring of clinical and hemodynamic parameters for objective assessment of the beneficial effects of infusion and for identification of adverse responses. According to their literature, there is *only one* indication for volume loading, namely, *hypovolemic.* However, this includes not only *absolute hypovolemia* but also *relative hypovolemia.* Absolute hypovolemia follows endogenous or exogenous loss of blood, fluid, and/or electrolytes. In cases of relative hypovolemia, the total intravascular volume may be normal or near normal but the capacity of the intravascular space is expanded. This, for instance, is the case after barbiturate intoxication

---

*Condensed from Starchuk E, Weil M, Shubin H: Fluid Challenge. *From* the Shock Research Unit, Center for the Critically Ill, Hollywood Presbyterian Medical Center, Los Angeles, California

or peritonitis. Temporary expansion of the intravascular volume may restore effective circulation.

The method of fluid challenge is as follows:

1. Determination of the initial CVP with a CVP line advanced from the internal jugular or the subclavian vein into the superior vena cava.
2. Selection of the fluid aliquot (specific portion). "The type of fluid used for challenge is contingent upon the nature of the defect. However, whole blood, washed red blood cells, crystalloid solution, or 5% albumin are commonly selected." Baseline clinical examinations form a basis for the judgment that underlies selection of the fluids to be administered. The technique involves administration of either 50, 100, or 200 ml of fluid over a period of 10 minutes. The fluid should be infused through *either* a peripheral or central venous route but *not* through the same catheter which is used for monitoring the effects of the fluid challenge.
3. The selected aliquot of fluid is infused over a 10-minute period.
4. The central venous pressure (CVP) is remeasured.
   A. If the CVP has increased 2 torr (mm Hg) or less, the infusion may be repeated over another 10 minutes.
   B. If the pressure exceeds 2 but is 5 cm or less, the fluid challenge is interrupted for a 10-minute wait period. At the end of this 10-minute wait period, the pressure is again evaluated.
   C. If CVP has declined to within 2 torr of the value prior to that period of challenge, the fluid challenge is resumed.
   D. However, if at any time the CVP increases by more than 5 torr during any one challenge or fails to return to within 2 torr after a 10-minute wait, the challenge is regarded as completed because the patient's cardiac competence is such that additional volumes would be likely to cause cardiac failure and pulmonary edema.

NURSING MANAGEMENT AND UNDERSTANDING SHOCK

Effective nursing management of the patient in shock or incipient shock depends on an understanding of the causes, monitoring techniques, and appropriate drug therapy as well as other supportive measures employed in the treatment.

HYPOVOLEMIC SHOCK

Hypovolemic shock (60%-70% of shock victims) is caused by the decrease in the intravascular volume relative to the vascular capacity, and is generally associated with the blood volume deficit of at least 15%-25%, and an even larger interstitial deficit. Although shock may follow trauma without coexisting hypovolemia, inadequate administration of fluid is the most frequent cause of its persistence.

In previously normal patients, the systolic pressure is often maintained relatively well until a blood volume deficit of at least 15%-25% has developed, but blood volume *loss* must be differentiated from blood volume *deficit*. If a patient *lost* 1500 ml of blood in 1 hour, about 400-600 ml of fluid might move from the interstitial space into the vascular space to partially correct the hypovolemia, thus, the actual blood volume *deficit* at the end of an hour might be only 900-1100 ml.

And again, in evaluating the patient with head injuries, look elsewhere for the cause of shock and maintain a high index of suspicion for occult bleeding.

MONITORING PARAMETERS

Close bedside monitoring of the shock patient is essential, noting and recording changes in mentation, pulse pressure, and skin changes, which will be a much better indication of blood flow and effective perfusion than systolic pressure alone.

Arterial Pressure

Arterial blood pressure may be difficult to obtain using the standard sphygmomanometer in patients with severe vasoconstriction and/or greatly reduced stroke volume. The most accurate arterial blood pressure reading can be obtained with a Doppler flow meter, which can provide accurate systolic pressure reading long after the sounds of Korotkoff are no longer audible.

Urine Output

Urine output is an extremely important measurement; a sudden decrease in renal blood flow or pressure will promptly result in a reduction of urine output; output may fall long before other signs of impaired issue perfusion become evident.

Output must be scrupulously monitored because it plays such an extremely significant role in evaluating the patient's status. Standard IV tubing may be connected to the Foley catheter and arranged to allow observation of the urine "drop by drop" into a closed collection system. With such tubing, about 15 drops usually equal 1 ml, thus it is possible to estimate urine output on a minute-to-minute basis. Obviously, this method will indicate changes in renal perfusion much sooner than an hourly record.

Urine should be recorded for hourly output, sodium concentration, and/or osmolality.

Acid-Base Status

Blood lactate determinations may be extremely helpful as an indicator of progress and prognosis. In the early phases of metabolic acidosis the acid-base abnormality can often be corrected by improving tissue perfusion. Later, however, sodium bicarbonate may be necessary, particularly if the arterial pH falls below 7.2. If the metabolic acidosis continues to progress, the amount of bicarbonate needed for correction increases almost geometrically.

If a combined metabolic and respiratory acidosis is allowed to develop, the chances for ultimate survival become extremely poor, even if the pH can later be restored to normal.

Serial arterial blood gases and electrolyte studies are necessary to monitor acid-base and blood lactate status, with sodium bicarbonate administered accordingly, as well as to correct electrolyte abnormalities, especially potassium and calcium.

DRUG THERAPY

Oxygen

Patients in shock or incipient shock should be given high flow oxygen during the initial 4-6 hours of resuscitation to maintain an arterial PaO_2 of at least 80 mm Hg. Oxygenating the tissues is the primary concern, and if possible, 100% oxygen should be given by mask (especially if the patient is cold, clammy, cyanotic, or if the PaO_2 is less than 80 mm Hg) and by endotracheal tube and ventilating unit if there is evidence of myocardial ischemia, and/or inadequate tidal volume, or minute ventilation. Liter flow and % of O_2 should be determined by method of administration.

Later, after the patient's cardiovascular status has been stabilized, concern can be directed to any potential pulmonary problems that may result from prolonged inhalation of concentrations of oxygen greater than 40%-60%.

Fluids

Fluids are administered according to the general clinical evaluation of the patient's status, as well as the results of the fluid challenge, with enough fluids given to correct hypovolemia without creating a circulatory overload. Pulmonary wedge pressure readings (PWP) are important if there is an acute myocardial infarction, sepsis, or respiratory failure.

Inotropic Drugs

Digoxin (Lanoxin) given when shock is accompanied by heart failure
Dopamine given to keep the mean arterial blood pressure high enough to perfuse heart, brain, and kidneys
Epinephrine given if dopamine is inefficient and the heart is not too irritable
Isoproterenol (Isuprel) given if the pulse rate is less than 110 and there is no myocardial ischemia
Glucagon occasionally given to help increase contractility

Corticosteroids

Physiological doses of steroids are considered by most to be beneficial although the use of pharmacological doses remains controversial.

Vasopressors

Consider vasopressors as potentially lethal drugs and give only as a temporary measure when there appears to be no other rapidly effective method of restoring adequate coronary or cerebral blood flow in patients who may have severe coronary or cerebral atherosclerotic narrowing.

Vasoconstrictor drugs should not be given to hypovolemic patients except, perhaps, very transiently (while other treatment is being initiated) to maintain coronary perfusion in the elderly or in those who may have marginal coronary artery circulation.

Diuretics

The most effective method for obtaining a satisfactory urine output is to administer adequate fluids. Diuretics are given as needed to maintain a urine output of at least 40 ml/hr once adequate hydration is established.

Narcotics

Narcotics given to patients to relieve pain following severe trauma (particularly morphine) will occasionally cause a severe drop in the blood pressure. Narcotics of this sort may increase vascular capacity by 1-2 liters or more; this can produce a sudden severe hypovolemia.

Before a narcotic is given to any patient with trauma or sepsis, it should be ascertained that the patient is not hypovolemic. An IV line should be established for rapid infusion of fluids if the blood pressure begins to fall. If a narcotic must be administered, it is given preferably in multiple small doses IV and is much more safely given in doses of 1-2 mg every 20-30 min than in doses of 8-15 mg every 3-4 hours.

OTHER SUPPORTIVE MEASURES

Autotransfusion

Autotransfusion is utilized by some of the larger EDs and trauma centers for selected cases of hemothorax and hemoperitoneum, with several systems available for general use. Returning the patient's own blood may be a life-saving factor with less risk than receiving blood from another with the inherent risks of error in crossmatching, hepatitis, and "shelf-life" of blood products.

If the blood remains uncontaminated and if the patient will require replacement of several units, autotransfusion is ideally suited, although there may be serious coagulation problems associated with defibrinization; in-line blood filters must be used to prevent microembolism.

The EDN should be familiar with preassembly and operation of the equipment and management of the procedure when it is indicated for a hemorrhaging patient, in order to prevent loss of valuable time and the commission of errors.

Military Anti-Shock Trousers (MAST)

MAST suits are seeing a wider acceptance now in the prehospital and ED phases of care; personnel must be familiar with their application and purpose, since the trousers are meant to *stay on the patient until* 1) a knowledgeable physician is present and has taken charge of the patient, 2) fluids are available for transfusion, and 3) anesthesia and surgical teams are ready for the patient if surgical intervention is indicated.

The MAST suit is a one-piece wrap-around trouser with Velcro fasteners and three inflatable compartments (abdominal and both legs), a 104-mm Hg pressure relief valve and a foot pump. The trouser is indicated in trauma and other situations with:

1. Hypotension with a systolic BP less than 90 mm Hg with evidence of decreased tissue perfusion (unless there is evidence of congestive heart failure [CHF]);

2. Hypovolemia with visual blood loss or history of same (GI bleed), or hemorrhage requiring direct pressure for control;

3. Injury that might cause either hypotension or hypovolemia (blunt trauma to abdomen, fractures, etc.)

The principle is the application of pressure with an encircling pressure of approximately 88-120 mm Hg around both legs and the abdomen when inflated, correcting or counteracting internal bleeding and hypovolemia by either preventing return flow to the lower portion of the body or returning pooled peripheral circulation beneath the pressure area to the upper portion of the body by way of the venous pathways.

The MAST suit is thought to have some important clinical applications and is indicated in 1) trauma with hypovolemia, 2) fractures (pelvis and/or femur with occult blood loss), 3) medical emergencies with volume depletion, 4) air embolus prevention, 5) DIC (disseminated intravascular coagulation), 6) retroperitoneal hematomas and now, even 7) cardiogenic shock.*

The MAST may be contraindicated, *relative to clinical circumstances,* in pulmonary edema; application of the abdominal segment constitutes fetal sacrifice in mid to advanced pregnancy. It is safe, however, to apply the leg sections for a pregnant woman in shock.

Removal of the garment must be done under controlled circumstances with slow deflation while the blood pressure is constantly monitored. Deflation should be balanced with maintenance of a systolic BP of 100 mm Hg.

SUMMARY

Shock continues to be associated with an extremely high mortality rate in most hospitals; frequently, the treatment was "too little, too late" as a result of lack of previous baseline data and clinical information, in addition to the lack of close observation in anticipation of severe problems. Patients who are candidates for shock or who are actually *in* shock must be closely monitored with *continuous nursing observations and care;* continual assessment of blood pressure and pulse pressures, continuous cardiac monitoring for heart rate and rhythm, continuous observation of the respiratory rate (noting depth and quality), and close attention to mental status and skin changes will all contribute crucial information on the clinical status of the patient and possibly prevent further deterioration by signaling the need for immediate intervention.

---

*Wayne MA: The MAST suit in the treatment of Shock. JACEP, Vol 7, No 3, pp 107-109, 1978

REVIEW

1. Define shock.
2. Identify the three factors that govern the maintenance of an adequate circulating blood volume.
3. List four situations in which altered perfusion should be expected.
4. Identify the four manifestations of inadequate tissue perfusion.
5. List five circumstances in which increased blood lactate from anaerobic metabolism is frequently seen.
6. List four simple classifications of shock.
7. Identify five monitoring parameters utilized in all kinds of shock.
8. Describe the difference between absolute hypovolemia and relative hypovolemia.
9. Describe the methodology of the fluid challenge.
10. Outline the nursing management guidelines for the patient in shock.
11. List seven precautions which should be taken when receiving a patient in shock in the ED.
12. Identify the indication, contraindication, and nursing responsibilities in autotransfusion.
13. Describe the rationale for use of the MAST suit and identify the contraindication for its use.

BIBLIOGRAPHY

Advanced Trauma Life Support (ATLS) Course Manual. ACS, Chicago, 1981

Budassi SA, Barber JM: Emergency Nursing: Principles and Practice. C.V. Mosby Co. St. Louis, Missouri, 1981

Cain HD: Flint's Manual on Emergency Treatment and Management. C.V. Mosby Co., St. Louis, Missouri, 1980

Cervera AL, Moss G: Dilutional reexpansion with crystalloid after massive hemorrhage: Saline versus balanced electrolyte solution for maintenance of normal blood volume and arterial pH. J Trauma, Vol 15, No 498, 1975

Civetta JM, Mussenfeld SR, et al: Prehospital use of military anti-shock trouser (MAST). JACEP, Vol 5, No 8, pp 581-587, 1976

Cohn IN: Blood pressure measurements in shock; mechanisms of inaccuracy in auscultatory and palpatory methods. JAMA, Vol 199, No 118, 1967

Dillman P: The biophysical responses to shock trousers. JEN, Vol 3, No 6, pp 21-24, 1977

Flint LM, Brown A, et al: Definitive control of bleeding from severe pelvic fractures. Ann of Surg, Vol 189, No 6, pp 709-715, 1979

Guyton A: Basic Human Physiology, 2nd ed. W.B. Saunders Co., Philadelphia, Pennsylvania, 1977

Hollingsworth PK: Autotransfusion in the emergency department. JEN, Vol 3, No 4, pp 9-10, 1977

Kelland D: Massive Blood Transfusions in the Emergency Department. Emergency Highlights. Emanuel Life Flight, Vol 2, No 2, Portland, Oregon, July 1981

McSwain NE: Pneumatic trousers and the management of shock. Trauma, Vol 17, No 9, pp 719-724, 1977

Starchuk E, Weil MH, Shubin H: Fluid Challenge. Los Angeles, Shock Research Unit, Center for the Critically Ill, Hollywood Presbyterian Medical Center, 1974

Warner C: Emergency Care: Assessment and Intervention, 2nd ed. C.V. Mosby Co., St. Louis, Missouri, 1978

Wayne MA: The MAST suit in the treatment of cardiogenic Shock. JACEP, Vol 7, No 3, pp 107-109, 1978

Webb WR: A Protocol for Managing the Pulmonary Complications of Patients in Shock. The Upjohn Co., Kalamazoo, Michigan, 1975

Wilson RF: Shock, Its Definition, Classification, Diagnosis, Pathophysiology, Monitoring, and Treatment. The Upjohn Co., Kalamazoo, Michigan, 1976

Wilson RF, Krome R: Factors affecting prognosis in clinical shock. Ann Surg, Vol 169, No 93, 1969

Wilson RF, LeBlanc LP, Walt AJ: Shock due to trauma. In The Management of Trauma: Practice and Pitfalls. Lea & Febiger, pp 56-75, Philadelphia, Pennsylvania, 1975

Wilson RF, Walt AF: Walt AF: Blood replacement. In The Management of Trauma: Practice and Pitfalls. Lea & Febiger, pp 136-148, Philadelphia, Pennsylvania, 1975

Wiley L: Staying ahead of shock. Nursing 74, April 1974

Wiley L: Shock, different kinds, different problems. Nursing 74, May 1974

MAJOR TRAUMA   15

KEY CONCEPTS

This chapter provides the EDN with an overview of recognition and management of chest and abdominal trauma and the problems that may be encountered in the patient with multiple injuries. Many of these basic concepts have been gathered from various physicians who have given their time to help develop these topics and have participated in an ongoing educational effort for emergency nurses. We are indebted to Adel Matar, M.D., and Aftab Ahmad, M.D., both cardiovascular surgeons in the Portland area; to Donald McNeill M.D., Joseph VanderVeer, M.D., Duane Bietz, M.D., John Schriver, M.D., and Regina Atcheson, M.D., all of the Portland area.

After reading and studying this chapter, you should be able to:

- Categorize the types of chest trauma and describe the priorities of management.
- Discuss the various types of lung injury, their complications and management.
- Describe needle and tube placements for decompression or drainage of the chest, explaining water seal and one-way attachment units.
- Identify the order of priorities in assessment of the multiple injured patient with the check points for a rapid and thorough 90-sec evaluation.
- Describe the diagnostic procedures employed in abdominal injury with the rationale for each.
- Discuss the most commonly injured abdominal organs and structures.
- Explain the possible extent of occult blood losses in pelvic and leg fractures and the threat posed by fat embolus.
- Describe the fluid of choice for replacement in massive blood loss and the precautions to be taken in blood replacement.

CHEST TRAUMA

An important concept in considering chest trauma is recognizing that very often there are other associated injuries and certainly, at a minimum, the involvement of other organ systems (skin, musculoskeletal, cardiovascular) as well as respiratory. Severe blunt trauma to the chest is one situation in which rapid and correct diagnosis within minutes of arrival can make the difference between survival and death. It is essential that ED personnel *guarantee an established airway immediately,* evaluate rapidly and accurately, alerting the physician, obtaining vital signs and preparing the patient for physical examination. These patients must be carefully monitored to detect early signs of deterioration with frequent auscultation of the chest and abdomen, continual assessment of consciousness, and serial blood-gas analysis. Alterations in blood gases always precede the onset of clinical changes of respiratory distress. Reliance on visual observations alone often delays therapy, and any patient who becomes *confused, restless,* or *violent* should have an immediate blood gas determination as a first step in the evaluation of these symptoms.

Chest trauma that will compromise the normally functioning lungs (Fig. 15.1) may be categorized as follows:

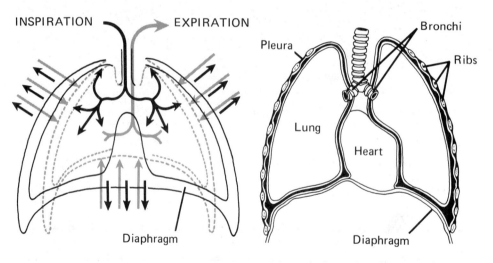

BREATHING RATE: 15-20 per minute
VOLUME OF AIR: 500 cc.

Figure 15.1. The lungs. (From Grant H, Murray R: Emergency Care, 2nd ed. Robert J. Brady Co., Bowie, Maryland, 1978)

Penetrating wounds—those that interrupt the chest wall and violate the intrathoracic organs. Examples are stab and bullet wounds, shrapnel, and violent trauma with associated rib fractures.
Nonpenetrating or blunt injuries—those that do not interrupt the chest wall. Examples are steering-wheel injuries, deceleration injuries, falls from

heights, crush injuries, blast injuries (high positive-pressure waves), and trauma associated with the forces of sheering and torsion.

PENETRATING CHEST TRAUMA

The essential points of priority consideration in a patient with penetrating chest trauma are:

1. Management of the airway, with immediate adequate oxygenation and prevention of aspiration. These patients must always be carefully evaluated for cervical spine damage before attempts are made at hyperextending the head for intubation.

2. Management of bleeding and shock in hemothorax (Fig. 15.2)

   A. Massive volume replacement of blood. The patient's own blood is sometimes administered by autotransfusion with blood from the chest cavity drained into citrated vacuum transfusion bottles and returned intravenously to the patient. Ringer's lactate solution can also be given for volume replacement, but the oxygen-carrying capacity of the blood will be diminished with too much crystalloid solution if large volumes are utilized.

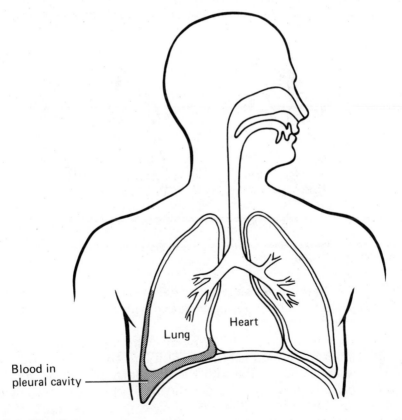

Figure 15.2. Hemothorax.

The lung beds are a reservoir of blood, with 900 cc readily available to the systemic circulation. Following trauma, the lungs can accommodate 3-5 liters of blood and one lung can hold as much as 3 liters. The approximate amount of blood needed to show on X-ray films of the lungs in an upright position is 500 cc. As much as *1 liter can be occult* in the supine patient on X-ray.

B. Placement of a chest tube through the *third, fourth,* or *fifth* intercostal space in the *midaxillary line* with attachment to a water seal drainage unit. Occasionally, bleeding points may tamponade and stop. However, careful monitoring of the amount of blood being lost is essential, and it is generally felt that 6 hours of bleeding of 200 cc an hour, or 12 hours of bleeding at 100 cc an hour is indication for operative intervention.

3. Emergency management of open pneumothorax with a sucking chest wound

A. Seal the wound with petroleum jelly (Vaseline) gauze or plastic (Saran) wrap because it is essential to stabilize the mediastinum and prevent shock caused by the side-to-side shift, distortion of the great vessels, and collapse of the remaining lungs, with decreased venous return and decreased cardiac output (Fig. 15.3). *The seal should be released periodically to prevent development of a tension pneumothorax, with the patient under continual close observation* (Fig. 15.4).

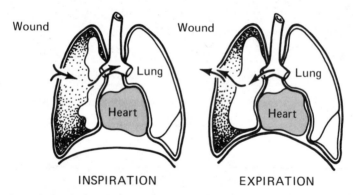

Figure 15.3. Pneumothorax. (From Grant H, Murray R: Emergency Care, 2nd ed. Robert J. Brady Co., Bowie, Maryland, 1978)

B. Place a chest tube or large-gauge needle at the *second* or *third* intercostal space in the *midclavicular line* with an attached flutter valve (Heimlich valve).

4. Evaluation for the possibility of other organ injury. The dome of the diaphragm is found normally at the fifth intercostal space with exhalation; any injury below the fifth rib, therefore, should be considered *abdominal as well as thoracic* since the liver, spleen, kidneys, and upper bowel content also lie within the rib cage. Operative repair of injured intraabdominal organs can be easily achieved through a thoracotomy (an

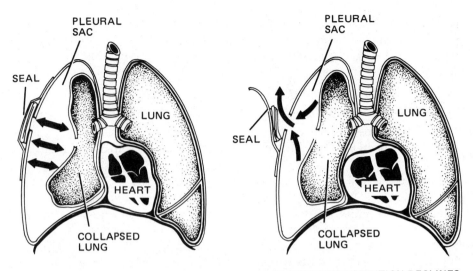

Figure 15.4. Tension pneumothorax. (From Grant H, Murray R: Emergency Care, 2nd ed. Robert J. Brady Co., Bowie, Maryland, 1978)

incision through the chest wall) for upper abdominal viscera, maintaining ventilation by endotracheal intubation and positive-pressure ventilation.

5. Continued close observation of the patient with chest X-rays taken every 4 hours for at least two series. The films should be inspiratory as well as expiratory.

6. Anticipation of infection from the open pathway. Empyema is commonly a late development in foreign body penetration. Although antibiotics should *not* be used indiscriminately, they *should* be given to treat specific anticipated infections. Tetanus toxoid, however, should *always* be given with contaminated wounds.

BLUNT CHEST TRAUMA

Initial management of the airway and prevention of aspiration are the priorities here. (Out of an annual motor vehicle accident fatality rate of 60,000, chest trauma accounts for approximately 12% and contributes to over 50%.) Data gathered at Detroit General Hospital since 1964 on 2000 trauma victims indicates that shock alone carried a mortality of 7.3%, while shock complicated by respiratory failure accounted for a 73.1% mortality.

Classification of Organs Damaged Singly or in Combination with Others in Blunt Trauma

1. Thoracic cage injury with fractures of clavicle, ribs, sternum, and ruptured diaphragm

2. Pleura with resulting hemothorax and/or pneumothorax
3. Lungs with contusion or bruising and damage without actual laceration or tearing of tissue (There is interstitial and intraalveolar hemorrhage and edema.)
4. Actual lacerations of lungs
5. Damage to main trachea and bronchi
6. Damage to esophagus
7. Damage to heart and pericardium, aortic arch, and major branches of the aorta
8. Ruptured diaphragm

Chest-injured patients must be triaged according to whether the injuries interfere with vital physiologic functions (10-15% of chest trauma) with no time to waste (these patients must go immediately to the OR), injuries that are severe but offer no immediate threat to the life with stable vital signs (allowing time for X-ray films and evaluation), or injuries that produce occult damage (aorta, spleen, liver, tamponade, etc.), and will require extremely close bedside monitoring.

General Signs, Symptoms and Treatment of Damaged Organs and Structures

Fractured Ribs. Fracture of the upper five ribs is an indication of serious trauma, and fracture of the first rib is especially serious since it has an associated mortality of approximately 36%. Approximately 90% of first-rib fractures are associated with esophageal and tracheal rupture as well as significant subclavian and aortic trauma and require very close nursing observation.

Symptoms. Pain and dyspnea secondary to the pain. Bruising may be visible, and crackling of ribs may be audible, as may subcutaneous emphysema.

Treatment:
1. Control pain to allow adequate ventilation and prevent atelectasis. It is important to realize that *secretions are increased in traumatized lungs,* as well as the fact that, as one physician put it, "The lung is dumb. It always responds to trauma by weeping (interstitial edema)." Strapping the chest can seriously compromise ventilation and should be avoided; local block of the intercostal nerves with bupivacaine hydrochloride (Marcaine) should be utilized.

    The intercostal block is done as far back toward the vertebrae as possible to anesthetize most of the nerve and generally should be placed about one hand's width from the vertebral column. Three intercostal blocks should be done for one rib (the rib above and the rib below) because an overlap of the nerve supply exists from rib to rib and the appropriate area must be prepped accordingly. Bupivacaine (Marcaine) with epinephrine will provide pain relief for a minimum 8-10 hours.

2. Take care of secretions with adequate tracheobronchial suctioning or by encouraging coughing. The patient should be made to cough every 15 min, depending upon the amount of secretions, with manual support or a pillow bolster given to support the chest and help decrease pain. If the patient is unconscious, aspiration of the secretions must be carried out by orotracheal or nasotracheal suction.

Flail Chest. Flail chest (Fig. 15.5) occurs as a result of multiple rib fractures with each rib fractured at two points, creating a "flail" segment. The flail segment "moves in" on respiration, and there is cross ventilation, with air moving from the lung on the affected side to the good lung. The patient is usually cyanotic and tachypneic.

Treatment. *Immediate* stabilization is required for adequate ventilation and oxygen administration. Intubation and positive pressure ventilation is the *most* effective therapy. Chest tubes should be placed, if surgical emphysema or pneumothorax is present, before placing on ventilator, to prevent tension pneumothorax. The concentration of oxygen to be used should be that required to produce a minimal PaO_2 of 70 mm Hg, decreasing as rapidly as feasible to 40% oxygen.* Remember that *hypoxia* is the commonest cause of combativeness.

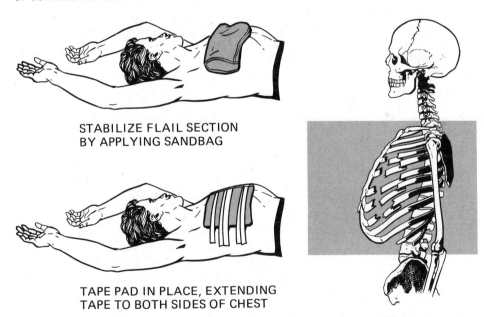

STABILIZE FLAIL SECTION
BY APPLYING SANDBAG

TAPE PAD IN PLACE, EXTENDING
TAPE TO BOTH SIDES OF CHEST

Figure 15.5. Flail chest. (From Grant H, Murray R: Emergency Care, 2nd ed. Robert J. Brady Co., Bowie, Maryland, 1978)

Fractured Sternum. Sternal fracture is difficult to demonstrate on X-ray films, but a lateral view will show whether fracture is present. There is a high

---

*Webb R: A Protocol for Managing the Pulmonary Complications of Patients in Shock. Upjohn Company, Kalamazoo, Michigan, 1975

mortality from associated injuries, and a fractured sternum may herald subsequent *severe* developments, again signalling the need for extremely close monitoring.

Ruptured Diaphragm. Crushing chest injuries and deceleration trauma occasionally cause rupture of the diaphragm. The common mechanism is a compressing force on the abdomen, such as a steering wheel or a high-riding seat belt driven into the abdomen. After a relatively asymptomatic period, the stomach or bowel may become distended; acute respiratory distress may develop with pain, which is usually referred to the shoulder.

Treatment:

1. Respiratory support
2. Insertion of nasogastric tube to decompress the distended stomach
3. Prompt surgical intervention

Lung Trauma. Usually injury to the lung accompanies chest trauma and is manifested in many ways. Pulmonary contusion is important because it may be initially asymptomatic (with no fracture of the bony cage in 50% of the cases). It may lead to *severe* respiratory distress; therefore, anticipate a developing problem if there is tachypnea, tachycardia, decreased PaO_2, decreased PCO_2, and a later rise in PCO_2.

Treatment. Endotracheal intubation with volume ventilator, steroids and diuretics to reduce septal edema of the lungs, control of fluids with strict intake and output (I and O). Along with the septal edema, there may be hemorrhage and in severe cases intraalveolar hemorrhage from rupture of pulmonary capillaries. When properly managed, pulmonary contusions will usually resolve in 3-10 days.

There *may* be laceration of the lung tissue with loss of surface continuity and leakage of air and blood causing pneumothorax and/or hemothorax.

Ruptured Esophagus. A sudden increase of intraluminal pressure may cause rupture of the esophagus in traumatic pneumothorax and should be suspected if mediastinal emphysema is present. This requires *immediate* surgical intervention and will frequently cause sepsis in the mediastinum. This is an extremely serious complication.

Rupture of the Trachea or Bronchi. This type of trauma is usually transverse, about 2 cm above the bifurcation of the trachea (corina), or one main bronchus may fear about 2 cm below the corina. It is diagnosed by bronchoscopy or bronchography. *Treatment is immediate* surgery and repair.

Damage to the Heart, Pericardium, and Aortic Arch. These injuries require massive amounts of blood replacement, so start blood type and cross-match immediately.

Ruptured aorta is caused frequently by deceleration injury. The most common rupture sight is distal to the left subclavian artery on the descending thoracic aorta. It accounts for nearly one-sixth of early deaths from motor vehicle accidents when associated injuries detract from early recognition and a chance at survival. The symptoms are upper limb hypertension, absent or delayed femoral pulse, and reduction in urine output. In full-thickness tears of the aorta, death from exsanguination will result immediately; if the tear is partial, the patient may survive for a period of time, allowing surgical intervention.

Cardiac contusion may vary from a simple contusion, with or without the ECG signs of infarction, to rupture of the atria or complete ventricular rupture. The most common cause is injury from the steering wheel, by sudden deceleration in vehicular accidents, and this should carry a high index of suspicion with continued close nursing observation.

The symptoms are retrosternal pain, anginal in character, refractory to nitroglycerin but frequently responsive to oxygen; tachycardia; conduction disturbances; and perhaps ECG alterations, depending on the location and extent of the trauma.

Treatment requires following up with serial ECG and enzyme studies. Acute hemopericardium producing tamponade requires immediate aspiration of the pericardial sac.*

Cardiac tamponade can result from massive trauma, extensive lacerations, or large-caliber gunshot wounds of the heart, which are quickly fatal as a result of sudden and voluminous blood loss. Small wounds, however, as from an ice pick or a small-caliber bullet should rarely cause immediate death. Since the pericardium is *inelastic,* the patient may suddenly go into shock or die if the volume of blood trapped in the pericardial sac reaches 150-200 cc.

The signs of cardiac tamponade include distant heart sounds, distended neck veins, a falling blood pressure, and advancing shock.

Treatment involves immediate aspiration of the pericardial sac as a mandatory first-aid measure. Aspiration of as little as 15-20 cc can save an apparently dying patient or at least buy time. The pericardial tap is done with a large gauge (16-18), short bevel 4-inch needle attached to a 50-cc syringe, with the needle inserted about 3 cm to the patient's left of the xiphoid process (Larrey's point) and aimed toward the left posterior shoulder. The usual depth of insertion should be about 4 cm (1.5 in.). The patient should be continually monitored by oscilloscope during the procedure with a V-lead attached to the needle hub with an alligator clip so that penetration of the myocardium or improvement in the cardiac function can be immediately ascertained. (Concerns over possible electrical hazard to the patient have made this technique somewhat controversial.) Bleeding is apt to recur, and the patient must be very closely observed for further deterioration, in which case thoracotomy for repair of the injury is immediately indicated.* A three-way stopcock should be attached to the needle after aspiration of blood so that repeated aspirations can be done if signs of tamponade persist.

A *ruptured diaphragm* is often a delayed diagnosis; however, a barium swallow will show gut in the chest cavity. This requires immediate insertion of a nasogastric tube and surgical intervention.

Aspiration is a common cause of severe respiratory distress and death. Victims of motor vehicle accidents vomit and aspirate frequently because they

---

*Adapted from Naclerio EA: Clinical Symposia. Vol 22, No 3, 1970 (with permission from CIBA-GEIGY Corporation)

have had a large meal or fluid intake several hours prior to the trauma. Aspiration of acidic gastric juices in the bronchial tree and lungs causes chemical pneumonitis, which seriously increases edema and respiratory insufficiency and rapidly leads to abscess formation and empyema. Particles of food in the bronchial tree can cause obstruction of some of the ventilatory units and absorption atelectasis results.

ADMISSION CRITERIA

Criteria for hospital admission following chest trauma include *increased probability* of the following:

1. Ruptured thoracic aorta if the MVA occurred at greater than 35 mph
2. Fractured first rib with associated subclavian and aortic trauma
3. Fractures of the ninth, tenth, and eleventh ribs, or of more than three ribs
4. Possible aspiration with atelectasis or chemical pneumonitis
5. Lung contusions (perfusion failure is likely to develop).

NURSING MANAGEMENT GUIDELINES

1. A well-cleared airway is always essential in chest trauma. Use suction, an oropharyngeal airway, intubation, or as a last resort, cricothyroidotomy or tracheostomy. Again, always listen to the apexes of both lungs following intubation to be certain the tube has not slipped into the right mainstem bronchus, causing nonexpansion and/or collapse of the left lung.
2. Draw ABG sample before oxygen administration, if possible, for baseline.
3. Oxygen should be given in carefully metered doses to meet the specific need of the patient. It should be heated to body temperature and fully humidified to 100% relative humidity at 37° C (98.6 F).
4. Start large-bore IV line with Ringer's lactate solution.
5. Anyone with a chest injury will have some degree of respiratory distress. With labored respiration, the accessory muscles are used, opening up the inferior constrictors and thus opening up the esophagus and creating a high negative pressure that allows air to be sucked down into the stomach. This almost invariably causes acute gastric dilatation, and passage of a nasogastric tube is important at the outset to prevent this. *(Remember that all tubes and catheters inserted in the patient must be clearly radiopaque.)*
6. Careful monitoring of intake and output is essential.
7. The EDN should anticipate the need for a volume ventilator in the following situations:
   A. A $P_{CO_2} > 60$ mm Hg
   B. A $Pa_{O_2} < 60$ mm Hg on an oxygen mask
   C. Flail chest with associated injuries

D. CNS depression

E. Generalized peritonitis (especially subdiaphragmatic)

F. Previous severe pulmonary disease

G. Severe prolonged shock

H. Severe smoke inhalation

8. Know the equipment, including the thoracotomy tray, the chest tube setup, and the water-seal chest drainage equipment available. The Pleur-o-vac (Deknatel) or Thoraklex (Davol), which are now marketed as a sterile and disposable unit, is often used in hospitals in place of the older three-bottle setup (Fig. 15.6). There is also a new four-bottle system, manufactured by the Sherwood Laboratory, that is available and in use in some hospitals.

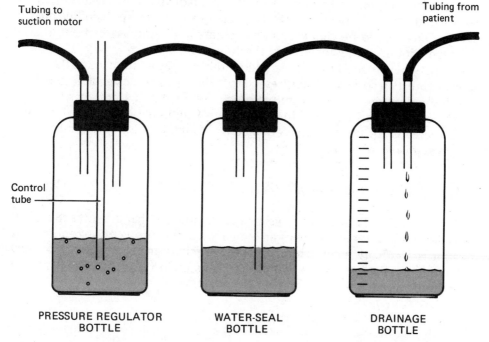

Figure 15.6. The three-bottle seal. The most commonly employed type of drainage system is the three-bottle system, a sterile procedure. It creates negative pressure, or vacuum, when attached to a low-pressure pump. This restores negative intrapleural pressure following interruption of integrity of lung surface or chest wall. (Adapted from drawing in Brunner LS, Suddarth DS: Lippincott Manual of Nursing Practice. J.B. Lippincott Co., Philadelphia, Pennsylvania, 1974)

9. Learn to evaluate your patient rapidly and effectively as you simultaneously:

A. Feel—Palpate pulse—Check for subcutaneous emphysema

B. Listen—Assess ventilatory exchange—Check for distant muffled heart sounds

C. Look—Note distended neck veins—Observe contour of chest—Check position of trachea (mid-line?)—Check for subcutaneous emphysema

MULTIPLE TRAUMA

Disaster has been defined as "a sudden and massive disproportion between the hostile elements of any kind and the survival resources which can be brought into action in the shortest possible time." This definition certainly applies to the individual with massive injuries and multi-organ trauma who is brought, in a critical state, to the ED.

The "survival resources which can be brought into action in the shortest possible time" are the skilled ED personnel, at least a basic minimum of life-support equipment, and the patient's remaining vital reserve.

Once the ABCs have been recognized and life support is underway, the skills of further assessment must be employed rapidly, since time is of the essence with the critically injured patient. The evaluation of abdominal trauma and the extent of the injury is, of course, the physician's area and responsibility, but the skilled EDN should be capable of an accurate and rapid assessment in conjunction with or in the absence of the physician.

The patient is triaged to an area adequately equipped to manage the problem and must be *completely* undressed to facilitate the quick evaluation of the injuries and permit further examination by the physician. Caution, of course, *must* be observed in undressing the severely injured patient in whom any movement may be contraindicated because of injuries. Clothing should be *cut away* whenever necessary.

THE INITIAL 90-SECOND EVALUATION

This is a rapid *head-to-foot* physical examination, which provides the initial overview of the patient and gives an indication of the intervention required. At best, it is a cursory examination for cardinal signs and symptoms that may require immediate action to stabilize and maintain the patient as well as a determination of laboratory and X-ray utilization.

Head

After the ABCs, look at and palpate the skull and posterior ligament of the cervical spine.

Ears

Look for CSF or blood. If an otoscope is used, the tympanic membrane should reflect light, move, and not be *blue* (indicating blood behind membrane). "Battle's sign" usually appears later.

Eyes

Look for orbital ecchymosis and conjunctival redness (goggle-like), grossly bloody conjunctiva (Pircher's sign) indicative of severe abdominal trauma and a surging venacaval injury, or rhinorrhea (CSF-like tears) with higher sugar count than nasal secretions. Carefully palpate facial bones and check for "blow-out" fractures of the orbital rim.

Mouth

Look for missing teeth and bleeding points or bleeding edematous tongue (airway danger).

Larynx

Uncommon injury but fracture may occur from steering wheel impact, wire injuries at shoulder height on bikes, or karate chops.

Neck Veins

Increased volume with distension is seen in tension pneumothorax, with displacement of the heart, myocardial tamponade, and myocardial contusion (with ST changes on the ECG).

Chest

Check stability of chest and rib cage with a sternal press and barrel push against sides of ribs toward the center. Feel for subcutaneous emphysema, commonly felt in the neck and subclavicular areas concomitant with pneumothorax and ruptured bronchus (prepare chest tube setup).

Breath Sounds

To be checked for quality and rate. Are they equal and normal? Are there rales? *Traumatized bronchi secrete more,* and atelectasis will develop if the patient is splinting and not expanding the chest normally.

Abdomen

Check breathing patterns. Is there a gentle rise and fall of the abdomen, or is the patient splinting? Check back for evidence of retroperitoneal bleeding or other damage. Again, the patient must be totally undressed and covered with warm blankets. Carefully logroll to examine the back. Always look for "exit" wounds when appropriate.

Pelvis

Press downward on both hips and on the symphysis. Even a semi-conscious patient will groan if he has a broken pubis. A pelvic fracture may cause a great amount of occult bleeding and may easily contribute to severe shock.

Urinary Meatus

Inspect for presence of blood from sheared urethra. Remember to document! Never pass catheter in presence of frank blood; call urologist.

Rectal

Examination is highly useful in pelvic trauma and should always be done for the presence of blood. Also highly indicative of spinal cord damage if flaccid sphincter is present.

Extremities

Check for pain, deformity, and range of motion (if no deformity is noted) by lightly running both hands along both aspects of extremities. If the patient is awake or semiconscious, make every effort as you work to reassure the patient in a positive, calm tone of voice and to explain, as you go, what you are doing. This will not only help reassure the traumatized patient who has just undergone a personal disaster but is also a means of evaluating the LOC according to the response received.

If at all possible, the same EDN should maintain constant observation of the patient throughout his stay in the ED so that while one obvious injury is being taken care of, a more critical one is not overlooked. *Remember that this nurse is the one with the flow of baseline observations and may be the first person to notice any significant change in the patient's LOC and general status.*

PATTERNS OF INJURY

As the patient is being admitted to the ED, transferred, and undressed preparatory to the initial assessment (beyond immediate airway requirements), there is an opportunity to obtain all the history possible from the ambulance crew, family, or the patient's doctor regarding the situation and the mechanism of trauma. The following questions should be covered:

1. The mechanism of injury?
2. Who did it? How did it happen?
3. Any drugs aboard now?
4. Any allergies?
5. Any medical problems?
6. Alcoholic withdrawal or DTs?
7. Time of last food or fluid ingestion?
8. Date of last tetanus booster?
9. Is patient a bleeder, or does patient take anticoagulants?

Think through the pattern of injury, and logic will help you in anticipating probable as well as possible findings. Some of the following points may help you, once you know the *mechanism of injury:*

1. Motor vehicle accident (MVA)
   A. Driver becomes missile on deceleration. Was seatbelt worn?
   B. Was shoulder harness worn?
   C. Look for soft tissue trauma on lower abdomen, with possible retroperitoneal injury.

  D. Look for steering wheel trauma with damage to the sternal area, frac-
     tured ribs, or facial bones with airway compromise and possible car-
     diac contusion or tamponade.
  E. Right front seat passenger may have been thrown through the
     windshield. Evaluate airway and facial compromise. Fractured femurs
     are common with lacerated knees as well as high-velocity impact frac-
     tures to the head of the femur.
2. "Pile driver" constellation of injuries from high falls and severe deceleration. Look for compression fractures of the spine from forward flexion,
   fractures of the heels, knees and hips. Suspect deceleration injuries to
   the liver (subcapsular hematomas) and spleen, and lacerations of aorta
   just distal to the left subclavian artery.
3. Motorcycle injuries. Anticipate head injuries with concomitant facial
   lacerations, neck and cervical spine injury, and fractured femurs.
4. Gunshot wounds (GSW). Always look for entrance *and* exit wounds.
   Again, it is essential that the patient's clothing be removed and a complete check made of the whole body.
5. Knife wounds. If a man wields the blade, the thrust will probably be
   upwards, whereas a woman tends to stab at a downward angle. If a knife
   wound is found at the costal margin delivered from a male assailant, it is
   probably confined to the chest and lungs. If, however, the assailant is
   female, suspect downward penetration of both lung and abdominal
   cavity.
6. Blunt abdominal trauma. This poses the major problems in the ED and
   commonly presents with evidence of contusions of lower chest wall,
   splinting of the abdominal wall, and localized tenderness. Be alerted to
   fractures of the lower third of the chest accompanied by pain in the
   shoulder or absence of peristalsis along with nausea, vomiting, and distention of the abdomen. Blood in the vomitus, stool, or urine is significant
   and frequently indicates intraperitoneal injury. (Abdominal trauma patterns will be dealt with later in more detail.)

TRAUMA TUBES

The tubes which must be employed in the management of severely
traumatized patients are discussed in order of priority:

Endotracheal Tube

The ET tube is available in French sizes (circumference of the tube in mm)
and millimeter sizes (inside diameter of the tube); in case of confusion, *use the
tube closest in size to the patient's little finger.* Always check for a patent cuff
and a universal adapter to fit the bag unit for ventilating the patient once the
tube is placed. If necessary, use mouth to tube (16% O_2 is better than *no* O_2). If
a rigid stylet is used to place the tube, it must *never* be used without a clamp or
a bend at the adaptor and must be positioned 1 cm back from the tip of ET

tube. Again, the intubation tray must be checked regularly for completeness and the assurance of a working light on the laryngoscope.

Nasogastric Tube

Any seriously injured person should have an N/G tube placed as soon as possible. This patient is likely going to be on oxygen or forced positive-pressure breathing which will inflate his stomach, hindering heart and breathing action. The N/G tube avoids the problem of acute gastric dilatation as well as unmanageable emesis. Put it down early.

Nasogastric intubation is a frequently employed procedure in the ED for the following purposes:

1. Decompressing the stomach contents (air, food, etc.)
2. Diluting and washing out ingested poisons
3. Removing blood in cases of GI hemorrhage and washing with iced saline

The procedure is a simple one and the equipment is minimal, as follows:

1. Nasogastric tube—usually a Levin, Ewald, or Salem Sump tube in various sizes. The Levin and Sump tubes are used in sizes 12-18 Fr, while the Ewald (red rubber) is used in 32-, 34-, 36-mm size for rapid lavage of gastric contents.
2. Water soluble lubricant, a towel and emesis basin, a glass of water with straw, and 0.5-in. adhesive tape.

It is important to have the patient understand the procedure, and he should be instructed to mouth-breathe and swallow as the tube is passed. Have the patient sitting with neck flexed and a towel across the chest. Dentures should be removed. Decide on a signal (such as raising a finger) to indicate "wait a minute" because of gagging or discomfort. If rubber tubing is used, it should be chilled on an ice bed to firm the tubing before passage. Plastic tubing may need to be dipped into warm water if too stiff.

Mark the distance the tube is to be passed by measuring the distance on the tube from the patient's ear lobe to the bridge of the nose, plus the distance from there to below the xiphoid process. Mark this spot on the tube with a piece of adhesive tape (which will usually fall between the second and third circular markings at the nares when the tube is in place).

Lubricate the tip of the tube for about 6-8 in., lift the patient's head and insert the tube into the nostril, gently passing it along the floor of the nose until it reaches the pharynx, at which time the patient may gag. Rest a moment and then with the patient holding his head in a normal position have him take several sips of water, advancing the tube as he swallows. Do not use force.

If there are signs of distress, such as gasping, coughing, or cyanosis, immediately pull the tube back to the nasopharynx and try again.

To check position of the tube when it is in the stomach:

1. Aspirate contents of stomach with a 50 ml asepto syringe;
2. Place end of the tube in a glass of water to check for air bubbles;

3. Place a stethoscope over the epigastrium and inject 20 to 30 ml of air into the N/G tube.

The only sure way to confirm the presence of the tube in the stomach is by X-ray unless you are obtaining a satisfactory return of stomach content.

Adjust the tubing to proper position and tape into place using a skin "tackifier" and hypoallergenic tape; being certain *not* to obstruct the patient's vision or cause any pressure against the nasal septum.

Intravenous Lines

Any severely injured patient with more than one organ system involved must be presumed to have some degree of hypovolemic shock, and measures must be taken to reverse it, regardless of the recorded blood pressure. A fair BP can disappear rapidly, and a venous catheter should be placed while the pressure is still good and the veins are full and stand out clearly. Use an upper extremity with a #14-gauge or #10-gauge angiocatheter, intracatheter, or IV tubing trimmed to a bevel for venous cutdown when massive volume replacement is indicated. Large bore lines in both arms are ideal in the severely traumatized patient.

Venous cut-down guidelines are as follows:

1. Indication: Need for administering large volumes of fluid rapidly
2. Site: Upper extremity preferred—cephalic vein in groove of bicep
3. Equipment
    A. *Prep agent:* Povidone-iodine solution
        70% isopropyl alcohol
    B. *Anesthetic:* 1% Xylocaine without epinephrine
        Small needle
    C. *Scalpel:*
        No. 15—skin
        No. 11—vein
    D. *Catheter:* Intravenous administration set tubing trimmed at oblique angle, or # 14-gauge intracatheter
    E. *Instruments:*
        Suture
        Toothed thumb forcep
        Curved scissor
        Straight and curved small hemostats
        Syringes, needles, and sponges
4. Precautions: Large amounts of cold blood given through venous tubing can cause ventricular fibrillation or irreversible shock. Attach several extension tubes, coil in pan, and run blood through tubing in *warm,* not hot, water.
5. Results: 1 unit of blood can be given in *1* minute when the blood bag is squeezed by hand.
    A. # 14-gauge catheter will take 5-10 minutes with drip method.

6. When massive amounts of blood are to be administered, an in-line filter should be used and changed every two units. One such filter, composed of a rigid plastic cylinder containing a nylon clot filter and patented dacron wool fibers, is the Swank Filter manufactured by Extracorporeal Medical Specialties, Inc., which will screen out 15 g of "garbage" in every unit of whole blood.

Central Venous Pressure Lines (CVP)

In the past there has been disagreement regarding the early use of CVP lines in the traumatized patient; the American College of Surgeons ATLS course advocates early use of CVP lines to monitor the candidate for shock, in order to manage an effective fluid challenge and evaluate adequacy of volume replacement. As the ATLS standards point out, the CVP line is *not* a primary IV resuscitation route and is initiated on an elective basis rather than an emergent one.

When used, the preferable sites are the jugular vein, the left antecubital with a long-line CVP, or the subclavian; ideally, the puncture should not be done on the injured side if chest trauma is present.

Initiation of subclavian lines is a high-risk procedure with complications which include infection, vascular injury, embolization, thrombosis, and, frequently, pneumothorax. Strict surgical asepsis should be the rule when preparing the site and placing the catheter in the hope of minimizing unnecessary complications.

Foley Catheter

This is indicated in all multiple system injuries *except when there is a straddle injury or blood evident in the urethral meatus.* An indwelling catheter is essential to monitor intake and output and kidney perfusion. A *minimum* output is 0.5 cc/kg/hour or 30-35 cc/hour for a 150-lb (70 kg) person. Placement of a Foley catheter also allows for total evacuation of all urine and gross observation of urine for blood. Be cautioned that when the catheter does not readily enter the bladder, or blood is evident at the meatus, a urethrogram should be done immediately to determine the status of the urethra before proceeding further, and a urologist should be called.

Chest Tubes

Positioned posteriorly (midaxillary line at 4th or 5th ICS) to drain fluid, and anteriorly (midclavicular line at 2nd ICS) to release air, with areas prepped accordingly.

Peritoneal Lavage

This technique is discussed on page 288.

LABORATORY TESTS

Initial laboratory tests should include basically the following on stat requisitions:

1. Hematocrit for indication of acute massive blood loss (decreased HCT) or hemoconcentration associated with shock (increased HCT).
2. Type and crossmatch blood. Typing can be done with a "hold" on the crossmatch if there is a question of need (less expensive for the patient).
3. The CBC is used primarily as a baseline and is of little value in the immediate situation.
4. A serum amylase may be of help but may also be confusing in the presence of head injury when the amylase may be elevated as a result of salivary gland trauma. A significantly elevated amylase without concurrent salivary gland involvement would probably be highly indicative of pancreatic trauma.
5. Blood sugar, and if indicated, a toxicology screen for barbiturates, salicylates, alcohol and abuse drugs.
6. Arterial Blood Gases (ABGs) for PCO_2, PaO_2 and pH
7. Electrocardiogram
8. Intravenous pyelogram and cystogram (defines kidneys, ureters and bladder and verifies the presence of *two* kidneys in case of anticipated surgery on a damaged kidney).
9. Urinalysis ASAP for presence of red cells.

TRAUMA DRUGS

The EDN must maintain a *current* knowledge of the drugs employed in management of trauma cases; the general groups are listed here as follows:

1. Oxygen
2. Cardiac drugs
3. Immunizations
4. Antibiotics (legitimately administered prophylactically) for: facial injury; skull fracture; open fractures; penetrating wounds; peritoneal wounds
5. Analgesics
6. Steroids specifically for: sepsis; aspiration; head trauma
7. Intravenous solutions
8. Blood products.

ABDOMINAL TRAUMA*

The initial overall evaluation of abdominal trauma depends upon, among other things, the examiner's knowledge of abdominal anatomy and topography. The abdomen is divided into four quadrants by a longitudinal and a

---

*Information adapted from Buckingham WB, Sparberg M, Brandfonbrener M: A Primer of Clinical Diagnosis. Harper & Row, 1971.

vertical line through the umbilicus. In addition, the epigastrium, suprapubic area, and flank designations are sometimes useful. The structures below the skin should be visualized in the mind's eye (Figs. 15.7, 15.8, 15.9).

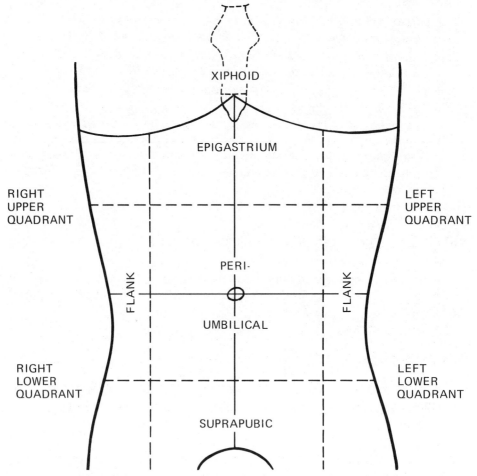

Figure 15.7. Topographic anatomy of the abdomen. The abdomen may be divided into quadrants, or specified areas: epigastrium, flanks, and suprapubic. (Adapted from Buckingham WB, Sparberg M, Brandfonbrener M: A Primer of Clinical Diagnosis. Harper & Row, 1971)

1. The right upper quadrant contains the hepatic flexure of the colon and the lower edge of the liver. The bulk of the normal liver lies within the right rib cage.
2. The left upper quadrant contains the stomach and the splenic flexure of the colon. These organs are normally not felt, nor is the normal spleen, which lies within the left rib cage.
3. The right lower quadrant contains the cecum and appendix.
4. The left lower quadrant contains the sigmoid of descending colon, often felt when filled with stool.
5. The epigastrium is the area between the xiphoid, two-thirds of the way to the umbilicus in the center of the upper abdomen, and contains the

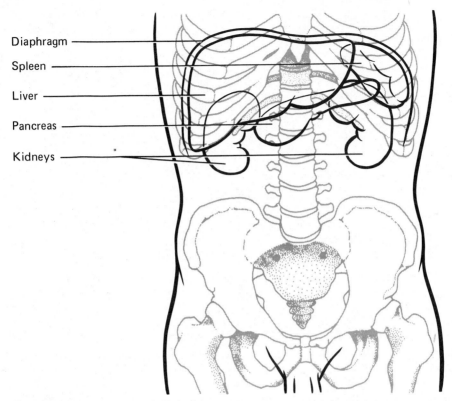

Diaphragm

Spleen

Liver

Pancreas

Kidneys

Figure 15.8. The solid organs. (From Grant H, Murray R: Emergency Care, 2nd ed. Robert J. Brady Co., Bowie, Maryland, 1978)

duodenum, pancreas, transverse colon, and descending abdominal aorta. Except for the aorta, these organs are not detectable in the normal person.

6. The suprapubic region normally contains intestine but may contain an enlarged bladder, ovary, or uterus.

7. The flanks are the lateral portions of the abdomen. The upper half contains the kidney and the lower half the ureter.

The abdomen should be examined from the patient's right side and should be carefully observed both from above and from the side with the light falling obliquely across the abdomen, so that minor changes in elevation will produce shadows and be more readily observed. Abdominal scars should be noted since the presence of scars may yield considerable useful information on the patient's past medical history.

The abdomen should be auscultated for bowel sounds before being palpated; palpating increases bowel sounds.

Palpation is considered the most important step in the examination of the abdomen, and although this is traditionally the area of the physician, the EDN, by observation, trial, and practice, can develop skills in the techniques of light, moderate, and deep bimanual palpation. Enlarged solid organs and distended

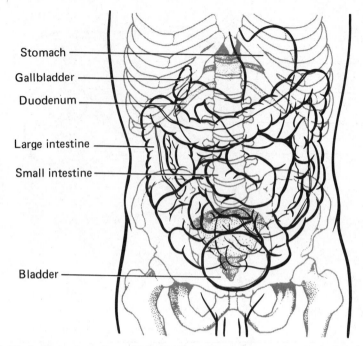

Figure 15.9. The hollow organs. (From Grant H, Murray R: Emergency Care, 2nd ed. Robert J. Brady Co., Bowie, Maryland, 1978)

hollow organs, as well as associated tenderness, may all be detected by this technique.

Some terms commonly used to describe reactions elicited by palpation are described here so that accurate documentation can be made of findings:

Guarding

Voluntary, or involuntary, tension (reflex contraction) of the abdominal muscles over an area of tenderness.

Rigidity

An extreme form of guarding, with the entire abdominal musculature tense and stiff. The term "boardlike rigidity" is sometimes used to indicate extreme stiffness of the abdominal muscles, and a silent abdomen with loss of bowel sounds, as a result of a paralytic ileus, will often accompany this degree of rigidity.

Rebound Tenderness

Indicates irritability of the parietal peritoneum, generally produced by peritonitis or irritation of the peritoneum adjacent to an inflamed organ.

Referred or reflected pain is that which may be present in an area separate from the site of examination. This may have definite localizing value.

As indicated before, blunt abdominal injuries pose the major problems in the ED, and they must always be suspected in every multiple-system injury. The prime examples are a ruptured spleen or other ruptured viscus. Perforating injuries to the abdomen or any obvious opening in the belly wall should be covered with sterile gauze soaked with normal saline solution, and bowel protruding through such a wound should not be replaced. The initial rapid assessment of a patient with abdominal trauma involves a simple format as follows:

1. *Look*—Note
   Breathing pattern
   Degree of distention
   Penetrating or blunt injury
   Bruises and scars
   Hematuria (full bladder on impact)
   X-ray signs
2. *Palpate*—for guarding, rigidity, rebound tenderness, and referred pain
3. *Listen*—Auscultate bowel sounds. This is the best screening for abdominal injury. If silent, be suspicious.
4. *Examine*—Perform
   Rectal exam for frank blood or flaccid sphincter
   Pelvic exam if indicated in a female patient
   Special examinations and procedures (abdominal pericentesis, peritoneal lavage, and stab wound injection)
5. *Observe*—Abdominal trauma victims should be observed carefully with a high index of suspicion for *occult damage* and bleeding. The early administration of fluids after trauma may dictate survival.

CLINICAL FINDINGS WITH SPECIFIC INJURIES

Spleen

The spleen is probably the most frequently injured organ in blunt trauma to the abdomen, and this injury is often associated with fractures of the left rib cage. The manifestations of splenic injury include signs of blood loss, abdominal pain localized to the left upper quadrant, and pain radiating to the left scapula and/or shoulder (Kehr's sign).

Liver

The clinical features of injury to the liver, probably the next most frequently injured abdominal organ, are localized pain in the right upper quadrant with radiation to the shoulder, absence of bowel sounds, and shock. Fifty percent of patients with liver injuries will exhibit signs of hypotension and 70% will have associated injuries. Since it is a solid fixed organ, lacerations of the liver are common in deceleration injuries.

Pancreas

Pancreatic injury is usually the result of blunt upper abdominal trauma and is often associated with trauma to other organs such as the stomach, duodenum, and liver. Occasionally, injury to the pancreas may be accompanied by damage to the major blood vessels, including the portal vein and the vena cava. Damage to the pancreas is manifested by abdominal tenderness, an elevated white blood cell count, and elevated serum amylase, with the diagnosis strongly supported by a history of an impaling force.

Blunt abdominal injuries indicate the need for special diagnostic studies, and if frank shock is present and a large blood loss is suspected, peritoneal lavage is frequently employed. Occasionally a four-quadrant tap is done.

SPECIAL DIAGNOSTIC PROCEDURES

The Peritoneal Lavage

The technique involved is no different from that of inserting a peritoneal dialysis tube with multiple holes. The lavage takes 20-25 min at best and carries a 96% chance of indicating significant injury if the results are positive. The procedure is indicated with altered consciousness, CNS injuries, spinal-cord injury, negative abdominal tap, shock, and multiple trauma. It is *contraindicated* with obvious penetration of the abdomen, adhesions, dilated bowel, pregnancy beyond the second trimester and massive abdominal distention. Some proponents advise lowering the bottle and waiting for the return flow while others advocate disconnecting the tubing and allowing the return flow to follow capillary action.

The American College of Surgeons Advanced Trauma Life Support (ATLS) program outlines an updated procedure for peritoneal lavage which should help standardize the approach when this diagnostic evaluation is indicated.

After it is certain that the patient's bladder has been emptied, the abdomen should be prepped, draped, and anesthetized in the low midline, one-third the distance from the umbilicus to the pubic symphysis using 1% lidocaine with epinephrine (to minimize bleeding and subsequent blood contamination from skin and subcutaneous tissues).

The skin and subcutaneous tissues are then incised vertically to the fascia; the fascia and peritoneum are incised and a peritoneal dialysis catheter is inserted and advanced, directing it toward the left or right pelvis. If aspirant reveals no gross blood, 10 ml/Kg Ringer's lactate is instilled into the peritoneum.

Gentle agitation of the abdomen distributes the fluid throughout the cavity and increases the mixing with blood, if present; the infused fluid should be allowed to remain 5 to 10 minutes before attempting to obtain return flow.*

An obviously bloody return will, of course, dictate the need for abdominal exploration, but in any case, the color of the return is significant. As little as 75

---

*American College of Surgeons Advanced Trauma Life Support (ATLS) Course Manual.

or 100 cc of blood within the peritoneal cavity will tint the fluid to a salmon or straw color, which would be interpreted as a weakly positive result. Gross blood (if you cannot read newsprint through the tubing) is strongly positive, but regardless of the findings visually, the fluid should be examined for white blood cells, bacteria, bile, and fecal content. An elevated fluid amylase suggests possible pancreatic injury (although the pancreas is retroperitoneal) and/or perforation of the duodenum or the upper small bowel.*

Stab-Wound Injection

A third procedure is employed as a method of exploring stab wounds. A knife or impaled object should *never* be removed until surgical support is available, but the area *around* the object is given a surgical prep whether or not operation is indicated.

After satisfactory prep to site of entry, a red rubber catheter is inserted into the wound as far as it will go and sewn into place tightly (after infiltration with local anesthesia) so that the "injection" will not leak. (If indication exists for an IVP, it should be done before injecting an abdominal stab wound.) The stab wound is then injected under pressure with Hypaque or some other radiopause IV medium. X-rays should be done, both AP and lateral, with the injection under pressure; the catheter is then removed, the wound irrigated, a drain placed, and the wound closed.

Retroperitoneal Bleeding

The existence of ecchymosis in the flanks signals a profound retroperitoneal bleed, which may originate from a torn aorta or other major vessel. Absence of one or both femoral pulses, even in the shock state, may be a valuable clue as to which artery is damaged.

VOLUME REPLACEMENT

Blood should be drawn immediately, of course, for type and crossmatch. But in the interim, massive fluids must be administered to restore circulating volume if indicated. The general choice of fluid in trauma resuscitation is Ringer's lactate since it closely mimics the extracellular fluid. The lactate is metabolized into carbon dioxide and water, providing 80-100 cc of free water, so there is no need to worry about providing water in addition to the resuscitation fluid.

OCCULT BLOOD LOSSES

Estimating blood loss is important in the assessment of the patient. Most of the time, the losses are underestimated. It is known, however, that severe fractures of the pelvis can result in *occult blood losses of up to 3000 cc (6 units)*, which will migrate into the retroperitoneal area as well as throughout the

---

*Gillespie: Sizing Up. Emergency Medicine, p 32, September 1975

pelvic areas. Another severe site of blood loss is a fracture of the femur, which can result in *occult blood loss of as much as 2000 cc (4 units)*, or a fracture of the tibia, with *a loss of 1000 cc (2 units)*. The normal blood volume in the average adult is 6000 cc (12 units), and the body can safely compensate for up to a 10% blood loss (600 cc) without progressing into a shock state.

The body can lose the first pint without any change at all in the pulse rate or blood pressure. *In trauma, however, a 120 pulse is by definition a 2-pint loss and if, addition, blood pressure is falling, it represents a 3-pint deficit.* *

Banked blood contains many ghost cells, small thrombi, and degenerating leukocytes which obstruct the pulmonary microvasculature. Again, when massive amounts of blood are being replaced, it is essential to use an in-line filter (Swank Filter) [Extracorporeal Medical Specialties] or a PALL filter [Johnson & Johnson] and to change the filter *every two units* to prevent the aggregates of platelets and microthrombi from passing into the patient's bloodstream, causing microemboli to be deposited in the lungs.

The American College of Surgeons ATLS Standards recommend that even though the majority of patients receiving blood transfusions do not need calcium supplementation, it may be necessary to offset coagulopathy. This is true particularly in patients receiving more than ten units of blood since normal existent intrinsic clotting factors have been exhausted. Binding of calcium by anticoagulants in banked blood is a problem with massive blood replacement. However, regardless of the volume given, if the infusion rate is less than 50-75 ml per minute, calcium mobilization is probably adequate. The patient should be monitored for duration of the Q-T interval during rapid infusion of citrated blood.

An appropriate dose, recommended in the Standards, is 0.2 grams of Calcium Chloride (2 ml of 10% Calcium Chloride solution) in a *separate* line for every unit (500 ml) of blood transfused. The total dose of calcium is not to exceed 2 grams unless there is objective evidence of hypocalcemia.**

Blood extravasated into peritoneal or pleural cavities is rapidly defibrinated and, therefore, incoagulable. Autotransfusion of intracavitary blood in trauma victims may minimize risk of microemboli and/or the need for systemic anticoagulation.***

ASSOCIATED PROBLEMS AND OTHER MANIFESTATIONS OF TRAUMA

Fat Embolus

Fat embolus is a more frequently recognized threat to the victim of multiple trauma than it was formerly, although it occurs 24-72 hours after trauma. It is seen in crush injuries and long-bone fractures, but the mechanism is obscure

---

*Freeark RJ: Excerpts from a talk. Emergency Medicine, p 29, October 1973

**ACS Standards for ATLS. ACS, Chicago, 1981

***Broadie T, Glover J, Bank N, et al: Clotting competence of intracavitary blood in trauma victims. Ann Emerg Med, Vol 10, No 3, pp 127-130, March 1981

since symptoms will not be produced by the intentional injection of fat globules into the bloodstream. However, it is believed that the incidence is probably reduced by early fixation of fractures to prevent manipulation. Stabilization of long-bone fractures will also minimize blood loss tremendously by allowing the fascia lata (muscle sheath) to tense and create a tamponade effect around the bone and bleeding points in the femur and hip. Again, remember that the upper thigh (cylindrical form) can accommodate 1-2 liters of blood with resulting shock.

Crush Injury

Crush injuries with massive tissue damage causing fat embolus, disseminated intravascular coagulation (DIC), and destruction of tissue with the release of potassium into the bloodstream can cause extreme problems. This type of trauma is frequently seen with MVAs, industrial accidents, beatings, etc. Decrease in the intracellular potassium with a rise in the serum potassium level can cause irreversible kidney injury, and the serum potassium level will continue to rise if kidney function is inadequate. (Remember that with abdominal crush injuries, probably fewer than 20% will have marks on the skin.)

Treatment involves initial resuscitation, management of shock, and exploration for abdominal injuries. The EDN should monitor these patients for signs of impending hypovolemic shock, pain, signs of peritonitis, fever, guarding, abdominal distention, and rebound tenderness (measure the abdominal girth and record with VS).

Diagnosis is confirmed by abdominal tap, X-ray films for air in the peritoneum, and signs of pancreatic or splenic injury. Hematuria requires IVP and kidney, ureter, and bladder X-rays (KUB). Kidney rupture is a frequent occurrence with a ruptured renal artery and tamponade or rupture of the capsule.

Disseminated Intravascular Coagulation (DIC)

Disseminated intravascular coagulation (also known as consumption coagulopathy or defibrination syndrome) is an intermediary mechanism of disease following shock, trauma with anerobic metabolism, burns, septicemia, snake bite, chronic metastatic Ca, malaria, heat stroke, obstetrical accidents, and intravascular hemolysis. Although rarely seen as a primary presentation in the ED, personnel should be familiar with its manifestations since it becomes rapidly fatal unless early intervention is undertaken.

The mechanism is that of normal clotting starting in an abnormal manner in small vascular areas; there is a rapid fibrin formation and then the liver lags in fibrinogen to maintain the clot mechanism. Paradoxical bleeding and clotting occur simultaneously, plasmin is activated, and the consumptive clotting factors are used up.

Diagnosis is made from an *unexplained drop in BP*, followed by petecchiae, ecchymosis, bleeding from at least 3 points at once (i.e., hemoptysis, epistaxis, hematuria, GI bleeding), local ooze at an injection site, and coma. Laboratory reports will show the platelets and prothrombin down, PTT increased, fibrinogen levels down, and a hemolytic anemia present with erythrocytes fragmented on a smear.

Treatment involves *early intervention* with anticipation of RAPID SHOCK, maintenance of BP, vigorous treatment of infection or bleeding, and administration of Heparin (2,500-5,000 sub-Q every 8 to 12 hours). This relieves the consumable factors and stops thrombin formation, breaking the paradoxical cycle.

NURSING MANAGEMENT REVIEW

Some final thoughts in reviewing the management of the multiple trauma victim include:

1. Areas of observation that should alert the EDN:
    A. *Hypotension is always a sign of hypoxia,* and if there is frank shock without heavy blood loss or the possibility of significant occult bleeding, suspect spinal cord injury, transection, etc.
    B. Cyanosis is a sign to check the airway again and be sure that the patient is ventilating adequately and getting a high enough concentration of oxygen.
    C. Anxiety and tachycardia should cause you to suspect blood loss and incipient shock.
    D. Delirium is an excellent indication of decreased cerebral blood flow and incipient shock.
    E. Skin changes are caused by the release of epinephrine in the shock state with resulting cool, clammy skin, pilo-erection, and mottled extremities. Check the lower legs.
    F. Distended neck veins with the patient in a 45° position indicate the likelihood of severe chest damage, tension pneumothorax, cardiac tamponade, or CHF.
    G. Flat neck veins (low CVP) accompany clammy, pale skin with major bleeding somewhere.
    H. Urinary output is the *major* monitor of visceral blood flow (the window of the viscera), and low output indicates the probable need for fluid. (Happiness is 30 cc/hr!)
2. All findings on vital signs must be carefully documented on a flow sheet for baseline information and evaluation, along with a closely monitored intake and output (I&O).
3. Learn to anticipate the needs of the patient *and* the physician. Time is of the essence.
4. Call for extra help when you really need it and make certain you have a "runner" for stat laboratory work, to make the necessary phone calls, and going ahead to hold the elevator for the critical patient who is being transferred from the ED to the ICU or the OR.
5. Provide portable oxygen and suction unit during transfer.

Before transferring the patient out of the ED be very sure that you have ruled out or know the patient's status regarding:

1. Hypoxia
2. Cervical spine fracture
3. Aortic tear
4. Pneumothorax
5. Hemothorax
6. Hemoperitoneum
7. Esophageal and/or bronchial trauma

PROCEDURE FOR TRANSPORTING A PATIENT WITH AN IV

1. *Before moving a patient* with an IV running:
   A. Make sure the infusion site is secure.
   B. Find out what kind and gauge of needle or intracath has been placed; identify on top piece of anchoring tape.
   C. Be certain IV bottle or bag is taped with starting time, how long it is to run, and at what rate of flow.
2. *Long trips:*
   A. Follow same procedure as before moving.
   B. Plastic needle should always be used if possible because of risk of trauma in moving.
   C. Try to keep tubing at stretcher level—tucked under pillow, for instance.
   D. Flush tubing every half hour for 15 sec, by turning the flow rate wide open and then resetting the drip rate.
3. *If the IV stops running:*
   A. Turn the bottle or bag upside down to let air obstruction out.
   B. Very carefully try to adjust the needle at insertion site by turning slightly.
   C. With extension tubing, try to milk the tubing to start fluid flowing again.
   D. Make sure that the arm in which the IV is inserted looks normal, since it is important to be certain that the infusion has not infiltrated. If the area around the infusion site is puffy, swollen, or discolored grossly, discontinue to the IV and remove the needle.
4. *Blood:*
   A. If two bottles are hung (one blood and one saline), only one should be flowing at one time. The procedure is the same as above before moving.
   B. As per flushing and on long trips, tubing should be flushed out at least every half hour.
5. *If everything fails* to make the IV run as it should, discontinue the infusion at once and apply a sterile light-pressure dressing.

REVIEW

1. In chest trauma, what differentiates the two main categories?
2. Identify the points of priority consideration with penetrating chest trauma.
3. Which organs and structures in the chest are likely to be injured with deceleration trauma and steering wheel injuries?
4. Identify *the* most common cause of combativeness and hypotension in an injured patient.
5. List five types of injury to the lung tissue itself and explain the severity.
6. List the types of injury likely to be sustained by the heart in trauma.
7. Identify the area for decompression of the chest wall in traumatic asphyxia and the area for placement of a chest tube for hemopneumothorax and the preparation required.
8. Describe the proper technique for passage of a nasogastric tube.
9. Explain the principle involved in closed drainage systems with an underwater seal.
10. Outline the procedure for setting up a closed drainage system with an underwater seal, either with a bottle and tubing set or a manufactured Pleur-o-vac or other unit.
11. Describe a flutter valve and the purpose it serves in specific chest problems.
12. Describe the pattern of associated-organ injury with a patient who has sustained a penetrating wound of the left chest wall at the level of the sixth intercostal space at the anterior axillary line.
13. Identify the order of priorities in intervention with the multiple injured patient.
14. Identify the tubes that are essential in treatment of the multiple injured patient, and give their order of importance.
15. Identify the basic initial laboratory procedures that should be ordered immediately and the rationale for each.
16. Describe the indications for venous cut-down and the equipment and procedure involved.
17. Define a disaster.
18. Locate the major abdominal organs according to the topographic divisions of the abdomen.
19. Describe the rationale and procedure for the most frequently employed diagnostic examination for internal abdominal bleeding.
20. Identify the most commonly injured abdominal organs and structures and explain the reasons for their susceptibility to injury.
21. Identify the solution of choice for fluid replacement in trauma and why.
22. Describe the amounts of occult blood loss possible in pelvic and leg fractures.

23. Describe the percentage of blood loss for which the body can compensate before the shock state becomes increasingly resistant to treatment.
24. Describe the immediate action to be taken if you had a heavily traumatized patient under close observation and the systolic BP dropped below 80 mm Hg.
25. What is the normal circulating blood volume in the average adult?
26. Describe what appears to be the most common cause of fat embolus and the associated symptoms and hazards to the patient.
27. Explain the pathophysiology of DIC and its recognition and management.

BIBLIOGRAPHY

Advanced Trauma Life Support (ATLS) Course Manual. American College of Surgeons, Chicago, Illinois, 1981

Barber JM, Dillman PA: Emergency Patient Care. Reston Publishing Co., Reston, Virginia, 1981

Bick RL: Disseminated intravascular coagulation (DIC), Parts I and II. Practical Cardiology, Vol 7, No 8, July 1981; Vol 7, No 9, August 1981

Brunner LS, Suddarth S: The Lippincott Manual of Nursing Practice, 2nd ed. J.B. Lippincott Co., Philadelphia, Pennsylvania, 1982

Buckingham WV, Sparberg M, Brandfonbrener M: A Primer of Clinical Diagnosis, 2nd ed. Harper & Row, New York, 1979

Budassi SA, Barber JM: Emergency Nursing: Principles and Practice. C.V. Mosby Co., St. Louis, Missouri, 1981

Cain HD: Flint's Manual on Emergency Treatment and Management. The C.V. Mosby Co., St. Louis, Missouri, 1980

Committee on Injuries, American Academy of Orthopedic Surgeons: Emergency Care and Transportation of the Sick and Injured, 3rd ed. George Banta Co., Menasha, Wisconsin, 1981

Cosgriff JH, Anderson DL: The Practice of Emergency Nursing. J.B. Lippincott Co., Philadelphia, Pennsylvania, 1975

Crossland S, Deyerle W: Compartmental syndrome. Nursing 80, Vol 10, No 11, pp 51-53, November 1980

Davis JJ, Cohn K, Nance FC: Diagnosis and management of blunt abdominal trauma. Ann Surg, Vol 14, pp 504-512, 1972

DeGowin E, DeGowan R: Bedside Diagnostic Examination. Macmillan, New York, 1981

Grant H, Murray R: Emergency Care, 2nd ed. Robert J. Brady Co., Bowie, Maryland, 1978

Himes VJ: Traumatic cardiac tamponade. JEN, Vol 6, No 2, pp 28-32, March/April 1980

Krome RL, Bock BF: Peritoneal lavage. Trauma Notebooks 6, JEN, Vol 3, No 3, 1977

Lance E, Sweetwood H: Chest trauma when minutes count. Nursing 78, pp 28-33, January 1978

Lockhart C, Mattox K, Philley C: A review of autotransfusion. JEN, Vol 5, No 2, pp 338-42, March/April 1979

Madoff IM, DesForges G: Cardiac injuries due to non-penetrating thoracic trauma. Ann Thorac Surg, Vol 14, pp 504-512, 1972

Meislin HW (ed): Priorities in Multiple Trauma (TEM). Lopen Systems Corporation, Gaithersburg, Maryland, 1980

Morris NS: Dissecting aortic aneurysms. JEN, Vol 5, No 5, pp 10-12, September/October 1979

Naclerio EA: Chest Trauma. Clin Symp, Vol 22, No 3, pp 86-109, 1970

Naclerio EA: Wounds of the Heart and Great Vessels in Thoracic Injuries. Grune & Stratton, New York, 1971

Olsen WR: The serum amylase in blunt abdominal trauma. J Trauma, Vol 13, pp 200-204, 1973

Romano T: Categories of hemorrhage assessment and treatment. Trauma Notebook 1, JEN, Vol 1, No 5, 1975

Spinella J: Clinical assessment of the shock patient. JEN, Vol 5, No 5, pp 34-37, September/October 1979

Starchuk E, Weil MH, Shubin H: Fluid Challenge. Shock Research Unit, Center for the Critically Ill, Hollywood Presbyterian Medical Center, Los Angeles, 1974

Sumner SM, Grau PA: To defeat hypovolemic shock, anticipate and act swiftly. Nursing 81, Vol 11, No 10, pp 46-51, October 1981

Therriault V: The trauma team: A nurse's perspective. JEN, Vol 1, No 6, 1975

US Public Health Service, DHEW: Physicians in Hospital Emergency Departments. Health Service and Mental Health Administration, Division of Emergency Health Services, Bethesda, Maryland, 1971

Warner C: Emergency Care: Assessment and Intervention, 2nd ed. C.V. Mosby Co., St. Louis, Missouri, 1978

Webb R: A Protocol for Managing the Pulmonary Complications of Patients in Shock. Upjohn Co., Kalamazoo, Michigan, 1975

White KM, DiMaio VJM: Gunshot wounds: Medicolegal responsibilities of the ED nurse. JEN, Vol 5, No 2, pp 29-35, March/April 1979

Wilson RF: Shock, Its Definition, Classification, Diagnosis, Pathophysiology, Monitoring and Treatment. Upjohn Co., Kalamazoo, Michigan, 1976

Wiley L: Shock: Different kinds, different problems. Nursing 74, May 1974

Wiley L: Staying ahead of shock. Nursing 74, April 1974

Zbilut JP: Disseminated intravascular coagulation. JEN, Vol 7, No 2, pp 213-215, September/October 1981

THE ACUTE ABDOMEN

16

KEY CONCEPTS

This chapter was developed to help the EDN recognize the potential significance of abdominal pain in the patient who presents to the ED and to provide an overview of acute abdominal problems with guidelines for assessment, evaluation, and intervention.

The bulk of the material in this chapter derives from lecture presentations by Don McNeil, M.D., Good Samaritan Hospital and Medical Center in Portland, Oregon, and William Krippaehne, M.D., Professor of Surgery, Oregon Health Sciences University, Portland, Oregon.

After reading and studying this chapter, you should be able to:

- Decribe the anatomic contents of the abdomen by quadrants.
- Define some of the specific terms used in relation to abdominal signs and symptoms.
- Identify some of the cardinal signs and symptoms and essential observations of the patient with abdominal complaints.
- Describe the pain patterns in various types of organs.
- Explain the significance of specific pain patterns and identify the priorities of treatment to be followed.
- List the important data base to be collected in specific situations and describe the supportive treatment that may be indicated.
- List the tubes that may be employed as monitoring devices, the important continued observations which must be made, and explain the diagnostic interpretations as they relate to history.
- Identify the three natural categories of abdominal diseases and explain the pathophysiology of each.
- Identify the nursing guidelines for managing the patient with severe abdominal pain.

The patient with complaints of abdominal pain is a frequent visitor to the ED and requires a thorough evaluation to rule out potentially serious disease before symptomatic treatment is instituted and the patient sent home with pain medication and instructions to call his physician in the morning.

The EDN is in a position to do some valuable screening and gathering of historical data to expedite further evaluation and diagnostic studies. This chapter deals primarily with disease processes rather than trauma of abdominal organs. As in the previous chapter, a working knowledge of abdominal contents and their anatomic locations in the assessment of a patient with abdominal distress is essential.

TOPOGRAPHY OF THE ABDOMEN

The abdomen is divided into four quadrants topographically as well as areas above, below, and lateral to the umbilicus (epigastrium, suprapubic area, and the flanks) (Fig. 16.1).

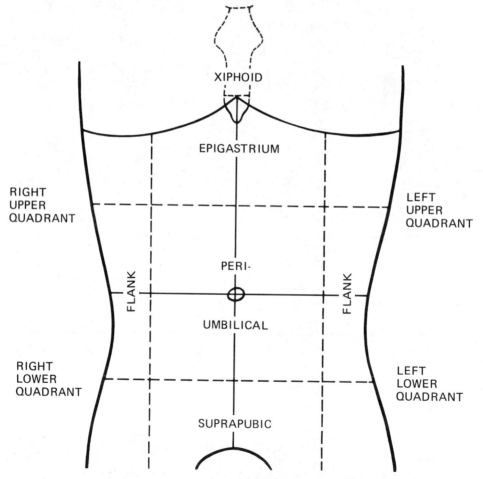

Figure 16.1. Topographic anatomy of the abdomen. The abdomen may be divided into quadrants, or specified areas: epigastrium, flanks, and suprapubic. (Adapted from Buckingham WB, Sparberg M, Brandfonbrener M: A Primer of Clinical Diagnosis. Harper & Row, 1971)

Epigastrium:

1) The subdiaphragmatic area; 2) stomach; 3) duodenum; 4) aorta; 5) pancreas; 6) transverse colon; 7) left lobe of the liver.

Right Upper Quadrant:

1) Liver and gallbladder; 2) duodenum and pylorus; 3) head of pancreas; 4) right kidney; 5) portal venous system; 6) hepatic flexure of the colon; 7) right lower lung; 8) possibly the cecum and appendix

Left Upper Quadrant:

1) Stomach; 2) spleen; 3) subdiaphragmatic area; 4) left kidney; 5) splenic flexure of colon; 6) tail of pancreas; 7) left lower lung

The *umbilicus* lies over the small bowel, mesentery, aorta, and vena cava.

Right Lower Quadrant:

1) Ilium; 2) cecum; 3) appendix; 4) ascending colon; 5) right ovary and fallopian tube (adnexa); 6) right kidney and ureter; 7) common iliac artery; 8) possibly the sigmoid colon; 9) testis and cord

Left Lower Quadrant:

1) Descending sigmoid colon; 2) rectum; 3) left kidney and ureter; 4) left adnexa; 5) testis and cord; 6) common iliac artery

Suprapubic (or Hypogastric) Area:

1) uterus; 2) urinary bladder; 3) appendix; 4) adnexa; 5) vagina or prostate

The right and left *flank* areas are controversial delineations but contain the kidneys and upper ureters.

SPECIFIC DEFINITIONS

Some definitions of specific terms are of value in standardizing interpretations and should include the following in the interest of accurate historical information:

1. *Vomiting* (emesis): forcible expulsion of gastric contents
2. *Regurgitation:* a backward flowing (as opposed to the *violent* expulsion of vomiting)
3. *Constipation:* infrequent or difficult fecal evacuation *or* hard and dry stools
4. *Diarrhea:* abnormal frequency *and* liquidity of feces

5. *Melena:* dark, pitchy and grumous (clotted or lumpy) stools stained with blood
6. *Hematochezia:* passage of bloody stools
7. *Hematemesis:* vomiting of blood
8. *Pain:* sensation of discomfort, distress, or agony
9. *Tenderness:* abnormal sensitivity to touch or pressure

RECOGNITION OF SIGNS AND SYMPTOMS

HISTORY

The history taken from the patient with an acute abdominal problem contributes 85% to the formulation of the diagnosis. The questions asked should not lead the patient to a desired response; they should allow a simple, easily worded choice of responses, like sharp or dull, steady or intermittent, etc. The occurrence of related symptoms such as malaise, nausea, vomiting, alteration in bowel or bladder regularity, or the status of menses may further aid in localizing the source of symptoms to a specific organ or area.

Pain Onset

Time: Day or night, with or without body functions/activity
Type: Superficial or deep in abdomen; sudden or slow onset; steady or crampy (colicky); sharp or dull; burning or aching. *Have patient point with finger to abdominal location of pain onset.*

Pain Progression

Location: Same place or new place; radiation or relocation of pain
Type: Same or changed (e.g., steady, dull or crampy, sharp); worse with body functions or lessened with body functions. *Have patient point with finger to where pain is the worse now.*

Previous Illnesses/Surgeries

This gives detail of organ misfunction or loss as well as a basis for understanding by what guidelines the patient can relate present abdominal pain to past painful episodes.

OBSERVATIONS

Observations by a skilled observer are an essential element in patient evaluation. The best opportunity to develop these skills is continued exposure to clinical situations. The EDN should learn to observe and evaluate many things, including:

1. *Complexion:* color, temperature of skin to touch, dry or moist skin, and facies (alert, tired, tense, worried, happy, sad, etc.)
2. *Body motion:* The patient is free and easy or guards specific sides of the body with certain usual body motions, for instance, slowness in raising the right leg, in lying down, and in placing hand over right lower abdominal quadrant where pain is located.
3. *Vital signs:* temperature, cardiovascular status (pulse and BP), and respiratory rate. (The pulse rate is generally the most sensitive parameter and is easily obtained to hypovolemic situations.)
4. *Abdominal contour:* scaphoid (depressed), flat, rounded. (This can be diffuse or in suprapubic area for pregnancy or "pregnoid" conditions.)
5. *Abdominal scars:* hints of previous organ removal

Skill in abdominal palpation is a valuable tool to develop. The patient's own relaxed nontender areas can give a baseline feel for the tender and possibly guarded areas through direct finger-hand inward pressure. The indirect finger tapped-to-finger percussion will elicit the so-called rebound tenderness and give a tonal quality to the abdomen, with a dull sound for solid organs and fluids and tympany for air-filled organs.

The auscultation of bowel sounds is a skill that must be developed through practice and continued application. It is necessary to listen to every abdomen as opportunity permits in order to become proficient in this technique. Bowel sounds are classified as none (or absent), hypoactive, normal, hyperactive, and excessive (if there are tinkles or rushes). *Borborygmi* are audible bowel sounds heard without the use of a stethoscope.

GENERALIZED SPECIFIC PAIN PATTERNS

It will be helpful to remember that the upper abdominal cavity contains both solid and hollow organs while the lower abdominal cavity contains organs which are *all* hollow except for the ovaries. A good rule of thumb, although generalized and simplistic, is that solid organs have steady, constant pain while hollow organs have colicky pain. Some of the generalized specific pain patterns which should be recognized are:

1. Bowel (stomach and small bowel). Crampy and sharp with 2- to 3-min repeat cycles, the large bowel is very slow and pain-free in most cases.
2. Capsulated organs (liver, kidney, ovary). Sharp and steady pain *without* relation to body functions.
3. Muscle-walled cavities (uterus, bladder, gallbladder). Sharp and crampy pain and *related* to function
4. Artery. Sharp, severe, and steady pain, with very sharp accentuations
5. Blood in abdominal cavity. Dull awareness and their sharp steady pain
6. Myocardium. All pain is referred. Dull, heavy ache is usual and worsens with activity.
7. Paired organs. Lateralized pain

ORGAN SYSTEM PAIN PATTERNS

Lactic Acidosis

As seen in diabetes mellitus patient on phenformin, the onset of lactic acidosis can be sudden, sharp, steady, and diffuse, and palpation shows rebound tenderness present with no bowel sounds or hypoactive bowel sounds.

Appendicitis and Terminal Ileitis

These are manifested with a diffuse, dull pain in the umbilical area followed later with crampy and sharp right lower quadrant pain.

Acute Myocardial Infarction

The pain of AMI is heavy, dull, and frequently vaguely localized to the epigastric or left upper quadrant.

Lower Lobe Pneumonitis

This causes steady full-to-sharp pain in the upper quadrant and, occasionally, the lower quadrant, frequently accentuated on deep inspiration.

Acute Cholecystitis

Generally, there is a diffuse, dull, slow onset of epigastric pain developing into sharp right upper quadrant pain on palpation, and there may be rebound tenderness in the right upper quadrant. There is usually pain in the right scapular area (referred pain that is steady and severe known as Kehr's sign).

Rupturing Aortic Aneurysm

Sudden, sharp lower-quadrant pain and testicular pain (referred) occurs, and there is palpation tenderness in the area of maximum pain and hypoactive or absent bowel sounds.

Ectopic Tubal Pregnancy Rupture

The pain is rather sudden, sharp, and steady in the lower quadrant (lateralized); usually bowel sounds are normal or hypoactive. There is deep palpation tenderness over the area of maximum tenderness and pain at the base of the neck and top of the shoulder (again referred pain from diaphragmatic irritation due to free blood in the abdomen).

Ileal/Jejunal Obstruction

This is marked by rather sudden and diffuse dull to sharp umbilical area pain, then crampy (colicky) sharp pains every 2-3 min; between cramps, pain is still present but dull and steady.

Reno-Ureteral Lithiasis

This is characterized by sudden and severe sharp lumbar (costovertebral angle) pain that can be colicky; pain then moves around the flanks toward the inguinal area and a colicky sharp pain persists; steady testicular pain is also present in the male.

CLASSIFICATION BY PAIN PATTERNS

Abdominal disease can be categorized in three general groups, although the signs and symptoms overlap. If the pain pattern description is complete, there is a high probability of placing the problem in the correct category and determining the optimum management regimen.

The categories separate naturally into *catastrophic, colic,* and *inflammatory.* It is important to be aware that the catastrophic category will have extensive blood volume deficit of either whole blood or plasma, and immediate replacement must be anticipated. Patients in this category are either in shock or will be shortly.

CATASTROPHIC ABDOMINAL DISEASE

The abdominal disease entities in the catastrophic category have a sudden onset, continuous pain, a boardlike abdomen, general tenderness, and a usually silent belly. There is shock with hemoconcentration and a variable temperature—low if in deep shock and febrile if the shock is compensated (general abdominal inflammation as in generalized peritonitis).

Etiology

The etiology is a perforated hollow viscus, ulcer, or appendicitis, hemorrhagic pancreatitis, perforated solid viscus, volvulus, mesenteric occlusion, or a ruptured abdominal aneurysm. An ECG and X-ray will rule out coronary occlusion, pulmonary embolism, and dissecting thoracic aneurysm, which can mimic abdominal organ pain.

Pathophysiology

The pathophysiology of the catastrophic group involves whole blood loss in vascular rupture, shock with hemoconcentration from plasma loss into the third space (high Hct) if inflammation is extensive, and bacterial sepsis in lower bowel areas of necrosis.

Management

Management begins with blood volume stabilization, utilizing whole blood, colloids, or Ringer's lactate (large losses can be equivalent to those of a 30%

total body area burn). Urgent surgery is needed to correct perforation or to excise devitalized tissue, and appropriate antibiotics should be administered.

COLIC

Organs with pain in the colic category are generally those of the gastrointestinal tract, all of which are hollow organs. The usual onset is sudden episodic pain, poorly localized, with hyperperistalsis if the gut is involved. There is lateralized pain if paired organs are involved.

Etiology

The etiology is hollow-organ obstruction (stomach, small bowel, colon, biliary tract, renal ureters, and tubal torsion).

Pathophysiology

The pathophysiologic conseqences are loss of water and electrolytes from vomiting or diarrhea and renal reciprocal electrolyte excretion to maintain the acid-base balance when H^+ is lost.

Management

Management of the colic category involves water and electrolyte replacement of gastrointestinal losses and urgent surgical correction of any obstruction or possible strangulation.

INFLAMMATORY ABDOMINAL DISEASE

Inflammatory diseases can be considered "minimodels" of the catastrophe group and manifest themselves with a gradual onset of steady pain, a visceral-to-parietal shift of pain with increasing severity and local tenderness and muscle spasm at the site of inflammation.

Etiology

The etiology of the inflammatory group includes cholecystitis, duodenal and gastric ulcer, interstitial pancreatitis, appendicitis, diverticulitis, and pelvic inflammatory disease (PID).

Pathophysiology

The pathophysiologic process involves plasma loss into the area of inflammation, which seldom exceeds 1 liter and is satisfactorily replaced with water-electrolyte solutions without colloid. There may frequently be a gut organism sepsis present.

Management

Management involves surgery (though it is less urgent than in the other groups), water and electrolyte replacement, and adequate antibiotic therapy when gut sepsis is present.

OBSERVATIONAL ALERTS FOR THE EDN

Some additional points are included here on the more frequently seen catastrophic abdominal disease states to facilitate an earlier recognition and more effective nursing management.

Perforated Peptic Ulcer

Most perforations of peptic ulcers (gastric or duodenal) occur in the anterior wall and allow leakage of gastric contents (highly acid) into the peritoneal cavity causing a "chemical" peritonitis. This results in copious secretion from the peritoneum, which rapidly develops into a purulent peritonitis. There is a 75-80% mortality associated with bleeding and/or perforated peptic ulcers, and these patients present as *critically ill* and *often hypovolemic.*

Gastric Lavage

With repeated emesis of bright blood indicating an active gastric bleeding point, an iced-solution lavage is frequently indicated. Whether iced water, saline, or Ringer's solution is best for lavage has not been critically studied and iced water is considered as safe, less expensive, and more readily available than saline, unless the patient has had prior gastric surgery.* A large-bore double lumen gastric tube should be passed and connected by a "Y" connector to continuous low suction so that lavage of 50-300 cc tidal wash of iced solution can be returned immediately. This repeated procedure can frequently hold or staunch a heavy, active gastric bleed.

Acute Pancreatitis

This disease is seen in varying degrees of severity and is usually associated with either *biliary tract disease* or *alcoholism* or both. The pancreas will begin digesting itself in the face of stimulation of secretions and duct obstruction. Alcohol is thought to have a stimulating effect on the production of pancreatic enzymes in an indirect way. Pancreatitis may also be associated with acute mumps, morphinism, and the effects of some other drugs and bacterial disease. Pancreatic autodigestion results in an outpouring of fluid into the retroperitoneal and peritoneal cavities. If large enough volumes are lost into these spaces, *hypovolemia and shock develop.*

---

*Tedesco FJ: Acute Upper Gastrointestinal Hemorrhage. Drug Therapy Hospital, p 27, July 1981

Relief of pain depends on meperidine (Demerol), since morphine is generally thought to cause *spasms of the sphincter of Oddi.* An NG tube will help relieve pancreatic secretion by drawing off gastric juice. A large-bore IV line is initiated with Ringer's lactate, to be followed with blood as necessary. Surgical intervention is urgent in pancreatitis associated with jaundice and in acute hemorrhagic pancreatitis.

Ruptured Spleen

Disease causing enlargement, delayed hematoma formation from trauma, or spontaneous rupture from straining, with production of intra-abdominal pressure may cause the spleen to rupture. A sudden onset of left upper-quadrant pain, again, sometimes refers to the left shoulder (diaphragmatic irritation) and is known as *Kehr's sign.*

Small Bowel Obstruction

Obstruction may occur at any site in the small bowel with proximal obstruction (the duodenum or jejunum) reflecting in emesis, while obstruction of the ileum will result in distention, with emesis following later. As the obstructive process persists, congestion occurs with edema and progressive compromise to the supporting circulation of the small bowel, eventually strangulation and perforation cause spillage into the peritoneum, and a severe chemical/bacterial peritonitis results.

Acute Appendicitis

Appendicitis is *the most common cause* of the acute abdomen and usually results from an obstructive process in the appendix. Anatomically, the appendix may lie in many varying positions, and inflammation of the appendix mimics many other acute abdominal conditions. The common denominator is *always* pain, usually periumbilical, which localizes to the RLQ and becomes increasingly sharper, with anorexia, nausea, and vomiting. The pain is usually constant, may radiate to the flank area, is aggravated by walking, straining, or coughing, and may be accompanied by a persistent, very strong urge to move the bowels.

Mesenteric adenitis commonly must be distinguished from appendicitis; the blood count is characteristically low, as in viral conditions, with a predominance of lymphocytosis, and pain is located along the route of the mesentery. With appendicitis, urinalysis shows a high specific gravity and blood cells may be present on microscopic examination.

Ruptured Aneurysm

One abdominal crisis which must be discussed is a ruptured aneurysm of the abdominal aorta or the splenic artery. This is indeed a catastrophic happening, seen mostly in *arteriosclerotic males over age 50.* There is a sudden onset of midline back pain, "constant and boring," which is unlike any back pain the patient has previously experienced. The abdominal pain is usually encircling or a sudden, sharp lower-quadrant pain with referred testicular or groin pain. Profound shock may be present, or the patient may be normo-tensive with a pulsatile mass in the periumbilical area, usually *to the left* of midline. Femoral pulses are present in most cases, but distal pulses depend on the peripherovascular status of the patient.

The immediate nursing management of this patient includes CBC, imme-diate upper airway care, CBC type and crossmatch. The patient is held NPO, with a large-bore IV line initiated for large amounts of Ringer's lactate. A Foley catheter is placed to closely monitor the output; a minimum of 8-12 units of blood is typed and crossmatched, and baseline ABGs are drawn if the patient is in shock. An ECG is done since most of these patients have arteriosclerotic heart disease. Abdominal X-rays are taken to demonstrate aortic calcification. Resuscitative measures are initiated as indicated, and immediate surgery for resection and prosthetic graft replacement is performed. A large majority of these aneurysms rupture *retroperitoneally* and are temporarily tamponaded until surgery can be performed. Still, there is a 50% mortality, and efficient management with minimal time loss may save the life.

PRIORITIES OF TREATMENT

The patient presenting with an acute abdomen is evaluated initially in the same manner as any other, in that the total patient must be assessed with re-gard to airway, adequate circulating blood volume to sustain the vital signs, and a satisfactory cardiac rate and rhythm.

Collecting a Data Base

In general, then, after these prerequisities are met, the EDN should proceed to collect a data base with a clinical impression of the organ system involved and a comprehensive history for the physician to build on, requisitioning the usual blood specimens (CBC, chemistry battery, serum amylase, possibly sugar or alcohol levels), urinalysis, surgical series of X-ray films (four-way of abdomen and chest: PA chest, PA abdomen in supine, upright, and lateral decubitus), blood pressure and pulse with possible "orthostatics" as indi-cated, and repeated serial VS with any bleeding.

Supportive Care

Supportive treatment initially, of course, depends upon the severity of the complaint, but a patient in severe abdominal distress should be held NPO, have an IV initiated to run TKO (to keep open) until fluid administration is indicated, possibly glucose or bicarbonate administered, blood at least typed with a "hold" on the crossmatch until indicated, and enough analgesia to re-lieve the "top edge" of pain. It is a simple matter for the physician to order meperidine (50 mg) or morphine (4 mg), and if all analgesic effect needs to be removed for diagnostic evaluation of pain, give naloxone (Narcan) 0.4 ml IV.

Tubes

The mechanics to be observed include a *Foley catheter* with a calibrated collection bag attached for accurate hourly output, an *NG tube* inserted (type of tube according to local preference), and a *CVP line* either inserted or by cutdown (if indicated).

Key Observation

Continuous observation of these patients is essential, with regular monitoring of VS and documentation on a flow sheet. "Hands on" evaluation is a valuable technique since a drop in blood pressure will cause the skin to become *cold* first at the ankles, then at the knees, calves, and, lastly, thighs. If all these areas are cold to the touch and the pulse rate is greater than 100 with a lowering blood pressure, there is probably severe trouble in store for the patient.

THE NURSE'S ROLE AND MANAGEMENT GUIDELINES

The nurse closely follows the patient's clinical status through repeated observations based on sound historical data. Observe what *needs* observing—*i.e.*, pulse rate, skin temperature, patient facies, posture, etc.; expect and anticipate change; anticipate the worst possible diagnosis so that you are prepared mentally to respond accordingly if a drastic situation develops.

The EDN should be able to expedite patient care by initiating basic systems support and monitoring parameters as well as clinical laboratory evaluations.

1. Learn supportive methods of airway control, including intubation.
2. Learn to draw ABGs.
3. Do catheterizations of the stomach and urinary bladder.
4. Learn insertion of Jelco-type catheters and angiocaths and become familiar with the assembly and use of CVP catheters, lines, and manometers.
5. Learn the assessment of cardiac rhythms and treatment methods.
6. Establish standing orders and procedures for the department, which your physician staff will help develop at a realistic level and allow those qualified to proceed confidently.

Above all, *listen, look,* and *observe* the patient who can tell the nurse so much about disease and acute abdominal situations. Strive to develop effective "focused interview" techniques, and give the patient simple direct choices in the interest of rapid and effective intervention in acute situations.

REVIEW

1. Describe the anatomic contents of the abdomen according to the topographic divisions used in medicine.
2. Define the following:
   - Vomiting
   - Regurgitation
   - Constipation
   - Diarrhea
   - Melena
   - Hematochezia
   - Hematemesis
   - Pain
   - Tenderness
3. List some of the essential areas of observation for the patient with an acute abdominal problem.
4. Describe the specific pain pattern for:
   - Bowel
   - Capsulated organs
   - Muscle-walled cavities
   - Arteries
   - Blood in the abdominal cavity
   - Myocardium
5. Explain the significance of a pain pattern.
6. List the priorities of treatment in the patient presenting with an acute abdomen and the supportive treatment to follow.
7. Identify the diagnostic procedures that are of value in determining the cause of distress in an acute abdomen.
8. Identify the three disease categories of classification for the acute abdomen.
9. Describe the signs and symptoms of each category of the acute abdomen and explain the pathophysiology involved with each group.
10. Identify the presenting symptoms, observations, assessment, and management guidelines for:
   - Perforated peptic ulcer
   - Ruptured speen
   - Acute pancreatitis
   - Acute appendictis
   - Small bowel obstruction
   - Ruptured aneurysm
11. Outline the general responsibilities of the EDN and the guidelines that should be employed in the management of a patient with acute abdominal distress.

BIBLIOGRAPHY

Buckingham WB, Sparberg M, Brandfonbrener M: A Primer of Clinical Diagnosis, 2nd ed. Harper & Row, New York, 1979

Budassi SA, Barber JM: Emergency Nursing: Principles and Practice. C.V. Mosby Co., St. Louis, Missouri, 1981

Cain HD: Flint's Manual on Emergency Treatment and Management. C.V. Mosby Co., St. Louis, Missouri, 1980

Cosgriff JH, Anderson DL: The Practice of Emergency Nursing. J.B. Lippincott Co., Philadelphia, Pennsylvania, 1975

DeGowin E, DeGowin R: Bedside Diagnostic Examination. Macmillan, New York, 1981

Guis JA: Fundamentals of general surgery. *In* The Acute Abdomen, Chapter 21, Year Book Publishers, Chicago, Illinois, 1966

Peterson CG: Perspectives in surgery. *In* The Acute Abdomen, Part V, Lea & Febiger, Philadelphia, Pennsylvania, 1972

Rudy EB, Gray VR: Handbook of Health Assessment. The Robert J. Brady Co., Bowie, Maryland, 1981

Smith C: Abdominal assessment—a blending of science and art. Nursing 81, Vol 11, No. 2, p 42, February 1981

Warner C: Emergency Care: Assessment and Intervention, 2nd ed. C.V. Mosby Co., St. Louis, Missouri, 1978

GENITOURINARY EMERGENCIES   *17*

KEY CONCEPTS

This chapter provides an overview of the genitourinary tract and the assessment and management of traumatic processes involving it, as well as the recognition and management of infectious disease processes, including those of the venereal or sexually transmitted disease (STD) types. The chapter is based on the concepts of recognition and management as presented to emergency nurses in lectures by James Pappas, M.D., and Arnold Rustin, M.D., both urologists in the Portland metropolitan area, and by Howard Kirz, M.D., emergency physician with Group Health Hospitals in the Seattle area, with background material researched and prepared by Sara Rich, R.N., M.Ed., Portland, Oregon.

After reading and studying this chapter, you should be able to:

- Describe methods of visualizing the GU tract.
- Explain externally evident bleeding as opposed to bleeding that occurs above the GU membrane.
- Describe the points of recognition and management for some common forms of external GU trauma.
- Identify some of the key factors affecting decisions in the management of renal injuries.
- Identify pathways by which bacteria enter the urinary tract.
- Describe the signs and symptoms of acute pyelonephritis, acute cystitis, and acute urethritis.
- Describe the pathophysiology of septic shock.
- Identify the signs, symptoms, and immediate intervention in septic shock.
- Outline management protocol for ED management of sexually transmitted diseases (STDs) including gonorrhea, body lice, venereal warts, herpes progenitalis and nonspecific urethritis (NSU).

REVIEW OF THE URINARY TRACT

The *normal* urinary tract is composed of two kidneys, two ureters, one urinary bladder, and the urethra (Fig. 17.1).

The kidneys are large bean-shaped glands located in the thoracolumbar region in the space behind the abdominal cavity (retroperitoneal) with the right kidney lying just anterior to the twelfth rib and the left kidney lying just anterior to the eleventh and twelfth ribs. The right kidney is slightly lower because of downward displacement by the posterior edge of the liver. The two ureters convey urine from the kidneys to the urinary bladder, where it is collected and voided via the urethra.

THE KIDNEY

The kidney functions to control extracellular fluids (volume of water, concentration of electrolytes, osmolarity, and concentration of hydrogen ion), to produce erythropoietin necessary for red blood cell maturation, and to indirectly control blood pressure by a hormonal mechanism called the renin-angiotensin system. The kidney is the site for excretion of the wastes of metabolism and derives its blood supply from the renal arteries, which are branches of the abdominal aorta. Occlusion of the aorta, whether due to thrombi, emboli, or obstruction secondary to trauma located above the origin of the renal arteries, may deprive the kidneys of adequate blood flow and predispose to renal failure.

THE NEPHRON

The unit known as the nephron (Fig. 17.2) does the work of the kidney, and there are probably a million or more nephrons in each kidney. The nephron is composed of the *glomerulus* or *Bowman's capsule* (in the cortex), the *proximal convoluted tubule,* the *loop of Henle,* and the *distal convoluted tubule* (penetrating down into the medulla). The glomeruli filter the blood as the first step in the formation of urine, depending on the hydrostatic pressure created by the pumping action of the heart, the volume of blood circulating through the glomeruli, and the resistance offered by the arterioles carrying the blood. The kidneys filter approximately 170 liters per day and reabsorb all but 1.7 liters, which are excreted as urine. Normally, with each heartbeat, approximately one-fourth of the blood pumped by the heart circulates through the kidney and is filtered through Bowman's capsule. The proximal tubule, loop of Henle, and distal tubule are the functional areas involved in filtering out the waste products of metabolism for excretion and regulating the water and salt balance of extracellular fluid. The kidneys eliminate all the excess water that is not lost through the gastrointestinal tract, lungs, or skin. It is necessary that there be some excess water for the kidneys to secrete because dissolved in the urine are substances that are toxic if not eliminated; therefore, we must take in daily more water than is lost by way of lungs, alimentary tract, and skin so that there

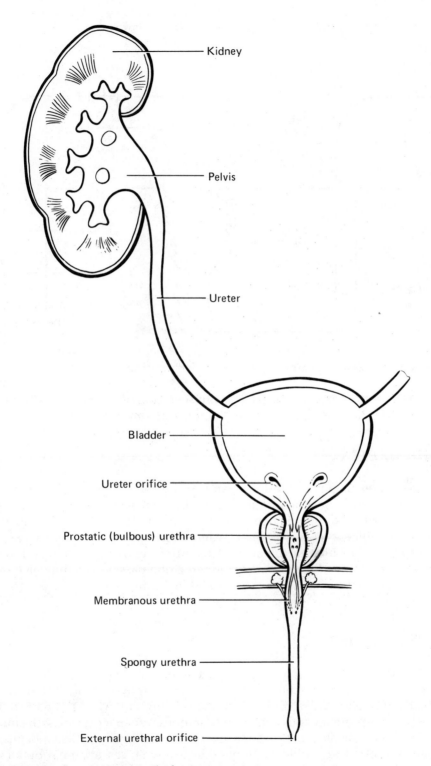

Figure 17.1. Outline of structures of urinary tract.

Proximal Convolution   Distal Convolution

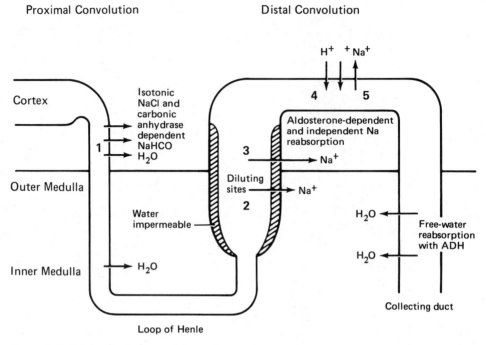

Figure 17.2. Schematic diagram of the nephron.

will be a sufficient amount to allow the secretion of urine. Normally, urinary output in a healthy adult should be approximately 1 cc/kg/hr.

THE URETER

The ureter begins at the lower end of the renal pelvis and normally lies behind the lower pole of the kidney with the average length of the adult ureter at about 10 in, depending somewhat on the height of the individual. The ureteric orifices of the bladder vary considerably in size, shape, and appearance. The internal urinary meatus and the two ureteric orifices form the three angles of the *trigone of the bladder.* Urine passes from the pelvis of the kidney, down the ureter, and into the bladder by means of a series of peristaltic waves.

THE BLADDER

The urinary bladder is a hollow muscular organ lying in the anterior part of the pelvis, behind and somewhat above the symphysis pubis. The bladder is chiefly muscular, with a complete mucous lining, and when the normal bladder is relaxed, the mucous coal is quite smooth. When it contracts, the muscle fibers bundle up all over the organ, except on the *trigone,* which remains perfectly smooth. The bladder is supplied by two main vessels, the superior vesicle and the inferior vesicle arteries, of which there is one on each side. The nerve supply to the bladder comes from the pelvic plexus on each side. The bladder is frequently torn in association with fractures of the pelvis or by blunt trauma, allowing urine to leak into the abdominal cavity.

THE URETHRA

The female urethra is about 2-3 cm long and is not liable to injury by the same forms of trauma as in the male. An accurate knowledge of the anatomy of the male urethra is important in appreciating the different types of injury, especially of the closed variety. The male urethra is approximately 20 cm or 8 in. in length in the average size adult and is divided into three parts: the first or proximal part is known as the *posterior* or *prostatic* urethra, lying above the genitourinary diaphragm (membrane) and, therefore, inside the pelvis. The *membranous uretha* is very short and transverses the diaphragm obliquely. The third or *anterior part* (sometimes referred to as the spongy urethra) reaches from just below the inferior layer of the genitourinary diaphragm to the external meatus.

VISUALIZATION OF THE GENITOURINARY TRACT

Injuries of the urinary tract are simple in nature, generally speaking, and it is an easy system to deal with because all parts of the GU tract can be visualized, as opposed to the general surgery involved in opening a belly and visualizing traumatized organs.

Radiologic visualization of the GU tract is accomplished by:

1. Intravenous pyelogram (IVP): provides a view of the collecting system and is nontraumatizing

2. Cystogram: provides a view of the bladder

3. Retrograde pyelogram: involves cystoscopy and catheterization of the ureters to visualize the tract

4. Cystoscopy: provides visualization of the bladder wall, prostate, and anterior urethra (vaginoscopy with cystoscope in young females is done for visualization of a foreign body or infection)

5. Renal angiogram: involves threading a catheter up the femoral artery to the aorta and selectively introducing dye for visualizing kidney vascularity (1-2% morbidity)

Contrast studies for visualization of the GU tract which will involve IV administration of radiopaque substances *should have an additional informed consent* signed by the patient, in case of untoward reaction to the injected dyes.

EVALUATION OF BLEEDING SOURCES

All of the urinary tract is *extraperitoneal,* an important concept to remember. Kidneys and ureters lie behind the posterior parietal peritoneum, and the bladder lies in the anterior part of the pelvis under the parietal peritoneum. The GU membrane (GU diaphragm, urogenital diaphragm) runs from the urethra, down along the perineum to the anus, and back to the coccyx to hook onto the sacrum, forming a complete envelope around the pelvic bone. *Any extravasation of blood within the pelvic floor will not be evident externally due to the barrier effect of the GU membrane, nor will any bleeding external to the pelvis be allowed to enter the pelvis.* If bleeding occurs in the urethra, blood will be evident at the meatus, but if blood is passed in the urine, look for a problem *in the bladder* or higher up the GU tract to the ureters and kidneys. If hematuria is present, be certain to ask the patient *where* in the stream the blood occurs. This information will likely give a general indication of the bleeding source. If blood is present throughout the stream, it is mixed in the bladder; if blood is present at the beginning of the stream, there is a bleeding point somewhere down the urethra.

TRAUMA TO MALE GENITALIA

Emergencies involving the external male genitalia are not uncommon and must be managed carefully and rapidly to avoid damaging consequences. Some of the more commonly seen problems with some very general guidelines for emergency intervention are as follows:

1. Phimosis (constricted foreskin) with or without balanitis. Treatment is a dorsal slit of the foreskin.
2. Adherent foreskin. Treatment is morphine sulfate or meperidine for the severe pain, local anesthesia, and retraction of the foreskin.
3. Paraphimosis with strangulation. Treatment is forceful drawing down of the foreskin, with a dorsal slit done if necessary to overcome the swelling. Hyaluronidase (Wydase), 1 cc, is sometimes injected locally to reduce swelling.
4. Ring constriction (frequently seen in children). Treatment is removal with a ring cutter or, if necessary, removal under general anesthesia.
5. Zipper injuries. Treatment is as follows:
    A. Sedate the patient as necessary to obtain cooperation
    B. Cut the zipper fabric from the clothing with scissors if necessary, but *do not bend or cut* the zipper with wire cutters since this may lock the teeth so that the slide cannot be pulled back.
    C. Holding the zipper firmly by both ends, close it a very short distance further and then gently disengage the entangled skin.
    D. A short inhalation anesthesia may be necessary, but most often a 2% lidocaine (Xylocaine) jelly or 4% lidocaine solution topical can be applied gently on the skin for some degree of a local anesthesia.

E. After removal of the tissue from the zipper teeth, an antiseptic ointment and dressing are applied, following with cold compresses for 12
hours. Adult male patients should use a suspensory until healed, to
reduce edema and to speed the healing process.

Local anesthetics should *not* be injected since this will add to the
problem of local edema, making the removal more difficult, and acute
toxic reactions may occur because of the extreme vascularity of the
tissues with subsequent rapid absorption. The skin should *never* be
cut free of the zipper teeth since this will produce a laceration requiring surgical closure, which may result in scar tissue with contraction
and permanent deformity.

6. Specific emergencies involving the scrotum and its contents include:

A. Scrotal tears, which are commonly seen in farming communities that
use power take-off equipment. Clothing is caught in the equipment,
and the skin of the scrotum is avulsed as a result. Treatment is accomplished with skin grafts; emergency treatment is to cover the
wounded scrotum with sterile saline packs and prepare the patient
for rapid admission to the operating room.

B. Scrotal hematomas are seen after delivery in newborns, in straddle
injuries, and, not infrequently, following vasectomies. There is no
treatment other than to watch for infection and treat for comfort.
These hematomas are *not* drained, unless there is a break in the skin,
because of the high infection risk.

C. Cryptorchidism (usually with testicular torsion) can be confused with
appendicitis. *Always* check for the presence of a testis in the scrotum
on the right side.

D. Scrotal *surgical* emergencies are:

- Indirect hernia or communication hydrocele with a palpable mass
in the scrotum, scrotal pain, and vomiting. This requires ruling out
an incarcerated hernia.

- Testicular torsion, which is a twisting of the supporting cord of the
testis, with pain, swelling, and tenderness. The majority of these
males (65%) are between the ages of 12 and 18, and 85% of them
experience an abrupt onset of testicular pain and testicular tenderness, with about half of them having had previous episodes. There
may be scrotal edema, fever, and abdominal pain as well. The testicular survival rate has been shown to be approximately 47% in
these cases. The major causes of the low salvage rate are a delay in
surgery or misdiagnosis. Generally speaking, there is surprisingly little morbidity of the testis up to 6 hours; up to 10 hours, a 70%
salvage rate. At more than 16 hours, the rate of testicular salvage is
extremely low. Rapid evaluation and surgical intervention are
required; *both* testes must be surgically fixed in place, or "pexed,"
within 6-12 hours for a significant salvage rate.*

*Kirz H: The tender testicle. Washington ACEP Scientific Assembly at SeaTac, Seattle, 1977

- Epididymitis is a most frequently seen scrotal pathology in the emergency department and it is essential to rule out 1) torsion in a young patient with resulting gangrene, 2) bleeding into a tumor, and 3) kidney stone, because the kidney, ureter, and testes basically have the same innervation (T_{11}, L_1). Epididymitis is an infection that is almost always secondary to prostatitis and is common over the age of 20, with a slow onset, and often following clearcut GU infections or instrumentation. Severe flank pain can be secondary to acute epididymitis. The treatment is bed rest, hot packs, and a scrotal "bridge." Prehn's sign (relief of pain in epididymitis when the scrotum is elevated) is useless in torsion of the testis.

SUMMARY OF GENERAL MANAGEMENT GUIDELINES AND NURSING ALERTS

The following are some of the general principles of management for genital and extrapelvic injury or pathology:

1. For wounds of the penis, preserve the tissue, divert the urine if necessary, and control bleeding with sutures and pressure.
2. Wounds of the penile skin and scrotum should be cleansed and debrided. Cover the sterile saline packs and prepare for the operating room.
3. Strangulation of the penis is managed by removing the constricting agent, diverting the urine, and preserving the maximal viable length surgically.
4. Priapism (sustained painful erection of the cavernous bodies of the penis) requires sedation, ice packs, and analgesia if necessary (after 12-24 hours). The etiology must be determined if possible (penile cancer, blood diseases, and psychological situations).
5. Testicular trauma. Minor trauma to the testes requires support and cold packs. Testicular mobility "mitigates" against injury in that it diminishes or lessens the chance of testicular trauma from entrapment.*
   A. Marked hematoma and swelling of the scrotum requires surgical exploration to drain, and lacerations must be ruled out or repaired.
   B. Remember that torsions can occur as a result of trauma.
   C. Explore, debride, and drain all penetrating wounds.
   D. Remember that "traumatic" epididymitis is rare and that tumor of the testis often presents after relatively minor trauma.
6. Hematuria is significant as an indication of a *stone* rather than torsion or epididymitis. In trauma, blood at the meatus requires a urethrogram before a Foley catheter is passed.

*Kirz H: The tender testicle. Washington ACEP Scientific Assembly at SeaTac, Seattle, 1977

7. When evaluating a scrotal "mass" or swelling, remember that fluid in the scrotum will *transilluminate* when a flashlight is held behind it; a solid mass will not. The presence of fluid indicates less likelihood of an emergency situation and is also less likely to be painful.

8. Torsion of the spermatic cord is surprisingly common. It is most likely to be found in a pubescent male who presents with abrupt onset of testicular pain, tenderness, vomiting, and often a history of previous episodes. Pathological and clinical studies indicate that *6-10 hours* is the critical time period; to avoid the problem of delay in surgery, patients with the appropriate clinical picture alone should immediately be treated for torsion.* The physician must be notified *without* delay.

EXTRAPELVIC INJURIES TO THE URETHRA

Urethral injuries are classified as extrapelvic (below the GU membrane) and intrapelvic (above the GU membrane). Most urethral injuries occur *below* the GU membrane, and some of the more commonly seen injuries are as follows:

1. Straddle injury (the most classic type seen) crushes the bulbous or prostatic urethra between the inferior border of the pubic arch and the object on which the patient falls, causing partial or complete tear of the urethra.
   A. The signs and symptoms include pain and the inability to void or a "stuttering" stream when voiding. The patient may void once but extravasation of urine from the damaged urethra will cause sphincter spasm, preventing further urination. Blood may be seen at the external meatus with extravasation of blood locally.
   B. Retrograde urethrography and pelvic X-ray films are indicated although the pelvis is not usually fractured. The patient should be catheterized in emergency situations with *meticulous* aseptic technique required. If the catheter cannot be passed, for any reason, either a suprapubic cystostomy and/or perineal exploration is indicated. (Fractured pelvis is associated with about 20% of injuries to the urinary tract.)

2. Perforated posterior urethra from instrumentation (iatrogenic, meaning physician-caused)

3. Crush injuries of the penis with protracted results.

4. Penetrating injuries with fairly obvious damage.

5. Periurethral abscess, seen generally in older diabetics.

6. Injury *within* Buck's fascia (the envelope of deep fascia surrounding the penile structure), which will manifest with blood in the voided urine.

7. Injury *outside* Buck's fascia will be seen as blood extravasated into the perineum, scrotum and up the abdominal wall.

*Kirz H: The tender testicle. Washington ACEP Scientific Assembly at SeaTac, Seattle, 1977

INTRAPELVIC INJURIES

Intrapelvic GU injuries (*above* the GU membrane) involve the same tract in the male and female, except for the prostate in the male.

URETHRAL PROBLEMS

It is less likely for the urethra to be torn off the GU diaphragm in females but fistulas *are* common in females. *Persistent* watery drainage from the vagina after a surgical procedure usually indicates a urethrovaginal (vesicovaginal) fistula *below* the GU diaphragm, and the patient will have water from the urethra and vagina on voiding.

Other intrapelvic genitourinary problems include cystocele, which is a prolapse of the bladder into the vagina, with stress incontinence; the presence of foreign bodies in the urethra and bladder; and, in the male, avulsion of the prostate (commonly seen in fractured pelvis), which may be found in conjunction with the bladder neck severed and floating free. The bladder neck will constrict, the bladder will distend with urine, and the patient will be unable to void. There may or may not be blood from the meatus. The patient has pelvic tenderness and although generally not in shock, must be watched closely, with vital signs carefully monitored. A KUB film shows lots of "hazy stuff" in the pelvis. The treatment is as little surgical dissection for primary care as possible; too much dissection or instrumentation threatens later sexual potency in the male.

BLADDER TRAUMA

Bladder injuries, like lung injuries, may be classified as penetrating and nonpenetrating (or blunt), with the mechanism of injury being a fractured pelvis, trauma to the abdomen, or deceleration injury from a seat belt (whether or not the victim has a full bladder at the time). The symptoms may include shock, pain, hematuria, and the inability to void as desired. However, remember that even with a ruptured bladder, hypotonic or isotonic urine may cause *little* pain initially in the peritoneal cavity and may remain asymptomatic for a period of time.

URETERAL TRAUMA

Ureteral injuries from penetrating or crushing trauma are rarely seen. These injuries may usually be repaired at operation, so a retrograde IVP is required for diagnosis and early definitive treatment is surgery. Hematuria may be absent.

RENAL TRAUMA

Renal injuries are rarely found singly, and 80% have associated chest or intraperitoneal injuries caused by direct force crushing against adjacent body structures of the spine and ribs, as well as by indirect injury from falls and violent muscular action. Some general considerations of renal injuries would include the fact that the kidneys lie in a protected position, and serious injuries are relatively uncommon, although minor trauma can produce severe renal injury, especially in diseased kidneys, which are more prone to injury. Definite diagnosis of renal injuries must be made by a urologist, and the initial diagnosis is usually made in the ED. Some of the key factors affecting decisions and the management of renal trauma are the following:

1. Unilateral renal agenesis is present in 1/500 people, and 10%-14% are born with *some* anomaly of the genitourinary tract. It is, therefore, mandatory to assess renal function and/or the presence or condition of the contralateral kidney.
2. One-third of patients with renal trauma may have major visceral injuries, one-half may have skeletal injuries, and one-third may have no other serious injuries.
3. Severe hemorrhage usually causes a tamponade effect, which occurs within Gerota's fascia (the capsule surrounding the kidney) after 800-1200 cc of bleeding.
4. Retroperitoneal bleeding, secondary to trauma, is almost impossible to stop immediately, and most physicians feel that administration of up to 20 units of blood is allowable before surgical intervention for a nephrectomy is mandated.
5. Urinary extravasations *must* be drained within a few days unless they are of minor degree and are transitory.

Signs and Symptoms

The signs and symptoms of severe renal trauma are flank pain, tenderness, possible hematuria, rigidity, fever, leukocytosis, paralytic ileus, shock, etc.

Intervention

Treatment comprises clinical assessment and resuscitation, including urinalysis, hemoglobin and hematocrit, renal function, urine culture and sensitivity tests (C&S), insertion of a Foley catheter with careful monitoring of output, and X-ray studies. The retrograde pyelogram is 90% diagnostic, but be wary of large doses of IV contrast media in situations favoring heart failure or volume overload, shock, or dehydration. These hypertonic radiopaque solutions *may* increase serum osmolality by 30%.

URETERAL STONES

Probably all stones found in the ureter come from the kidney. The majority pass down to the bladder after one or several attacks of colic, although a smaller number are arrested in their passage because of their size or irregular shape. It is rare for the stone to pass through the ureter without pain, usually starting in loin, passing through to the front, reaching the scrotum in the male and the vulva in the female. The pain is extremely severe, causing the patient to double up and writhe about in bed, sweating and groaning. There may be anuria, occurring when a stone blocks each of the ureters or only the functioning side. Hematuria may be present or absent depending upon the degree of blockage. If there is a partial obstruction of the ureters, red blood cells will be found in the urinalysis. A total obstruction will usually reveal no red blood cells.

Nursing Responsibilities

Immediate treatment includes generous medication for the severe pain, *filtering all urine* for stones, urinalysis, and culture and sensitivity in case of an obstruction with infection, as well as continued close observation. Diagnosis is confirmed by an intravenous pyelogram and/or KUB. The indications for intervention with renal or ureteral calculi are 1) infection, 2) obstruction, and 3) intractable pain.

URINARY RETENTION

There are many causes of urinary retention in the male patient, the most common being prostatic hypertrophy, followed by obstruction from various causes. Other causes include strictures of the urethral meatus, foreign bodies, retention associated with trauma, gonococcal infections, and various drugs, including the belladonna alkaloids, amitriptyline HCl (Elavil), desipramine HCl (Pertofrane), and imipramime HCl (Tofranil). The management of the severely distended bladder involves observing great caution when decompressing a bladder that has sustained insult in a patient who has *cardiovascular* complications. The following is a *guideline* for safe decompression:

> The maximum amount of urine to be removed at any time should be 500 cc. Clamp the catheter. Wait 1 hour and remove another 100 cc. Remove 100 cc/hour until the bladder is empty, and then remove 200 cc/hour as the bladder regains normal function and capacity.

INFECTIONS OF THE GU TRACT

Apart from the distal centimeter or so of the anterior urethra, the urinary tract is normally sterile, and it is abnormal for organisms to be present in the bladder. Infections do occur, however, in the kidneys, ureter, bladder, and the urethra—some together and some separately. Any part of the genital system, the prostate, vesicle, vas, epididymis, and testes may also be affected. The treatment for acute infection of the urinary tract requires accurate diagnosis of the infection, and before any definitive treatment is started, a clean catch specimen must be obtained in a sterile container for laboratory analysis and culture. Any urine specimen going to the lab should be marked, for safety's sake, "hold for C&S" until the physician decides whether culture and sensitivity tests are needed.

The bacteria commonly responsible for infections of the urinary tract are *Escherichia coli,* one or more species of *Klebsiella, Enterobacter, Proteus, Pseudomonas,* and various enterococci, all normal constituents of the bowel flora. *Escherichia coli* is the positive organism in about 85% of acute infections of the bladder and kidneys in patients who have not been subjected to instrumentation and in whom no obstruction exists. Patients who have been treated with antimicrobial drugs and those who have been subjected to urologic procedures are more likely to have *Proteus, Pseudomonas,* or *enterococci* as the invading organisms.

PATHWAYS OF INFECTION

Pathogenic organisms invade the urinary tract by four pathways: 1) the ascending route, 2) urethrovesical reflux, 3) instrumentation and, 4) blood and lymph channels.

1. Invasion of pathogenic bacteria within the urethra represents the most common pathway of infection of the urinary tract. In the male, the length of the urethra and the antibacterial properties of prostatic secretion are thought to be effective barriers against invasion by this route, explaining why males have a much lower incidence of urinary tract infections than females. The high incidence of urinary tract infections (UTI) at the time of marriage, in association with sexual activity, clearly implicates the ascending urethral pathway in urinary tract pathology in females. Probably the major way in which most bacteria are introduced into the urinary tract, both in children and in adults, is by fecal soiling of the urethral meatus.

2. Urethrovesical reflux occurs when intrabladder pressure increases suddenly in normal women, as during coughing, resulting in urine being squeezed out of the bladder into the urethra. The urine may then flow back into the bladder when pressure returns to normal, and in this way washes bacteria from the anterior portions of the urethra into the bladder.

3. The spreading of potentially pathogenic bacteria via instruments is an important cause of infection because it is commonly done, and it is usually preventable. Typical acute UTI and pyelonephritis *often* follow the use of a catheter or a cystoscope.

4. Infection of the kidney via the bloodstream is unusual but is to be strongly suspected in cases of staphylococcus urinary infections (kidney infection is likely to be secondary to an infection elsewhere in the body), as well as invasions of *E. coli* subsequent to severe gastrointestinal disturbances.

NONSPECIFIC INFECTIONS OF THE KIDNEY AND URETER

Pyelonephritis

This fairly common disease is a frequent cause of chronic renal failure and hypertension. In acute pyelonephritis, multiple inflammatory foci are scattered through the parenchyma of the kidney with sudden onset of a general feeling of malaise, backache, shivering, fever, and an aching in one or both loins. Within 24 hours of onset, there is usually some disturbance of urination, usually with increasing frequency, burning, and occasionally frank hematuria. The temperature may go as high as 105° or over, and examination of the urine will show pus and organisms with a few red blood cells and the organisms grown on culture. This is probably the commonest of all kidney diseases, and it may occur in association with renal stones although more frequently no actual cause for the infection is found.

Cystitis

A common occurrence, cystitis affects all ages and is especially prevalent in the female, in childhood, in pregnancy, after the menopause, and is frequently recurrent. The most common cause is a bacterial infection, and the most common affecting organism in the initial attack is *E. coli*. Acute inflammation usually starts quite suddenly with a little irritation in the bladder region and a desire to pass urine. Severity of the symptoms rapidly increases until there is an almost constant desire to urinate, and scant amounts are passed which burn and cause pain, especially severe at the end of micturition. The patient may appear flushed with a dry tongue and exhibit tenderness in the suprapubic region. Urinalysis will show an acid state, hazy in appearance, and containing pus, bacilli, and a few red cells. Again, culture will show the commonest organism to be *E. coli*. If treated promptly and adequately, the symptoms rapidly subside. However, if therapy is insufficient, the situation may quickly relapse or recur in a short period of time.

Acute Urethritis

Acute inflammation of the urethra will occur within a few hours of exposure when the organisms have gained a firm foothold on the first part of the urethra. In the course of several days, pus forms and is discharged from the urethra. The symptoms, which may develop with 24 hours of exposure, at first consist of an itching, tickling, or burning sensation at the external meatus, which soon becomes red, feels hot, and burns on passing urine. There is increased frequency of urination, and a discharge soon appears, which may be watery or frankly purulent. There may also be hematuria. Acute urethritis is often associated with coitus.

SEPTIC SHOCK

Perhaps the major difference between the course of hypovolemic shock and that of septic shock is *time*. In hypovolemic shock, the progress from hypotension to ischemia to anoxia usually takes several hours, time enough to stop the bleeding and institute treatment in most patients. In septic shock, stagnant anoxia may develop in a very short period of time, depending on the amount of endotoxin released by gram-negative bacteria and the susceptibility of the patient. The overall prognosis (mortality between 70% and 90%) can be improved, and often the patient's condition, before shock develops, is the key to the possibility of survival. With the possibility of survival so low, prevention of shock is far superior to the best treatment. The susceptible patients must be identified: for instance, newborns, patients over 60 years old, all debilitated patients, diabetics, cancer patients who have undergone tumor chemotherapy or whole-body radiation therapy, patients with open wounds or abscesses, surgery patients, patients on immunosuppressive medications, and *catheterized* patients.

NURSING RESPONSIBILITIES

Once susceptible patients are identified, the nurse must watch for subtle changes that may indicate sepsis. A patient may have normal skin temperature, normal pulse, and normal urine output, and still go into shock. If a susceptible patient develops headache, fever or a subnormal temperature, if breathing becomes rapid and shallow, if a *change is noted in the patient's mental state,* or *if the urine output decreases slightly but steadily,* don't wait any longer before calling the physician and getting treatment started.

Treatment must be directed against the cause of sepsis as well as the shock. Usually the cause is a gram-negative organism (*E. coli*). If the focus of infection is not known, antibiotic therapy should be started immediately with a powerful broad-spectrum agent until culture results are available. At the same time supportive treatment must be started as follows:

1. *Support respirations.* More septic shock patients die with respiratory problems than with perfusion failure. If an airway is needed, put it in early and supply enough oxygen to augment hemoglobin levels and reduce tissue hypoxia. Shunting is common in septic shock and should be suspected if the patient's extremities continue to be cold and pale and obliguria continues despite oxygen and fluid replacement.

2. *Provide adequate circulating volume.* As endotoxin is released in the bloodstream, it causes intense vasospasms in small vessels, particularly in the liver, kidneys and lungs. This effect is so similar to that of anaphylaxis that many suggest endotoxic shock is an anaphylactic reaction. Whatever the mechanism, the result is a pooling of blood in the affected capillaries, fluid flows into the interstitial space, and circulating blood volume is further reduced. Compensating for this loss of circulating blood volume calls for fluid infusion, either blood or other colloids if the patient is

anemic, crystalloid if he is not. The amount must be titrated on the basis of the patient's response (CVP, blood pressure, urine output, pulse, and sensorium). Two points must be emphasized. First, the fluid must often be rapidly hyperreplaced in the patient with septic shock—sometimes 8-12 liters are required in a few hours. Second, obliguria is *not* an indication for decreasing fluid infusion.

3. *Give pharmacologic support.* Although it is highly controversial in the treatment of shock, many physicians are now recommending a single massive steroid dose at the first sign of sepsis. Others give repeated doses during the first 24 hours of treatment, and still others reserve steroid administration for patients who do not respond to treatment with fluid replacement, oxygen, and antibiotic therapy. The number of physicians who believe steroids have no place in shock therapy is diminishing, and every ED should have the capability of administering massive doses of steroids when ordered by the physician.

VENEREAL (SEXUALLY TRANSMITTED) DISEASE

The term venereal disease has been replaced with the usage of sexually transmitted disease (STD), as adopted by the World Health Organization (WHO). This section of the chapter will deal with more frequently seen STDs in this country and those that are posing a public health problem of almost epidemic proportions in many areas.

SYPHILIS

Although syphilis has not regained epidemic proportions as yet, it is making a "comeback," according to epidemiologists, and there has been an eightfold increase in primary and secondary syphilis cases. *Treponema pallidum* is the causative organism and is a delicate spirochete found in lesions and in the bloodstream. Moisture and warmth of the body temperature are necessary for survival and the organism is therefore transmitted by direct contact with infectious lesions of early syphilis.

Primary Stage

Following an incubation period of approximately 10-90 days (the average is 21 days), the lesion of *primary syphilis* begins as an indurated papule that breaks down rapidly to form a single, relatively painless, clean-based indurated ulcer. This chancre forms at the site of treponemal penetration. Common sites for the chancre include the genitalia, rectum, mouth, and lips, but it is important to remember that the chancre may occur anywhere on the body.

Secondary Stage

Approximately 6 weeks to 6 months (the average is 6-8 weeks) following the onset of syphilis, the patient enters the *secondary stage*. This is marked by a great variety of dermatologic manifestations, which are present either as a generalized eruption or may occur on only a small area of the skin. Macular lesions are a raw ham color and blanch on palpation. Papular lesions are usually reddish infiltrated lesions, approximately 0.5 cm in diameter, and are the commonest lesions seen, occurring on flexor surfaces of the palms and soles. Mucous patches found in the mouth, rectum, and vagina are highly contagious.

Lymphadenopathy is generalized, and the character of the enlarged lymph nodes is the same as is found in primary syphilis: firm, freely movable, nontender, round, and rubbery, without erythema of the overlying skin.

In addition to dermatologic manifestations, secondary syphilis is a systemic disease, that is, possible subacute meningitis and a mild, transient asymptomatic proteinuria may develop.

Latent Stage

In the absence of treatment, the lesions of secondary syphilis heal in approximately 4-12 weeks, and the patient enters the *latent stage*. Latent syphilis is defined as the absence of clinical lesions. Early latent syphilis (less than 4 years' duration) is considered potentially infectious following relapse to secondary. Late latent syphilis (greater than 4 years' duration) is considered noninfectious, although it is transmitted congenitally. Adequate treatment of the mother during the first 18 weeks of gestation prevents infection of the baby, adequate treatment after the 18th week cures the baby *in utero*.

Treatment for primary and secondary syphilis is:

1. Benzathine penicillin G, 2.4 million units total, into one or two intramuscular injection sites, or
2. Aqueous procaine penicillin G, 600,000 units daily intramuscularly for 8 days to total 4.8 million units.

In the event of allergy to penicillin, erythromycin or tetracycline may be given, 500 mg qid × 15 days, but should not be attempted on an outpatient basis because of difficulty in follow-through.

CHANCROID OR SOFT CHANCRE

This is a less frequently seen disease manifested by an ulcer that is usually situated on the external genitals but may occasionally be intrameatal in position, causing considerable pain on voiding. The incubation period varies between 1 and 3 days, and the ulcer first appears as a small reddish papule, which soon becomes pustular and breaks down to form a painful, nonindurated ulcer with undetermined edges. The base is dirty gray or yellow in color; the lesions are invariably multiple fresh areas, often with a linear distribution, developing by autoinoculation. Papules, pustules, and ulcers are often seen on the same day, which is a helpful diagnostic point, and pain is a marked feature. The inguinal glands become enlarged and tender, and the lymphatics leading to the groin may stand out as red painful threads. Treatment of choice is administration of sulfonamides.

GONORRHEA

The causative organism of gonorrhea is *Neisseria gonorrhoeae,* commonly called the gonococcus. It is a gram-negative diplococcus of the genus *Neisseria* and does not possess spores, true capsules, or flagella; it is aerobic but grows best under stimulation of carbon dioxide. The organism has fastidious growth and survival requirements; it needs a medium on the alkaline side and dies on exposure to the weakest acid, requires a temperature of 35 to 36° C, (95 to 96.8° F) and dies if the temperature is raised or lowered by 3 degrees. It must have moisture and dies immediately on drying.

Symptoms may occur as early as 1 day or as late as 2 weeks after contact. The average incubation period for males is 3-5 days; in the female, it is difficult, if not impossible, to know when symptoms first begin. There is a history of sexual exposure within the prior 2 weeks, and the early symptoms include uncomfortable sensations along the course of the urethra (a tickling sensation) followed by frequency of urination. In the male, this is commonly followed in a matter of hours by a purulent urethral discharge, dirty yellow in color. Infection is localized to the anterior urethra for the first 2 weeks or so and then spreads backward to the posterior urethra, involving the prostate and often the seminal vessels; from here the infection follows the vas to the epididymis, resulting in a painful, usually unilateral epididymitis.

In a female, acute gonorrhea usually involves the urethra, Skenes glands, Bartholin glands, and the cervix. The vagina is never affected after the age of puberty. Pelvic inflammatory disease (PID) may follow immediately after an acute infection or may be delayed for several months and, as a rule, during the childbearing years. When it occurs, both fallopian tubes are frequently affected; resulting scar tissue may block the lumen or trap purulent discharge to form a pyosalpinx which may in turn provoke peritonitis. Proctitis, when it occurs in males, is almost always a result of homosexual contact. In women, it may be caused by direct spread from vaginal discharges as well as genital-rectal exposures. A 50% failure rate in the treatment of pharyngea gonococcal infections has been documented, with an increased rate of pregnant women with pharyngeal gonococcal infections. It has been recommended, therefore, that cultures of the cervix and the pharynx both be done in pregnant women with gonococcal infections.

Diagnosis

To diagnose gonorrhea in women, culture specimens should be obtained from the endocervical and anal canals and inoculated on separate Thayer-

Martin (TM) culture plates or in separate Trans-grow (TG) bottles. Again test-of-cure cultures are recommended for all women treated for gonorrhea, and specimens should be obtained from the endocervical and anal canals as well as the pharynx if the woman is pregnant. Gram-stain smears are *not* adequately sensitive to rule out the presence of gonorrhea.*

In diagnosing gonorrhea in men, microscopic demonstration of typical gram-negative, intracellular diplococci on smear of a urethral exudate *does* constitute sufficient basis for a diagnosis of gonorrhea. When gram-negative diplococci cannot be identified under a smear of a urethral exudate or when urethral exudate is absent, a culture specimen should be obtained from the anterior urethra and inoculated on TM or TG medium. In homosexual men, additional culture specimens should be obtained from the anal canal and the oral pharynx, and inoculated on TM or TG medium.

FOLLOW-UP AND TREATMENT

Syphilis

It is desirable that follow-up urethral cultures be obtained from males 7 days after completion of therapy; cervical and rectal cultures should be obtained from females 7-14 days after completion. It is recommended that gonorrhea patients have a serologic test for syphilis at the time of diagnosis. Patients receiving recommended parenteral penicillin need not have follow-up serologic tests. However, patients treated with ampicillin, spectinomycin, or tetracycline should have a follow-up serologic test for syphilis each month for 4 months to detect syphilis that may have been masked by treatment for gonorrhea. Patients with gonorrhea who also have syphilis should be given additional treatment appropriate to the stage of syphilis. While long-acting forms of penicillin are effective for treatment of syphilis, they have no place in the treatment of gonorrhea.

Gonorrhea

Untreated gonococcus will progress into disseminated gonococcal infection (DGI), and this accounts for *greater than 50%* of the arthritics seen between 15 and 30 years of age. There are characteristic skin lesions seen in DGI, with hemorrhagic or pustular lesions on the extremities more than on the trunk. There may be papules or petechiae and hemorrhagic bullae (usually seen in meningococcemia).

The drug therapy of choice in uncomplicated gonococcal infections in men and women is the administration of *aqueous procaine penicillin* G (APPG), 4.8 million units, intramuscularly, divided into at least 2 doses and injected at different sites at one visit, together with 1 g probenicid by mouth just before the injections. (*Whenever* penicillin is given parenterally, the patient *must* be observed for at least 30 min to be certain an anaphylactic reaction will not occur.)

*Taken from Criteria and Techniques for the Diagnosis of Gonorrhea, DHEW, Center for Disease Control, Atlanta, Georgia, 1973

The alternate regimen for patients for whom oral therapy is preferred is *ampicillin,* 3.5 g by mouth, together with 1 g probenicid by mouth, administered at the same time. There is evidence that this regimen may be slightly less effective than the recommended APPG regimen. Patients who are allergic to penicillin (penicillin G, ampicillin) or probenicid are treated with tetracycline HCl, 1.5 g initially by mouth, followed by 0.5 g by mouth 4 times per day for 4 days for a total dosage of 9.5 g. Other tetracyclines are not more effective than tetracycline HCl. All tetracyclines are ineffective as single-dose therapy.

Spectinomycin hydrochloride (2 g IM) in one injection may be given as the last alternative. However, the Venereal Disease Control Advisory Committee of the National Center for Disease Control recommends that spectinomycin be held in reserve for treatment of failures of other therapies. A small percentage of gonococcal infections have been refractory to treatment with penicillin and on a second positive culture were found to be *penicillinase* producing Neisseria gonococcus (PPNG). Penicillinase (Neutrapen) is an enzyme produced by certain bacteria, which converts penicillin to an inactive product and thus increases bacterial resistance to the antibiotic. Therefore, it is essential that this strain be eradicated as rapidly as possible. For this reason, spectinomycin is being held as the specific treatment for PPNG, and it becomes imperative that repeat cultures be obtained to identify persistently positive cultures.

BODY LICE

Body lice (Phthiruspubis or "crabs" as they are called on the street) are frequent visitors to the ED and are found in the pubic hair areas, although other hairy areas should be inspected as well for nits (eggs). The lice have a 7-day egg cycle during which time the larvae hatch, grow to maturity, and lay their eggs. Gamma benzene hexachloride (Kwell), the treatment of choice, is a prescription item and is a liquid which should be applied liberally over the genital area and any other hairy areas that may be infected, left on for 12 hours, reapplied and left on for another 12 hours, and then showered off. This treatment should be repeated every 7 days for several weeks in order to be effective. Patients under treatment for body lice will become reinfected unless their immediate personal environment (bedding, clothing, etc.) is treated concurrently with an over-the-counter preparation called RC Spray (not for human use). There are several other over-the-counter preparations for body application although they are not as effective as gamma benzene hexachloride (Kwell). In order of potency they are "A-200," "Dolex," and "Triple X;" instructions should be carefully followed on each individual medication.

VENEREAL WART

The venereal wart (condyloma acuminatum) is viral in orgin and has an incubation period of up to 6 months. The warts are found in the anal area, foreskin, and vaginovulvar region, with chronic discharge. Venereal warts have been treated with trichloracetic acid and, most effectively, topical application of a 25% solution of podophyllin in compound tincture of benzoin. The podophyllin solution is liberally applied to the *warts only,* since it may be toxic to normal skin, and is allowed to remain for 4 hours; it should then be washed off. The patient should return in 1 week for a retreatment. Podophyllin is known to be keratogenic and is capable of causing congenital abnormality and should not be used on pregnant women.

GENITAL HERPES

The *herpes 2 virus* (progenitalis) is being seen in epidemic proportions. The female patient may present with multiple small vesicular ulcerations of the skin and mucous membranes in the vulvovaginal area, which are extremely painful, and there may even be an enlargement of the inguinal lymph nodes. The primary episode may last from 14 to 21 days, and as the primary lesions heal, the virus travels up to the *presacral ganglia,* where it lies dormant between recurrences, which will flare about every 2 months in approximately half the patients. Diagnosis is made by a Pap smear showing multinucleated giant cells recovered from the endocervix. Male partners will have a high virus titer in their semen.

Congenital malformations as well as *neurologic defects* can develop during the first month of life in *30% of newborns* exposed to the herpes virus, which is either swallowed in the birth canal or acquired from the mother's milk. There is also thought to be a possible relationship to hearing defects and, indirectly, to damaged IQs. There has been enough concern expressed to generate the medical judgment that the presence of herpes on the labia is an indication for a caesarean section.*

The treatment for the herpes 2 virus is for the most part palliative, with frequent sitz baths, local soothing ointments and analgesics. No consistently-effective treatment has been found although some believe that idoxuridine (Stoxil) will help to control the infection in spite of recurrences; others advocate the use of proflavine, a dye that is applied topically and then exposed to light. Proflavine, however, is known now to be carcinogenic beyond certain dosage levels. Acyclovir has been found effective in initial cases with a shortened viral shedding time and accelerated healing of lesions.

NONSPECIFIC URETHRITIS

Nonspecific urethritis (NSU) or nongonococcal urethritis (NGU) is frequently seen in males following administration of penicillin with bacterial overgrowth of Chlamydia trachomatis.

---

*Holmes K: An Overview of STD, Oregon ACEP Spring Seminar on STD, Portland, Oregon, 1975

Chlamydia is known to be the causative agent in trachoma (a chronic infectious disease of the conjunctiva and cornea) and lymphogranuloma venereum, as well as nonspecific urethritis.

The symptoms may resemble those of gonorrhea and frequently are mistaken as such until a negative GC culture is obtained. About 50% of problems with male urethritis are, in fact, NSU.

Treatment should consist of:

1. Tetracycline 500 mg qid $\times$ 7 days for both partners since about 75% of female partners have been found to have Chlamydia present in the endocervix.

2. Urinalysis and C&S with sulfisoxazole (Gantrisin) as drug of choice if urinary tract infection is present.

3. Phenazopyridine hydrochloride (Pyridium) 100 mg given for urinary anesthesia if no bacteria are present on microscopic examination of urine.

Table 17.1 Genital Ulcerations

DISEASE	ULCER	PAIN	BUBO
Syphilis	3+	0	2+
Chancroid	4+	3+	3+
Herpes 2	2+	4+	0
Granuloma Inguinale	3+	1+	0
Lymphogranuloma Venereum	2+	1+	0
Chlamydia (NSU/NGU)	0	1+	0

CATHETERIZATIONS IN THE ED

Catheterization of the urinary bladder in most instances is a nursing procedure and one that requires great attention to technique and accountability. The patient who is suffering from trauma, debilitation, or illness may easily undergo extensive and even devastating complications if scrupulous aseptic technique is not exercised while introducing the catheter to avoid contamination and sepsis, especially with gram-negative organisms.

Too often, details of sterile technique are lost or neglected in the frequently harried efforts to get "all the tubes going" with a critically ill or injured patient, and the use of antibiotics is relied upon to make up for all of the "violations." It *still* remains the primary nursing responsibility to safeguard the patient's well being by following every careful step of the procedure, as well as the following ones:

1. Discarding contaminated catheters or gloves if technique is broken

2. Prepping the meatus properly

3. Introducing the catheter with strict aseptic technique and minimal trauma

4. Immediately attaching a sterile one-way drainage unit, irrigant, or plug if the catheter is to remain indwelling

5. Taping the catheter carefully to the inner thigh with a chevron tape to prevent pulling or undue pressure on the retention bulb.

Only sterile *disposable* catheters should be used in the ED, and most now are either silicone-treated or Silastic to minimize traumatic irritation to the meatus. The Tieman Foley catheter is recommended by many urologists for male catheterizations because the configuration of the tip reduces trauma to the prostatic urethra and facilitates passage of the catheter.

REVIEW

1. Explain the procedures available to visualize the GU track.
2. List six major functions of the kidney.
3. Explain the reason external bleeding is evident as opposed to internal bleeding in relation to the GU membrane.
4. Describe the symptoms, observations, and management protocol for the following traumas:
   A. Straddle injury of the urethra
   B. Testicular torsion
   C. Wounds of penile skin and/or scrotum
   D. Severe renal trauma
   E. Kidney stone
5. List the five key factors affecting decisions in the management of renal trauma.
6. In relation to the abdominal peritoneal cavity, where does *all* of the urinary tract lie?
7. Identify the structure that defines the division between intrapelvic and extrapelvic urinary tract injuries.
8. Explain a KUB showing "hazy stuff" in the pelvis, accompanied by anuria or hematuria and borderline shock following a fractured pelvis or deceleration injury from seat belts.
9. Identify a very helpful diagnostic aid for a swollen and/or edematous scrotum and explain the rationale.
10. Identify four pathways by which bacteria enter the urinary tract.
11. Describe the signs and symptoms of the following:
    A. Acute pyelonephritis
    B. Acute cystitis
    C. Acute urethritis
12. Describe the pathophysiology of septic shock.

13. Outline the signs, symptoms, and steps to be taken for immediate intervention in septic shock.
14. Explain the importance of the time element in rapid intervention.
15. Explain the diagnostic criteria of gonorrhea for males and females.
16. Describe the recommended ED management of the following:
    A. Gonorrhea
    B. Body lice
    C. Venereal warts
    D. Herpes progenitalis
    E. Nonspecific urethritis in males

BIBLIOGRAPHY

Badenock AW: Manual of Urology. Year Book Medical Publishers, Chicago, Illinois, 1974

Brunner S, Suddarth DS: The Lippincott Manual of Nursing Practice, 2nd ed. J.B. Lippincott Co., Philadelphia, Pennsylvania, 1982

Budassi SA, Barber JM: Emergency Nursing: Principles and Practice. C.V. Mosby Co., St. Louis, Missouri, 1981

Cain HD: Flint's Manual on Emergency Treatment and Management. C.V. Mosby Co., St. Louis, Missouri, 1980

Center for Disease Control: Criteria and Techniques for the Diagnosis of Gonorrhea. Center for Disease Control, USPHS, Atlanta, Georgia, 1973

Center for Disease Control: Gonorrhea Recommended Treatment Schedules. Center for Disease Control, DHEW, USPHS, Atlanta, Georgia, 1974

Committee on Injuries, American Academy of Orthopedic Surgeons: Emergency Care and Transportation of the Sick and Injured, 3rd ed. American Academy of Orthopedic Surgeons, Chicago, Illinois, 1981

Cosgriff JH, Anderson DL: The Practice of Emergency Nursing. J.B. Lippincott Co., Philadelphia, Pennsylvania, 1975

Curran JW, Schrader MV, Moyer JK, et al: Gonorrhea in the emergency department. JEN, Vol 7, No 2, pp 209-213, September/October 1981

DeGowin E, DeGowin R: Bedside Diagnostic Examination. Macmillan, New York, 1981

Freeman PB: Gonorrhea. JEN, Vol 6, No 3, pp 17-22, May/June 1980

Guis JA: The acute abdomen. Fundamentals of General Surgery, Chapter 21, Year Book Publishers, New York, 1966

Holmes K: An Overview of STD. Oregon ACEP Spring Seminar on STD, Portland, Oregon, 1975

Kirz H: The tender testicle. Washington ACEP Scientific Assembly at SeaTac, Seattle, Washington, 1977

Livingston WK: Visceral pain. Clinical Aspects of Visceral Neurology, Chapter III, Charles C. Thomas, publisher, Springfield, Illinois

Miles PA: Sexually transmissible diseases. JEN, Vol 6, No 3, pp 6-12, May/June 1980

Oill PA: Herpes virus type 2 infection of the genital tract. JEN, Vol 6, No 3, pp 13-16, May/June 1980

Symposium on venereal diseases. Med Clin N Am, Vol 56, No 5, 1972

Warner C: Emergency Care: Assessment and Intervention, 2nd ed. C.V. Mosby Co., St. Louis, Missouri, 1978

OBSTETRIC/ GYNECOLOGIC EMERGENCIES *18*

KEY CONCEPTS

This chapter should provide the EDN with an overview of pelvic and obstetric emergencies with general guidelines for assessment and intervention in the ED setting.

After reading and studying this chapter, you should be able to:

- Outline the presenting signs, symptoms, and management for:
  Vaginal bleeding
  Pelvic inflammatory disease
  Postabortal infection
  Ectopic pregnancy
  Adnexal pathology
  Mittelschmerz
  Intrauterine device (IUD) complications
  Vaginal discharges.
- Describe the evaluation and management of a pregnant woman in the last trimester of pregnancy presenting with signs of toxemia.
- Describe the evaluation and management of a woman during precipitous childbirth.
- Explain the APGAR scoring method for newborns.
- Describe the management of a breech delivery.
- Describe the management of a presenting prolapsed cord.
- Describe the management of a premature placental separation.
- List the contents of an emergency OB pack.

in the ED, the pelvic problems of females can be effectively managed by a logical and cautious approach, ruling out the possibilities step by step. The most common obstetric and gynecologic emergencies seen in the emergency setting are 1) bleeding, 2) pain, 3) infections, 4) complications of pregnancy, and 5) trauma.

VAGINAL BLEEDING

When a female presents with a complaint of "vaginal bleeding," it is always a sound concept to *assume that she is pregnant* until proved otherwise. Menstrual cycles vary widely, as do amounts of menstrual flow (normally between 70 and 100 cc per period); the advent of the oral contraceptive (OC) and the intrauterine device (IUD) bring many other variables into the picture.

The patient may complain of vaginal beeding with or without pain and should be closely observed for the amount of bleeding and for general complexion. Since this "bleeding" can be a relative description from the patient, safeguard your observations by placing a clean perineal pad in position to obtain a baseline of accuracy in your description while you proceed with assessment. The nursing history should include an evaluation of the vital signs, the date of last menstrual period (LMP), number of pregnancies, number of living children, use of IUD, use of the OC, any treatment for infection or other problems, number of pads saturated per day, and any signs of urinary tract infection.

Determine pregnancy by a gravid index of the urine and draw blood for a CBC (including hematocrit), type and hold on crossmatch. An IV line should be initiated if there is significant bleeding, and the patient should be prepared for pelvic examination.

PELVIC INFLAMMATORY DISEASE

Pelvic inflammatory disease (PID) generally results from chronic gonorrheal infections and frequently occurs from irritation of an IUD. The patient with PID presents with two rather typical signs that are almost diagnostic by themselves: 1) the "shuffle," a characteristic bent-over shuffling gait of the PID patient who cannot endure the pain of standing upright, or the jarring of a normal gait because of exquisitely tender pelvic organs secondary to the inflammatory process; and 2) the "chandelier sign," a term used when the PID patient experiences such incredible pelvic tenderness during the pelvic examination that the slightest lateral torsion exerted against the cervix will trigger even greater pain on the stressed adnexa, causing the patient to "go for the chandelier."

The patient generally complains of pain and vaginal discharge with or without bleeding and on examination will usually have severe bilateral nonradiating pelvic pain, often following cessation of menses, with an elevation of temperature and some vaginal spotting. A CBC and sedimentation (sed) rate should be done and will usually show a very high WBC (20,000-30,000) and an elevated sed rate. A gram stain may be positive, and culture and sensitivity tests will be positive.

Hospitalization should be strongly considered for women with suspected salpingitis who are severely ill, to administer antibiotics and analgesics, to drain cul-de-sac abscesses if necessary, and to intervene surgically. A ruptured pelvic abscess is an indication for immediate abdominal hysterectomy and bilateral salpingo-oophorectomy. Mortality runs high if postponement is as much as 12-24 hours. Adequate treatment of women with acute gonococcal salpingitis must include appropriate treatment of their male sex partners because of the high prevalance of nonsymptomatic urethral gonococcal infection in such men. Failure to treat male sex partners is a major cause of recurrent gonococcal salpingitis. Follow-up of patients with salpingitis is essential, and all patients who have been treated in hospitals should return for repeat pelvic examinations and cultures for N. gonorrhoeae after treatment.

POSTABORTAL INFECTION

The symptoms are chills, fever, *severe* lower abdominal pain with foul vaginal discharge and dark, scant urine. Observations will reveal abdominal distension, hypoactive bowel sounds, and lower abdominal tenderness with rebound. The vaginal discharge is extremely offensive, and the entire pelvic area is extremely sensitive, with a dilated cervix.

Assessment of this patient would include a culture and sensitivity check of the endocervix for both aerobic and anaerobic organisms. Gram-stained smears, CBC (marked leukocytosis—a leukopenia means a poor prognosis), a BUN and creatinine for baseline of renal function, platelets, serum fibrinogen and clotting time for assessment of clotting ability (DIC?), whole blood type and crossmatch (hold on crossmatch), and a surgical abdominal X-ray series for the presence of free air under the diaphragm, which would indicate perforation of the uterus.

NURSING RESPONSIBILITIES

The patient must be admitted for massive antibiotic therapy and surgical evaluation of the uterine content. Nursing responsibilities include continuous monitoring of vital signs, arterial blood gases, CVP, intake and output, and close observation of the patient. Be prepared to manage septic shock and peritonitis.

ECTOPIC PREGNANCY

Ectopic pregnancy bears a 13% mortality and should be suspected in any woman in the reproductive age group with acute abdominal pain of sudden onset. A woman who becomes pregnant with an IUD in place has a 1:25 chance that the pregnancy is ectopic. Even women who have undergone tubal ligation present occasionally with this abnormality.

Abdominal pain and intermittent slight brownish spotting are frequent occurrences after a missed menstrual period. Profuse bleeding is seen in only about 5% of patients. *Unilateral* pain, cramping that is mild or sharp and excruciating is seen in over 90% of these patients. Occasionally, there is lateral lower abdominal pain with reflex shoulder pain from subdiaphragmatic irritation resulting from the massive intraperitoneal hemorrhage. In some, the sudden onset of pain is associated with syncope. In 40-60% of patients, a palpable pelvic mass is present, but *repeated examinations* can lead to *rupture* of the mass with resulting intraperitoneal hemorrhage and shock. In 20-30%, there is no history of amenorrhea, but most do have a history of one or more periods missed. These women appear acutely ill and usually have a marked pallor and a distinctly "shocky" look about them. *Immediate* assessment includes a CBC (including Hct and Hgb), type and hold for crossmatch. Cul-de-sac aspiration, using a 10-cc Luer-lok syringe and an 18-gauge spinal needle, is sometimes done; the return of fresh nonclotting blood indicates intraabdominal bleeding.

Immediate management is to institute an IV line for volume replacement with Ringer's lactate followed by whole blood (type-specific), oxygen at a high flow rate, and preparation for emergency surgery to perform laparotomy and salpingectomy with resection of the involved tube.

ADNEXAL PATHOLOGY

Adnexal pathology includes torsion of the adnexa, ruptured ovarian cyst, and intraabdominal bleeding associated with ovulation.

Torsion of the adnexa is most common in ovaries with cystic or solid tumors and is related to unusual mobility. There is a sudden onset of severe lower abdominal pain, usually unilateral. Tachycardia, signs of pelvic peritonitis, and a slightly elevated temperature will be observed. Examination will show an exquisitely tender pelvic mass. The CBC and temperature, which may be normal during the first 12-24 hours, will elevate as the ovary becomes gangrenous. Intervention requires immediate laparotomy and excision of the involved adnexa.

Ruptured ovarian cyst can be caused by trauma (including a pelvic examination), or it may be spontaneous. The onset is sudden, with unilateral low abdominal pain of a prominent nature and, on examination, local abdominal tenderness, rebound tenderness, and exquisite adnexal tenderness. A CBC should be done and the temperature checked. The latter will usually be elevated, as will the WBC. The treatment is with simple analgesics and observation at home. The symptoms will usually subside within 3-7 days.

MITTELSCHMERZ

Mittelschmerz is one of the most common causes of abdominal pain in young women and occurs *mid-cycle* (as the term implies), during ovulation as the ovum is released. It is localized to one adnexa (often confused with appendicitis when the right ovary is involved) and is self-limiting. Mild to severe pain and rebound tenderness may be present, and the WBC may be slightly elevated. The treatment is palliative. The important clue is the anticipated date of the next menstrual period.

INTRAUTERINE DEVICES

The IUD can cause many complications. For every 100 women who have an IUD inserted, about 11 will expel it in the first year. An additional 12 will have the device removed because of difficulties. (These problems, however, decline with parity.) The most commonly used types are Lippe's loop, the Saf-T-Coil, and the Copper 7. Complications from IUDs are most commonly 1) pain and bleeding, 2) PID in about 2%, and 3) perforation of the uterus in about 0.4%, at time of insertion or later working through the wall of the uterus.

VAGINAL DISCHARGE

Vaginal discharge has many causes, but the most common ones seen in the ED are gonococcal, trichomoniasis, moniliasis, or candidiasis, and retained, forgotten tampons.

1. Cultures for GC, both cervical and rectal, should be done routinely in the ED on any woman presenting with vaginal discharge. The treatment is as outlined in Chapter 17 under Venereal and Sexually Transmitted Disease.

2. Trichomoniasis presents as a frothy, watery, yellow discharge with pruritus and punctate hemorrhages of the vagina. Diagnosis is made by a hanging loop, and treatment is metronidazole (Flagyl), 1 tablet TID for 10 days. The partner must also be treated with metronidazole to prevent reinfection. When metronidazole is prescribed, the patient must be *carefully instructed* on the many significant precautions to be observed, as well as the adverse reactions to recognize. Nystatin-neomycin sulfate-gramicidin-triamcinolone acetate (Mycolog cream) is sometimes helpful in soothing the irritated vulvovaginal areas.

3. Moniliasis or candidiasis is prevalent in patients with diabetes (high sugar in the vaginal flora), those on OCs, pregnant women, those with venereal disease, and patients following an antibiotic regimen. Symptoms are local edema, discharge, and pruritus. Treatment is with nystatin (Mycostatin) vaginal tables for females and cream for males.

4. Forgotten retained tampons can account for extremely foul odor and discharge. If one is to be removed in the ED, have deodorant spray on hand

for the sake of other patients as well as staff, and dispose of the offending tampon as soon as possible in the hopper or in a sealed, plastic bag.

OBSTETRIC EMERGENCIES

Obstetric emergencies addressed here include toxemia of pregnancy, breech delivery, prolapsed cord, premature placental separation, and emergency childbirth.

TOXEMIA OF PREGNANCY

Toxemia of pregnancy is a term applied to a group of diseases that are manifested by hypertension, proteinuria, edema, convulsions, and/or coma, all of which may occur singly or in combination. Acute toxemia of pregnancy is an acute hypertensive disease of pregnant or puerperal women, called in its nonconvulsive stage, *preeclampsia,* and in its convulsive stage, *eclampsia.* The patient will complain of abdominal pain, nausea and vomiting, headache, and swelling of the fingers, stating that her rings don't fit. Observation will reveal elevated blood pressure, edema of the extremities, hyperactive reflexes, and albuminuria.

The etiology is not known, but there is an increased incidence associated with twins, primiparity, diabetes mellitus, hydatidiform mole, underweight, hydramnios, vitamin B deficiency, emotional conflict, essential hypertension, and renal disease. Among the other hormonal alterations during pregnancy, there appears to be a markedly abnormal rise in the antidiuretic hormone (ADH) in preeclampsia and eclampsia.

Nursing Management Guidelines

A CBC, urinalysis (clean catch), and evaluation of the edema are done, with continual monitoring of the blood pressure. An IV line should be initiated (heparin lock), and oxygen (at 6 LPM if indicated) with suction should be on standby. Strict intake and output must be maintained (with daily intake usually restricted to 1000 cc over output). Admission for absolute bed rest and sedation is indicated during the last trimester of pregnancy, with anticonvulsant protection at the bedside, including a padded tongue blade, airway management equipment, and intravenous magnesium sulfate.

BREECH DELIVERY*

In a breech delivery, the buttocks and trunk of the infant should be allowed to deliver spontaneously, while the legs and trunk are supported as they de-

*Adapted from Committee on Injuries, American Academy of Orthopaedic Surgeons. George C. Banta, pp 201-202, Menasha, Wisconsin, 1971

liver, letting the legs dangle on each side of your arm with your palm under the trunk. Usually the head follows; however, there are times when the head does not deliver within 2-3 min. Traction must never be applied unless it is done by the physician. Gentleness is the watchword, and since the infant must be provided oxygen if the umbilical cord is compressed by the head in the birth canal, you can try to create an airway for the baby by putting the middle and index fingers of your gloved hand along the face of the infant with your palm toward the face. Extend your hand into the vagina until your fingers reach the area of the infant's nose and form an airway by pushing the vagina away from the baby's face until the head is delivered. Do not allow the head to be delivered forcefully, but slowly as with a normal delivery. *Do not* attempt to pull the baby out. After delivery administer the same care as described for the umbilical cord, placenta, baby and mother in the section on Emergency Childbirth on page 342.

PROLAPSED CORD*

If a *prolapsed* cord becomes evident during delivery, immediately place the mother in shock position with legs elevated, give oxygen at high flow, and keep her warm. With sterile-gloved hand reach into the vagina and push the baby's head up 3-4 in., to allow blood flow through the compressed cord. Continue exerting enough pressure against the baby's head to keep the cord from compressing until the physician arrives, and do not try to replace the cord or apply any pressure to its surface.

PREMATURE SEPARATION OR ABRUPTIO PLACENTA

A premature separation of the normally implanted placenta, or abruptio placentae, presents with vaginal bleeding and uterine pains of varying degrees. Bleeding may be occult and should be suspected if there are signs of impending shock or if there is a rapid increase in the height of the fundus or excessive uterine irritability.

This is a catastrophic situation with two lives at stake. The premature separation of the placenta may be classified in three divisions as mild, moderate, and severe, depending on the stage of labor, the parity of the mother, and the amount of blood lost.

General guidelines for care include estimation of the degree of bleeding, typing and crossmatching for at least 4 units of blood, a CBC (including hematocrit), and an IV line running with an 18-gauge needle. Urinalysis, intake and output, and frequent monitoring of vital signs and the fetal heart are necessary, marking the height of the fundus to determine whether the uterus is enlarging with hemorrhage. If the fetus is at term and a rapid labor cannot be

---

*Adapted from Committee on Injuries, American Academy of Orthopaedic Surgeons. George C. Banta, pp 201-202, Menasha, Wisconsin, 1971

precipitated with oxytocic stimulation, intervention is indicated by means of cesarean section.

EMERGENCY CHILDBIRTH

Precipitous labor or emergency childbirth is a situation requiring quick thinking and a fast evaluation on the part of the EDN as to the time allowance prior to actual delivery of the child. There are several check points that will help in making the correct decisions, and if at all possible, the patient should be transported rapidly to the delivery suite, where the child can be managed in a relatively protected and adequately equipped environment. The initial check points which must be covered are as follows:

1. Is the woman a primipara or multipara? This generally determines the length of the stages of labor unless the fetus is posterior, transverse, or breech.
2. Are the membranes intact? If so, time is on your side.
3. Is there any bright red "show?" This indicates active cervical dilatation and generally is seen in the *last* stages of dilatation.
4. Does the woman feel as though she has to "push" or "bear down?" This indicates delivery is imminent. Instruct the patient to "breathe like a puppy," with short fast respirations and *not* to bear down or push. A forceful expulsion untended can result in extensive lacerations to the mother and damage to the child.
5. Is there "crowning?" This is the presenting part of the baby, as it begins to bulge through the vaginal orifice. In a primipara, this may still leave enough time to get the patient to the delivery room if the pains are not too intense (depending on the distance involved).
6. How long do the pains last? A labor contraction must last at least 45-60 sec to be effective, and the pains should be 1-2 min apart. Anything less than this is not likely to produce a baby in the ED (but don't bet on it!).

If you find yourself in the position of having to manage a precipitous birth, the following are some simple guidelines:

1. Drape and prep the patient as time allows, making every effort to provide the infant a "sterile field" for delivery.
2. Use a sterile gloved hand and sterile towel to push against the infant's head gently as it presents, so that the head does not "explode" from the vagina.
3. When the head is delivered, look and feel to see whether the umbilical cord is wrapped around the neck. If so, slip the cord gently over the baby's upper shoulder, being careful not to tear the cord!
4. As the shoulders deliver, carefully hold and support the head and shoulders while the body delivers, which is usually rather sudden. The baby will be slippery, so be prepared and support the head and neck with one hand while holding the feet with the other hand.

5. Immediately place the baby on its side, with the head lower than the body, and gently suction the nostrils and mouth with a sterile rubber suction bulb to be certain that the airway is clear of mucus and blood. *This is essential. Clear that airway!* It is good practice to lay the baby up on the mother's abdomen with the head slightly lowered while the airway is cleared.

6. It is also essential to *cover the baby immediately* with warm blankets (sterile if possible) to offset a rapid heat loss and possible ensuing acidosis (especially if the Apgar score was low).

7. Clamp the cord with two clamps after cessation of "pulsation," 2-3 in. apart, about 6-8 in. from the navel, and cut between the clamps. An OB nurse can apply cord clamp closer to the navel later in the nursery under controlled circumstances.

8. Record the baby's time of birth and the Apgar score according to chart in Table 18.1.

Table 18.1 Apgar Score Chart

SIGN	APGAR SCORE		
	0	1	2
Heart Rate	Absent	Below 100	Over 100
Respiratory Rate	Absent	Slow, irregular	Good, crying
Muscle tone	Limp	Some flexion of extremities	Active motion
Reflex irritability (response to catheter in nostril)	No response	Grimace	Cough, sneeze, or cry
Color	Blue, pale	Body pink Extremities blue	Completely pink

Sixty seconds after the *complete* birth of the infant (disregarding the cord and placenta), the five objective signs are evaluated and each given a score of 0, 1, or 2. A score of 10 indicates an infant in the best possible condition. Infants with scores of 5-10 usually need no treatment. A score of 4 or below indicates the need for prompt diagnosis and treatment. Approximately 90% of normal infants should score 7 or more 1 min after birth.

The two most important things to remember after the child is delivered are 1) immediately place the baby on its side with the head lower than the body and gently suction the nostrils and mouth to *be certain the airway is clear* of mucus and blood, and 2) *keep the baby warm* at all times and prevent loss of body heat.

Admit the infant to the isolation nursery as soon as possible, with the time of birth and the APGAR score recorded and accompanying the child to the nursery.

Delivery of the Placenta

Following birth of the child, the placenta is delivered. The placenta *usually* separates from the wall of the uterus in a few minutes after delivery of the child, but it may take as long as 15-30 min. The EDN should have oxytocin (Pitocin), 5 units, or methylergonovine maleate (Methergine) 1 ampule, ready for IV administration after the placenta delivers, noting whether the placenta appeared intact or not. Then place a sterile perineal pad between the patient's legs and massage the fundus to speed involution of the uterus and the reduction of bleeding.

Keep the mother warm, the fundus firm, and admit her to OB as soon as possible.

Baptism in Emergency Situations

Baptism is traditionally the responsibility of clergy. However, in emergency situations with no clergy present, exceptions are made. In the event of an apparent "stillborn" infant or of imminent death of the infant following birth, emergency personnel of any religion may baptize the newborn child of Christian parents, either upon their request or because of personal religious convictions. The procedure is to put a drop or two of water on the bare head of the baby while saying "I baptize thee in the name of the Father, and the Son, and the Holy Ghost." This exact wording should be followed.

THE EMERGENCY OB PACK

A simple emergency OB pack should be kept in every ED and need not contain anything more than the following:

Sterile pack:

- 2 infant blankets
- 2 surgical towels
- 2 cord clamps (plastic disposables)
- 2 OB perineal pads
- 12 gauze sponges (4 × 4)

The sterile pack should be wrapped separately, rotated and re-autoclaved regularly, and kept in plastic wrap with a 3-month shelf date.

Additions to top of the pack, which need not be re-autoclaved are:

- 1 sterile, disposable, suction bulk for infant
- 1 sterile, disposable, No. 15 surgical blade
- 2 pair sterile surgical gloves
- 2 plastic sacks (for placenta, soiled garments, etc.)

REVIEW

1. Describe the presenting signs and symptoms of the following entities and outline the management for each in the ED.
   A. Vaginal bleeding
   B. PID
   C. Ectopic pregnancy
   D. Mittelschmerz
   E. Vaginal discharges

2. Identify the one assumption that must be made about a woman who presents with vaginal bleeding, until proven otherwise.

3. If a pregnant multiparous woman in the third trimester presents in your ED with complaint of swollen extremities and a persistent headache, describe your first questions to her and your first approaches to physical assessment.

4. Identify six checkpoints of importance in evaluating the stage and speed of labor process.

5. Describe the Apgar scoring method of the newborn infant and explain its purpose.

6. Evaluate the Apgar score for an infant following a rapid precipitous delivery when the fetal heart tones had been depressed (100), there were no visible respiratory efforts, some flexion of extremities was present, the infant grimaced in response to a catheter in the nares, and the body was pink with blue extremities.

7. Evaluate the Apgar score for an infant born with an HR of 148, a good loud spontaneous cry, active motion, good reflex irritability, and a pink body with blue extremities.

8. Identify the priority of intervention in a breech delivery with a prolonged delivery of the after-following head and describe what action you would take.

9. Describe the immediate intervention to be taken if a woman presents in hard labor with a prolapsed cord and the infant's head crowning, and why.

10. Describe the immediate action to be taken with a suspected premature placental separation.

11. Identify the two essential priorities of management with a newborn infant regardless of time, place or situation.

12. Describe the baptismal procedure for a stillborn infant.

13. Describe the contents of an adequate emergency OB pack.

BIBLIOGRAPHY

Apgar V: Apgar method of scoring. Cur Res Anesth Analg, Vol 32, p 260, 1953

Avila S, Blinik G: Emergency management of vaginal bleeding. JEN, Vol 1, No 6, 1975

Barber H, Fields DH, Kaufman SA: Quick Reference to Ob/Gyn Procedures, 2nd ed. J.B. Lippincott Co., Philadelphia, Pennsylvania, 1979

Budassi SA, Barber JM: Emergency Nursing: Principles and Practice. C.V. Mosby Co., St. Louis, Missouri, 1981

Cain HD: Flint's Manual on Emergency Treatment and Management. C.V. Mosby Co., St. Louis, Missouri, 1980

Committee on Injuries, American Academy of Orthopaedic Surgeons: Emergency Care and Transportation of the Sick and Injured, 3rd ed. American Academy of Orthopaedic Surgeons, Chicago, Illinois, 1981

Cosgriff JH, Anderson DL: The Practice of Emergency Nursing. J.B. Lippincott Co., Philadelphia, Pennsylvania, 1975

Manisoff MT: Intrauterine devices. Am J Nurs, pp 1188-1192, July 1973

Talbert LM: Lady in pain. Emergency Med, pp 194-196, February 1974

Warner C: Emergency Care: Assessment and Intervention, 2nd ed. C.V. Mosby Co., St. Louis, Missouri, 1978

ORTHOPEDIC EMERGENCIES

19

KEY CONCEPTS

The purpose of this chapter is to identify the problems that exist in the recognition and management of fractures, dislocations, and sprains and to promote the ability to intelligently assess these problems as they present in their varying degrees of severity and involvement.

Much of this material is based on lecture content presented to emergency nurses by John Blosser, M.D., a Portland orthopedic surgeon who has devoted much of his time to teaching emergency personnel.

After reading and studying this chapter, you should be able to:

- Identify the true orthopedic emergencies and describe fractures and dislocations with their classifications and commonly used terminologies.
- Describe the history typical to the fractured bone and explain two areas of concern with long bone fractures.
- Identify the most common dislocation seen, the three types, and describe the positioning of a patient with shoulder dislocation.
- Describe the general management for dislocations.
- Describe the management procedures taught to EMTs with regard to fractures of both the upper and lower extremities.
- Explain the phases of healing after bone injury and the rationale of management.
- Describe the equipment and materials needed to stock a cast room and explain the correct method of dipping plaster.
- Outline the instructions that should be given to patients after casting.
- Identify the important management guidelines when receiving patients with bone and ligament injury in the ED.

Orthopedic injuries are, by and large, rather straightforward in their involvement unless associated with other organ systems following trauma. Trauma to the axial skeleton is rarely considered an emergency situation but frequently does require attention on an urgent basis. The two orthopedic emergencies that *do* exist, so far as the axial skeleton is concerned, are fractures and/or dislocations of the elbow or knee, since these are not only exquisitely painful but can easily cause permanent damage to nerves and vessels distal to the injury if not attended immediately.

A predisposition to fractures does exist in some people. The strength of skeletal bones in each individual is determined by several factors and the absence of these factors predisposes to fractures with very little trauma as a causative agent. However, bone that is stressed over a long period of time—for instance, the os calcis (heel) in gymnasts—develops a denser deposit of calcium to withstand the repeated impacts sustained on landing without resultant fracture. Nutritional factors, such as the amount of protein ingested (to supply the protein collagen fibers) as well as adequate amounts of calcium and vitamin D in the diet, are important to building strong bones. Hormonal levels of estrogens play a part in offsetting osteoporosis, which is seen in the pathologic fractures of elderly people.

FRACTURES AND DISLOCATIONS

A *fracture* is defined as the *breaking* of a part, especially a bone, or a *break* or *rupture* in a bone, with numerous specific fractures defined further in Dorland's Medical Dictionary, some of which will be discussed here as they relate to the most commonly seen fractures in the ED.

A *dislocation* is defined in Dorland's as the *displacement* of any part, more especially of a bone and is called also *luxation,* with 28 varieties defined. Although not as numerous in description, dislocations *can* be incredibly more painful than fractures because of the disruption of tendons, nerves, and vessels traversing the jointed areas.

FRACTURES (See Fig. 19.1)

Fractures are most generally classified as closed and open, although they used to be identified as simple and compound according to how many bones were broken. The current terminology assigns synonymity to closed and simple and to open and compound. In other words, if the skin is unbroken the fracture is *simple* technically, regardless of how many bones are in how many pieces; conversely, a fracture is *compound* if the skin is broken, even though the fracture may be single and minor in nature. A compound fracture is considered to be more serious because of the risk of infection.

There are some additional terms applied to specific fracture sites and types which may be of interest:

1. An *avulsion* fracture is an indirect fracture caused by avulsion or the pull of a ligament at the point of attachment.

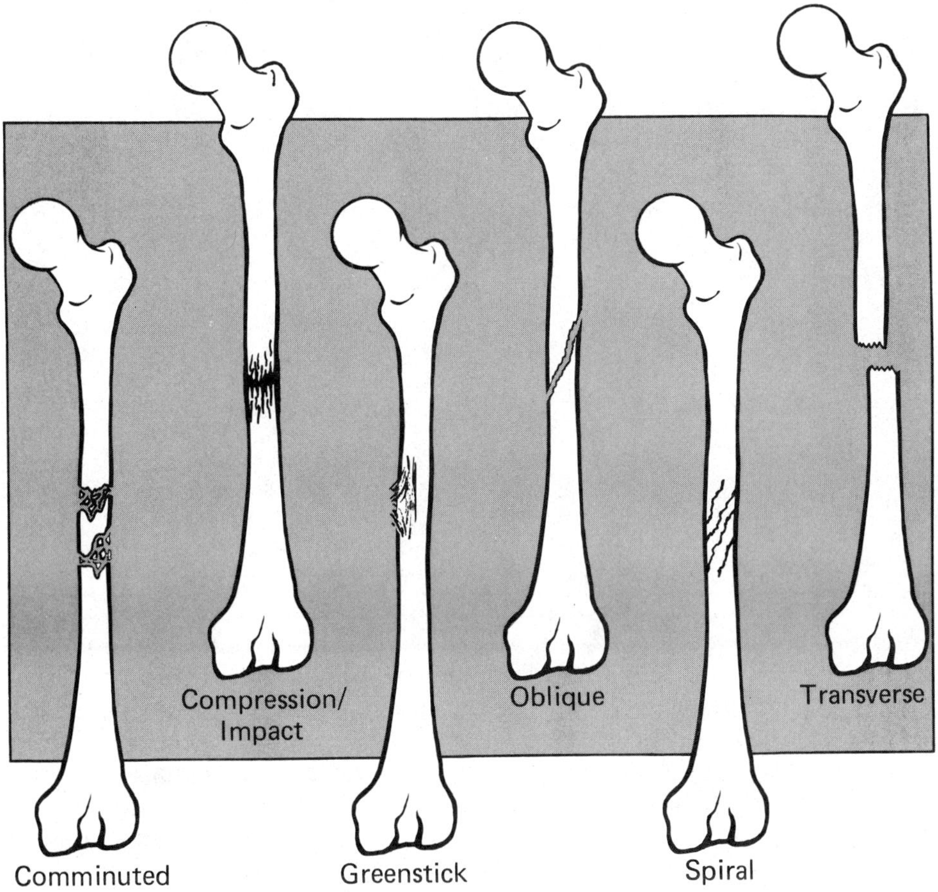

Figure 19.1. Fractures.

2. *Colles* fracture is of the lower end of the radius in which the lower fragment is displaced posteriorly. If the lower fragment is displaced anteriorly, it is a *reverse Colles* or *Smith's* fracture.
3. *Comminuted* fracture is one in which the bone is splintered or crushed.
4. *Compression* fracture is caused by compression, e.g., vertebral fracture.
5. *Direct* fracture is fracture at the point of injury.
6. *Dislocation* fracture is fracture of a bone near an articulation with concomitant dislocation of that joint.
7. *Double* fracture is fracture of a bone in two places—also called segmental.
8. *Epiphysial* fracture is fracture at the point of union of an epiphysis with the shaft of a bone.
9. *Fatigue* fracture is attributed to the strain of prolonged walking or exercise (march or stress fracture usually seen in foot and tibia).
10. *Greenstick* fracture is one in which one side of the bone is broken, the other being bent; an infraction; called also *hickory-stick* or *willow* fracture.

11. *Indirect* fracture is one occurring at a site distant from the site of injury.
12. *Oblique* fracture is one in which the break extends in an oblique direction.
13. *Pathologic* fracture is one occurring from mild injury due to preexisting bone involvement with tumor, cyst, infection, absence of estrogens, etc.
14. *Silver-fork* fracture is of the lower ends of the radius; so called because of the shape of the deformity that it causes.
15. *Spiral* fracture is one in which the bone has been twisted apart; called also *torsion* fracture.
16. *Transverse* fracture is one at right angles to the axis of the bone.

Fracture History

Fractures present in a variety of ways, but if the patient provides a *history of trauma* followed by sudden pain, tenderness, swelling, and discoloration, as well as any degree of deformity and grating (or crepitus) caused by broken bone ends rubbing together, the injured part should be treated and regarded as a fracture site until ruled out by X-ray films.

Fractures of the long bones are apt to produce a steady, slow bleed which, in time, may bleed occultly to the extent of as much as two units (1 liter) in the lower leg and four units (2 liters) in the thigh. These patients must be closely watched for incipient shock, with the long bone fracture immobilized for comfort and to allow the fascia lata to function as a splinting mechanism.

Bony fragments protruding through the skin are obviously indications that the fracture is angulated, contaminated, and no doubt compromising the local nerve supply and circulation. These require immediate attention, realignment under controlled circumstances, and care to the wound to prevent further contamination with a resulting long-term infection of the bone itself and to restore the integrity of vessels and nerves supplying areas distal to the fracture site.

Fractures may or may not (depending on severity) involve either loss of use or at least a guarded motion in adjacent joints.

DISLOCATIONS

Dislocations are commonly referred to in the following terms:
1. *Complete* dislocation is one that completely separates the articulating surfaces of a joint, tearing the ligaments.
2. *Complicated* dislocation is one associated with other important injuries.
3. *Compound* dislocation is one in which the joint communicates with the external air.
4. *Habitual* dislocation is one that often recurs after replacement.
5. *Incomplete* dislocation is a subluxation; a slight displacement.
6. *Pathologic* dislocation is one resulting from paralysis, synovitis, infection, or other disease.
7. *Simple* displacement is one in which the joint is not penetrated by a wound.

The most common complaints with a dislocation are severe pain and inability to move the joint involved, as well as obvious deformity. The most frequent site of dislocation is the shoulder; 95% of such dislocations are anterior and subcoracoid. The first time a shoulder dislocates, it should be splinted for 6 weeks; the second occurrence should indicate the need for surgical correction since the problem tends to become chronic if not taken care of. Elbows, fingers, hips, ankles, jaws, and less commonly, the wrist or knee, can all dislocate, but the shoulder is seen most frequently. The shoulder may dislocate anteriorly, posteriorly, and very rarely, inferiorly. Pain is extremely severe in all three, and the patient should be supported and transported in the most comfortable position, which is usually that of sitting up with the arm and shoulder supported in whatever position is the least painful.

Dislocations of the elbow are usually caused by a fall that "jams" the elbow and causes a deformity that is very apparent and exquisitely painful. These injuries should always be splinted and immobilized in the position as found and should be seen immediately by a physician for evaluation and reduction before damage is done to the nerves and vessels. Any numbness or paralysis distal to the dislocation is an indication of pressure on the nerves, while loss of pulse or coldness of the distal part indicates pressure on the arterial vessels, requiring immediate medical intervention.

SPRAINS

Sprains occur when *ligaments* are torn by a forcing motion beyond the range of the joint involved. The damage to the ligament will vary in severity, and the more seriously injured ligaments may well resemble a fracture or dislocation since they all manifest with pain, swelling, discoloration, and impairment of motion. Sprains do not manifest with deformity, however, and in this way are differentiated from dislocations but require X-ray to rule out fracture. The two most commonly seen areas of sprain are the ankle and knee, and both should be immobilized for comfort until seen by a physician for further evaluation.

STRAINS

A strain is injury to *muscle* from overextension or overexertion and may cause intense pain, some swelling, and difficult movement. Strains are most frequently seen in the muscles of the back and arms and rarely are truly serious.

PRE-HOSPITAL CARE OF FRACTURES AND DISLOCATIONS

Rationale

Emergency medical technicians and ambulance personnel across the country are now being taught to deal with fractures and dislocations in a manner that will *do no harm*. They are taught that, short of open fractures with massive bleeding, most fractures do not require speed in either treatment or transportation and, in fact, should be treated and transported slowly and deliberately, with the realization that the manner in which initial care is given determines in many instances whether there is a favorable patient outcome.

They are taught that no matter how short the distance to the hospital, all injuries to bones and joints must be splinted as if they were known fractures until proved otherwise since the patient may not be treated immediately upon arrival in the ED. The exception is dislocations, which should never be straightened since movement of the displaced bones may damage nerves and vessels that have already been displaced. These are splinted *as they are found.**

Splints

Emergency department nurses should be familiar with the various types of splints employed in the prehospital phase of care and should understand the rationale involved with the application of each type. Splints are applied for protection of the injury, with an attempt to minimize damage and prevent further trauma to the tissues involved, as well as to lessen pain and provide some degree of relative comfort. Any material or appliance that can be utilized to immobilize traumatized bones and tendons qualifies as a splint. Many varieties are commercially made, such as wooden splints, soft wire splints, cardboard splints, padded plastic and metal splints, plastic inflatable air splints, and various types of traction splints which include the Thomas, Hare, and Sager traction splints.

Rigid splints, when applied, are effective only if they are long enough to allow the entire fractured bone to be immobilized; if they are padded sufficiently; and if they are secured firmly to an uninjured part.

Air splints are limited in their effectiveness to fractures of the lower leg and forearm. When they are applied in cold weather, they must be carefully monitored since air in the splint will expand as it warms and may exert potentially dangerous pressure. An air splint should be inflated only by mouth and to the point at which an indentation in the splint can be made easily with the thumb. Distal toes and fingers must be carefully monitored for perfusion, just as circulation is checked with a new cast, and the air splint should be deflated periodically and/or removed as soon as possible to prevent macerated tissues under the moist pressure. One of the distinct advantages of the air splint is that it immobilizies as it also *tamponades* the bleeding site and allows visual access to the injury.

Traction splints are applied not to reduce the fracture but to align it and immobilize the bone ends to prevent further damage during movement and transportation to the hospital. If on arrival, the circulation, color, and sensation of the distal parts are within normal limits, the splint should be left in place until definitive treatment takes place. For this reason, hospitals and ambulance

---

*Grant H, Murray R: Emergency Care. Robert J. Brady Co., Bowie, Maryland, 1971; Committee on Injuries, American Academy of Orthopaedic Surgeons: Emergency Care and Transportation of the Sick and Injured. Chicago, Illinois, 1971

companies should have *interchangeable rotating equipment* that can be left with one patient while a replacement is obtained for the next time of need.

With upper extremity injuries, EMTs are taught the following:

1. Fractured humerus should be immobilized with a short splint and bound to the body with a sling and swathe arrangement.
2. Injured elbows are to be immobilized in the position in which found, and the patient transported without delay to the nearest medical facility.
3. Angulated fractures of the forearm are to be straightened carefully with manual traction before splinting, and pillow bolsters may provide comfort.
4. Injured hands are to be splinted in position of function, while injured fingers can be splinted with a padded tongue blade.

With hip and lower extremity injuries, EMTs are taught the following:

1. Fractured or dislocated hips should be immobilized with a long board splint or by simply padding between the legs, tying both legs together, and placing the patient on a long backboard for transport. Dislocated hips manifest with marked deformity at the joint with some flexion and inward rotation of the leg. Once transferred to bed in the ED, the patient will be more comfortable with the leg on the injured side slightly flexed and supported with pillow bolsters.
2. Severe angulation of the femur must be corrected by steady traction after the femur has been placed into neutral alignment, using traction splinting, a well-padded board splint, a full backboard, or again tying the legs together with adequate padding between the thighs, knees, and ankles.
3. Knee fractures or dislocations must be *immobilized in the position found* with a well-padded splint or possibly a pillow molded around and tied much like a Manchu cotton compression dressing.
4. Lower leg fractures should be placed in neutral alignment and immobilized with air splints, pillow bolsters, or traction splints.
5. Foot and ankle injuries can be immobilized with a pillow splint molded around the injured foot with pins and cravats securing it in place. There is also an air-splint boot in some sets, which is effective but must be watched carefully for circulatory shutdown.

HEALING PHASES OF BONE

The process of bone healing is very similar physiologically to soft tissue healing with a lag phase of about 5-7 days, which peaks at about the fourth day.

During this time, the phagocytes function in their role of cleaning away the dead cells of bone and tissue so that the actual healing can take place with vascularization of the clot formation which then modifies and forms bone matrix. The average healing time is 6-16 weeks, depending, of course, on the extent of the bone injury, with callus formation, an unorganized meshwork of woven bone developed on the pattern of the original fibrin clot following fracture of the bone, to be ultimately replaced by hard cortical bone about 1 year later.

Many orthopedic physicians prefer to allow up to a week after a fracture before attempting to set and cast a fracture, since this delay will allow soft-tissue swelling to reduce and the lag phase to complete. Frequently ED personnel are required to apply a nonabsorbent cotton compression wrap (sometimes called a Manchu wrap), or some type of rigid padded appliance with Velcro or buckle closures, specifically designed to immobilize that injured part, to be worn by the patient until swelling has subsided and the physician is ready to reduce and set the fracture. It should be appreciated that Manchu cotton compression splints can stay in place for *many* days or even 1 or 2 weeks without causing skin problems, while air splints will macerate the skin after several hours.

THE CAST ROOM

In cast application, although the basic equipment and rationale still apply, many physicians have their own personal preferences in casting materials. The EDN should strive to be proficient in the knowledge and application of all materials in stock as well as the use of the basic tools.

Several types of instruments are usually necessary including cast knives, cutters, and saws needed for removing old casts. Bandage scissors are necessary for removing bandages under the cast, and a heavy pair of shears should be available for cutting heavy felt padding. Sheet wadding or a thin nonabsorbent cotton web covered with starch to hold it together is commonly used for padding. Piano felt, cut in suitable sizes, is used to provide additional protection against pressure on bony prominences, and sponge rubber padding is also occasionally used. Materials for reinforcing the cast at stress points will include aluminum strips, yucca board, and even plywood, with additions of walking heels and wedges for leg casts. Tubular stockinette in assorted widths is used for the cast lining.

HANDLING PLASTER

Assisting in cast application can be a very enjoyable and satisfactory experience if the materials are properly handled. Gloves and gowns should be on hand for physician and assistant, and a deep bucket of water between 95° F and 105° F is essential. Water cooler than this will delay the setting of the plaster.

Some of the newer forms of plaster casting set in a matter of minutes, while some of the older ones take up to 24 hours, depending on the extent of the cast. They should all be handled in the same manner, however, submerge the roll of plaster on edge until the bubbling ceases, lift it vertically from the water, and hold it horizontally with the ends secured in the palms. Water is expelled by very gently compressing the roll in a short twist, no more than it takes to supinate the right hand a single time, keeping the left hand in pronation. The roll should not drip when handed over but also must not be wrung so dry that the physician will have difficulty in incorporating it into the cast. The end of the plaster roll is unrolled 2-4 inches before handing it to the physician, and only one roll should be submerged at a time. Care should be taken to pour plaster residue in the bottom of the bucket down sinks that have *plaster traps* and not down plumbing with a standard trap. The faucet should be wide open to assist in washing the plaster down rapidly. A very good practice is to line the plaster bucket with a plastic bag and after plaster residue has settled, the water is poured off and the plastic bag with residue is lifted out and deposited in the waste container. This minimizes plumbing problems.

INSTRUCTIONS TO PATIENTS

Patients leaving the department with *any* sort of orthopedic appliance that might possibly affect or hinder circulation must be instructed carefully regarding danger signals and proper care of the wounded part. The patient should be instructed to:

1. Keep the injured part elevated (at least 6 inches above heart level) for the next 48 hours.
2. Check for pink, warm-feeling fingers and toes continually. If fingers or toes become dusky or even pale, if there is numbness and severe tingling, and if the extremity becomes cold, the physician should be notified immediately.
3. Realize that pain should begin to subside and the physician will prescribe medication as he determines the need. Persistent pain unresponsive to medication should be reported to the physician.
4. Release tensor bandages and adjustable splints and reapply if circulation is compromised or pain is too severe from the compression.

GENERAL MANAGEMENT GUIDELINES

Again, any patient arriving in the ED with fracture and/or dislocation of either the knee or the elbow must be considered a real emergency, as well as the patient with a fracture of the femur. This person may be having significant *occult blood loss* and may require rapid evaluation for swelling of the part as well as vital signs. If a traction splint has been applied, this should be left in place until assessment is completed, including *evaluation of distal pulses*, sensory perception, and motor power of the toes, fingers, and circumferential measurement of the part, if appropriate.

1. Always immediately assess the *whole* patient. Be sure the airway is open, checking LOC, range of motion, etc.
2. Deformities should be noted, and an assessment of circulation is essential. A *pulseless extremity* is a serious emergency.
3. Always supervise transfer of the patient to the appropriate stretcher, gurney, or X-ray table.

4. Always assume the possibility of cervical injury in an unconscious patient with head injury. Be prepared to manage airway and vomitus without endangering the cervical spine.

5. If the patient is severely injured, start a flow sheet for vital signs and initiate an IV line. A large-bore catheter or needle should be inserted into an appropriate vein, particularly one in the upper extremity or an opposite uninjured limb to draw blood for CBC, type and crossmatch, and start volume replacement with Ringer's lactate. *Remember the potential for occult bleeding in long bone and pelvic fractures!*

6. *After* the patient has been stabilized and the limb completely immobilized, the appropriate X-rays may be requisitioned and obtained.

7. Lacerations may be washed and covered with moist sterile dressings of normal saline solution.

8. Refrain from cutting off clothes unless necessary, but *don't* refrain from getting them *off*.

9. Be alert for associated injuries and common combinations, such as the following:

   A. Patient falling from a great height with obvious fracture of the calcaneus may also have a compression fracture of the spine.

   B. Patient with injuries to the spine or pelvis may develop a paralytic ileus.

   C. Commonly associated injuries are

   - Kidney injuries with blows to the spine
   - Spleen or liver injuries combined with rib fractures
   - Genitourinary injuries combined with pelvic fractures
   - Injury to a joint adjacent to an obvious fracture
   - Fractured patella from MVA combined with a fractured or dislocated hip or femur.

10. When ordering X-rays (*most* radiology departments observe these points)

    A. Have joint above or below the fracture included in the films

    B. Always have at least two planes filmed

    C. Knees require AP, lateral, *and* a patellar or "sunrise" view

    D. Ankles require AP, lateral, and oblique, rolling leg inward 10-15° for visual alignment.

    E. Wrist injuries in young adults should routinely include the *navicular* view since fractures of the fossa navicularis do not displace.

11. If general anesthesia is anticipated for an immediate reduction, enforce NPO, and be certain of time of last ingestion (record), height, weight, and obtain operative consent.

12. Remember that elevation and cold packs to injured areas can minimize congestion of the returning venous circulation.

13. As a general rule, pain from musculoskeletal injuries can be controlled within reason by proper immobilization, elevation of the injured part, and application of cold packs. If the patient continues to be in great discomfort, the whole problem should be reevaluated for complications requiring immediate attention (entrapment of a nerve or improper splinting of a joint or fracture). Generally, the main problem is anxiety and not pain.

14. When applying splints:
   A. Be certain injuries are splinted with adequate padding over pressure points.
   B. *Carefully check extremity pulses* with deformity injuries. If pulse is not obtainable, assess the capillary filling by compressing and then quickly releasing pressure on the nail bed. Extremities must be closely monitored to assure adequate blood supply.
   C. Before applying any splint that will exert pressure (air, Manchu, or plaster reinforcements), carefully assess and document the absence or presence of motor and sensory status to avoid having someone later contend that the splint caused it.

15. Pelvic fractures may not be obvious until full evaluation is done and the pelvic girdle has been stressed by pressure over the symphysis. The patient will complain of pain in the groin without much deformity, if any. Remember that pelvic fractures can account for occult bleeding of up to 6 units (3 liters).

16. Fracture of the clavicle (collar bone) is one of the commonest fractures seen, with pain, deformity, and the tendency to support the arm on the injured side. A "figure-8" splint is applied with shoulders back and squared, checking carefully for *quality of distal pulses.*

REVIEW

1. Identify three true orthopedic emergencies.
2. Define fracture and dislocation.
3. Explain the classifications of fractures and the way in which they are identified.
4. List at least 12 fractures that are commonly seen, by type rather than by location.
5. Describe a typical history that might be given by a patient with a fractured radius.
6. Explain the two main areas of concern when long-bone fractures occur.
7. Describe the way in which a patient with a joint dislocation presents and the management that is indicated.
8. Identify the most common type of dislocation seen, and describe three types.

9. Explain the difference between a sprain and a strain.

10. Describe the philosophies of management which are taught to EMTs regarding fractures and dislocations.

11. Explain the phases of healing after a bone injury and the reason for delayed reduction of some fractures.

12. Describe the manner in which you would equip a cast room and the procedures you would observe in assisting with cast application.

13. Outline the instructions that must be given to a patient after casting or the application of any constricting sling or wrapping.

14. Identify the important management guidelines in order of priority when receiving patients with bone and/or ligament injury in the ED.

BIBLIOGRAPHY

Barber JM, Dillman PA: Emergency Patient Care. Reston Publishing Co., Reston, Virginia, 1981

Brunner S, Suddarth D: The Lippincott Manual of Nursing Practice, 2nd ed. J.B. Lippincott Co., Philadelphia, Pennsylvania, 1982

Budassi SA, Barber JM: Emergency Nursing: Principles and Practice. C.V. Mosby Co., St. Louis, Missouri, 1981

Chipman C (ed.): Orthopaedic emergencies. TEM, Aspen Systems Publications, Rockville, Maryland, Vol 2, No 4, January 1981

Committee on Injuries, American Academy of Orthopaedic Surgeons: Emergency Care and Transportation of the Sick and Injuried, 3rd ed. Chicago, Illinois, 1981

Cosgriff H, Anderson DL: The Practice of Emergency Nursing. J.B. Lippincott Co., Philadelphia, Pennsylvania, 1975

Grant H, Murray R: Emergency Care, 3rd ed. Robert J. Brady Co., Bowie, Maryland, 1982

Rodi M: Emergency Orthopedics, Emergency Care: Assessment and Intervention, 2nd ed. C.V. Mosby Co., St. Louis, Missouri, 1978

Schneider FR: Orthopaedics in Emergency Care. C.V. Mosby Co., St. Louis, Missouri, 1978

Stephenson H: Immediate Care of the Acutely Ill and Injured, 2nd ed. C.V. Mosby Co., St. Louis, Missouri, 1978

Weeks PM: Acute Bone and Joint Injuries of the Hand and Wrist: A Clinical Guide to Management. C.V. Mosby Co., St. Louis, Missouri, 1981

FACIAL TRAUMA AND EYE, EAR, NOSE AND THROAT EMERGENCIES 20

KEY CONCEPTS

This chapter is designed to help the EDN understand the basic concepts involved in the recognition and management of EENT problems and those of maxillofacial trauma as they present in the ED, with a brief review of the anatomy of the eye and ear and some working guidelines for management of the most frequently seen problems.

The material presented in this chapter is based on lectures developed and presented to emergency nurses by Craig T. Smith, M.D., an otolaryngologist practicing in Oregon City, OR, and covers a broad spectrum of practical management techniques for the working EDN with many valuable suggestions included.

A review of the anatomy of the eye and terminology used is reprinted with permission of Ethicon, Inc. from their teaching manual, the Human Body manual.

After reading and studying this chapter, you should be able to:

- Describe the recognition and treatment for various types of eye injuries, including foreign bodies, chemical burns, superficial injuries, penetrating/perforating injuries, and nontraumatic medical emergencies.
- Describe the guidelines, procedure for treatment, and danger areas in the management of epistaxis.
- Describe the general principles for management of maxillofacial trauma including nasal fracture, orbital fracture, orbital blowout fracture, and maxillary and mandibular fractures.
- Identify the most common ear problems seen in the ED and the general management indicated for each.
- Describe the symptoms and treatment of laryngotracheal trauma.
- List the equipment necessary for adequate management of epistaxis.
- Describe the correct method of applying eye patches.
- Describe the correct procedure for "dropping eyes."
- Describe the correct method of assessing and recording visual acuity.

ANATOMY OF THE EYE

The eye (Fig. 20.1) is a sensory organ that functions to give man sight. The structures of the eye are the globe or eyeball and its contents: the bony orbit (socket), muscles and tendons, conjunctiva, eyelids, tear ducts and glands, the optic nerve, and that portion of the occipital lobe of the brain that is concerned with vision. Terminology relating to the eye is presented in Table 20.1.

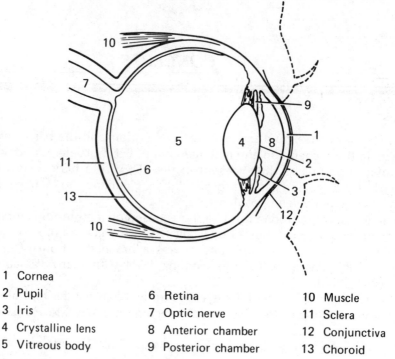

1 Cornea		
2 Pupil	6 Retina	10 Muscle
3 Iris	7 Optic nerve	11 Sclera
4 Crystalline lens	8 Anterior chamber	12 Conjunctiva
5 Vitreous body	9 Posterior chamber	13 Choroid

Figure 20.1. The eye. Eyes convert light rays into nerve impulses enabling humans to see. (Reprinted with permission of Ethicon, Inc., Somerville, New Jersey)

TESTING VISUAL ACUITY

Eye injuries can be classified as superficial, penetrating/perforating, or nontraumatic medical emergencies. Regardless of the classification, it is essential to use common sense as your guide to treatment. Any patient seen in the ED with trauma to the facial region is a candidate for some degree of damage to one or both eyes, and a thorough check is required.

All patients with eye problems should be questioned for a complete history of injury or cause, as well as the presence of a glass eye. *Visual acuity should be checked,* with the patient wearing glasses if they are normally worn. The Snellen eye chart should be used to check both eyes and the findings recorded. Recording is done as OD (oculus dexter or right eye) 20/? and OS (oculus sinister or left eye) 20/?.

Every ED should be equipped with a wall-mounted Snellen eye chart, as well as a smaller version to be used for patients who must remain on a stretcher. The small Snellen chart is used while holding it 14 in. from the eyes.

Table 20.1 Terminology Relating to the Eye and Its Function

TERM	PURPOSE AND/OR FUNCTION
Anterior chamber	Frontal space in eyeball, bounded by cornea, iris, and lens
Aqueous humor	Watery, transparent fluid found in anterior and posterior chambers of eye, helps maintain conical shape of front globe and assists in focusing light rays on retina
Bony orbit	Rounded socket in cranium, in which eyeball is partially sunk
Conjunctiva	Mucous membrane that lines eyelids and covers anterior surface of globe except for cornea
Cornea	Transparent frontal layer of eyeball
Crystalline lens	That part of eye just behind anterior chamber which, in addition to the cornea, refracts light rays and focuses them on the retina
Extraocular	Adjective meaning *outside* the globe of the eye
Globe	Eyeball
Intraocular	Adjective meaning *inside* the globe of the eye
Iris	Colored membrane of eye separating the anterior and posterior chambers; contracts and dilates to regulate entrance of light rays
Lacrimal ducts & glands	System of ducts and glands that secrete and conduct tears
Occipital lobe	Posterior section of brain, where mental images are formed of what is seen
Optic nerve	Second cranial nerve with special sense of sight
Posterior chamber	Space between iris and lens, filled with aqueous humor
Pupil	Opening at center of iris
Retina	The "seeing" membrane lining inside of posterior eye where images are focused by lens and cornea, then transmitted to brain via optic nerve
Sclera	White outer coat of eye which extends from optic nerve to cornea
Sensory receptors	Rods and cones in retinal layer which are stimulated by light rays to conduct nerve impulses to brain via optic nerve
Vitreous humor	Transparent substance having consistency of raw egg white which fills posterior cavity of eyeball; also called hyaloid

THE EYE TRAY

An eye tray should be available in every ED which contains a minimum of the following items:

Small eye chart
Ophthalmoscope
Flashlight or penlight
Pair of magnifying eye loupes

Small suction bulb for removing hard contact lenses, and disposable lens
   storage cases
Sterile irrigating solutions (ophthalmic isotonic buffered solution)
Fluorescein strips (solution will support *Pseudomonas* growth)
Clean 4 × 4 gauze pads
Sterile applicators
Sterile eye pads
Clear tape (1 in.)
Assorted medications in single (unit) dose-dispensing packages
   Topical anesthetic such as procaracaine HCl (Ophthaine) (must be kept
     under refrigeration)
   Antibiotics
   Cycloplegics (for paralysis of accommodation)
   Mydriatics (for dilating the pupil)
   Miotics (for constricting the pupil)
A sterile lid retractor should be readily available

Anesthetizing the Eye

If the patient is in too much pain to be examined adequately, wait until topical anesthesia has been administered and then check for the visual acuity
bilaterally. Frequently errors occur during this procedure, so the following
"suggested" procedure is given as a guideline:

Suggested Equipment

The eye tray
Anesthetic drops (procaracaine HCl [Ophthaine], or tetracaine [Pon-
   tocaine], 0.5%)
Cleansing tissues

Suggested Procedure

1. Have patient lie on back.
2. *Carefully* inspect for contact lenses. *Always* ask! Lenses can be identified
   by shining a beam of light from the side.
3. Remove contact lenses if necessary
   A. Hard lenses are removed with small suction bulb and placed in
      container
   B. Soft lenses are removed by sliding downward on eyeball and "pinch-
      ing" lens gently between thumb and forefinger. NB: Soft lens *must* be
      placed in *normal* saline solution (NSS) or special soft lenses disin-
      fecting solution only! Any other solution containing buffers can ir-
      revocably damage a soft lens.
   C. Place lenses in container with appropriate solution and *label* R
      and L.

4. Gently pull lower lid of eye downward, instruct the patient to look up, and place two drops of the anesthetic solution in the pouch of the lid.
5. Instruct the patient to close eyes and try to relax. Explain that the topical agent may sting for a few seconds, causing the eyes to water heavily. Have cleansing tissue handy.
6. Write the medication, number of drops, R, L, or OU (*oculus uterque—each eye*), and time administered on paper tape and apply to patient's forehead *upside down* so that the next person on scene will notice, read the message, and *not* repeat the medication.
7. Record the same information immediately on the ED chart.
8. Have the eye tray on a stand at the head of the table in readiness for the examination.

Remember that depth perception and reflex responses are seriously affected if the eyes have been dilated and/or anesthetized for examination and that any patient who has had an anesthetic instilled should have that eye patched until the effects of anesthesia wear off. This precaution will protect the eye from foreign body invasion or further trauma.

EYE INJURIES AND EMERGENCIES

SUPERFICIAL INJURIES

These are the most commonly seen eye problems in the ED and include corneal abrasions (scraping injuries that denude skin or membrane), foreign bodies, chemical burns, and heat and flash burns.

Corneal Abrasions

Corneal abrasions are common and present with copious tearing, spasms of the eyelid, and squinting. A complete history is extremely important and visual acuity (VA) must be checked for present management as well as medicolegal implications that may arise in the future. Topical anesthesia will usually be required before the VA can be obtained.

The abrasion is defined by the use of fluorescein strips and a few drops of normal saline solution or ophthalmic irrigating solution which will show the denuded surface epithelium under the cobalt blue diffuse light. An antibiotic ophthalmic ointment of choice (usually neomycin or a sulfa preparation) is applied, and the eye is patched and kept at rest for 24 hours, at which time it should be seen again for follow-up by an ophthalmologist.

When patching an eye, use as many patches as necessary to fill the orbital depth, bringing the height of the patch to above the frontal ridge. In some patients with deep-set eyes, it may be necessary to fold one eye patch in half to build up a base and then proceed with other layers. The important thing is to patch with enough pressure to keep the lid from moving across the corneal surface, as well as to exclude light and keep the eye at total rest. The patch should then be firmly taped with clear and highly adhesive 1-in. tape high on the forehead and down across to the cheek, taping as many times as necessary to anchor the patch and exclude light.

Foreign Bodies

Foreign bodies (FB) are probably the most common ocular injury, although most are relatively simple in nature. The history is *extremely* important because if the eye has been penetrated by an oxidizing metal (ferrous metals, copper, leaded glass, etc.), late problems can develop with scarring which may cause blindness of the afflicted eye. These patients should be referred to an ophthalmologist directly from the ED.

The VA is checked, the eye anesthetized, and then examined. The presence of a small puncture wound and point of entry would indicate the necessity to rule out perforation of the orb, and the leakage of humor or blood would be indictive. The lid must be everted for a thorough examination to determine whether the foreign body is imbedded in the lid and riding over the cornea with every blink of the eye.

Eversion of the upper lid is accomplished by having the patient look downward toward the feet as the lashes of the upper lid are grasped to exert downward and outward pull away from the eye, gentle direct pressure is applied against the lid (at about the "fold" line) with an applicator stick as the lid everts back over the stick. Having the patient look up will readily flip the lid back to its normal position.

If a foreign body is successfully removed, apply antibiotic ointment or drops and patch. The patient should be seen by an ophthalmologist in 24 hours. If, however, the object is *not* successfully removed, the patient should go to the X-ray department with full instructions to the technician for special views if indicated and an ophthalmologist should be called.

Chemical Burns

Chemical burns are treated by retracting the lids and irrigating immediately and copiously with normal saline at body temperature. Use ophthaine anesthetic topically if necessary but *irrigate*.

1. Acid burns require irrigation for a minimum of 10-20 min, depending on the severity of the exposure.
2. Alkali burns are more serious and will continue to burn into the tissue so that irrigation must be done for a *minimum* of 20-30 minutes and longer if indicated.

These patients *must* be referred immediately to an ophthalmologist for evaluation and treatment.

Heat and Flash Burns

Heat and flash burns from welder's arcs, ultraviolet light (sunlamps), and flash heat are fairly common in the ED. A history is taken, VA checked before or after the eyes have been anesthetized, and antibiotic drops or ointment is applied. Patch both eyes for 24 hours.

Antibiotic ointments should always be applied by everting the lower eyelid and spreading the ointment from the inner to the outer canthus of the conjunctival sac. Drops are applied in the same manner, dropping medication in the conjunctival sac.

PENETRATING OR PERFORATING INJURIES

This group of injuries from blunt trauma or foreign body penetration (sticks, glass, rocks, metal, etc.) require essentially the same initial management as those of simple foreign body. The history of penetration is important, as discussed before, including the time of the accident and the mechanism of injury, type of pain, and VA. If the anterior chamber of the eye is bloody (hyphema), an ophthalmologist should be called. This is a very serious sign and an emergency condition. A ruptured globe (ocular rupture) may involve retinal detachment, diagnosed by poor vision, a soft orb, and severe pain. In examining this eye, touch only *once* if the eye is soft, or touch lightly and gently with two fingertips over the lid and press lightly. The emergency treatment is to protect the eye with a *loose* eye shield and keep the patient flat and at rest until the ophthalmologist arrives.

NONTRAUMATIC MEDICAL EMERGENCIES

This group of acute eye problems includes glaucoma, iritis, and keratoconjunctivitis.

Acute Glaucoma

Acute glaucoma can precipitate blindness in hours. The pupil is dilated and fixed, the eye is red and *hard* (press lightly), and there is very severe pain. This requires fast attention, and an ophthalmologist should be called for a pilocarpine order, diuretics, etc. It is necessary to open the iris and diurese fluids to shrink the pupil.

Acute Iritis

Acute iritis may be of bacterial, viral, or autoimmune disease (lupus) origin. Diagnosis is made from a red iris (limba flush) where white meets iris and a small pupil. Treatment is the use of a cycloplegic agent, pain medication, and dark glasses for the relief of severe photophobia.

Keratoconjunctivitis

This general inflammation of the outer coating of the eye is caused by virus or bacteria, and diagnosis is made from pus in the eye, pink eye, a matted eye with discharge, redness, swelling, etc. Treatment depends on the causative agent! Cultures should be taken for bacterial presence and sensitivity as a baseline study.

1. *"Pink eye"* is generally thought to be a viral infection but is really bacterial in origin and responds to sulfa drugs. It is highly contagious among children, and those who are in the acute phase should be kept out of school. Hands should be very carefully washed after examination.
2. *Herpes simplex* is viral and responds to idoxuridine (Stoxil).
3. *"Gooey"* eyes with purulent exudate are usually bacterial infections, and antibiotics are indicated (neomycin or sulfa).

GENERAL GUIDELINES FOR MANAGEMENT

1. Suspect a detached retina if the patient complains of loss of vision without a history of trauma, fuzzy vision (also present with an elevated blood sugar), and a halo effect around lights.
2. *Never* put cortisone, steroids, or any medication that has any steroids in it into an inflamed eye! Ulcerations from herpes will "go crazy" with steroids applied, and some fungal infections will do the same.
3. *Always* check for contact lenses before "dropping" eyes (instilling medications).
   A. Remove hard lenses with a suction device or have the patient remove them and store appropriately in a safe place.
   B. Soft contact lenses must be removed in a different fashion. If the lenses have been in the eye for some time, they will dry out and adhere to the cornea unless irrigated with normal saline to allow them to be "pinched" gently off the surface of the eye with the thumb and index or middle finger. Soft lenses are porous and will absorb solution, therefore, anything other than normal saline solution will be harmful to the lenses. They are *very* costly to replace! Again, if the lens does not lift easily off the surface, it must be irrigated until it moves easily without denuding the cornea to *any* extent.
4. Learn to use the slit lamp for eye examinations if your department has one.
5. Learn to use and care for the tonometer (for testing intraocular pressure in glaucoma) and know where it is kept in case it is needed in the middle of the night.
6. When eyes require irrigation, always retract the lids after anesthetizing the surfaces. A bent paper slip makes a good retractor if all else fails or no retractor is available.

7. Remember that generally both eyes should be patched, if an eye injury is of any real significance, to keep the injured eye *completely* at rest.

8. Remember to always check the eyes for trauma and injury after any head and/or facial injuries.

9. Lid lacerations should have both eyes covered with sterile saline dressings, until treatment by the ophthalmologist, with no manipulation in the interim.

10. Remember that eye injuries generally repair well if infection is controlled.

EPISTAXIS

Probably the most common ENT emergency is epistaxis that is either refractory to simple treatment or has not received the proper initial simple treatment prior to the patient's coming to the ED. Most nosebleeds (80-90%) are anterior bleeding from the nasal septum, which is known as Little's area. Many also occur from the lateral side of the nose and bleed profusely.

These patients should be kept sitting in an upright position and leaning slightly forward to let the blood drip out of the nose rather than being swallowed. Reassurance is needed, and special attention must be paid to the cardiovascular status with careful monitoring of the blood pressure, especially in *elderly* patients, since hypertension frequently co-exists. Hypotension, on the other hand, may develop insidiously due to lack of oxygen if the nostril has been packed for a period of time.

ESSENTIAL EQUIPMENT

The basic equipment necessary for the management of epistaxis includes the following items:

1. Headlamp of a quality that will allow two free hands to work (Goode-Lite or Storz-Lampert are two good examples)

2. Tray containing:
   - Nasal speculums—one short and one long
   - Frazier suction tip (small metal angulated tip with suction port)
   - Bayonet forceps
   - Petroleum jelly (Vaseline) gauze (0.5 × 36 in.) packs, applicators, cotton balls, sterile cotton pledgets
   - Sterile medicine cup
   - Silver nitrate sticks (must be held *firmly* over bleeding point for 3-5 min; 2 min is adequate over very small vein)
   - Topical adrenalin
   - Topical xylocaine 4%

3. Back-up tray containing:
   - Assortment of sterile ENT instruments—pharyngeal mirrors; assorted speculums; forceps; suction tips

- Selection of posterior packs
- Electrocautery tips
4. Electrocautery unit

IMPORTANT POINTS OF INITIAL MANAGEMENT

1. Three essentials that must be ready and in working order for the physician are:
   - Good light source
   - Nasal speculum
   - Adequate suction with the proper tip
2. *Always* have a cover gown ready for the physician and wear one when working with epistaxis.
3. If the patient is bleeding heavily, send blood to laboratory for hemoglobin, hematocrit, and type. Hold for crossmatch.
4. Caution must be used when administering hypotensive drugs (morphine, chlorpormazine HCl [Thorazine], etc.); keep a close watch on the blood pressure.
5. Use of topical cocaine (4% or 10%) may precipitate an adverse reaction, so always have resuscitation equipment close by and diazepam (Valium) at hand for reversal of seizures (10 mg slow IV push).
6. Clots *must* be removed to treat bleeding sites.
7. A posterior bleeding point is *trouble* and requires a posterior pack to exert pressure. A Foley catheter with 10-15 cc water in the balloon, tension as needed, and anchored securely is effective, or string packs can be placed. *Never* tie strings *around* the septum, but tie separately on a dental roll placed *between* the nares to avoid pressure.
8. Antibiotic ointment should be used on nasal packing to avoid infection and complications as well as an overpowering stench on removal.
9. Always *document* the number of packs and the types placed in the nose.
10. Remember that probably 20% of patients with bilateral posterior nasal packs and a history of cardiorespiratory disease will be significantly morbid with precipitating heart attacks from the progressive anoxia. Be alert for increased CO_2 and decreased O_2 levels (dry mouth, confusion, tachycardia, restlessness, and even belligerence).

EPISTAXIS TELEPHONE INSTRUCTIONS

When patients call the ED about nosebleeds, the following instructions may be very helpful and fall within a sensible range of telephone advice:

1. Blow nose gently to remove clots.
2. Hold pressure by pinching the nose as far back on the nostril as possible for a *full 5 minutes* by the clock.

3. Remove pressure.
4. If bleeding starts again, repeat steps 1, 2, 3.

Probably 50% of nosebleed patients can avoid coming to the ED if this procedure is used. Instruct the nosebleed patient in this manner on discharge, should the bleeding start again.

NASAL PACKING TECHNIQUE

An anterior nasal pack should be placed from the top to the bottom and left in place *no more than 1-2 days.* Do not start the pack on the floor of the nose, for it will obscure your vision. Place a finger on the tip of the nose to anchor the speculum and with a bayonet forceps take one strip of petroleum jelly (Vaseline) gauze with *antibiotic ointment applied* and place one loop to the back of the nostril. Use the speculum *under* the packing to lift and pack it into place and keep feeding the strip gauze with bayonet, packing to the top of the space until it is filled. Tape the end of the packing at the external nares.

Posterior packing should be removed in 3-5 days. Usually the posterior pack is placed and then followed with an anterior pack, but both must be covered with antibiotic ointment to minimize sinusitis from occlusion of the nasopharynx.

Carefully monitor these patients for *hypoxia* and if *signs of restlessness or confusion begin,* administer oxygen by mask with the flow rate to be determined by the physician.

MAXILLOFACIAL TRAUMA

Victims of motor vehicle accidents frequently present with some degree of facial trauma, and the following general principles of management can be applied to all:

1. Airway obstruction and hemorrhage are the most important initial considerations. The patient may require intubation, cricothyroidotomy, or tracheotomy if the airway is compromised from trauma. In the patient with a fractured jaw, the tongue will swell and fall back into the throat.
2. Stop bleeding, where possible, with pressure on vessel(s). Spurting arteries should not be clamped with anything other than vascular clamps.
3. Associated injuries must be *thoroughly* and systematically evaluated (CNS, LOC, cervical spine, eyes, chest, abdomen, extremities).
4. Diagnostic examination involves feeling the head with both hands as if giving a shampoo, all over the scalp. A gloved finger in lacerations can define fractures. Ask the patient about
   A. Dental malocclusion
   B. Sensory loss

C. Double vision

Look closely for asymmetry of the face and skull, and feel carefully for discontinuity of the orbital rim and crepitation.

5. Lacerations should be closed with careful plastic technique, after cleaning thoroughly, debriding carefully, and irrigating copiously. The wound should be kept moist with saline gauze after the prep.
6. Tetanus immunization status must be assessed.
7. Facial nerve and parotid duct injuries require initial repair.

NASAL FRACTURES

With nasal fractures, the bony nose can be repaired in 7-14 days, but the cartilaginous nose should be repaired in 2-3 days. Deformity is usually observed, and there is crepitation and mobility on palpation. Edema ensues rapidly, and it is best to wait 3-4 days to evaluate the extent of deformity because of swelling. A septal hematoma may develop, which dissects the mucosa off the septal cartilege and robs the blood supply. If the hematoma becomes infected, the septum will necrose in *24 hours!* This *must* be drained, and the nose packed firmly with antibiotic ointment and gauze packing. These patients must be instructed *not* to blow the nose because of the danger of transmitting infection to the brain or eyes. Patients presenting with *any* history of nasal trauma should be carefully examined for the presence of a septal hematoma.

ORBITAL FRACTURES

Orbital fractures (malar, zygomatic, etc.) are often associated with eye injuries when the orbital floor fractures. There may be diplopia caused by entrapment of the eye muscles, a limitation of the upward gaze from entrapment of eye muscles, and V_2 anesthesia (upper lip, second division of the fifth cranial nerve, the trigeminal). Again, visual acuity and mobility of the eyes must be checked and recorded, but if the patient is unable to see clearly for the small Snellen chart, use two, three, or four fingers directionally for acuity and response (LOC).

An *orbital blowout* fracture, as opposed to a palpable fracture of the bony orbital rim, results from heavy trauma or pressure against the eye, pushing it in, exerting equal pressure all around and blowing out the orbit in the weakest part (the floor) downward into the maxilliary sinus. The maxillary midface, malar and lateral inferior orbital rim usually all break in a "step-down" displacement process with numbness of cheek, teeth, and palate. There is depression of the malar eminence and a flattened facies, swelling, malocclusion of the jaw, spasm of the jaw muscles (trismus), and mobility of the maxilla. Prop the jaw open with a stack of tongue blades placed *way back* across the molars and the base of the tongue, and *then* grasp the palate with fingers. Pain on motion usually indicates fracture (floating maxilla), but this is often missed.

MANDIBULAR FRACTURES

Mandibular fractures are the most common. Usually there are two or more fractures in the arch, with malocclusion, pain with chewing, deformity, deviation upon opening, and again, trismus. Check the ears for blood, as there may be a communicating fracture of the tympanic bone. Torn, blue, or red ear drum may indicate a basal skull fracture.

The treatment is with a simple splint on the jaw to stabilize for pain. If there is anterior dislocation, place a stack of tongue blades at the back of the molars crosswise for protection, place thumbs inside the mouth in the angle of the jaw, *pull down* and then *push back*. Jaws in severe spasm can bite fingers off, so be certain to use the protection of a *heavy* tongue blade "bolster!" Morphine and diazepam, sometimes given for pain and spasm, are effective, although general anesthesia is sometimes required to reduce the dislocation of the mandible. If the patient has been heavily traumatized and is in borderline shock, the administration of morphine may precipitate severe hypotension so the situation must be closely monitored.

THE MOST COMMON EAR PROBLEMS

Ear problems are not frequently seen on an urgent or emergent basis, but it is appropriate here to review the anatomy of the ear as depicted in Figure 20.2.

The most commonly seen ear problems and some of the therapeutic measures are given here:

1. Wax or foreign body against the tympanic membrane is painful. This is usually irrigated out with warm saline and a control syringe.
2. Acute otitis media is usually treated with decongestants to open the eustachian tubes, and with antibiotics, although sometimes myringotomy is done.
3. Chronic otitis with perforation and drainage is managed much the same. A culture and sensitivity test should be taken on any draining condition.
4. Labyrinthitis, whether toxic, drug-induced, or viral, is generally treated with mild sedatives, analgesia, antivertigo agents, and low-sodium diet. Deafness or hearing loss with "head noises" may accompany the other symptoms of unsteady gait, dizziness, and nausea, with occasional head pain.
5. Hematoma of the ear may occasionally be seen, and this will dissect the perichondrium off the cartilage, causing rapid necrosis of the external ear structure. Treatment is incision and drainage (I & D), pack with moist cotton, and apply a mastoid pressure dressing.
6. Water trapped in ears after swimming may be relieved with a mixture of *4 parts 70% isopropyl alcohol and 1 part vinegar* poured into the ear and swished around. This forms a weak acetic acid, breaks the surface tension, allowing the ear to drain, and produces an acid environment.

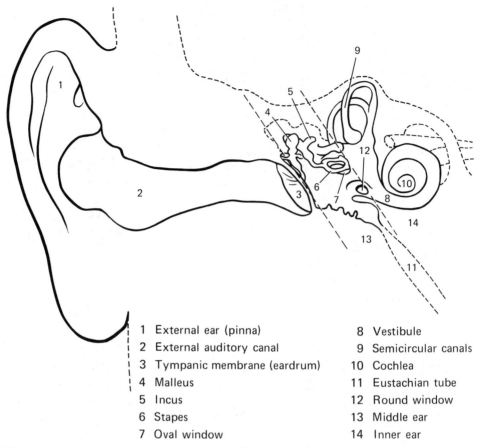

1 External ear (pinna)
2 External auditory canal
3 Tympanic membrane (eardrum)
4 Malleus
5 Incus
6 Stapes
7 Oval window

8 Vestibule
9 Semicircular canals
10 Cochlea
11 Eustachian tube
12 Round window
13 Middle ear
14 Inner ear

Figure 20.2. The ear. Sound waves, transmitted to the hair cells of the inner ear, stimulate the cells by displacement or distortion to send impulses to the brain so that man may hear. (Reprinted with permission of Ethicon, Inc., Somerville, New Jersey)

7. Vegetable foreign bodies in the ear canal should never be irrigated with warm water because of the possibility of causing the material to swell in the external ear canal, greatly complicating removal.

LARYNGOTRACHEAL TRAUMA

The EDN should never lose sight of the fact that laryngotracheal trauma is present to some degree in 10% of MVAs and can be a rapidly fulminating emergency situation. The signs and symptoms are subcutaneous emphysema, pain or swallowing, coughing, blowing nose, aphonia or hoarseness, and loss of landmarks in the neck. Evidence of a normal voice is not a guide to the severity of the trauma, however.

Treatment is to hospitalize for close observation of the airway, X-ray films of the cervical spine to rule out fractures, preparation to intubate, if necessary, and establishing the capability to perform tracheostomy if intubation is contraindicated because of cervical fractures.

SORE THROAT

The sore throat tends to be relegated to a "garden-variety" category and frequently gets very little attention in the ED. The patient with an acute pharyngeal infection is in great distress and pain, however, and may be having systemic reactions. The alert EDN should examine the throat, palpate the cervical and sublingual glands, and obtain a throat culture for sensitivity while preparing the patient for examination by the physician. Septic sore throat from acute streptococcal infection, diphtheria, Vincent's angina, infectious mononucleosis, and even pharyngeal gonorrhea are not infrequently seen. These patients are in real distress and need careful evaluation and immediate comprehensive management.

EPIGLOTTITIS

Very recently a surprising increase has been noted in the numbers of epiglottitis cases seen in adults; one theory proposes a diminished resistance to the Hemophilus influenzae organism after a generation of widespread ampicillin usage.

These patients will present with the classic symptoms of difficult swallowing, toxic appearance with high temperature, and tendency to hold head forward and very still coupled with the usual history of a URI several days prior. The typically swollen and "cherry red" epiglottis can readily cause a total airway obstruction if manipulated during an examination. Therefore, it is *essential* to have emergency airway management equipment on hand and in readiness before beginning any examination. If a lateral neck film for soft-tissue swelling is indicated, it should be done in the ED or with airway management personnel and equipment accompanying the patient to X-ray.

REVIEW

1. Describe the treatment of a superficial foreign body in the eye.
2. Describe the management of a corneal abrasion.
3. Identify the two important items in the evaluation of an eye injury.
4. Describe the method for everting the upper eyelid.
5. Describe the method for "dropping" eyes.
6. List the equipment that should be contained in an ED eye tray.
7. Describe the proper technique for removal of a soft contact lens and the reason NSS irrigation may be necessary.
8. Describe the emergency management of an eyelid laceration.
9. Identify the three cardinal points of the initial management of epistaxis.
10. Itemize the basic equipment necessary for the management of epistaxis.

11. Describe the telephone instructions that may be helpful to a patient with a nose bleed.

12. Identify the two most important initial considerations in the general management of maxillofacial trauma.

13. Explain the danger of a septal hematoma and the time limit before permanent damage is sustained.

14. Describe the mechanism of an orbital blowout fracture and the associated signs.

15. Describe the labyrinthitis and the manner in which it is manifested.

16. Describe the method for releasing water trapped in the external ear canals after swimming.

17. Identify the eventualities that should be prepared for in laryngo-tracheal trauma.

18. Identify five causes of septic sore throats that are seen not infrequently in the ED.

19. Name the one procedure which should always be carried out for any draining wound or lesion with exudate, whether it be in the eye, ear, nose, or throat.

BIBLIOGRAPHY

Anderson D, Cosgriff J: Epistaxis. JEN, Vol 2, No 4, 1976

Benenson AS: Control of Communicable Diseases in Man. The American Public Health Association, New York, 1970

Boyd-Monk H: Examining the external eye, Part 1. Nursing 80, Vol 10, No 5, Horsham, Pennsylvania, May 1980

Boyd-Monk H: Examining the external eye, Part 2. Nursing 80, Vol 10, No 6, Horsham, Pennsylvania, June 1980

Brunner LS, Suddarth D: The Lippincott Manual of Nursing Practice, 2nd ed. J.B. Lippincott Co., Philadelphia, Pennsylvania, 1982

Budassi SA, Barber JM: Emergency Nursing: Principles and Practice. C.V. Mosby Co., St. Louis, Missouri, 1981

Cain HD: Flint's Manual on Emergency Treatment and Management. C.V. Mosby Co., St. Louis, Missouri, 1980

Cosgriff JH, Anderson DL: The Practice of Emergency Nursing. J.B. Lippincott Co., Philadelphia, Pennsylvania, 1975

Ingram NM: Trauma to the ear, nose, face, and neck. JEN, Vol 6, No 4, pp 8-12, July/August 1980

Kelly CA: Ocular trauma. JEN, Vol 4, No 2, pp 23-28, March/April 1978

Lee B, Hansen E, Poppell M: Facial fractures take a special kind of nursing care. Nursing 80, Vol 10, No 8, pp 42-46, August 1980

Warner C: Emergency Care: Assessment and Intervention, 2nd ed. C.V. Mosby Co., St. Louis, Missouri, 1978

THE BURN PATIENT

21

KEY CONCEPTS

This chapter is provided to help emergency personnel develop a working knowledge of the pathophysiology of burns and to understand the essential considerations involved in assessment and intervention in the ED setting, as well as the preparation involved for the safe and orderly transport of the burn patient to an organized burn unit. Much of this material was contributed by Carolyn Wecks, R.N., and personnel of the Burn Unit at Emanuel Hospital and Medical Center in Portland, OR.

After reading and studying this chapter, you should be able to:

- Define the functions of the skin.
- Explain how a determination is made of the extent and severity of a burn.
- List the immediate priorities of assessment and intervention in order.
- Describe the pathophysiology of the burn injury and the systems involved.
- Define the nursing role and responsibilities in immediate intervention.
- Describe the steps to be taken in the stabilization and disposition of the burn patient.
- Explain and discuss the "Rule of Nine."
- Explain the customary analgesia for the severely burned patient.
- Describe the best methods of cleansing wounds and removing tar and asphalt.
- Explain the standard fluid replacement formula commonly used.
- List the emergency equipment that should be on hand for problems with a seriously burned patient.
- Describe the procedure that should be followed in transporting a patient by ambulance to another facility.

A severe burn is one of the most physically and psychologically devastating injuries that can occur. Dr. Carl Jelenko, of the Georgia Burn Unit, describes a burn injury as trauma turned inside out. This is helpful in realizing the ramifications involved for each specific burn patient. A burn injury greater than 20% *total body area* (TBA) of an adult and greater than 12% TBA of a child is a *pansystemic* injury involving other organ systems that are essentially worked overtime to eliminate the toxins and debris, as well as to produce the means of fighting infection and stabilizing the fluid balance of the body.

The goal in care of the burn patient, then, is to direct all efforts toward restoring integrity to the skin and to preserve life, function, and appearance. It is the responsibility of the ED personnel to begin the establishment of these goals through a calm and organized system of care.

DETERMINING THE EXTENT AND SEVERITY OF BURN

The skin is the largest organ in the body and has seven basic functions:

1. Protects against infection
2. Prevents loss of body fluids
3. Controls body temperature
4. Functions as an excretory organ
5. Functions as a sensory organ
6. Produces vitamin D
7. Determines identity

There are two anatomic layers to the skin: the epidermis and the dermis. The epidermis consists of epithelial cells that form a barrier against the environment. The dermis consists of epithelial cells and connective tissue, and contains blood vessels, hair follicles, nerve endings, sweat and sebaceous glands—all of which contribute significantly to patient function and survival.

DEPTH OF THE BURN

A first-degree burn is a superficial burn involving only the epidermis. It is red in color and somewhat painful, but it is not a serious burn and will heal within a few days without scarring.

There are two types of second-degree burns: superficial and deep. The superficial second-degree burn involves the epidermis and superficial dermis. It is reddened and has blisters that continue to increase in size; this is the most painful type of burn because the nerves have been damaged but not destroyed. This burn heals within 10-14 days and may have some discoloration (which is probably temporary) or minor scarring. It does not require skin grafting.

The deep second-degree burn involves the epidermis down to the deep dermis and is very similar in appearance to the third-degree burn. This burn is usually whitish in color and may have a leathery feeling. It is somewhat anesthetic, and it often takes as long as 7 or 8 weeks to heal. A skin graft is not necessary to heal this wound since even in deep dermis there are epithelial cells around the hair follicles that will regenerate and form skin; because of the prolonged time involved, a skin graft is occasionally done to speed up the heal-ing process. Heavy scarring may occur with the deep second-degree burn.

The third-degree burn involves the epidermis and all of the dermis, destroy-ing all epithelial cells that can regenerate skin. This burn has a whitish or charred appearance, is anesthetic, and has a tough, leathery feeling. It does require a skin graft to heal unless it is a very small area that can heal in from the sides. The third-degree burn is the most serious of the burns.

The terminology now used more frequently to describe the depth of a burn is 1) superficial partial thickness burn (first-degree and superficial second-degree), 2) deep partial thickness (deep second-degree), and 3) full thickness (third-degree). This method of classification is more accurate in describing the depth of a burn.

EXTENT OF A BURN

The *Rule of Nines* is a fast and easy way to determine the amount of body surface burned (Fig. 21.1). The body is divided into multiples of 9, as shown in Table 21.1.

Table 21.1 Rule of Nines in Burns

BODY PART	AREA (%)
Arms (shoulders to fingertips) each	9
Head (adult)	9
Each leg (adult)	18
Anterior trunk	18
Posterior trunk	18
Perineum or neck	1

It should be remembered that the percentage of body surface for the head and legs of a newborn is *reversed* from that of an adult (the child's head is 18% and the legs are 14%). This ratio slowly changes until, at approximately 15 years, the percentages are the same as an adult.

For small burns, a good rule of thumb is that the palmar surface of the patient's hand is approximately 1% of that patient's body.

OTHER FACTORS TO CONSIDER

Though the depth and extent of burn are two of the most important factors in determining the severity of the injury, there are other factors to consider. One of the most important to take into the evaluation is age. The very young

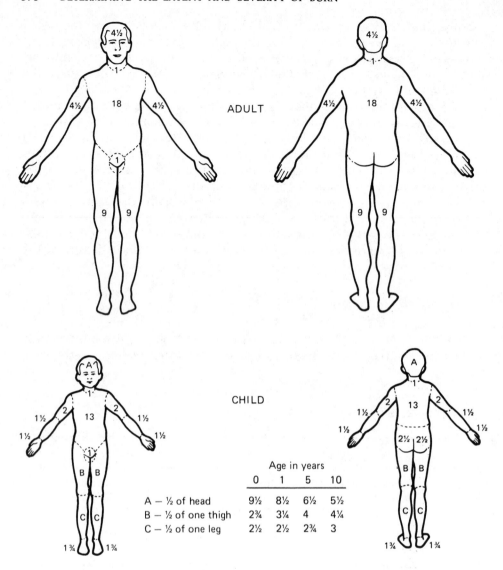

ADULT

CHILD

	Age in years			
	0	1	5	10
A — ½ of head	9½	8½	6½	5½
B — ½ of one thigh	2¾	3¼	4	4¼
C — ½ of one leg	2½	2½	2¾	3

Figure 21.1. The Rule of Nines for adults and children.

and the older patients do not tolerate even the minor or moderate burn, and the mortality for these age groups is high.

The past medical history can significantly affect the patient with a burn, especially the patient with diabetes or with cardiac, renal, respiratory, GI, and/ or cerebral problems.

Associated injuries along with the burn, as well as the area of the body burned, are also factors to consider. Burns of the 1) hands, 2) face, 3) feet, and 4) perineum are serious in terms of 1) functional problems, 2) cosmetic problems, 3) inactivity problems, and 4) infection.

CLASSIFICATION OF BURN INJURY

Burns caused by exposing a small part of the body to a heat source (a finger, small part of the hand or arm, hot water splashing on a very limited area of the trunk, etc.) are considered nonserious burns and can often be treated at home with no complications (Fig. 21.2). Those that could, or do, require the attention of a physician are categorized in the following way:

Minor Burns
    2° Adult 15% TBA or less
        Child 10% TBA or less
    3° 2% or less
Moderate Burns
    2° Adult 15-25% TBA
        Child 10-20% TBA
    3° Less than 10% TBA
Major Burns
    2° Adult 25% TBA or more
        Child 20% TBA or more
        Burns involving hands, face, feet, eyes, ears, or perineum
    3° 10% TBA or more
        Burns from electrical injury or involving inhalation of heat or chemicals

One common question asked by ED personnel is, "What type of burn requires hospitalization?" Basically, any burn of 10% TBA that is superficial partial thickness should be considered for admittance, and any burn of 3% TBA that is deep partial or full thickness should also be considered for admission. A patient with questionable problems (very old, very young, infirm, inhalation injury, other injuries) should also be evaluated for hospitalization. Those patients with a major burn belong in an organized burn center.

PATHOPHYSIOLOGY OF BURN INJURY

LOCAL CHANGES

Three major local changes occur with burn injury. These must be remembered when caring for the patient in the ED: 1) the loss of the microbe barrier, which opens the way for massive infection; 2) loss of the fluid barrier so that exudate is allowed to seep from the wound (this is not the cause of the massive fluid shift that occurs following burn injury); and 3) the loss of temperature control can cause the patient to become hypothermic if he is exposed to subnormal temperatures.

RENAL CHANGES

Following the burn injury, the glomerular filtration rate is reduced as a result of hypovolemia and decreased renal plasma flow, which continues for 24-72

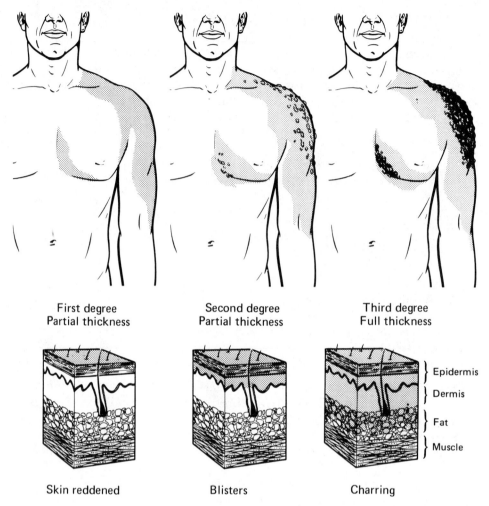

First degree
Partial thickness

Second degree
Partial thickness

Third degree
Full thickness

Skin reddened

Blisters

Charring

Figure 21.2. The classification of burns. (Reprinted from Grant H, Murray R: Emergency Care, 2nd ed. Robert J. Brady Co., Bowie, Maryland 1978)

hours. The kidneys receive 20-25% of the cardiac output per minute normally, but after a burn they may only receive 10%.

Tubular damage may also be caused by free hemoglobin from extensive red cell damage that forms casts in the tubules. An inflammatory reaction develops around the casts, interstitial edema ensues, and there may be necrosis of the tubules.

RESPIRATORY CHANGES

Not infrequently, the patient with a burn also sustains inhalation injury. The first problem that arises stems from the fact that the patient may have inhaled CO, which can rapidly displace O_2 on the hemoglobin and cause severe hypoxemia.

The second problem is the formation of edema in the upper respiratory tract. This is due to the chemical or heat injury and to the tremendous amount of fluids required to resuscitate the patient. Both contribute heavily to occlusion of the airway with edema.

The third problem is that the lower respiratory tract may be injured from smoke and/or chemicals and foreign particles that may have been inhaled. Note that this injury is almost always chemical and not a thermal (heat) injury to the tract. The pharynx is very moist and will tend to cool down any flame or heat that has entered the mouth; at the same time, the glottis will rapidly close if heat advances that far.

The last problem is eschar (burn tissue) restriction of the chest. With deep circumferential burns, the patient may have trouble expanding his lungs; the tight leathery burn tissue around his chest will not allow normal inhalation.

CARDIOVASCULAR CHANGES

Very shortly after a major burn injury, there is a decrease in the cardiac output, secondary to hypovolemic shock due to extensive capillary leakage. There may also be approximately 10% destruction of red blood cells due to hemolysis, but it is usually not enough to warrant whole blood to resuscitate the patient.

The real cause of burn shock is a capillary leak, which allows the plasma to leak out into the tissue. If the burn is less than 30%, the capillary leak is localized in the area of the burn. If the burn is over 30%, there is a generalized leak throughout the body. The patient may lose up to 50% of the plasma volume within the first 3 hours after a burn, if he has a major burn.

PRIORITIES OF CARE

NONSERIOUS BURN INJURY

When a patient enters the ED with a small burn from a household injury or minor work injury, the wound should be cleaned with saline and a mild soap or antiseptic solution. If there is blistering, the intact blisters should be left alone, as they provide a comfortable clean dressing for the wound. If the blisters are broken, *only* the very loose skin should be removed. Apply an antiseptic ointment or cream like silver sulfadiazine (Silvadene) or an antiseptic gauze impregnated with 1% bismuth (Xeroform), and cover with a sterile bulky dressing, which is to serve basically as a protective dressing. Have the patient return to the ED or his doctor's office for a dressing change every 1-3 days until the wound is healed, and be certain that he understands that the wound and dressings must be kept clean and dry! Instruct him to watch for signs of infection: e.g., purulent drainage or a foul odor from the dressing, redness around the edges of the wound, an increase in temperature, or a wound that will not heal. If these signs or symptoms occur, the wound should be cultured and treated with a topical agent specific to the causative organism.

TREATMENT OF THE SEVERE BURN INJURY

When the ED is notified that a severe burn victim is on the way, a clean room that is as isolated as possible should be set up with the emergency equipment listed on page 386. Gowns, masks, caps, and gloves should be available so that some semblance of protective (clean) isolation is established.

Initial Nursing Management

As the patient arrives in the ED, any smoldering clothing should be immediately removed (though it is unlikely that the patient will still be burning after the paramedics or firemen have treated him). Once the heat source has been removed or cooled, the patient should be checked for *respiratory* involvement. A *history* of where the burn occurred is important, since any patient with a burn that involves smoke occurring in an enclosed space has a significant chance of developing some respiratory complications. The nose and mouth should be examined for soot and singed hairs, and blood should be drawn to determine *carboxyhemoglobin level* and *arterial blood gases.* It is also important to include a *chest X-ray;* this initial chest film should be normal because the lower respiratory tract injury (which includes the lung infiltrates, pulmonary edema, etc.) does not become evident for a few days. Thus, if the X-ray film shows abnormality, there is probably another problem not related to the burn injury.

If any respiratory involvement is suspected, oxygen should be started at 2-4 LPM. Since major problems with smoke inhalation may not show up for 6-24 hours after injury, the patient should be under close hospital observation for 24 hours if there is any question of the severity of the smoke inhalation.

Signs of Severe Respiratory Involvement

The most common signs of more severe respiratory involvement include *singed nares* and *sooty mouth,* a *high carboxyhemoglobin level* (normal is about 0-5), ABGs with a *low* PO_2 and a *high* PCO_2, *sooty sputum, increasing hoarseness, difficulty swallowing, shortness of breath,* and *cyanosis* (a rather late sign). These patients are probably developing an upper-airway obstruction due to chemical (smoke) injury and edema. The treatment is endotracheal intubation with O_2 mist until the edema has subsided (probably 24-72 hours later). An upper-airway obstruction could also be caused from a circumferential deep burn of the neck, and an escharotomy (incision into the eschar) may be needed. This is always done parallel to the circulatory path but a safe distance from major vessels. If suctioning is needed, it should be done with extreme caution, since the tissue has already been traumatized by the toxic gases and soot particles; careless suctioning could easily cause considerable further damage to an already compromised airway.

Lower Respiratory Complications

The complications that occur with a lower respiratory injury may not be seen in the ED since they usually occur 24-72 hours after the burn, but they will be mentioned here as they frequently occur in patients who have had upper-airway injury. As was mentioned before, the lower respiratory tract is never thermally injured. It can be chemically injured (even down to the alveoli) as a result of toxic gases. This will begin to manifest on chest X-ray films in a few days as possible atelectasis or infiltrates caused by the edema that forms. Patients with severe respiratory injury are candidates for respiratory distress syndrome due to the damaged alveoli and tremendous fluid loads. These patients are treated with an *endotracheal tube, oxygen, a volume ventilator with PEEP,* and sometimes *steroids* for a very short time. Even as the patient improves, vigorous pulmonary care is given to insure movement of secretions and to prevent pneumonia.

The patient with a circumferential deep burn of the chest will have trouble expanding his chest (as was mentioned earlier), and this tightness will usually have to be relieved with an escharotomy.

Fluid Replacement

Stabilizing circulation is extremely important when you consider how much fluid the patient is losing. An IV should be started on an adult patient with (minimally) a 20% superficial partial thickness burn or a 10% deep burn, and on a child with a 10% burn of any depth, or if there is any nausea or vomiting. The formula that is most commonly accepted for fluid replacement is:

4 cc Ringer's lactate / kg body wt / % of burn in first 24 hrs

Half the amount is to be given in first 8 hours, the balance in next 16 hours. The formula is only a guideline, however, and the *chief indicator of adequate fluid replacement is the urine output.* Intravenous tubes are adjusted to keep the urine output at 30-50 cc/hr for an adult and 1.5 cc/kg/hr for a child. If there is hemoglobin in the urine, the rate is increased until the urine clears, to prevent tubular necrosis.

Note that there is no dextrose in the Ringer's lactate. Dextrose given to the severely burned patient will significantly increase the blood sugar and can cause an osmotic diuresis, thus giving an inaccurate evaluation of fluid replacement.

Colloids are not used to resuscitate the patient in the first 24 hours except in some small children or in patients with very large burns, because the albumin will leak out into the tissue and hold fluid in the tissue instead of in the circulatory system, where it is needed. After the vessels have sealed up again, plasma may be used to replace that which was lost initially. The Ringer's lactate will also leak out into tissues, but it is mobilized more easily, and the resultant edema will subside faster.

Because of the amount of fluid needed to resuscitate the patient, it is important that the patient's body weight be obtained soon after admission since these patients will gain a great deal of fluid weight in the first 24-48 hours. This can be done on the burn unit, and it *does* need to be done, somehow, within the first 3 hours to be accurate.

Tubes

Foley catheters are inserted in all patients with a 30% or more burn and in any other patient with less burn if there is a questionable renal or cardiac problem. Patients over 60 years of age, especially, should be evaluated for the need of an indwelling Foley catheter.

All patients should be kept NPO while in the ED, because it is not uncommon to develop a paralytic ileus due to the stress of injury. Patients with burns over 30%, or deep facial burns (because of swelling), should have an *NG tube* connected to low intermittent suction (Gomco) for 12-24 hours. Any patient who is nauseated or vomiting should also have an NG tube.

Initial Laboratory Evaluations

Initial laboratory studies should include the following:

1. Complete blood count every 6 hours (increase in Hct and Hgb, possible increase in WBC)
2. Electrolytes (probably will be normal initially)
3. Blood urea nitrogen (probably will be normal initially)
4. Creatinine (should be normal)
5. Albumin and total protein (may be slightly low)
6. Arterial blood gases (carboxyhemoglobin will be increased if patient was burned in a closed space.)
7. Blood sugar (may be elevated initially from stress)
8. Urinalysis should include a test for hemoglobin as well as myoglobin, which can help monitor for renal problems, and there may be an elevated glucose.
9. An ECG should be done on patients with any question of cardiac problems and especially elderly patients; chest X-rays should be done on any questionable respiratory injury.
10. Photographs should be taken ASAP in ED to document initial involvement as baseline information for later comparison.

Wound Care

After primary care has been given, ED personnel can turn their attention to the burn wound. All clothing articles should be removed to be sure that all burn areas have been accounted for, and the size of the burn should be reevaluated. It is helpful to estimate first the amount of burn area and then the amount of unburned area, which should add up to 100%. If not, you have over or underestimated the size of the burn, and it should be reassessed. All gross debris should be cleaned away with sterile saline and a clean cloth, and any very loose hanging skin should be removed. *Do not,* however, debride intact blisters or peel off sheets of intact epidermis. Initial wound management should be limited to *cleaning,* using bland soap (Ivory), plain normal saline solution, or povidone-iodine (Betadine) as necessary. Commercial cleansers, available in automotive supply stores, will remove heavy grease and oils, while tar and asphalt deposits may be removed with heavy applications of polymyxin B-bacitracin-neomycin ointment (Neosporin ointment) topped with saline compresses and applied every 4 hours or less expensively with mineral oil applications. Most will lift off of burned surfaces in about 24 hours, and although this has no particular ED application, it may be helpful as general information.

As for application of topical agents to the wound, it is best to contact the facility to which the patient will be transferred to find out what the routine is. In some cases, if the transfer is to a close facility, they will ask that the wound simply be covered with a clean or sterile sheet and no topical agent be applied. If it is to be a long transfer, the facility may have you apply the agent of their choice, wrap in a dressing, and transfer.

In any case, the patient should be kept warm and not transferred in cold, wet dressing, as loss of ability to control body temperature will cause the patient's body to adjust to the outside temperature. The only exceptions to this are a superficial partial-thickness burn that is less than 20% or a chemical burn. In those cases, the burn area may be kept moist for the patient's comfort; *in all* other cases the patient should be transferred *warm* and *dry.*

Analgesia

In attempting to control the burn victim's pain, the EDN should remember that in a serious burn, the fluid is flowing from the circulatory system to the tissue, not from the tissue to the circulatory system. Thus, the patient will not absorb an IM injection until the vessels seal and the fluid is mobilized. All medication on a major burn must be given IV, except that for tetanus, which should be given IM! It should also be remembered that the patient with deep or full-thickness burn will suffer less pain than will the patient with a superficial partial-thickness burn. Intravenous morphine is an effective drug in controlling pain, but it should be diluted in 10 ml NSS and given in 2- to 4-mg increments to prevent respiratory depression, as a slow IV push; meperidine is also effective IV.

A tetanus booster should always be given (IM) to any patient who has not been recently immunized.

Continued close observation of the respiratory status, monitoring of VS every hour, temperature every 2 hours, and urine output with specific gravity every hour should be maintained.

THE PATIENT AND FAMILY

Remember that underneath all that soot and char, there is a very frightened person. Somewhere not far behind, there are probably some very frightened family and friends. As much as possible, keep *both the patient* and *those with him* informed of what is going on and why. They are at the beginning of what could be a very long and trying stay in the hospital for the patient, and their initial impression will stick with them.

STANDBY EMERGENCY EQUIPMENT

Every ED should have at least the following equipment on hand for the initial management of burned patients as they are received, whether the equipment and materials are kept in one designated area or stocked on a portable cart.

1. Oxygen and suction
2. Endotracheal intubation tray
3. Heavy-duty scissors to remove clothing
4. Cart with the following items:
   A. 2 ABG setups
   B. 1 CVP tray and 1 CVP manometer
   C. 1 cutdown tray
   D. 4 liters Ringer's lactate
   E. Sterile gloves and clean gloves
   F. 1 Foley catheter set and drainage bag with one ounce measurement for determining urinary output per hour (Urimeter)
   G. 1 NG tube (sump type)
   H. 1 Toomey syringe
   I. Various blood tubes
   J. Isolation supplies (caps, masks, gowns)
   K. Sterile
      • Gauze sponges
      • Instrument sets
      • Scalpels with #15 blades
      • Mosquito clamps
      • Chromic suture
      • Razors (for removing hair from burned areas)
      • Ring basins
      • Normal saline

TRANSFERRING THE PATIENT

The care of a burn patient is difficult and time-consuming. It involves a whole team of people, not just a physician and nurse. Because of the specialized care that a burn patient requires, any major burn should be transferred to an organized burn unit if one is not available within the local hospital.

If the decision is made to transfer, the burn unit should be contacted so that transfer guidelines can be established. The following outline is a review of what has been previously covered but can serve as a standard guideline in preparing for the transfer:

1. Establish the airway; intubate if necessary.
2. Identify the source and circumstances of the burn and get medical history.
3. Cut away clothes and evaluate entire patient for other trauma.
4. Keep as warm as possible while:
    A. Estimating extent and severity of burns
    B. Initiating a large bore IV line above the waist with Ringer's lactate
    C. Drawing blood for laboratory analysis
    D. Placing an indwelling Foley catheter with urine gauge (Urimeter)
    E. Placing an NG tube PRN (keep patient NPO).
5. Observe consistent, clean, protective technique.
6. Cleanse gross debris and debride loose *hanging* skin only, as time allows, and reevaluate burn. *Do not peel the patient!*
7. Contact the burn unit for specific instructions on burn care and transfer.
8. Monitor VS and urine output.
9. Maintain fluid intake via IV line.
10. Give analgesics IV, PRN, for pain and anxiety, and be certain tetanus status is adequate.
11. Send complete concise documentation with an appropriate transfer form.

CONCLUSION

With the development of emergency medical services systems across the United States, we have seen the emergence of well-equipped and expertly staffed burn units who receive patients from whatever areas the units serve; critically injured patients are transported to them in vehicles that are fully equipped with life-support hardware and staffed by trained nurses and paramedical personnel. The chances for survival and return to a relatively normal life style have increased greatly in recent years for the seriously burned patient but depend heavily on the integrity of care in each phase of management. Nursing care of the burned patient is a highly skilled, specialized, and demanding area—demanding physically, emotionally, and professionally; this is all too obvious to those of us who receive burned patients initially and feel a total sense of loss at first impact. Emergency personnel are not necessarily expected to know all the fine points of advanced burn care but must certainly be expected to know the essential management philosophy and protocols while the patient is their responsibility.

REVIEW

1. Define the classifications of burns as they relate to depth.
2. List five factors having a direct effect on determining the severity of a burn.
3. Explain the role of the "Rule of Nine" in determining severity of a burn.
4. In general terms, explain the pathophysiology of a burn injury.
5. Describe the immediate priorities of treatment when a burn patient presents.
6. Define the nursing role and responsibilities with the care of a burn patient in the ED.
7. Explain the rationale of the customary drug therapy employed in the care of a severely burned patient.
8. Describe what you feel should be admission criteria for a burn patient.
9. Using the standard replacement formula, how much Ringer's lactate would be given to a 40-lb child with a 40% TBA burn in the first 8 hours?
10. Explain why D5/W should not be given to burn patients.
11. Using the standard replacement formula, how much Ringer's lactate would be given to a 188-lb woman with a 60% TBA burn in the first 24 hours? How much in the first 8 hours?
12. What percent of TBA burn is required to necessitate admission of a burned child?
13. When approximating the percent of TBA, the width of one hand represents what percent?
14. What is always the first priority when receiving a burn patient?
15. What technique should ED personnel observe when handling a burn patient?
16. Describe two methods of removing tar and asphalt from burned tissue.
17. Describe a properly equipped burn cart.
18. Describe the proper procedure for preparing and transporting a severely burned patient to another facility by ambulance.

BIBLIOGRAPHY

Barber JM, Dillman PA: Emergency Patient Care. Reston Publishing Co., Reston, Virginia, 1981

Brunner S, Suddarth D: The Lippincott Manual of Nursing Practice, 2nd ed. J.B. Lippincott Co., Philadelphia, Pennsylvania, 1982

Budassi SA, Barber JM: Emergency Nursing: Principles and Practice. C.V. Mosby Co., St. Louis, Missouri, 1981

Cosgriff JH, Anderson DL: The Practice of Emergency Nursing. J.B. Lippincott Co., Philadelphia, Pennsylvania, 1975

Committee on Injuries, American Academy of Orthopaedic Surgeons: Emergency Care and Transportation of the Sick and Injured, 3rd ed. Chicago, Illinois, 1981

Dyer C: Burn care in the emergency period. JEN, Vol 6, No 1, pp 9-16, January/February 1980

Frank HA, Wachtel TL (eds.): Thermal injuries. TEM, Vol 3, No 3, October 1981

Grant H, Murray R: Emergency Care, 2nd ed. Robert J. Brady Co., Bowie, Maryland, 1978

Jelenko C: Initial burn management. Third Annual Rocky Mountain Regional Conference on Emergency Medicine and Nursing, Keystone, 1977

Jones C, Feller I: Burns: Emergency care of burn victims. Emergency Nurs, May/June 1975

Myers MB: Sutures and wound healing. Am J Nurs, Vol 71, No 9, 1971

Noe JM, Kalish S: Wound Care. Cheesebrough Ponds, Inc., Greenwich, Connecticut, 1975

O'Brien K: Care of the burn patient. Emergency Highlights, Vol 2, No 1, Emanuel Life Flight, Portland, Oregon, April 1981

Simmons R: Emergency management of electrical burns. JEN, Vol 3, No 2, 1977

Thompson RV: Primary Repair of Soft Tissue Injuries. Melbourne University Press, Melbourne, Australia, 1969

Warner C: Emergency Care: Assessment and Intervention, 2nd ed. C.V. Mosby Co., St. Louis, Missouri, 1978

SURFACE TRAUMA AND WOUND MANAGEMENT 22

KEY CONCEPTS

This chapter has been compiled to help the EDN understand the structure of the human skin and the various types of soft-tissue injuries that result from trauma, and to provide detailed guidelines for initial wound management, including evaluation, preparation, closure, and dressing, as it relates to the appropriate skills level of the nurse.

The bulk of this text is based on lecture content and wound repair skills taught by Howard Kirz, M.D., a Seattle emergency physician, and Michael Turman, P.A. of Portland, Oregon.

After reading and studying this chapter, you should be able to:

- Identify and describe the three layers of the skin.
- Define open and closed soft-tissue injuries and give examples of each.
- Identify the three phases of healing.
- Define primary, secondary, and tertiary intention healing.
- List at least eight factors that affect optimum primary healing.
- Identify at least six basic points in good preliminary wound management.
- Describe the characteristics of the three layers of the skin and how they relate to the formation of scar tissue.
- Identify the two essential prerequisites to uneventful healing of a wound.
- Describe the preliminary considerations of wound evaluation.
- Describe the proper method of cleansing and preparing a wound for repair.
- Explain the formula for wound irrigation.
- Identify the key to proper wound cleansing and describe the best method.
- List at least six guidelines to follow for infiltrating the wound with local anesthesia.
- Explain the Kirz Square Rule for wound repair.
- List the situations in which the nurse should never close the wound.

- Explain the rationale for administering tetanus toxoid boosters.
- Explain general management protocols for rabies prophylaxis.
- Describe the three-layer concept of dressing a wound, and explain the rationale as well as the function of a dressing.

An essential area of assessment and management that falls to the EDN is that of surface trauma and subsequent management of the resulting wounds. Experience in this regard varies widely, as does interest on the nurse's part. However, whether or not a nurse *ever* performs a wound closure, it remains a primary nursing responsibility to carefully evaluate the wound, exercise the correct initial management, and prepare the wound adequately for surgical closure. This chapter will attempt to develop a new awareness of the varieties of problems involved, the best avenues of management, and the basics of wound closure as applied to uncomplicated superficial wounds, which would be appropriate for an EDN to close.

Dr. Kirz has proposed that in the presence or absence of a physician, the properly trained EDN should be capable of evaluating minor soft-tissue trauma for the degree of severity, impairment of neural or circulatory function, and the need for immediate definitive attention. Further, the EDN should be expert in the irrigation and preparation of wounds, in the recognition of the presence of foreign material and of unusual circumstances such as those involving tendons, nerves, vessels, etc. In the absence of a physician, the EDN should be capable of making an independent judgment as to the need for suturing, steri-stripping, etc. In the absence of a physician *but* in the presence of appropriately prepared standing orders, the EDN should be capable of applying such treatment to minor lacerations, including suturing. In the presence of the physician and subject to prior approval of that physician, the EDN should be capable of and responsible for performing the same competent act of minor suturing, with expert follow-up on proper wound dressing, splinting, and instructions to the patient regarding post-repair care and recognition of complications.

We support these concepts and urge every reader to commit this chapter to memory and strictly adhere to the guidelines that are spelled out. Wound care and closure has traditionally been the physician's area, and as nurses broaden their roles and capabilities in the ED, they must do so with caution and the continual exercise of sound judgment. Any wound that is not a superficial, uncomplicated laceration or that falls into the high-risk category, as outlined in this chapter, is *not* appropriate to the EDN's skills for closure and must never be attempted. This lack of caution and judgment could easily harm the patient, jeopardize the privileges of other EDNs, and stifle the development of an area where nurses can expand their skills and capabilities.

THE SKIN

Skin, the major organ of the integumentary system, is remarkable and versatile (Fig. 22.1). Skin, which makes up about 15% of the dry weight of the body, acts as the principal barrier between man and his environment and at the same time is a means of communication between the two. Human skin is never static but undergoes constant change, renewal, and adaptation to meet man's needs. Consider the difference in skin appearance in various body sites: it is smooth and soft in some regions but rough and furrowed in others. Thick, coarse hair grows in areas such as the eyebrows, axillas, and pubis, but only downy fuzz is visible on the forehead. Skin appearance varies with age and race, as well as from place to place on the same individual's body.

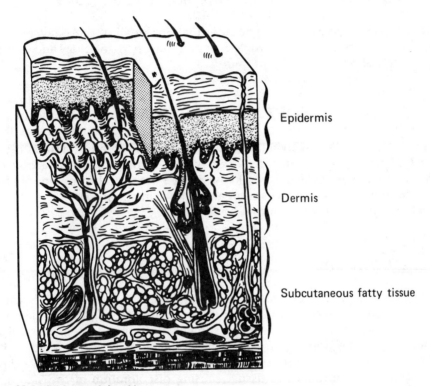

Epidermis

Dermis

Subcutaneous fatty tissue

Figure 22.1. Anatomy of the skin.

Wide variations in skin thickness exist also. The skin of the eyelid is almost paper-thin, for instance, while the soles of the feet are perhaps 10-20 times thicker. Skin is made up of three layers: the epidermis, dermis (corium), and subcutaneous tissue. The outer layer, *epidermis,* contains stratified epithelial tissue. The second layer, the *dermis* or corium, is connective tissue with both elastic and collagen fibers and contains structures of the integumentary system: hairs, nails, oil glands, sweat glands, and ducts. Hairs are dead structures composed of protein cells firmly cemented together to form a solid shaft. Nails grow upon the dermal skin layer and take their nourishment from it. Oil and sweat glands are also located in the dermal layer, under which lies the *subcutaneous* tissue, composed primarily of fatty tissue and vascular networks.

The skin has several functions that are vitally important to man. Skin is the largest single body organ and, as such, performs the following functions:

1. Holding the body tissues and fluids together in a shape with acceptable visual form.
2. Holding water in the body tissues, except for the insensitive water loss from the lungs of about 500 cc/day.
3. Protecting the underlying tissues from invasion by infection.
4. Serving as principal regulator of body heat.
5. Metabolic regulation of salt, glucose, water, and fat.
6. Providing perception of heat, cold, touch, pressure, pain.

When evaluating wounds, remember that any or all of these layers, structures, and functions may be involved, depending on the etiology and physical factors operating at the time of injury.

SOFT TISSUE INJURY

Soft-tissue injuries involving the skin and underlying muscle beds can be classified generally as open and closed. A *closed* wound or bruise is one with soft-tissue damage involving the skin without a break in the continuity of the skin. An *open* wound involves a break in the skin surface or in the mucous membrane that lines the external body orifices.

CLOSED INJURIES

Closed injuries to soft tissue, sustained from blunt force to the tissues, can be extremely painful and temporarily disfiguring to the patient. This damaged area, called a *bruise or contusion,* is subject to varying degrees of swelling, depending on the depth of tissue injury and, generally, is accompanied by enough capillary damage to result in extravasation of blood, with blood pigments migrating through the tissue, causing discoloration of the skin, generally referred to as "black and blue" marks. The full extent of discoloration may take 24-48 hours to materialize and will be very dark in color. As the healing process takes place and the dead cells resorb, the bruised area becomes paler, greenish-brown, and finally yellowish, as the tissues return to normal. A yellowish bruise is an old bruise.

When larger vessels are disrupted secondary to contusion, there may be rapid formation of a pocket of blood collecting within the damaged area; this is referred to as a *hematoma.* These are generally well-defined subcutaneous lumps of varying dimensions and will show discoloration almost immediately. Hematomas occasionally require incision and drainage to allow the healing process to proceed without infection and complication. The presence of hematoma should always be noted and taken into consideration in overall wound management.

OPEN INJURIES

Open wounds of the soft tissues, which are highly susceptible to hemorrhage and infection, are classified as 1) abrasions, 2) lacerations, 3) avulsions/amputations, and 4) puncture wounds.

Abrasions

Abrasions (Fig. 22.2) involve the loss of a partial thickness of skin from a friction rub against the skin surface, with a resultant denuding. These are sometimes referred to as friction burns, mat burns, or sliding burns, and frequently there will be embedded foreign material present. This material must be removed to prevent not only infection but permanent tattooing. Frequently, this can be accomplished by first anesthetizing the surface area with a topical application of 4% lidocaine (Xylocaine), which should be allowed to remain on the wound for a period of 10-15 min. This is done by simply saturating gauze with the medication and laying it across the abraded area. Since some of the lidocaine is absorbed systemically, care should be taken not to exceed toxic levels (see later discussion) in cases of large abrasions or small patients. Local injection with lidocaine may also be used to insure anesthesia. Following anesthesia, it is a relatively simple matter to cleanse the wound with a soft sponge surgical scrub brush and lift out deeply embedded materials with a needle point or pointed blade (a No. 11 Bard Parker blade works well), followed by irrigation. A light film of antibiotic ointment may be applied to the abrasion, followed by a layer of porous nonadherent material, topped with a gauze dressing to absorb seepage. The dressings may be changed daily until the surface has formed an eschar.

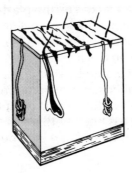

Figure 22.2. Abrasions.

Lacerations

Technically, a laceration (Fig. 22.3) is a tear in the skin, involving the full thickness, and may be the result of many causes. Lacerations from sharp objects are referred to as "incisional" but may also be jagged tears and pressure splints. They vary in size, type, shape, amount of associated contusion, and depth. This presents other problems, including the involvement of the underlying structures of tendons, nerves, vessels, fascia, and muscles. Patients with deeply penetrating wounds are often assigned immediately to the operating room, where adequate exploration and cleansing can be carried out under general anesthesia. It must be remembered that the deeper the laceration and the more structures it involves, the more painstaking the efforts must be to achieve satisfactory wound closure while preserving function and cosmetic integrity.

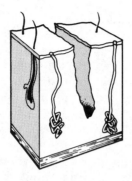

Figure 22.3. Lacerations.

Avulsions/Amputations

An avulsion (Fig. 22.4) is a loss of tissue. This may involve skin that has been totally torn away or left hanging as a flap. Avulsed tissue (especially structures such as ears, nose, fingers, and large areas of skin) should be handled in special ways in an effort to preserve the viability and structure of the tissue, if any salvage is to be realized. Rather than placing tissues into sterile saline solution as was done in the past, we are asked by the plastic and replantation surgeons to place the avulsed tissue or part in a gauze wrap which has been *moistened* with sterile, normal saline solution, seal it in a plastic bag, and place the bag in a bath of iced, normal saline. In this manner, the severed nerves, tendons, and vessels will not become macerated by soaking and will be more readily identifiable under the electron microscope at operation. In many instances, tissues have been replaced surgically as long as 6-10 hours later when this procedure was followed, and the result has been both a functional and cosmetic success. Steps for home care of an amputated part include 1) *not* putting it in water, 2)

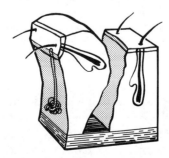

Figure 22.4. Avulsions.

rolling it up with fat on the inside, and 3) protecting it from drying and heat. The area from which tissue has been avulsed should be protected with moist, sterile, normal saline-soaked gauze pads, with bleeding controlled in the appropriate manner.

Puncture Wounds

A puncture wound (Fig. 22.5) occurs when the skin is penetrated by a sharp or blunt object and most commonly is sustained by stepping on nails, staples, thumb tacks, needles, and broken glass. It may also be the result of an intentional assault with a sharp instrument. Again, if wound depth and organ involvement are apparently significant, these patients are candidates for the operating room. The main concerns with wounds of this sort are not only damage to underlying structures and the risk of infection but the fact that puncture wounds are particularly prone to tetanus. It is especially important to be certain of the immunization status of patients with these injuries, and if the wound is extensively contaminated, prophylactic antibiotics are frequently prescribed.

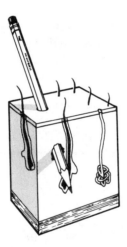

Figure 22.5. Puncture wounds.

Embedded Foreign Bodies. Embedded foreign bodies present further problems and can be difficult to manage. Unless the patient can describe the angle of entry and is certain what the foreign body is and its present location, disposition is tedious. If an embedded foreign body is a certainty, the wound *must* be explored, whether in the ED or OR. Occasionally, an X-ray film is helpful in locating the object if it is metal or glass, but wood splinters rarely show up unless they are coated with lead-base paint, and that is relatively rare. Wooden foreign bodies commonly cause infection, and some fulminate rapidly especially redwood, hemlock, and cedar, and can become quite serious unless taken care of immediately. These are urgent situations!

Deeply *impaled foreign bodies* with penetrating injury should never be removed except by the physician, for the entry may have severed a vessel and the foreign body itself is possibly tamponading a heavy bleeder. The EDN can only prepare the wound for surgery or further evaluation. Emergency medical technicians are taught specifically to leave the impaled foreign object in place to stop bleeding by use of direct pressure above the point of bleeding without exerting pressure on the impaled object or directly adjacent tissue, and to use a bulk dressing to stabilize the object before attempting to transport the patient to the ED. The same guidelines hold true until the physician is present to make further decisions.

Foreign bodies with shallow penetration can usually be removed gently with steady, careful traction exerted. Once the object has been recovered, it should be attached with cellophane tape as part of the patient's permanent medical record.

INITIAL MANAGEMENT

Initial wound management upon presentation to the ED involves control of the bleeding, prevention of further contamination, and immobilization of the injured part. The best way to control a bleeding wound is by application of pressure directly over the wound with a bulk dressing, either held by hand or bound into place with a pressure bandage, a dressing held under pressure by an inflated air splint, or by direct pressure with the bare hand if no dressing is available. Virtually, all bleeding wounds can be controlled with these simple pressure measures. Uncontrolled bleeding may, in rare cases, require using the arterial pressure points of the body, or in the most extreme cases when the patient is threatened with exsanguination, a tourniquet is indicated, but *only* then! If heavy bleeding is stemming from a spurting artery, it should be clamped with vascular clamps or pinched shut with the fingers (if the end has not retracted), again to avoid traumatizing the fragile structures and preventing anastamosis under microscopic surgery.

HEALING PHASES

An understanding of the healing phases involved in overall wound management is important to any nurse who is involved in wound care or who wishes to be able to instruct the patient intelligently about the time elements involved in the healing process. Wound healing takes place in three phases.

Lag Phase

The lag phase (catabolic or autolytic stage) is the time during which edema is present; white blood cells migrate into the wounded tissue to phagocytize the area in preparation for regeneration. This period of 5-7 days is the *weak* period for the wound. For this reason, suture lines should be reinforced with skin strips prior to suture removal if done in less than 10 days to 2 weeks, depending on the size of the wound and location.

Anabolic Phase

The anabolic phase follows and overlaps the lag phase with a migration of fibroblasts and collagen fibers into the fibrin network that has been laid in the wounded tissue to bridge the defect. The wound edges take on a reddened color as the blood supply increases to the area, and the tissue in the area is referred to as granulation tissue. Fibroblasts continue to increase in number, adding strength to the wound as it heals, and scar tissue gradually forms. As the wound heals from below, the epithelial cells regenerate and gradually cover the surface of the defect. This phase lasts from 2 to 3 weeks, and depending on the depth and location of the wound, it is generally safe to remove sutures in 7-10 days, reinforcing carefully, when indicated, with skin strips.

Maturation Phase

The maturation phase may last from 3 months to 2 years. A pink scar is seen during this period as more collagen is laid down with other interlaced fibers of collagen. The scar will fade further and mature with some degree of retraction and/or contraction. These facts should be carefully explained to patients and especially to parents of children who are concerned about poor cosmetic results that are seen in the early stages of healing but that will likely mature to the desired result in time.

HOW WOUNDS HEAL

Wound healing may occur in three ways: 1) primary intention, 2) secondary intention (granulation), and 3) tertiary intention (delayed closure or secondary suture).

Primary Intention

Primary intention (first or primary closure) is a desirable means of closing wounds and is possible in most cleanly incised type wounds, which have been debrided and revised as necessary. The underlying structures are reapproximated with care to make certain that no dead spaces exist for collection of serum and formation of hematomas, as well as to provide support for the surface closure. Then the opposing wound edges are reapproximated as precisely as possible to restore function and integrity of the surface structures.

Secondary Intention

Secondary intention (granulation) is indicated in wounds that involve a relatively extensive loss of tissue and either cannot or should not be closed, such as gaping avulsions, gunshot wounds, and burns. When a wound is allowed to "granulate in," there will be a substantial scar formation with subsequent contraction of the scar, which may lead to greater deformity and further loss of function in the area involved.

Third Intention

Third intention (tertiary) closure is the method of delaying closure for a specific time to combat infection or gross contamination. While the wound remains open, it is continually cleansed and debrided, as a minimal amount of granulation tissue is allowed to form. Subsequently, the wound is closed surgically (usually about a week later), resulting in a scar formation greater than primary closure but generally far more cosmetically acceptable than healing by secondary intention with unsightly granulation tissue scar formation.

SCAR FORMATION

To understand the technique of obtaining the best possible cosmetic results with wound closures, the nurse must understand how scarring occurs. Scars come from lacerations, avulsions, contused lacerations, and perforating wounds. There is nothing in *skin* that can scar, however. Scarring comes from the subcutaneous layer with the upward migration of fibroblasts. Simply put, a *gap* left open in the dermis will allow free migration of fibroblasts to the surface, forming a scar with which the patient lives the rest of his life.

The epidermis is made up of epithelial cells and has *no* tensile strength, but it *does* regenerate. It is multitalented and covers whatever lies underneath it like tissue paper. A surface of epidermis approximated to a surface of epidermis, however, will not heal.

The dermis has tensile strength, but *no* other talents. The dermis is physiologically inert and does *not* regenerate or resorb. It stays layered and is the *key to repair* of all lacerations, since results of interference with the dermis remain forever unless plastic repair is done. Examples of this include acne pits, chickenpox scars from scratching, and poorly closed or poorly approximated wounds.

The subcutaneous tissue is similar paper and will not hold stitches since it, like the epidermis, has no tensile strength. *Fibroblasts* come from this layer and migrate to the surface through poorly approximated layers of dermis and cause *scarring.*

Meticulous hemostasis (with the elimination of dead spaces and bleeding) and *precise approximation of wound edges* are the two essential prerequisites to proper healing with minimal scarring. Perpendicular edges of the dermis must be brought together precisely and sutured in apposition to close the wound and prevent the upward migration of scar-forming materials. This is the key to rapid healing and optimal cosmetic results for all wounds.

FACTORS AFFECTING HEALING

The overall objective of wound care is to achieve primary healing with an uneventful course, restoring the area to full function, and preserving the tissues in cosmetically acceptable fashion. There are several key factors that affect the way in which wounds heal and the rates at which they heal:

1. The condition of the patient
   A. Status of overall health
   B. Circulatory status
   C. Age (affects the rate of laying down collagen)
   D. Nutritional status
   E. Preexisting disease (diabetes, renal disease, etc.)
   F. Temperature
   G. Dependence on medication (aspirin, anticoagulants, steroids)
2. Type of wound
   A. Vascular supply
   B. Injury to associated structures (vessels, nerves, tendons)
   C. Presence of crush injury or hematoma
   D. Location on the body (face versus leg, etc.)
3. Degree of contamination
   A. Type of possible contamination
   B. Age of the wound

PRELIMINARY WOUND MANAGEMENT

The basic elements of management for which the EDN is responsible are:

1. Control of bleeding with the use of pressure, cold applications, elevation of the injured part, and splints if necessary
2. Prevention of further contamination of the wound; cover with a sterile pad
3. Preservation of the blood supply as well as possible
4. Handling the wound gently with inspection and cleansing, since tissue cells are easily destroyed
5. Shaving as little as possible, since shaving increases desquamation of the epithelium and increases contamination of the area. *Never* shave eyebrows, since they do not always grow back and are expensive items in court.
6. Decreasing the edema of the area, however possible, since edema will cause tissue tension.
7. Preventing dryness and keeping the wound moist with sterile saline pads.

Preliminary Considerations

As Dr. Kirz pointed out for several years while conducting the wound management workshops for ACEP/EDNA Scientific Assemblies, the nurse who sutures *must* be acutely aware of whether the wound to be closed is appropriate for his or her level of skill. Wounds must be carefully examined and evaluated before closure, and many considerations need to be taken into account. If, in the first place it is acceptable practice in the nurse's place of employment, and the State Nurse Practice Act permits, the wound must still qualify further as being suitable for someone other than the licensed physician to repair.

Any one of the following criteria would be reason enough (for the patient's sake, the nurse's sake, and medicolegal savvy) for the nurse to *not* close the wound:

1. Presence of concomitant injuries requiring further evaluation
2. Any mechanism of injury which could have produced trauma to underlying structures with resulting complications:
    A. Crushed finger with underlying fractures
    B. Sliced finger with possible nicked tendon sheath
    C. Laceration from broken glass with possibility of embedded foreign body
    D. Embedded foreign body of wood
    E. *Bites of any sort,* whether animal or human, deep or superficial. Human bites are by far the more serious because of the multiplicity of organisms in the human mouth, and infections from these bites may be unusually severe. These require the full attention of a physician.
3. Allergies to local anesthetics, tetanus antitoxin, epinephrine, or antibiotics
4. Questionable tetanus immunization status which may make the wound high risk
5. Inadequate immobilization of patient or wound. "If it won't hold still, it won't hold stitches." (Howard Kirz)
6. Again, is the repair of the laceration appropriate to the current skills of the nurse? Legs, arms, scalp, abdomen, and back are areas where the nurse might be able to close superficial lacerations that are linear or slightly jagged but do not involve loss or involvement of deeper structures. Wounds located over joints can be complicated and need careful consideration. Be aware also that the areas most prone to scarring and keloid formation are the anterior chest and the anterior thigh. They all overlie large active muscle bellies that will additionally stress the closure line. The face and neck, because of their cosmetic impact, are probably best sutured by very experienced persons.
7. Any wound over 6 hours old must be considered high risk, and the patient must be questioned specifically as to exact time of occurrence. Many physicians will not do a primary closure on wounds over 10 hours old and generally observe the tertiary approach to safeguard against infection.
8. Wounds with extensively crushed tissue along the edges *must* be revised and unless the revision is very minor in nature, it should be the physician's responsibility.
9. Any wound that compromises circulation or affects sensory perception, motor function, or range of motion should be documented accordingly and considered a high-risk wound. Sensory perception may be tested

with a cotton-tipped applicator or a light prick with a sterile needle distal to the wound.

Consideration of the Patient

While preparing to carry out a wound repair, give the patient some thoughtful consideration by using the best psychological tools. Combine your repair techniques with a thoughtful use of language, avoiding as much as possible the obvious reference to stitches, needles, knives, cutting, etc. Try to establish a comfortable chatting rapport with your patient as you set about your repair and be prepared to give the local anesthesia time to work, providing as calm and quiet an atmosphere as possible. Reassure as necessary and reinforce your actions with positive statements, being honest but not afraid to say "this may hurt a little."

PREPARATION OF THE WOUND

In the initial treatment of wounds, cleansing and preparation can make the difference between a clean, healed wound and an infected one. Techniques for preparation should be adhered to rigidly. After the initial thorough evaluation of the wound, the surrounding area of skin may be shaved (except the eyebrows) but no more than necessary. Many authorities currently advise avoiding shaving if possible. After this preparation, a thorough cleansing of the skin surrounding the wound is done. This should take 5-10 min by the clock (depending on the extent of the area), observing surgical protocol and using a surgical scrub soap of choice, preferably one of the povidone-iodine group. The skin is then flushed with sterile water or saline, and then the wound itself should be copiously irrigated with a Toomey or control syringe and sterile NSS and a No. 18 needle to create an effective "hydraulic action."

The key to proper wound cleansing is *mechanical action,* and if foreign material is present, it must be scrubbed out with a surgical scrub sponge and then reirrigated. Wounds must also be debrided of loose and torn tissue before closure.

A guide for adequate irrigation of wounds is the Kirz rule:

Irrigate with *50 cc NSS per inch of wound per hour of age of wound*

This will be sufficient in most open gaping wounds, but use more irrigant when flushing dirty, ragged, older wounds and less with clean little kitchen-knife type cuts. In small wounds, a 5-cc syringe with a No. 22 needle works well to force an irrigating jet into the wound and cleanse effectively. If the patient cannot tolerate the irrigation and cleansing, anesthetize the wound first, and then cleanse.

Anesthesia may be accomplished with several agents, but there are some guidelines which must be carefully followed:

1. You may use 1% lidocaine (Xylocaine) with epinephrine 1:200,000 *only* on the leg, forearm, upper arm, back, chest, abdomen, and scalp. The

epinephrine gives some hemostasis but should be avoided unless bleeding is heavy.

2. Use only PLAIN lidocaine on fingers, toes, penis, nose, ears, and elderly people.

3. Use a 5- or 10-cc syringe with *no larger* than a No. 27 needle (preferably a No. 30) for infiltration. The pain of lidocaine injection is related to both the amount and rate of infiltration.

4. Infiltrate through the wound edge under the dermis (not through the skin), injecting ahead of yourself and reentering the edge of the injected area where anesthesia is accomplished.

5. Limit to 20 cc in adults (usually only 2-3 cc are necessary).

6. Limit to maximum of 3 mg/kg in children.

7. Be alert to the side effects of lidocaine, which might include:
   shivering, tremors, euphoria, convulsions,
   respiratory depression and arrest, cardiac
   arrest and vascular collapse
   In event of serious side effects, administer high-flow oxygen immediately and have IV diazepam (Valium) 10 mg ready if convulsions begin. Stay calm!

8. Several alternatives are available if the patient is allergic to the "caines":
   A. Pack with ice for 10-15 min.
   B. Use of diphenhydramine HCl (Benadryl), 50 mg diluted in 2-3 cc sterile water or normal saline and infiltrate.
   C. Infiltration of sterile NSS.
   D. Various forms of systemic anesthesia, including narcotics and general anesthesia. Wound repairs that require anesthesia other than standard lidocaine infiltration should *not* be attempted by the EDN.

9. Give the anesthesia adequate time to be effective before further exploration or closure.

10. Carefully inspect the wound, looking for foreign bodies, dirt, clots, wood bits, hair particles, grass, etc., and reevaluate for damaged structures, such as tendons, nerves, and blood vessels, irrigating and flushing copiously as outlined.

PHYSICAL ARRANGEMENTS, PREPARATIONS, AND TECHNIQUE

Before committing yourself to a sterile field and a satisfactory wound repair, be certain you have extricated yourself from the other activities of the department. Turn over the keys (if they're in your pocket), make any necessary phone calls, arrange your stool at the proper height, adjust the light over the field, and have a runner within earshot for standby.

Nurses who accept the responsibility of wound repair in the ED *must* use scrupulous sterile technique and should consider wearing a surgical mask. The

Communicable Disease Center in Atlanta (CDC) states that 30-40% of normal people may shed coagulase-positive *Staph. aureus* in their nasal secretions, and the EDN must rule out that possibility of contaminating the patient's wound. The field must be adequately draped and a scrupulous effort made to keep the fall of the suture within a well-draped sterile field. The technique must be impeccable.

HANDLING TISSUES

Wound revision must be taught under direct supervision by the physician, but in preparation for learning the techniques, the EDN should be aware that issues must be handled gently, and when using a grasping tool for managing the skin edges, use only one side of a mouse-toothed forceps or a skin hook merely as a lifting tool. Do not puncture the skin with your forceps! Skin edges must be perpendicular for precise approximation, and edges may be revised with iris scissors, No. 15 blade or blade-breaker technique, to trim ragged edges and those without circulatory support. An exception to this is in the hairy areas, where the wound should be parallel to the hair follicles. Test alignment and skin tension, undermine tissue if necessary to approximate *without tension*. When in doubt, *always* ask your physician.

SUTURE

Choice of suture primarily depends on the tissue being repaired. Closure is done in layers (muscle, fascia, fat, skin) to obliterate dead space and prevent collections of serum or blood that may interfere with healing. Selection of suture material is a matter of individual choice, since there is a large variety of absorbable and nonabsorbable types of suture in most emergency facilities. In general, absorbable sutures are used to approximate the deeper layers of wounds, and nonabsorbable sutures are used for the skin, to be removed at specific times.

Chromicized catgut is stronger and takes longer to be absorbed by the body than plain catgut; however, it is more irritating to the tissues and produces a greater inflammatory response. Synthetic absorbable suture (Polyglactin 910 or polyglycolic acid suture) is now available and may be preferred. Nonabsorbable sutures in common use for skin closure include silk and a variety of synthetic materials (Mersilene, Prolene, Dermalon, Ethilon). The smallest suture and finest needle adequate to accomplish the closure should be used, provoking a minimal tissue response while promoting good healing.

Subcutaneous closure of muscle and fascia, if needed to reduce dead space prior to skin closure or to support surface sutures, usually calls for a 4-0 chromic type suture or synthetic absorbable, and 5-0 chromic is used for the face, if suturing is unavoidable. Particular attention must be paid to strong closure of the deep layer in the scalp (galea) if it has been interrupted, and this requires 4-0 chromic suture, tying at least double knots and cutting the suture close.

Skin closure generally calls for 4-0 nylon (Ethilon or Dermalon) or polypropylene (Prolene) with a P3 needle for extremities, scalp, or trunk. In areas under less tension and on fingers and fingertips, 5-0 nylon or polypropylene may be used, with 5-0 and 6-0 suture usually suitable for the face.

Preparation of the Wound Edges

Closure of superficial wounds involves careful cleansing and inspection of the wound edges. Many wounds have undergone a certain amount of crushing, which creates additional edema and will lead to more pronounced scarring because of the additional fibroplasia which develops. It is necessary, then, to excise the crushed tissue. One method used by Ira M. Dushoff, M.D., author of "A Stitch in Time," is to prep the wound edges with peroxide and follow with aqueous benzalkonium (Zephirin). The peroxide produces a white patch wherever the wound edges were crushed, and then a careful excision is done, using whatever edge revision method has been taught. The wound edges are carefully undermined and approximated without undue tension, and the wound closed with the appropriate suture material.

Placement of Sutures

Skin edges should always be slightly everted in apposition (Fig. 22.6), and in order to achieve a smooth, even closure, without bunching of edges, you must sew the skin the same distance along each side of the wound; i.e., if the stitches are 3 mm apart on one side, they must come out exactly the same distance on the other side to avoid diagonal tensions, which will readily distort the wound edge.

Just as there is a relationship between the depth and the width of the stitch, there is also a relationship between tension on the wound, the distance between stitches, and the distances of the stitch from the wound edge. The principle involved is that the more tension on the wound, the closer the stitches

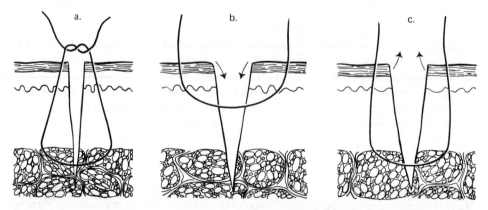

Figure 22.6. Suture placement. a) A suture placed angling away from wound edges is bottle shaped and produces a closing with everted edges. b) A suture placed with its width greater than its depth will invert the wound edges. c) A suture placed with depth greater than its width will evert the wound edges.

should be to each other; the more tension on the wound edge, the closer the stitches should be to the wound edge.*

When closing superficial wounds, if the stitch is unevenly placed or distorts the wound edge, *remove it and place another stitch!*

The Kirz "Square Rule" for Suturing

The Kirz "Square Rule" (Fig. 22.7) is as follows:

1. Hold the needle *squarely* and properly in the needle holder between the middle and the proximal one-third (Fig. 22.7a).
2. Hold the needle *square* (perpendicular to the skin) and rotate the wrist after the needle has pierced the tissue downward (Fig. 22.7b).
3. Use the *square* stitch method to accomplish *eversion* of edges (placing the stitch deeper than it is wide, with a squared or "bottle bottom" configuration) (Fig. 22.7c).
4. Tie *square* knots and throw a minimum of two *full* square knots (Fig. 22.8), cutting the suture ends slightly less than 0.5 in. long (Fig. 22.7d).

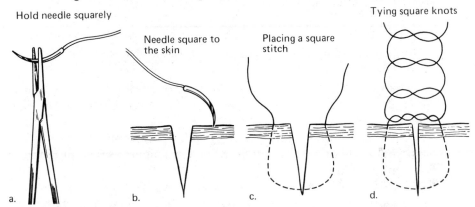

Figure 22.7. The Kirz Square Rule of suturing.

The Kirz Instrument Tie

The technique for the *instrument tie* (Fig. 22.9) should be practiced until a high degree of proficiency is achieved. A fresh pig's foot is an excellent object on which to practice, but if one is not available, try rolling a towel bolster and placing a few stitches, which can be easily cut and removed before the towel goes to the laundry.

The steps in performing the square-knot instrument tie are as follows:

1. Place suture through wound edges, one side at a time, testing for approximation.
2. *Always* place needle holder on top of *long* end of suture.

---

*Dushoff I: A stitch in time. Emergency Medicine. p 3, January 1973

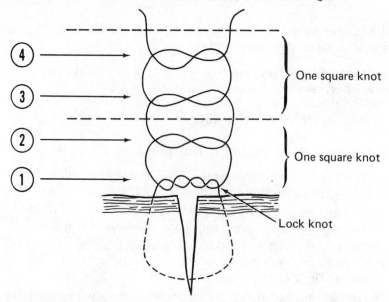

Figure 22.8. The square knot detailed. Use "double throw" lock knot on *first* loop only. Follow this with a minimum of three more single throws for two full square knots.

3. With needle holder in right hand, hold one end of suture with left hand.

4. With needle holder lying on top of suture, form a double loop around needle holder.

5. Reach over and pick up free end (*at the better end*) with needle holder and pull it through loop, laying knot flat by crossing left hand over right and laying out long end of suture to your right.

6. Lock first half of this square knot by pulling short end of suture (still being held in your needle holder) back to the right in same direction as long end of suture.

7. Now tie the second "throw" of square knot by placing holder ON TOP of LONG end of suture to right and make one loop around needle holder.

8. Reach over and pick up free end (*at the bitter end*) with needle holder and pull it through loop.

9. Lay knot flat by pulling on strands in opposite directions. This completes *one* square knot.

10. Repeat square knot (two throws) at least once, always tying a minimum of two complete square knots regardless of type of suture used.

DRESSINGS AND INSTRUCTIONS TO THE PATIENT

Too frequently patients are sent out of emergency department with inadequate dressings, improperly applied and temporary at best. A well-constructed dressing has many functions and should be considered from that standpoint. It provides protection to the wound, with antisepsis, pressure, immobilization, absorption capability, support, comfort, and an esthetic appearance.

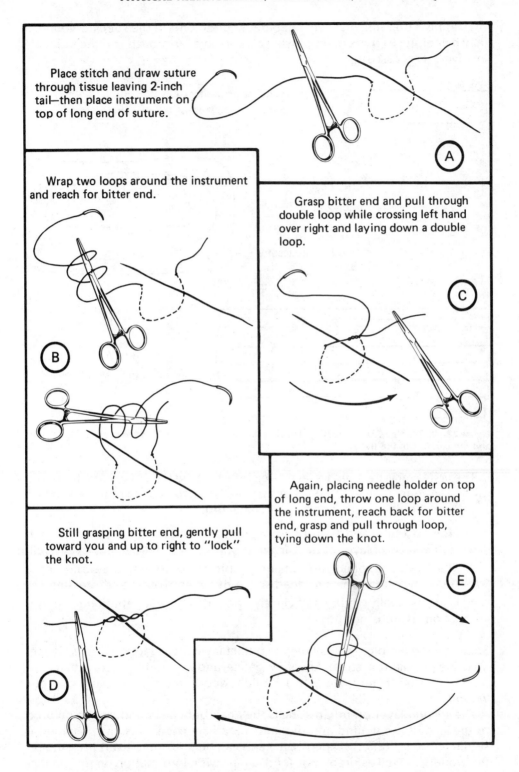

Place stitch and draw suture through tissue leaving 2-inch tail—then place instrument on top of long end of suture.

A

Wrap two loops around the instrument and reach for bitter end.

B

Grasp bitter end and pull through double loop while crossing left hand over right and laying down a double loop.

C

Still grasping bitter end, gently pull toward you and up to right to "lock" the knot.

D

Again, placing needle holder on top of long end, throw one loop around the instrument, reach back for bitter end, grasp and pull through loop, tying down the knot.

E

Figure 22.9. The Kirz method square knot instrument tie.

To apply a dressing that can meet the requirements of the specific wound, it may be helpful to think of employing a three-layer approach and the rationale involved (Fig. 22.10).

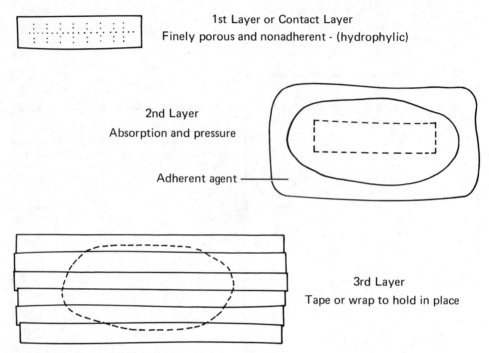

1st Layer or Contact Layer
Finely porous and nonadherent - (hydrophylic)

2nd Layer
Absorption and pressure

Adherent agent

3rd Layer
Tape or wrap to hold in place

Figure 22.10. The three-layer dressing. The dressing should be tailored to the needs of the wound and the comfort of the patient.

The *first* layer is the contact layer. Regardless of the type of wound, there will always be some exudate that seeps into the contact layer. For this reason, the first layer should have the following characteristics:

1. Nonabsorbent and hydrophilic to permit wound exudate to pass through to the second layer of dressing without wetting the contact layer itself.
2. Sterile when applied and soft and pliable, to conform to the surface contours, avoiding gaps and dead space between wound and dressing.
3. Clinging quality but of sufficiently fine mesh that penetration by granulation tissue is not possible.

Some good examples of this type of contact layer are Adaptic, Owens Gauze, Vaseline petrolatum gauze, Aquaflow gauze, and Xeroform gauze, which contains 3% bismuth impregnation to mildly deodorize a potentially odorous wound.

The *second* layer of the dressing is the absorbent layer and can be tailored to the size of the wound and the anticipated seepage. This layer should be sterile (4 × 4's, fluffs, ABD pads, etc.) and can be utilized to exert pressure on the wound, as well as protection, and can provide information on the character and amount of drainage.

The *third* layer of the dressing is simply the outer wrap, which binds the dressing in place and maintains its contour. It should be conforming and stretchable, in case severe edema should result, and capable of allowing some degree of motion, unless the area is to be splinted and immobilized.

If these simple concepts of wound dressing are understood, it becomes relatively easy and highly satisfying to send patients out with well-dressed wounds.

Frequently, there is the need to apply small dressings in the facial area. Several alternatives are available for face and scalp including:

1. Spray dressings
2. Collodion (which requires ether or acetone for removal)
3. Thin mesh gauze and paper tape (beige preferably). Whenever paper tape is applied, the skin should be painted first with tincture of benzoin or other adherent to provide a tacky surface for optimum adherence. This will keep the dressing in place until removal is indicated.
4. Whenever skin strips are applied, either as primary closure or as reinforcement to the suture line, care should be taken to use tr. benzoin or other adherent for the same reasons.

TETANUS IMMUNIZATION STATUS

The EDN is responsible for checking the date of the patient's last tetanus booster and applying the guidelines from the Committee on Trauma of the American College of Surgeons as follows:

1. To the great majority who have been actively immunized within the past 10 years, give 0.5 cc of absorbed tetanus toxoid as a booster, unless it is certain that the patient has received a booster within the previous 5 years. Public health departments advocate the use of diphtheria-tetanus toxoid to maintain control over diphtheria outbreaks.
2. To those with severe, neglected, or old (more than 24 hours) tetanus-prone wounds, give 0.5 cc of absorbed tetanus toxoid unless it is certain that the patient has received a booster within the previous year.
3. When the patient has been actively immunized more than 10 years previously, to the great majority give 0.5 cc of absorbed tetanus toxoid. To those with severe, neglected, or old (more than 24 hours) tetanus-prone wounds or those who have *never* been immunized:
   Give 0.5 cc of absorbed tetanus toxoid (or Dip/Tet Toxoid).
   Give 250 units of tetanus immune globulin (human).
   Consider providing oxytetracycline or penicillin.

RABIES PROPHYLAXIS

Some general management measures for patients needing evaluation for rabies prophylactic treatment have been made available recently by CDC in

Atlanta. It is recommended that all bites and wounds be immediately cleansed thoroughly with soap and water and irrigated copiously, followed by application of 70% alcohol or preferably one of the quartenary ammonium compounds (Aq. Zephirin 1:1000) which are rabicidal.

If vaccine treatment is indicated, both rabies immune globulin (RIG) and human diploid cell rabies vaccine (HDCV) should be given as soon as possible, regardless of interval of exposure. (The administration of RIG is the more urgent procedure. If HDCV is not immediately available, start RIG and give HDCV as soon as it is obtained.) If either RIG or HDCV is unavailable, substitute antirabies serum equine (ARS) and/or duck embryo vaccine (DEV), respectively. Do not exceed recommended RIG or ARS dose. Common local reactions to DEV do not contraindicate continued treatment. Vaccine use should be *discontinued* if tests of animal tissues for rabies antigen, using fluorescent reagents, are negative.

Table 22.1 Rabies Postexposure Prophylaxis Guide*

ANIMAL SPECIES	CONDITION OF ANIMAL AT TIME OF ATTACK	TREATMENT OF EXPOSED PERSON
Household Pets: Dogs and Cats	Healthy and available for 10 days of observation	None unless animal develops rabies. At first sign of rabies in animal, treat patient with RIG and HDCV. Symptomatic animal should be killed and tested as soon as possible.
	Rabid or suspect unknown (escaped)	RIG and HDCV Consult public health officials. If treatment indicated, give RIG & HDCV.
Wild Animals: Skunks, bats, foxes, coyotes, raccoons, bobcats, other carnivores	Regard as rabid unless proved negative by laboratory tests. If available, animal should be killed and tested ASAP.	RIG and HDCV
Other animals: Livestock, rodents, lagomorphs (e.g., rabbits, hares)	Consider individually. Local and state public health officials should be consulted on the need for prophylaxis. Bites by the following almost never call for antirabies prophylaxis: squirrels, hamsters, guinea pigs, gerbils, chipmunks, rats, mice, and other rodents, rabbits, and hares.	

*Adapted from Morbidity and Mortality Weekly Reports, Center for Disease Control, USPHS, Atlanta, June 13, 1980.

PATIENT INSTRUCTIONS

If a *tetanus booster* is administered, record the dosage and date on the patients' written instruction sheet so that a record can be maintained at home. Instruction sheets to the patient should include the key points of wound care, when to have the stitches removed, and symptoms to observe for the first signs of infection.

If *pressure dressings* have been applied, especially on fingers with tubular gauze (Tubegauz), instruct the patient on checking circulation and sensation to be certain circulation is not being compromised, make certain it is understood that fingers are kept splinted in physiologic position (never straight), and that the part should be kept elevated above heart level for the first 24-48 hours to avoid local congestion.

The patient should return to the physician or outpatient facility for *suture removal* according to the following *general* guidelines:

1. Facial sutures should be removed in 4-5 days to keep the scarring to a minimum. Skin closure strips should be applied with an adherent before suture removal.
2. Scalp sutures should be removed in 5-7 days, and the same applies for head and neck.
3. Palm, trunk, arm, and dorsum of hand sutures are removed in 7-10 days.
4. Sutures in legs and in lacerations crossing flexures or over moving parts should be removed in 10-14 days.
5. If you have occasion to remove sutures on a patient's return to your department, always test the wound line before removal to be sure the wound does not separate. If there is any doubt, apply a skin adherent and skin strips between sutures before removing them. Also retest and record range of motion and sensory perception after suture removal.

The patient should understand that he must see his physician immediately if any signs of infection occur, and these should be provided on the instruction sheet, read aloud, and explained. Watch for:

1. Unusual redness or swelling
2. Increased pain
3. Red streak starting up arm or leg
4. Foul drainage or odor from wound
5. Elevation of temperature

REVIEW OF THE BASICS FOR GOOD CLOSURE AND MINIMAL SCARRING

1. Meticulous hemostasis and precise approximation of wound edges are essential to uneventful healing and minimal scarring.
2. Scrupulous surgical technique must be employed with all wound closures.

3. The key to proper wound preparation is mechanical irrigation.

4. To minimize tissue reaction to sutures, learn to use the least amount and smallest size suture consistent with the holding power of the tissues.

5. The number of "throws" you make to tie the suture securely will vary according to the material used. Generally speaking synthetic suture materials (nylon, polypropylene, polyester fiber) have very smooth surfaces. Unless careful attention is paid to knot security, synthetic materials may have a greater tendency to slip than surgical gut or silk.

6. Shadow and color will show a poor scar. A wound with matched planes will not be generally visible, even if it is wide, so long as it is flat, flexible, and does not have an overly reddish cast.

    A. A scar elevated above its surroundings will cast a shadow and be noticeable.

    B. A deep scar, no matter how narrow, will stand out like the Grand Canyon.

7. Wound edges are everted by holding the needle square to the skin and passing the needle at an angle slightly away from the wound, giving a bottle-shaped stitch, which offsets the tendency of the wound edges to become depressed with the usual scar shrinkage.

    A. A stitch placed so that its width is greater than its depth will *invert* the wound edges, retarding healing and creating a scar.

    B. A stitch placed so that its depth is greater than its width will *evert* the wound edges.

8. Matching skin heights perfectly (precise approximation) with slight eversion of skin edges is essential!

9. Stitches must be placed evenly and in juxtaposition to provide close approximation and equalized tension.

10. The more tension on the wound, the closer the stitches must be to each other *and* to the wound edge.

11. A properly constructed dressing tailored for the specific wound will facilitate healing and provide comfort to the patient.

REVIEW

1. Identify and describe the three layers of the skin and their characteristics.

2. Describe a closed soft-tissue injury and the structures involved.

3. Define an open soft-tissue injury and give four examples of the types.

4. Identify the three phases of healing and the time periods involved with each.

5. List at least eight factors which affect optimum primary healing.

6. Identify at least six basic points in good preliminary wound management.

7. Explain how scarring occurs.

8. Identify the two essential prerequisites to uneventful healing.

9. List five points of consideration for wound repair by the EDN.

10. Explain the Kirz formula for irrigating a wound prior to closure.

11. Identify the key to proper wound cleansing and preparation.

12. Describe the proper method of cleansing a wound in preparation for repair.

13. List at least six guidelines to follow for infiltration of a wound with local anesthesia.

14. Explain the Kirz Square Rule for wound repair.

15. Identify the situations in which the EDN should not undertake wound closure.

16. Explain the rationale that applies to administration of tetanus toxoid boosters.

17. Explain the placement of a stitch to evert the skin edges.

18. Under what circumstances may a nurse suture a wound resulting from an animal or human bite?

19. List the functions of a suitable dressing on the wound.

20. Explain the rationale for applying a three-layer dressing.

21. Describe the proper method of applying tape or skin strips.

22. Explain the instructions that should be sent with the patient in writing as well as given verbally on discharge.

BIBLIOGRAPHY

Ault M et al: Wound healing. Nursing 72, Vol 2, No 10, 1972

Barber JM, Dillman PA: Emergency Patient Care. Reston Publishing Co., Reston, Virginia, 1981

Budassi SA, Barber JM: Emergency Nursing: Principles and Practice. C.V. Mosby Co., St. Louis, Missouri, 1981

Cain HD: Flint's Manual on Emergency Treatment and Management. C.V. Mosby Co., St. Louis, Missouri, 1980

Clostridia when it's clean. Emergency Med, Vol 8, No 5, 1976

Cosabb W, Smith JW: Plastic Surgery. Little, Brown & Co., Boston, Massachusetts, 1973

Cosgriff JH, Anderson D: The Practice of Emergency Nursing. J.B. Lippincott Co., Philadelphia, Pennsylvania, 1975

A cut for a bite. Emergency Med, Vol 6, No 8, 1974

Dushoff I: About face. Emergency Med, January 1973

Dushoff I: A stitch in time. Emergency Med, January 1973

Emergency Care and Transportation of the Sick and Injured, 3rd ed. Committee on Injuries, American Academy of Orthopaedic Surgeons, Chicago, Illinois, 1981

Ethicon, Inc.: The Human Body. Ethicon, Inc., Somerville, New Jersey, 1972

Frank IC: Avulsed scalp replantation. JEN, Vol 5, No 4, pp 8-11, July/August 1979

Guyton AC: Textbook of Medical Physiology, 3rd ed. W.B. Saunders Co., Philadelphia, Pennsylvania, 1977

Hass J: Emergency management of soft tissue injuries. JEN, Vol 6, No 5, pp 20-25, September/October 1980

Hienrich J, et al: Human bites. JEN, Vol 2, No 1, 1976

Myers MB: Sutures and wound healing. Am J Nurs, Vol 71, No 9, 1971

Noe JM, Kalish S: Wound Care. Cheesbrough-Ponds, Greenwich, Connecticut, 1975

Reagan L: Care of simple wounds. *In* Physicians in Hospital Emergency Departments. U.S. Dept of Health, Education, and Welfare, Rockville, Maryland, 1971

Roberts N: Hand injuries. JEN, Vol 6, No 6, pp 8-13, November/December 1980

Schaeffer M: Guide to the treatment of animal bites. Hosp Med, May 1971

Stevenson T et al: Cleansing the traumatic wound by high pressure syringe irrigation. JACEP, Vol 5, No 1, 1976

Thompson RV: Primary Repair of Soft Tissue Injuries. Melbourne University Press, Melbourne, Australia, 1969

Tindall JP, et al: Pasteurell multacida infections following animal injuries, especially cat bites. Arch Dermatol, Vol 105, 1972

Warner C: Emergency Care: Assessment and Intervention, 2nd ed. C.V. Mosby Co., St. Louis, Missouri, 1978

When the dog bites. Emergency Medicine, pp 62-71, September 1981

Zimmer B: Animal and human bites. JEN. Vol 5, No 8, May/June 1979

PEDIATRIC EMERGENCIES 23

KEY CONCEPTS

This chapter will help EDNs to refresh their knowledge of general pediatric assessment and to manage nonacute pediatric problems; to become familiar with the recognition and management of the "battered child" syndrome; to competently assess and effectively intervene when the more commonly seen pediatric emergencies present.

Much of this material derives from lecture content developed and presented to emergency nurses by Mary Ann Zimmer, R.N., PNP, Michaelle Ann Robinson, R.N., M.S., Marilyn Redick, Medical Social Worker, Clair Messenger, R.N., Pediatric Critical Care Specialist, and Frank McCullar, M.D., Emergency Physician, all of whom practice in the Portland Metropolitan Area.

After reading and studying this chapter, you should be able to:

- Outline the pertinent questions that should be asked the mother of a sick child in order to focus the interview.
- Identify the signs of a child with serious head injuries.
- Outline the areas of evaluation in the pediatric physical examination.
- Identify areas of specific teaching that can benefit parent and child.
- Explain the instructions that should be given parents for care of the child in various situations, including elevated temperature, clear liquid diets, recognition of dehydration, and contagious skin diseases.
- Describe the age group in which most child abuse occurs and the retardation and mortality associated with physical abuse of children.
- Identify the characteristic reactions and attitudes that may be observed in the abusive parent.
- Describe the most common physical manifestations of child abuse.
- Define the new whiplash "deceleration traction" syndrome.
- Describe the procedural guidelines that should be followed when child abuse is suspected.
- Identify the special situations requiring immediate assessment and treatment as pediatric emergencies.
- Identify the special pediatric airway considerations.

417

- Describe the cardinal signs of airway obstruction in a child.
- Identify the cardinal signs of respiratory failure.
- Describe the signs, symptoms, and intervention for croup, epiglottiditis, and acute asthma.
- Define the pediatric norms for BP and urinary output.
- Describe the immediate intervention for anaphylactic shock.
- Define the priorities of treatment with a coma or seizure and the key areas to check for diagnostic clues.
- Identify the immediate steps of intervention and management in coma or seizure.
- Explain the percentages of weight loss found in the three stages of dehydration.
- Describe the classic symptoms found with intussusception and the manifestations of congenital anomalies of the GI tract, including tracheoesophageal fistula, pyloric stenosis, intestinal obstruction, volvulus, and inguinal hernia.

COMMUNICATION

A few very important points about communication with children must be presented at the outset. Busy personnel in busy emergency departments do not always take time to realize that the child who is brought to the ED for care is more than likely "spastic with fear" at the sight of all those strangers and the unknown "hurts" that lie in store. For most children, people in white uniforms stir up disturbing memories of "shots" and painful experiences.

The crying, hysterical child can usually be calmed down one way or the other, given a little time, but there are some sound, realistic, and helpful guidelines to follow when talking to the child:

1. Move down to the child's eye level.
2. Hold his hand—if the child will let you.
3. Talk slowly.
4. Speak in a low tone of voice.
5. Be truthful with explanations and never tell a child it won't hurt if it *will* hurt. Rather, say, "This might hurt a little bit but it's all right to cry if you want to."
6. Speak in terms and words that the child will understand and take time to be certain the child *does* understand.

If the parent seems supportive and the child relates well, it is sometimes best to allow the parent to stay in the room during procedures if desired. Otherwise, it is probably best to ask the parent to wait outside and deal with the child alone in a reassuring and straightforward manner.

NONACUTE PEDIATRIC PROBLEMS

The EDN is frequently called upon to evaluate a child who is not acutely ill, as well as to answer all manner of inquiries over the telephone at any hour of the day or night. These children must be carefully evaluated so that more serious problems are not overlooked. Any advice given over the telephone from the ED must be well reinforced with instructions to the parent to bring the child in to be checked by a physician should any untoward symptoms develop.

There are some good general guidelines to follow and some specific questions to ask about the various problems, which will aid in assessing and managing the situation. Always use simple direct questions and paraphrase the response, to be certain you understand what the parent (who is frequently excited) is trying to communicate. If you are dealing with the child present in the ED, know the age and address of the child by name. In questioning the chief complaint, chart it in the mother's words, in quotes. Question the present illness as follows, remembering that symptoms are relative and change rapidly under 6 months of age.

1. When was the child last well?
2. Has he/she been playing normally?
3. Has he/she been acting normally?
4. Are there any physical problems? How is the general health?
5. Has he/she been eating and drinking normally?
6. Are there any sick playmates in the neighborhood?
7. What has been done so far? Any medications? How much? Any results? Has anything helped?
8. What other advice has the mother been given? (Mother-in-law, neighbors, etc.)
9. What is the mother most concerned or worried about?

A card file with indexed symptomatology should be developed for the ED telephone inquiries. There is a Quick Reference Guideline, which was printed in Nursing '74, June issue, which is very explicit in covering abdominal pain, colds and coughs, diarrhea, earache, fever, rashes, sore throat, and vomiting. It states the conditions in which the child should be seen by a physician, as well as home treatment and follow-up.

ADVICE ON HEAD INJURIES

There are specific criteria for head injuries when parents call the ED for advice and when there is difficulty equating the injury. The parent may be instructed as follows:

1. The head injury is considered trivial or mild if the child falls, hits head, cries a few moments, and resumes normal activity.

    A. No loss of consciousness, no vomiting, or change of color is present

    B. May complain of a mild headache

If the abrasion is minor, clean with antiseptic. If necessary, come in for sutures. Apply cold compresses to slight swelling and observe closely for 24 hours.

2. The head injury is moderate if:

    A. There is a *brief* loss of consciousness and return to normal alert state.

    B. There is a decreased level of consciousness for some time and the child needs rousing.

    C. There are one or two episodes of vomiting shortly after the injury. The decision of whether the child should be seen depends on how far the child is from the hospital and whether the mother is competent to observe accurately for a 48-hour period for:

      • Persistent vomiting

      • Unequal pupil size

      • Excess drowsiness or lethargy

      • Weakness of an arm or leg

      • Continuous crying

      • Change of color from normal to pale

    If any of these signs develop, the child is to be seen immediately!

3. The severe head injury that requires immediate hospitalization is one in which the child has:

    A. Loss of consciousness and remains unconscious

    B. Persistent vomiting

    C. Convulsions

    D. Irregular respirations

    E. Pale color

    F. Bleeding from the external ear canal (basal skull fracture)

    G. Worsening of any of the symptoms of moderate head injury.

GUIDELINES FOR ASSESSING THE PEDIATRIC PATIENT

Some general points of value to the EDN in doing physical examinations of children are:

1. If the child is over 6 months of age, do the exam on the table, and if under 6 months, leave the child on mother's lap. A child over 3 years of age should be standing or sitting.

2. Do the examination as quickly as possible with the least amount of trauma and upset to minimize crying.

3. A head-to-toe checkup should take (with practice) 1-8 min without interference.

4. *Feel* all parts of the body as well as looking.

5. Leave the area of the chief complaint for the *last* part of the examination.

6. If the child is under 6 months, leave the head, mouth, and ears till last.

7. Casually observe the relationship between the mother and child during the examination.

8. Describe the child as alert, active, well-developed, well-nourished, etc., or as screaming painfully, crying, lethargic, disturbed, etc.

9. For more specific points of evaluation, study the following section on the physical examination.

THE PHYSICAL EXAMINATION

It is usually not feasible to examine babies in the same routine as adults, beginning at the head and going downward, because certain procedures, such as examination of the eyes, ears, nose, and throat, will frighten most children and initiate crying. An initial approach on a friendly basis will allow observation and general inspection, followed then by examination of abdomen, lungs, and heart. The frightening and/or painful parts of the examination are left to the end; however, the findings should be recorded in the following form:

1. Height, weight, and complete vital signs, with blood pressure checked in both arms and both legs if heart disease is suspected.

2. Measurements of head circumference and chest circumference in infants and children under 2 years old and in others where indicated.

3. General appearance should be noted with description of development and nutritional and mental status. Note any pertinent observations, such as pain, restlessness, abnormal posture, paralysis, abnormal respiratory pattern, or skin tone.

4. Observe and record turgor, color, and texture of skin, mucous membranes, and lymph nodes if adenopathy is present.

5. Head and neck should be checked for skull conformation, size, fontanelles (anterior fontanelle closes at 6-18 months and posterior closes at 2 months), condition of scalp and hair.

   A. The eye, ear, nose and throat check should include nasal and buccal mucosa, teeth, tongue, tonsils, adenoids, postnasal drip.

   B. Neck should be checked for position, flexibility, position of trachea, and lymphadenopathy (if not previously noted).

6. Chest is checked for general conformation, symmetry, depth, and regularity of the respiratory pattern, noting any retraction of intercostals.

   A. Lungs: inspection, palpation, percussion and auscultation

   B. Heart: location of point of maximal impulse, quality and intensity of heart sounds, murmurs, rate and rhythm of pulse, and quality comparison of radial, femoral, and pedal pulses if possible to obtain.

7. Check the abdomen for general conformation, herniations, scars, visible peristalsis, and tenderness. Auscultate for intestinal sounds.

8. Anus and genitalia: note any abnormalties in form; in female, check the condition of vulva, urethral meatus, presence or absence of vaginal discharge or labial adhesions; in the male, check descent of testes, condition of prepuce, presence of hydrocele or hypospadius.

9. Back and extremities are checked for length and general conformation of extremities, edema, clubbing of fingers, ridging of nails, scars, color of nailbeds, simian crease, etc. Any gross abnormalities of the axial skeleton, swelling or joint tenderness, curvatures or spasms should be noted.

10. Neurologically, the child should be encouraged to demonstrate status of cranial nerves by "making faces," looking from side to side, up and down, wrinkling forehead, sticking tongue way out, etc. Sensory and motor status can be evaluated by testing levels of response, coordination, strength, or weakness of muscle groups and noting gait, general posture, dystonia, or involuntary jerky movements.

11. Developmental evaluation will include what you objectively observe, as well as your opinion of the child and whether he/she falls within normal limits, taking into account the physical stature of the parent. In children under 6 months, estimate relative maturity; the ability to hold the head up and follow objects with the eyes; grasp capability; hearing response; musculoskeletal tonus; and a general evaluation of whether the child impresses you as a "well baby," developing within normal limits.

12. The important and pertinent findings should be very briefly summarized.

SPECIFIC AREAS IN WHICH
TO TEACH PARENTS

Frequently, the EDN has the opportunity to accomplish some worthwhile teaching of the parents before discharging the child following treatment. A good deal of preventive medicine can be taught at this time, and the following are some of the points to be effectively made:

1. The importance of keeping immunizations current and *recorded* as boosters are received.

2. Instructions on ear infections:
   A. There is a high incidence of tooth decay and a very high correlation of eustachian tube inflammation with *night bottles*. (Formula runs into the naso-oropharynx and seeps into the eustachian tubes.)
   B. Nose drops are given to open the eustachian tubes, and the mother should be taught the correct method of administration, holding the child supine across the lap with the nostrils perpendicular to the ceiling and maintained in that position for 3-5 min following administration of drops, to allow penetration.
   C. When antibiotics are prescribed, *all* of the medication is to be given until gone.

    D. The child's ear should be *rechecked* in 2 weeks to be certain the infection is resolved.

3. The importance of realizing that antibiotics are *not* effective in viral infections and are prescribed only to fight secondary bacterial infections.

4. Instructions for high temperature (over 103° F) include aspirin or acetominophen (Tylenol) every 3-4 hours, as directed for age and weight, and a tepid sponge bath for 20-30 min every 3-4 hours as necessary.

5. The danger of allowing any child to handle *any* medications, bottles, or boxes, and of playing with grandma's, or *anybody's,* purse. Most purses contain medication such as digitalis, nitroglycerine, oral contraceptives, tranquilizers, headache medicines, etc. *Danger* area!

6. Explanation of the correct method of taking a rectal temperature.

7. With elevated temperatures, the importance of pushing *clear* liquids like 7-Up, liquid jello, apple juice, etc., and *avoiding* milk because lactose "sloughs" in the GI tract. Ice chips and popsicles frequently work well.

8. The recognition of dehydration and indications that the child should be seen by a physician without further delay (dry tissues, no tearing in the eyes, scant urine, and sunken fontanelles with gray color to skin).

9. Awareness of community health regulations regarding contagious skin diseases that allow the child to return to school when under treatment with medication as follows:
    A. Impetigo—polymixin B-bacitracin-neomycin (Neosporin) ointment (over-the-counter drug)
    B. Ringworm—tolnaftate (Tinactin) ointment (over-the-counter drug)
    C. Scabies—gamma benzene hexachloride (Kwell) (still a prescription drug, although this may change)

10. Care of diaper rash to prevent a secondary infection as well as to provide general comfort for the child

11. Tendency (normally) to constipation when the child is breastfed

12. The importance of learning to evaluate the child effectively and accurately and to use the ED properly.

CHILD ABUSE

The EDN is usually the first member of the staff to receive the child and to evaluate the situation before the child and parent(s) have had significant time to react to the sights, smells, sounds, and inquiring glances of hospital personnel. This is an important time for the EDN to gather preliminary data and observe the interaction between the child and parent, hopefully, with an awareness of the statistics involving injuries in small children as well as "failure to thrive" states. When dealing with the possibility of child abuse, one is required to complete an accurate assessment, differentiating willfully, inflicted injury from authentic, accidental injury, and if indicated, to proceed with an appropriate reporting to provide protection for the child and bring the abusive parent into contact with needed help. This will certainly require some astute reasoning and a fair amount of determination.

In the mid 1940s a pediatric radiologist, Dr. John Caffey, observed that healing and healed multiple long-bone fractures, unexplained by any history of trauma, were often present in infants whose principal disease was chronic subdural hematoma. Caffey at first thought that fractures of the long bones were a complication of infantile subdural hematoma. In 1953 Dr. Silverman acknowledged Caffey's observation and concluded that the origin of these injuries was trauma unrecognized or not admitted by the infant's custodian. Dr. C. Henry Kempe, pediatrician at the University of Colorado, coined the term "battered child syndrone" in 1962.

NATIONAL FINDINGS

Since child abuse awareness has developed across the country, there have been some shocking statistics generated:

1. The average age of the abused children reported has been under 4 years, with most under 2 years.
2. It is estimated that probably 10% of childhood accidents are, in reality, abuse.
3. The average age at death with these children is just under 3 years, and there does not appear to be any sex differentiation.
4. About 45% of abused children are of premature birth.
5. Abused children with no intervention in their behalf reflect a 30-40% retardation rate and a 5-10% mortality.
6. Physical abuse may be a greater killer (at 6-12 months of age) than any specific cancer, malformation, or infectious disease.
7. After the age of 1 year, physical abuse is second only to true accidents as the cause of death.
8. Of the "accidents" seen in the ED, 10% are associated with gross neglect.
9. An abused child returned to his home without therapeutic precautions runs a 50% chance of repeated abuse and a 10% chance of death.
10. One year after abuse, approximately 33% of abused children manifest hard signs of CNS damage, and another 20% will show "soft" signs.
11. Permanent damage *can* be avoided if appropriate steps are taken with early signs of abuse.

Professionals who have worked with abused children concluded that it is axiomatic that when one form of abuse exists, other forms usually coexist, such as:

- Nutritional neglect (sometimes to the point of frank starvation)
- Drug abuse (as in chronic sedation)
- Medical care neglect

- Sexual abuse
- Safety neglect

Once abused, these children are high risk for repeated abuse and the consequences of permanent disability, brain damage, developmental lags, personality disorders and death.

SIGNS OF ABUSE

The most frequently seen manifestations of physical abuse are bruises and welts, burns ("punched-out" appearance from cigarettes, burns of perineum, buttocks, and hands and feet from being dunked into scalding water), abrasions, bizarre-shaped lesions, subdural hematomas and other head injuries manifesting in convulsions and coma, soft-tissue swelling, dislocations and fractures, lacerations and contusions around mouth from forceful feeding, and limited motion of extremities with loss of function and tender painful areas.

Some valid criteria for identifying a case of suspected abuse are as follows:

1. Multiple injuries, clustered and on different body surfaces. Example: soft-tissue swelling on one shoulder with several bruises on the opposite anterior chest wall. (Document location, size, shape, and color of bruises.)
2. Multiple lesions in various stages of healing. Example: two fresh and weeping, two crusty and pustular, and one dry with pink edges and dark center (cigarette burns?)
3. Injuries that reflect the outline of an object or mode of infliction. Example: belt buckles, looped electric cords, patterns of heater grids, radiators, etc.
4. Explanation of cause that is implausible or not fitting with the child's age. Example: A 9-month-old-child "climbed" into a bathtub of hot water (?) and burns were clearly outlined 1 inch above both ankles.

Less obvious injuries will require more astute observation, and data must be gathered that will be as significant as the overt physical signs and should include an assessment of the history, behavior of the parents, and behavior of the child in response.

The general pattern seems to be delay in seeking treatment till the morning after or several days later. The parents are then likely to exhibit indifference to treatment, prognosis, and the child in general.

If your suspicions are raised for any reason, keep your eyes open. Upon investigation, findings in the truly physically abused children will usually reveal:

1. Skull fractures, 80% of which are linear and the others depressed (ping-pong type).
2. Signs of skull fracture, with tympanic membrane discoloration and CSF leaks from the nose and ears.

3. Bleeds into the brain, which carry the highest mortality:
   A. Epidural hematoma from injury to the temporal area, with laceration of the middle meningeal artery developing within 12 hours. This carries a high mortality.
   B. Subdural hematomas most commonly seen and most commonly found on postmortem examination, often in a child who does not appear injured. They are usually bilateral, causing increased intracranial pressure with ultimate brain-stem depression and death. Seizures, lethargy, coma, and vomiting are easily attributed to other causes.
   C. Chronic subdural bleeding, which is slow in developing, with an enlarging head and bulging fontanelle and hyperirritability, retinal hemorrhages, lethargy, coma, and occasionally occult bruises.
   D. Subdural bleeds occurring with associated fractures, which are frequent.
   E. A new syndrome, which has been defined now as a whiplash "deceleration traction" (acceleration/deceleration). Violent shaking of a child's head can cause subdural hemorrhage without any further extraneous trauma. This is now thought to be a *major* unrecognized cause of brain damage!

CONTRIBUTING FACTORS

As difficult as it may be to imagine a parent willfully harming a child, it should be remembered that many factors contribute to this tragic event. Parents are not always bottomless pits of love and understanding but *are* human beings faced with conflicts of temperaments, daily pressures, and unexpected crises. They were possibly abused themselves as children. Many believe in physical punishment and lack the necessary knowledge of child development. Not all of them love their children all the time—16 hours a day but not 24. Further, it is known that a woman with a low opinion of herself is more apt to dislike her children.

Remember, too, that there are limited options for the poor and economically deprived members of our society. Boarding schools and weekend escapes are for the more affluent; abortions are not easy to obtain in spite of changes in the laws; and these families are not properly counseled to put unwanted babies out for adoption.

NATIONAL REPORTING LAWS

All 50 states have laws now making it mandatory to report child abuse, and though the details vary, the laws all contain two basic principles:

There is a mandate to report any injury suspected of being caused by neglect or being willfully inflicted by the caretaker.

There is exemption from liability for any professional person reporting suspected child abuse.

It is suggested that every EDN become familiar with the specific laws of the state regarding reporting, as well as hospital policy for management of the suspected child-abuse case.

AFFECT ON THE CHILD

The child will often manifest a rather typical behavior that readily correlates with physical signs of possible abuse, and the behavior should be carefully observed and evaluated. There is usually no protest when the parent leaves the room, and the child just lies there looking rather like a discarded object. Children under 6 years tend to be excessively passive while those over 6 years are apt to be excessively aggressive; both appear to be constantly on the alert for danger, drawing back with physical contact.

EXAMINATION TECHNIQUE

Examination of this child requires *complete* examination of all body surfaces and parts, including genitals. It must be done gently to prevent further pain, fear, and distrust of adults. Simultaneously assess the child's behavior and reactions to examination. It is considered good objective practice to conduct the exam and assessment with another nurse or physician since a sounder and more comfortable decision is made with a professional peer sharing the opinion. This also lends credence and validity to the assessment and provides support to the person doing the examination. Recordings must be scrupulously objective; do not record anything that you would not want read back in court!

INTERVIEWING THE PARENTS

When interviewing the parents, the following guidelines must be remembered and adhered to:
1. Do not alienate the parents, making them hostile and defensive.
2. Try to be tolerant and nonjudgmental of whatever the parent says.
3. Show an attitude of caring, concern, and understanding.
4. Avoid taking "sides" with the child.
5. Get as much detail as possible.
6. Record the parent's exact words. Recounting details reduces anxiety for most parents but will produce anxiety if the injury is not accidental.
7. Note and record (objectively) the parent's behavior toward the child.

When a question of child abuse is real, action should *always* be taken in favor of the child, and the child should be admitted or detained for observation, permitting an opportunity for further evaluation. If the family insists on taking the child, report it to the appropriate protection agency without delay.

Any fears about reporting should be heavily outweighed by considering the magnitude of the fear and danger experienced by the child who must return to a hostile environment in which he has no protection from physical, emotional, or spiritual abuse.

PEDIATRIC EMERGENCY SITUATIONS

In dealing with pediatric emergencies, there are several points to always remember: 1) If there is ever any doubt in the assessment of a sick child, it is always wise to admit him; 2) Children are not just small adults; they are little individuals, who are affected by their own sets of hereditary and environmental factors, who become ill rapidly and return to normal with proper management just as rapidly; and 3) *Children have special airway considerations, which must be kept in mind: a child's tongue is larger, his airway smaller and softer, and his chest wall is softer and more pliable.*

TRIAGING CHILDREN

When triaging the pediatric patient, the EDN must rely strongly on the initial impression and whether the child appears in real distress. There are some guidelines for children requiring immediate attention which include:

1. Airway difficulty of any degree
2. Dehydration
3. Coma
4. Convulsions
5. Possible meningitis
6. Anaphylaxis
7. Ingestion of toxic substances
8. Rectal temperature of over 103° in a child under 1 year of age

As the child is being undressed and quickly evaluated for vital signs, the parent should be asked:

- Age of the child
- How long child has had respiratory difficulty (if present)
- How long child has been sick
- What the fluid intake has been (retained fluids) in the past 24 hours
- What the approximate output has been in terms of wet diapers or trips to the bathroom
- What has been done for the child and whether child is better or worse now?

It is wise to include a general background of information on the child under age 2, relating to birth weight, health status during infancy, allergies, and family history of diabetes, seizure states, cardiac problems, and any other suitable pertinent data that might be indicated in the particular situation. If you are dealing with a high-risk child, it is well to know it at the outset.

If an accurate and thorough assessment is to be done, the child must be stripped down to diaper or panties and evaluated for respiratory pattern, peripheral perfusion, general color and neuromuscular status, and general response to the environment. A really sick child will *look* like a really sick child: apathetic, pale or gray in color, lack-luster eyes, shallow respiratory pattern, and poor peripheral perfusion.

RESPIRATORY DISTRESS

The dyspneic child is apprehensive, restless, and has expiratory stridor and wheezing and retractions, both intercostally and sternally. Airway obstruction results from myriad causes in children, including congenital anomalies, peritonsillar abscess, laryngeal obstruction, elevated diaphragm, cardiac failure, cystic fibrosis, drug intoxication, and pneumothorax. A history of sudden onset usually is indicative of foreign-body obstruction or spasms somewhere along the respiratory tract. Gradual onset of respiratory distress indicates pulmonary or cardiac insufficiency with coughing and perhaps hemoptysis. Allergies and exposures to disease processes must be ruled out. When the child is mouth-breathing and/or has heavy nasal secretions, consider adenoids or foreign-body infections. Pharyngeal infection will produce dysphagia.

Initial laboratory work should include a CBC, blood culture, and culture and sensitivity tests on tracheal aspirate and throat swabs, and X-ray films of the chest and lateral neck.

Croup (Laryngotracheobronchitis)

Croup is a complex of symptoms that manifest as hoarseness, a barklike cough, changing voice, dyspnea and tachypnea, and inspiratory retractions. Usually these children become stricken between 11 P.M. and 2 A.M., exhibiting anxiety and restlessness accompanied by cough and dyspnea, with the severity decreasing and the cough loosening after several hours. They may run a low-grade temperature, and these bouts may recur two or three nights in succession.

Croup is considered a mild viral infection that may sound far worse than it is but must be considered a serious illness when it persists for several days, and the child begins to slowly deteriorate. Frequently, the distress will ease with steam inhalations *or* cold mist. Very often a child who is taken out on a foggy night en route to the hospital appears significantly improved on arrival. Corticosteroids and antibiotics are usually given as indicated, but this child should be admitted and carefully evaluated to rule out the possibility of further obstruction and/or epiglottitis. An increased heart rate and depressed respiratory rate are danger signals!

Epiglottitis

The child with epiglottitis will typically present in an anxious state, with respiratory distress, frequently drooling because of difficulty in swallowing and breathing, and sitting forward with neck extended. He may have audible respiratory sounds and generally appears flushed and toxic with a high temperature. The epiglottis is typically swollen and "cherry red" and can readily cause a total airway obstruction *if it is manipulated* during examination. About 50% of children with acute epiglottitis require intubation, cricothyroidotomy, or tracheostomy, so it is *mandatory* to have the necessary equipment on hand and in readiness before any examination is done. If a lateral neck film for soft-tissue swelling is indicated, it should be done in the ED, and an acutely ill child should *never* be sent to the X-ray department without airway management personnel in attendance. With this situation, as with all others involving respiratory compromise, do not wait too long before intervening with a child who has been slowly deteriorating into severe hypoxia. You *may* be too late! The responsibility for this critical evaluation will frequently fall to the EDN, who must then alert and expedite the physician's presence. Laboratory specimen procurement should be deferred until the airway is safeguarded.

Foreign-Body Aspiration

The aspiration of small objects, such as parts of toys, beans, peanuts, buttons, etc. will cause choking, gasping, and dyspnea alternating with silent periods and episodes of coughing. (An upper airway obstruction is usually worse on inspiration, causing "inspiratory stridor."). There is, of course, concern, but complete airway obstruction is unlikely, and the item can be removed by laryngoscopy or bronchoscopy. X-ray films will almost always be diagnostic of the cause and location of the foreign body.

Asthma

Asthma is discussed in the chapter on respiratory emergencies, but asthma in the very small child requires even more delicate evaluation and management. Large and small airway obstruction with wheezing, dyspnea, and coughing results from increased production of thick mucus with edema of the respiratory tract and bronchospasm. Asthma in the very small child is thought to be an allergic reaction aggravated by emotional and psychological factors. Toddlers with allergies to milk, wheat, fruit juices, peanut butter, etc., frequently exhibit a "failure to thrive," bouts of vomiting, excessive mucus secretion, frequent URIs, a tendency to bronchitis, skin rashes, and infantile eczema.

Treatment of these children consists of low-flow-rate oxygen, administration of epinephrine (Adrenalin) 1:1,000 0.01 ml/kg or epinephrine 1:10,000 0.1 ml/kg, bronchodilators, and antibiotics with cautious use of sedation. Suppositories should never be used because of the uncertainty of uptake, and antibiotics are indicated only if there is 1) pneumonitis, 2) persistent attack over 24 hours' duration, and 3) a WBC over 15,000. If sedation is necessary, chloral hydrate should be used with a respirator on standby; opiates are used *only* if the child is on a respirator. Acidosis must be correctd, and if the child is febrile, hypothermic measures must be instituted.

Status asthmaticus in children mandates hospital admission and requires arterial blood gases every 4-8 hours, electrolytes, CBC, throat culture, upper-airway care, and X-ray films of chest and lateral neck for soft-tissue swelling.

Respiratory failure is manifested with:

1. Increased P_{CO_2} (55-65 mm Hg)
   Decreased P_{O_2} (40-60 mm Hg)
   Low pH (7.2 or less)
2. Onset of cyanosis in 50% oxygen
3. Increased dyspnea or distress
4. Severe retraction and use of accessory muscles of respiration
5. Decreased breath sounds
6. Decreased level of consciousness
7. Decreased response to pain

Treatment must be *immediate* intubation and ventilatory support. Curare or succinylcholine (Anectine) is usually administered to the awake child prior to intubation. USE A TEAM APPROACH WITH INHALATION AND ANESTHESIA PERSONNEL.

Some further complications of asthma can be pneumonia, convulsions from a rapidly decreasing PaO_2, aspiration of stomach contents (use NG tube), GI bleeding, stress ulcers, and pneumothorax.

Pneumonia

Both viral and staphylococcal pneumonia are common problems in infants and children; 75% of pediatric cases occur in the first year of life, with more than 50% in the first months. Peak incidence is in winter and spring. Pneumonia is a prime example of lower respiratory tract infection leading to obstruction following a history of URI, a gradually developing anorexia, irritability with lethargy, vomiting and diarrhea (a common symptom), tachypnea at rest over 50-60/min with grunting and nasal flaring, temperature over 101° rectally or subnormal (less than 97° rectally in infants), peripheral cyanosis, impaired breath sounds, dullness to percussion, and rales. The "pneumonia triad" to look for is fever, tachypnea at rest, and a significant cough.

Diagnosis is made by CBC and differential count, a blood culture, nasal aspirate culture, and a chest X-ray film. Significant findings include:

- Leukocytosis greater than 20,000 (common)
- Leukopenia (a bad diagnostic sign)
- Condition tending to deteriorate rapidly, making hospitalization mandatory

Intravenous therapy is instituted with aqueous penicillin or other antibiotic of choice, and inhalation therapy provides percussion, drainage, and suctioning. Children of 6 months to 1 year are usually given oxygen mist therapy and rest, being kept NPO for 24-36 hours with IV lines providing hydration and nutritional requirements.

CARDIOVASCULAR EMERGENCIES

These situations, fortunately, are rarely seen but involve treatment aimed at restoring or maintaining adequate tissue perfusion. Arrhythmias are rare and usually not that severe in children although ventricular fibrillation is occasionally seen after surgery or as a terminal manifestation.

Emergency department personnel must periodically review the CPR techniques to be used with infants and children:

1. Infants: use the thumb or two fingers to compress the sternum 100-120 times per minute.
2. Small child: use the heel of the hand only.
3. Older child: use one hand on top of the other as with an adult.
4. Remember to use restraint and *refrain from too vigorous* a resuscitation.

In children cardiac arrest is generally secondary to respiratory arrest. When resuscitating, be careful not to hyperextend the head and neck *too far,* or the airway will be closed; always listen for bilateral breath sounds and watch for symmetrical chest expansion. If an ET tube is placed, check its position with X-ray, checking as well for atelectasis and/or pneumothorax. Correct acidosis with sodium bicarbonate, 1 mEq/kg body weight.

If countershock is required, pediatric or adult paddles should be used as follows:

- Infant (10-12 lb) 10-15 w/s
- Child, 1-3 years 50-150 w/s
- Child 3-10 years 150-300 w/s

Digitalis intoxication would elicit a prolonged PR interval greater than 0.2 sec, vomiting, and diarrhea, which increases with the severity of the intoxication. Treatment is to stop the drug and if it has been ingested, lavage the stomach immediately. Give potassium chloride PO or IV, monitor with ECG, and have a pacemaker on hand if the intoxication is severe.

Severe congenital anomalies such as the "Four Terrible Ts" (transposition of the great vessels, tetralogy of Fallot, truncus arteriosis, and tricuspid atresia) are not dealt with here except to review the fact that they all produce cyanosis with a low pulmonary blood flow, right-to-left shunting with decreased PaO_2 and increased PCO_2, which can rapidly result, during severe bouts of crying or stress, in a deterioration leading to convulsions, brain damage, and death. These children must be carefully handled, pacified, and carefully medicated to avoid disastrous developments.

SHOCK

Shock may present itself in the pediatric patient as 1) hypovolemic, which is the most common (from third space loss); 2) septic (from gram-negative organisms); 3) anaphylactic (from allergy shots, insect stings, and penicillin); and 4) cardiogenic (rare in children).

Septic shock fulminates rapidly, and death can occur in 24 hours without timely and effective intervention. Blood cultures, UA, tracheal smear and culture, and a lumbar puncture are indicated diagnostically, with airway support, oxygen administration, and volume replacement the keys to initial therapy.

Anaphylactic shock is, unfortunately, an all-too-frequent occurrence following injections of penicillin, allergy preparations, and various "boosters," as well as insect stings. There is a mass outpouring of histamine and a hormonal type substance called the Slow-Reacting Substance in Anaphylaxis (SRSA) which cause vasodilatation, local edema, hives due to the increased capillary permeability, and bronchial constriction, which rapidly deteriorates into a shock state followed by collapse and sudden death.

Immediate treatment is as follows:

1. Give epinephrine 1:1000 0.1-0.2 cc IM, in side opposite injection or sting.
2. Place a tourniquet above site of injection or sting.
3. Give epinephrine 1:1000 0.1-0.2 cc, injected into site of injection or sting.
4. Summon help.
5. Start oxygen at high flow rate.
6. Start IV, if possible, with Ringer's lactate and pediatric drip chamber. Employ venous cutdown approach if a vein cannot be cannulated routinely.
7. Have airway management equipment in readiness, including ET tray, tracheostomy tray, and bag/mask unit with a pediatric mask.
8. Diphenhydramine HCl (Benadryl) and cortisone may be helpful although their action is slower.

Blood Pressure

Determination of blood pressure in a shock state is extremely difficult in infants and very small children. The "flush" method is sometimes employed where a hand or foot is elevated and squeezed firmly and steadily to cause blanching; an appropriately sized cuff is inflated proximally without releasing the hand pressure until inflation is above the anticipated systolic pressure. As the cuff pressure is slowly released, the hand or foot will flush with arterial blood flow at a point corresponding to the systolic blood pressure ± 10 mm Hg. Arterial palpation is an alternative if the pulse is palpable.

Normal limits of blood pressures and urinary outputs in children are given in Tables 23.1 and 23.2. Urine output must be monitored in the shock patient. Dry mucous membranes in cheeks and poor skin turgor indicate dehydration.

Table 23.1 Blood Pressure Levels in Children

AGE	SYSTOLIC BLOOD PRESSURE (NORMAL LIMITS)
Birth to 3 months	60- 80 mm
3 months to 1 year	80-100 mm
1 to 12 years	Add 2 mm for every year + 100

Table 23.2 Urinary Output in Children

AGE	URINARY OUTPUT
Normal	
Birth to 1 year	1 cc/kg/hr (or a "norm" of 5 wet diapers/day)
1 year and over	0.5 cc/kg/hr up to 35 cc/hr
Low (poor kidney perfusion)	
< 3 years	10-15 cc/hr (poor)
5-12 years	20 cc/hr (poor)

General Management

The treatment, in general, for *hypovolemic shock,* whether it is caused by hemorrhage or hypotension in children includes the following steps:

1. Establish airway immediately, with oxygen support
2. Insert IV or CVP lines through the external jugular by cutdown if necessary and administer 10-20 cc/kg/hr, using a pediatric volume control and drip chamber to avoid overload. (*Never* hang more than 500 cc over a child and always with a pediatric volume control.)
3. Monitor the heart.
4. If whole blood is given (10-30 cc/kg), use the freshest blood possible to avoid electrolyte imbalance or hypokalemia.
5. Give albumin for third space loss.
6. Laboratory evaluations should include BUN, urea, ABG, electrolytes, CBC.
7. Treat shock according to the specific etiology.
8. Give sodium bicarbonate to correct acidosis (1 mEq/kg).
9. If a CVP line is initiated, watch the "trends" rather than the absolute values, with 0-6 cm being low and 15 cm being high.
10. If sepsis is suspected, do a full septic work-up, with cultures and a lumbar puncture.

COMA AND SEIZURES

Coma and seizure states are commonly seen in the ED and are commonly seen in the same patient. The etiology ranges from birth injuries, developmental anomalies of the brain, meningitis, fluid and electrolyte imbalances, general trauma, and subdural hematomas to inborn errors of metabolism in infants. With toddlers, consider, additionally, poisonings and febrile seizures. With pre-school children, add the possibility of brain tumor or diabetes. From ages 5 to 10 add the possibility of head trauma, diabetes, epilepsy, brain tumors, and glomerulonephritis. For children over 10, rule out diabetes, epilepsy, and coarctation of the aorta. Other causes can be kernicterus (high serum bilirubin), sickle cell anemia, hypoglycemia, and poisonings from lead, atropine, salicylates, and thallium.

Priorities of treatment include:

1. Provide a patent airway with oxygen support.
2. Insure adequate cardiopulmonary function.
3. Treat seizures with either diazepam (Valium) or phenobarbital given IV.
4. If poisoning is suspected, do gastric lavage.
5. Treat shock as previously discussed.

The history, of course, is essential. Has there been any recent trauma? Previous seizures? Febrile episodes? Ingestion? Environmental exposure to carbon monoxide, insecticide, lead? Any recent infection? Any inadequate treatment with antibiotics? Type of onset? How long? Any weakness or paralysis? Any family history of this same problem?

Laboratory Indications

Diagnostic procedures should include all routine laboratory work-ups including a type and crossmatch if bleeding is suspected and a toxicology screen for barbiturates, alcohol, and salicylates, along with X-ray films of the skull and chest. Lumbar puncture should be done only if there is *no* evidence of papilledema or increased intracranial pressure.

General Management

The immediate steps of management are to keep the airway patent with oxygen flow at 4 LPM until ordered otherwise, keep patient warm if not febrile, combat shock if present, avoid use of depressant drugs, keep IV fluids at 75% of maintenance to prevent cerebral edema, draw blood for blood sugar analysis and then give IV glucose 50 g, terminate seizure activity with IV diazepam (Valium) or phenobarbital (2-3 mg/kg), be prepared to intubate and ventilate, prevent injury by placing child on his side with a bite block in place, elevate the head of the bed 30° to reduce cerebral edema if it is possibly present, and institute hypothermic measures as necessary if child is febrile.

The criteria for admission should be:

1. Any alteration of the level of consciousness (LOC)

2. Symptoms of impending shock and/or apathy
3. Persistent headache
4. Nausea and vomiting or both
5. Bleeding from the nose or mouth
6. Blood or CSF behind the ear drums
7. Any evidence of skull fracture
8. Visual disturbances and/or paralysis

DEHYDRATION

Gastroenteritis is common in infants and children and can be very serious through the loss of fluid and electrolytes in stools (third space loss) leading to severe dehydration, metabolic acidosis, shock, and death. Fever, vomiting, diarrhea, and decreased intake can all rapidly precipitate a state of dehydration for the small child. An infant at 2 weeks of age will require *150 cc/kg/24 hours for adequate hydration,* and a baby should have a normal weight gain of 2 lb per month. An infant or small child presenting with gastroenteritis or signs of dehydration must be *weighed,* and on the basis of the child's weight on its last examination, the percentage of weight loss is computed. Dehydration can be classified by these percentages as follows:

2-4% weight loss—mild dehydration
5-9% weight loss—moderate dehydration (child should be hospitalized)
10% or more weight loss—severe dehydration, carrying a significant mortality in infants

Serious gastroenteritis in children is infectious in origin and is generally caused by *E. coli,* salmonella, or shigella. The child appears with the classic symptoms of dehydration:

1. Dry skin and mucous membranes
2. Sunken eyes
3. Pinched and anxious expression
4. Depressed anterior fontanelle
5. Absence of tears or salivation
6. Ashen gray color
7. Obliguria or a concentrated urine of greater than 1.025 specific gravity

Further symptoms of really severe dehydration are:

8. Abnormal neurologic signs with decreased deep tendon reflexes (DTR)
9. Lethargy progressing to coma with Kussmaul breathing
10. Cherry red lips
11. Smooth muscle irritability, abdominal distention, weakness, and—rarely—paralysis.

Laboratory Indications

Diagnostic laboratory procedures indicated are: BUN, electrolytes, creatinine, ABG, hematocrit, and a stool culture for etiology.

General Nursing Guidelines

Treatment is directed at correcting the cause of the dehydration and replacing fluid and electrolyte losses by oral (if tolerated) or IV solutions. When vomiting has been identified as a nonspecific gastroenteritis, the treatment of choice is small amounts of clear liquids for 24 hours, gradually increasing the diet while eliminating milk. Vomitus is high in potassium, so this should be replaced with clear fruit juices and "flat" 7-Up. If potassium must be replaced parenterally, the maintenance dose is 3-4 mEq/kg, to be added *after* voiding and with a maximum of 40 mEq/liter. The nursing responsibility here is to obtain an accurate weight and accurate records of intake and output, with documented observations of the child's clinical response to the rehydration regime.

CONGENITAL ANOMALIES OF THE GI TRACT

Diaphragmatic hernia presents with symptoms of dyspnea, cyanosis, vomiting, absent breath sounds unilaterally, a scaphoid abdomen, and loops of bowel visualized in the thorax on X-ray films. The prognosis is good if there is no respiratory distress, and the treatment is immediate surgery.

Tracheoesophageal fistulas in newborns are recognized by excessive salivation, choking on feedings, cyanosis, and dyspnea. The treatment is immediate surgery.

Pyloric stenosis is generally seen in first-born males. Symptoms are the onset of projectile vomiting from 2-3 weeks of age to 2 months, with a constant hunger despite vomiting, peristalsis that can be seen from left to right and a palpable, smooth, olive-shaped epigastric mass. Treatment is a medical regimen of thick formula with phenobarbital added, followed up with early surgery.

Intestinal obstruction presents with symptoms of green, scant vomitus, and sometimes an absence of stools. An upright X-ray film shows dilated loops of bowel. The treatment is to watch for peritonitis and fluid levels in the abdomen. Gastric suction and fluid replacement (cc for cc) with 0.5% NSS/dextrose is the regimen until the decision is made for surgery.

Intussusception is a telescoping of one section of bowel into another; it may be small bowel into small bowel, small bowel into colon, or colon into colon. Most frequently, the small bowel inserts into the colon (ileocolic intussusception), and it usually occurs in the very young in the first year of life but may be seen in the older child. The contributing factors are thought to be diarrhea, constipation, cathartics, URIs, or allergies. After age 3 it is thought that other factors may be responsible. An occasional polyp, tumor, or Meckel's diverticulum may form the starting point for the process.

The symptoms are classic and include:

1. Severe spasmodic pain, explosive in onset
2. Vomiting present in a previously healthy infant
3. A characteristically "startled" look

4. Knees flexed and relaxing as the pain eases
5. "Currant-jelly" stools usually 12 hours after the initial pain
6. A tender sausage-shaped mass, which can usually be palpated in the ascending colon or transverse colon
7. The RLQ may feel empty
8. There may be blood on the examining finger

Surgical intervention is usually indicated; the intussusception is manually reduced and the bowel examined for compromise of the blood supply. Recurrence is unusual.

Volvulus is a twisting of the bowel upon itself causing an obstruction, and it constitutes a surgical emergency. The symptoms are abdominal distention, occasional blood in the stool, vomitus of all feedings, subnormal temperature frequently, and X-ray films show a "ground glass" appearance as the bowel loops are edematous and filled with fluid.

Inguinal hernia, commonly seen in males in the first year of life, may be either unilateral or bilateral, with swelling in the inguinal canal. The swelling is usually reducible by applying steady, gentle pressure and elevating the legs. Sedation may be required, cold packs to the swelling. Remember, however, that an incarcerated hernia is irreducible and is a surgical emergency!

It must be concluded that seeing these children early and carefully evaluating them may lead to early successful treatment; much of this initial assessment will fall to the alert EDN.

Specific doses, weights, amounts, tube sizes, etc., for pediatric patients can be found in the *Handbook of Pediatrics,* by Harriet Lane (see Bibliography), which should be available on the bookshelf of every emergency department.

Again, whenever IV fluids are administered to children, a micro-drop chamber *must* be used with no more than 500 ml hung in a single bottle and observing a drip rate of 10 ml/kg/hr for two to three hours in order to avoid cardiac overload.

REVIEW

1. List at least eight questions to ask the mother of a sick child in order to focus the interview.
2. Identify the signs of a serious head injury in a child.
3. Explain the problems associated with night bottles for children.
4. List the instructions that should be given to the parent of a child for elevated temperature, a prescribed diet of clear liquids only, recognition of dehydration and management of contagious skin diseases.
5. Identify the age group in which most child abuse occurs.
6. Describe the retardation rate and mortality associated with physically abused children.

7. List at least six fairly characteristic reactions and attitudes that the EDN may observe in the abusive parent.
8. Describe some of the characteristic responses of an abused child.
9. Identify at least four of the most common physical manifestations of abuse.
10. Define the new whiplash "deceleration traction" syndrome.
11. Identify the guidelines that should be followed by ED personnel when there is suspected child abuse.
12. List five special situations requiring immediate assessment and intervention with children presenting in the ED.
13. Identify at least eight cardinal signs of airway obstruction that can be observed in a child.
14. Describe the classic symptoms of croup.
15. Describe the classic symptoms of epiglottitis.
16. Identify the precautions that must be taken with epiglottitis.
17. Describe the protocol for the initial management of an asthmatic child in an acute attack.
18. Identify at least eight cardinal signs of respiratory failure.
19. Specify the pediatric norms for BP for birth to 3 months, 3 months to 1 year, and 1 year to 12 years.
20. Specify the pediatric norms for urinary output for birth to 1 year and for 1 year and older.
21. Outline the immediate steps of intervention for anaphylactic shock.
22. Define the priorities of treatment in coma or seizure.
23. Identify at least eight key areas to question for diagnostic clues in a coma or seizure.
24. Identify the criteria for hospital admission associated with coma or seizure.
25. Define the percentages of weight loss found in the three stages of dehydration.
26. Describe seven symptoms of early dehydration.
27. Describe six symptoms of further deterioration into severe dehydration.
28. Describe the classic symptoms presenting with intussusception.
29. Identify at least six congenital anomalies of the GI tract that are manifested in the early years and that the EDN should be able to assess.

BIBLIOGRAPHY

ACLS for infants and children: Drugs and doses, standards for CPR & ECC. JAMA, Vol 244, No 5, p 488, August 1980

Advanced cardiac life support for neonates, standards for CPR & ECC. JAMA, Vol 244, No 5, pp 495-500, August 1980

Budassi SA, Barber JM: Emergency Nursing: Principles and Practice. C.V. Mosby Co., St. Louis, Missouri, 1981

Cohen SA: Pediatric Emergency Management: Guidelines for Rapid Diagnosis. The Robert J. Brady Co., Bowie, Maryland, 1982

Cosgriff J, Anderson DL: The Practice of Emergency Nursing. J.B. Lippincott Co., Philadelphia, Pennsylvania, 1975

Gaffney K: The pre-schooler in the ED. JEN, Vol 2, No 6, 1976

Gray M: Neonatal resuscitation. JEN, Vol 6, No 6, pp 29-32, November/December 1980

Hansen M: Accident or child abuse? Challenge to the ED nurse. JEN, Vol 2, No 1, 1976

Korting GW: Diseases of the Skin in Children and Adolescents, 3rd ed. W.B. Saunders Co., Philadelphia, Pennsylvania, 1979

Lane H: Handbook of Pediatrics, A Manual for Pediatric House Officers, 9th ed. (edited by DL Headings). Year Book Medical Publishers, Chicago, Illinois, 1981

Pascoe D, Grossman M: Quick Reference to Pediatric Emergencies. J.B. Lippincott Co., Philadelphia, Pennsylvania, 1973

Pierog J, Pierog L (eds): Pediatric emergencies, TEM. Aspen Systems Publications, Rockville, Maryland, Vol 3, No 1, April 1981

Schultz C: Grieving children. JEN, Vol 6, No 1, pp 30-36, January/February 1980

US Public Health Service, DHEW: Physicians in Hospital Emergency Departments. Health Services and Mental Health Administration, Division of Emergency Health Services, Bethesda, Maryland, 1971

Vaughn VC, McKay RJ: Nelson's Textbook of Pediatrics, 11th ed. W.B. Saunders Co., Philadelphia, Pennsylvania, 1979

Warner C: Emergency Care: Assessment and Intervention, 2nd ed. C.V. Mosby Co., St. Louis, Missouri, 1978

MEDICAL EMERGENCIES 24

KEY CONCEPTS

This chapter presents an overview of the pathophysiology, recognition, and management of most of the more commonly seen medical emergencies and is based on lecture presentations to emergency nurses by Cameron Bangs, M.D., Belle Slesh, R.N., Marc Bayer, M.D., Paul Blaylock, M.D., Earl Showerman, M.D., and Gideon Bosker, M.D.

After reading and studying this chapter, you should be able to:

- Describe the mechanisms of heat stroke, heat exhaustion, and heat cramps and to be able to explain the recognition and management of each.
- Identify the five mechanisms of heat loss from the body and some of the metabolic abnormalities that may cause hypothermia.
- Describe the nursing responsibilities in the management of hypothermia and frostbite.
- Identify the metabolic causes of coma, and describe the cardinal signs, symptoms, and the essential steps of management.
- Identify the mnemonics useful in going through a differential diagnosis with the comatose patient and the two conditions that produce flaccid paralysis and reactive pupils.
- Describe the pathophysiology associated with diabetes mellitus and the recognition and management of the various associated emergencies.
- Describe the pathophysiology associated with hypothyroidism and hyperthyroidism and the emergencies which they present, as well as immediate management.
- Explain anaphylactic reaction and describe the immediate steps of intervention.
- Identify the subdivisions of seizure states and describe each.
- Identify the significant information that should be gathered relating to the patient with severe recurrent headache and some important axiomatic guidelines to evaluation.

HYPERPYREXIA

Body temperature is controlled by a cerebral "thermostat" located in the hypothalamus. The hypothalamic point of body temperature can be elevated either by endogenous pyrogens or by a neurologic lesion that produces direct hypothalamic lesions. The mechanisms of fever production (body temperature in excess of the normal 98.6° F or 37° C) are 1) the cessation of diaphoresis, which is controlled by the hypothalamic center; 2) peripheral vasoconstriction; and 3) increased heat production via muscle exertion when shivering.

In adults, fevers of 104° F are generally well tolerated physiologically, but fevers above 105° F are associated frequently with convulsions. Fevers above 108° F produce irreversible damage to the adult brain.

Emergency treatment is indicated therefore in:

1. Any fever above 105° F (CNS cannot function normally with temperatures over 106° F)
2. Elevated temperature associated with disorientation
3. Fever greater than 103° F with any clinical suspicion of heat stroke
4. High fever with associated shock or congestive failure

The three clinical hyperpyrexic syndromes associated with exposure to environmental temperatures are:

- Heat stroke
- Heat exhaustion
- Heat cramps

All three tend to occur early during a period of rising temperature before the victim has become acclimatized. Acclimatization usually results after 8-10 days of exposure to high temperature; however, fully acclimatized persons may also suffer. These syndromes are more severe in children and older individuals. *Heat stroke* occurs in individuals with underlying chronic circulatory, renal, or cerebral disease including alcoholism and/or a history of heat or sun stroke.

Heat exhaustion is more commonly seen and occurs in those persons involved in strenuous exercise in warm and humid weather. Some people with certain conditions are predisposed to heat exhaustion: those who are hypertensive, those taking potent diuretics or suffering from diarrhea, and the elderly, who may not have adequate intake of liquids.

Fluid loss through perspiring can amount to as much as 3-4 liters an hour in extreme temperatures, and the salt content of sweat increases 0.2-0.5% as the temperature rises.

HEAT STROKE

Heat stroke is a medical emergency caused by a shutdown or failure of the heat-regulating mechanisms in the hypothalamus. This is a rare happening but is an extreme emergency!

Recognition

The symptoms are headache and visual disturbances, dizziness, nausea, hot and flushed dry skin, a weak, rapid and irregular pulse, and a sudden loss of consciousness. The temperature may rise to 106° to 112° F, with a cessation of perspiration and severe muscle cramping.

Initial laboratory evaluation will show:

- Increased serum potassium due to muscle necrosis
- Other electrolytes probably within normal limits
- Normal hematocrit

Guidelines for Nursing Intervention

Immediate and vigorous intervention is necessary, as this syndrome carries a very *high mortality* (50%) even with timely and adequate management. The most important factor is reduction of body temperature by immediate immersion in a cool bath, hypothermia blankets, ice packs, or sponging with cool water. Do NOT lower the temperature *below 102°* however.

Treatment is as follows:

1. Small, diluted doses of chlorpromazine (Thorazine) IV may be given to control delirium and shivering.
2. Small doses of morphine sulfate (2-4 mg IV increments titrated) may be given to decrease shivering and increase vasodilation. Both chlorpromazine and morphine sulfate may precipitate hypotension, so watch the BP carefully.
3. Acetylsalicylic acid, 10-15 gr, may be given orally or rectally in small temperature elevations.
4. Oxygen, under pressure if necessary, will help to maintain an adequate airway and, at high enough flow, to maintain perfusion.
5. Avoid sedatives unless patient convulses, since convulsions will create further disturbance of the heat-regulating mechanisms.
6. Diazepam (Valium) IV is the drug of choice to offset convulsions.
7. Hypotonic solution is given IV very slowly (run TKO) to avoid danger of pulmonary edema.
8. All intake and output must be carefully monitored, so a Foley bladder catheter is indicated. (Acute tubular necrosis is a complication.)
9. Monitor all VS and the LOC very closely, especially during rapid changes of temperature. Both shock and/or congestive failure frequently occur in association with heat stroke.
10. Avoid immediate reexposure to heat. Hypersensitivity to high heat may remain for a considerable time.

Complications

The complications of heat stroke are severe and include shock (pressor agents are *inadvisable*), hypernatremia, acute tubular necrosis, disseminated intravascular coagulation (DIC), arrhythmias without infarction, acute cerebral thrombosis, and hyperkalemia with acute muscle necrosis and finally death. There is no hope for survival in untreated cases of heat stroke; a 50% chance of survival in treated cases, and surviving patients may have permanent mental damage.

HEAT EXHAUSTION

Heat exhaustion is the inadequacy or collapse of the peripheral circulation secondary to a profound salt depletion and the loss of an effective circulating blood volume. It frequently occurs with underlying cardiac, cerebral, or systemic disease.

Recognition

The symptoms include weakness, dizziness, stupor with or without muscle cramps, a cool pale skin, profuse perspiration, oliguria, tachycardia, hypotension, mental confusion, and muscle incoordination.

Laboratory findings will show a low serum sodium and hemoconcentration. Electrocardiographic tracings may show arrhythmias without infarction.

Guidelines for Nursing Intervention

Treatment is simple and straightforward:

1. Place the patient at rest in a cool place.
2. Elevate the feet and massage the legs.
3. Give sodium chloride either PO or IV (1-2 liters NSS) unless patient is in danger of cardiac failure.
4. Treat shock if present.
5. Avoid immediate reexposure to heat.

HEAT CRAMPS

Heat cramps are painful spasms of involuntary muscles of the abdomen and extremities due primarily to salt depletion. With a large intake of water, salt loss is disproportionate to water loss, and there is intracellular overhydration.

The symptoms are a cool moist skin, muscle twitching, and a normal or slightly increased temperature. Laboratory evaluation will show a low serum sodium and a hemoconcentration.

The treatment is sodium chloride, 1 g every 0.5-1 hour, with large amounts of water. Physiologic saline solution by mouth or IV usually relieves attacks promptly. Place the patient in a cool place and massage the sore muscles gently. Rest should be continued for 1-2 days depending upon the severity of the attack.

HYPOTHERMIA

Heat loss is regulated by altering body insulation such as clothing or, as long-term measures, by increasing subcutaneous fat or effecting neurovascular changes mediated by the hypothalamus. The mechanism of heat production is most important in maintaining body temperature in the face of exposure to cold. In a cold environment, shivering mediated by the hypothalamus increases muscular heat production.

The mechanisms of heat loss are:

1. *Radiation,* the indirect transfer of heat through the air
2. *Conduction,* the direct transfer of heat from one object to another (Water conducts 240 times faster than air.)
3. *Convection,* the removal of the air blanket from around the body, as with the chill factor
4. *Evaporation,* the conversion of water from liquid to gas
5. *Respiration,* the loss of body heat during exhalation

The body's major heat loss is from the head and back of the neck.

LOWERING CORE TEMPERATURE

The normal body core temperature is 99° F. The cardinal signs and symptoms of a lowering core temperature and the degree of hypothermia are:

99-91.5° F   Shivering and an impaired ability to perform complex tasks, followed by more violent shivering, hyperventilation, difficulty in speaking, sluggish thinking, and beginning amnesia

91-86° F   Decrease in shivering as strong muscular rigidity sets in, the exposed skin becoming blue and puffy, comprehension dulled, possible total amnesia but posture still maintained, as is appearance of psychological contact with environment

85-81° F   Irrationality, loss of contact with surroundings, stupor, continued muscle rigidity, slow pulse and respirations, possible onset of supraventricular arrhythmias

80-70° F   Unconsciousness, no response to spoken word (most reflexes cease to function at this temperature level; heart beat becomes erratic)

68-0° F   Failure of cardiac and respiratory control centers in the brain, cardiac fibrillation, probable edema and hemorrhage in lungs, death

Contributing Factors

Hypothermia resulting from *metabolic abnormalities* is generally mild and responds to treatment of the underlying problem including uremia, hypothyroidism, adrenal insufficiency, hypoglycemia, shock from any cause, lesions in or near the hypothalamus, infarcts, and arteriosclerosis.

Without any predisposing causes, it is most frequent in the elderly population and occurs even in absence of exposure to extreme cold. Survivors in this group have been shown to have *impaired hypothalamic function*, presumably as a result of arteriosclerosis.

Some *drugs* that can contribute to hypothermia include general anesthetics, alcohol (since it both suppresses the hypothalamus and acts directly as a cutaneous vasodilator), barbiturates, phenothiazines, opiates, and more recently, methadone and marijuana; street people and "winos" are often victims of this problem by virtue of their unprotected environment.

Clinical Findings

Laboratory findings are as follows:

1. Blood gases show a metabolic acidosis (pH ↓ HCO_3 ↓ PCO_2 ↓)
2. There is a high hematocrit secondary to hypovolemia
3. Potassium may be high
4. Creatine phosphokinase (CPK) may be markedly elevated
5. Blood urea nitrogen (BUN) is increased
6. Blood sugar can go as high as 500 to 600 mg/100 ml
7. Electrocardiograph shows bradycardia and lowering T wave (with K^+ shift), a wide complex, J wave developing in terminal 0.04 sec of QRS complex, resembling a notched R wave. The origin has been ascribed to current injury, anoxia, delayed ventricular depolarization, or "early" repolarization.

Intervention

Immediate treatment starts with the warming process. There is a current controversy over 1) *active* internal warmth (warm inhalation, warm IVs, warm blood bypass, warm enemas), 2) external warmth (warm blankets) and 3) *active* external warmth (hyperthermic blankets and tub immersion).

Nursing responsibilities include:

1. Initial vital signs, including rectal temperature using a thermocoupler
2. Cardiac monitoring, with arrhythmias treated as indicated. Without ECG evidence of ventricular fibrillation or standstill, well-intended but totally unnecessary cardiac massage will almost surely precipitate ventricular fibrillation in the cold, slowly-beating heart. Injudicial patient handling or manipulation may also bring on this fatal arrhythmia, Ventricular fibrillation should be prevented at all costs because the customary methods of defibrillation are almost totally ineffective below 86-87° F (30-32° C). Prevention depends on the exercise of extreme caution in moving, transporting, manipulating, intubating, etc.
3. An IV and possibly CVP line to monitor blood volume. Warm NSS or Ringer's lactate with dextrose; run in 2-3 liters rapidly.
4. Foley catheter with urimeter to monitor output

5. Warm blankets continually reinforced after patient is removed from tub (if used)

6. Continual observation and monitoring of VS every 15 min. Report any ECG changes to physician.

7. Watch temperature of patient and remove from tub (if used) when the temperature reaches 99° F or 37° C.

8. If using the tub procedure, maintain the water temperature at 104° F, and remain with the patient constantly. If the procedure involves a partial immersion, use a basin of water at 100-110° F.

Warm water immersion has been shown to be a very rapid form of rewarming. However, because of the potentially hazardous effects of possibly precipitating an increased after-drop of temperature, ventricular fibrillation, and rewarming shock, this technique must be employed with extreme caution. It must also be understood that the warm water bath setting complicates the use of ECG monitors, cardiac massage and defibrillators, endotracheal intubation, and mechanical ventilation.

Preferred Method

Inhalation of warm, saturated oxygen (active internal warmth) may prove to be the method of choice in rewarming victims of all types of hypothermia. It has been demonstrated in animals that the greatest heat gain with this method is to the heart and that since the distribution of heat was essentially limited to the core, peripheral heating and vasodilation was very slow to develop. In studies by a research group at the Naval Regional Medical Center in Bremerton, WA, the least average after-drop in core temperature in nine subjects occurred with inhalation rewarming, which has the added advantage of being adaptable at the scene of rescue, en route to the hospital, and in the ED, while ECG monitoring and positive pressure inhalation is being administered to the severely hypothermic patient.

FROSTBITE

Superficial frostbite is similar to sunburn but a little deeper. There is a redness followed by branny desquamation and blister formation in 24-36 hours, which is followed by sheet desquamation. Face, hands, and feet are the most common areas involved, and one should NEVER RUB the area with anything, especially snow or slush.

Deep frostbite—for example, the whole foot—may appear yellowish and waxy, even "wooden" to palpation. These patients are not necessarily stretcher cases, as a rule, but still should *never* be allowed to walk on the frostbitten feet.

The treatment is rapid thawing, but the frostbitten part should be *kept frozen* until this can be done. The body core temperature must be maintained; no alcohol (ethanol) is allowed until the core temperature is restored to 97°, no friction is applied, no anticoagulants are given, and no vasodilating drugs (including alcohol) are given. *The frostbitten areas are treated as gently as a severe burn, and sterile technique is essential!*

The important points to be remembered in the management of the frost-bitten patient are 1) restore circulation as rapidly as possible; 2) use sterile technique; 3) treat all extremities if one is frostbitten; 4) curare may be effective in controlling shivers; and 5) be ready to manage cardiac arrest if patient is hypothermic as well.

METABOLIC EMERGENCIES

COMA

When a comatose or near-comatose patient arrives in the ED with no explanation for the crisis situation, a rapid differential diagnosis must be made by the physician. Is the coma or near-coma 1) metabolic, 2) structural (supratentorial or subtentorial), or 3) of psychiatric origin (hysteria, catatonia, etc., which are frequently confused with coma)?

Causes of Coma

Consciousness "shuts down" when any of the following events occur:

1. Loss of oxygenated hemoglobin at a rate in excess of 750 cc of blood/min. Oxygen is lost in two ways: when there is enough blood with too little oxygen or when there is only a little blood with enough oxygen. It makes no difference either way because without oxygen, the brain cannot support energy demands and coma results.
2. Decrease in blood sugar to less than 40 mg/100 ml. Glucose is the major and virtually the *only* brain substrate (substance on which an enzyme acts). A good blood flow with good oxygenation but low glucose produces coma.
3. A temperature rise to above 105° or fall to lower than 92°.
4. Drastic alterations of serum sodium, potassium, or calcium concentrations.
5. Flooding the brain with CO_2, drugs, and poisons, including those that cannot be handled by defective kidneys and liver.
6. Presence of a large, expanding mass inside the head, increasing pressure and shutting off blood flow, or severe meningitis or encephalitis destroying brain cells directly or indirectly.

When coma becomes severe, major controls over temperature, blood pressure, food regulation, response to stress, and survival are abolished. Life cannot continue without support and rapid reversal of the underlying cause of the coma.

Metabolic diseases that cause coma or near-coma are 1) ischemia; 2) anoxia; 3) hypoglycemia; 4) diabetic acidosis; 5) vitamin deficiency; 6) hepatic failure; 7) uremia; 8) pulmonary insufficiency; 9) hypertensive encephalopathy; 10) Addison's disease; 11) myxedema; 12) ethanol abuse; 13) drugs; 14) poisons; 15) shock; 16) hyperosmolar and hypoosmolar states; 17) hypercalcemia and hypocalcemia; 18) meningitis; 19) encephalitis; and 20) postictal states, among others.

A metabolic cause should be suspected if

1. There is an absence of lateralizing signs, ruling out a supratentorial structural lesion.
2. Pupils are reactive to light (*barbiturate intoxication* and *hysteria* are two specific conditions that produce flaccid paralysis and reactive pupils).
3. Initial laboratory studies indicate an abnormality known to cause metabolic encephalopathy, *i.e.*, electrolyte abnormalities, elevated BUN, hypoglycemia, hyperglycemia, hypoxia, hypercapnia, hypocapnia, or an acid-base disturbance.
4. There are signs of drug abuse and intoxication (needle tracts and miosis).
5. There are signs of liver failure or portal hypertension. Asterixis is seen most commonly in hepatic failure but also in other forms of metabolic encephalopathy, such as uremia and respiratory acidosis. (Squeeze the forearm while holding it at a 90° angle and watch the hand twitch; the reaction is called "liver hand," "liver flap," or asterixis.
6. Multifocal myoclonic jerks are evident.
7. There is a history of a seizure disorder.

Immediate Nursing Intervention

In dealing with the seriously ill patient, first things must come first, and this means, again, check for a patent airway and rapidly evaluate how well the patient is perfusing. Next check for bleeding or signs of hypovolemia and shock, which would indicate the need for IV fluids immediately. A further rapid clinical assessment is done with full vital signs, eye signs, and an evaluation of the LOC.

Once these areas have been covered, the next step is to obtain as thorough a history as possible from whoever accompanied the patient to the ED. The history is of tremendous importance, and *all* personnel should be aware of the fact that police and family or friends must be detained for information. Valuable history is lost when these people are allowed to wander away. Make every effort to obtain information directly and not through second parties, and if medications accompany the patient, attempt to reach the druggist or prescribing physician if necessary to determine why the medication was prescribed, how long, and how much.

The patient in coma or near coma has passed through *earlier stages,* and it is important to note the time elements, tracking the level of consciousness before and during admission, to obtain this crucial information. The earliest changes in metabolic comas are:

• Decreased awareness
• Decreased orientation and "grasp"

- Decreased attention and memory changes
- Apathy, withdrawal, and an anxious fearful attitude

These are all signs of incipient changes, and *when the patient becomes agitated, he will tend to become worse faster.*

Review of the Levels of Consciousness

LOC I	Alert and wakeful, well oriented and responsive
LOC II	Altered state with such descriptive terms as "drowsy," "apathetic," "confused," "agitated"
LOC III	"Lethargic" and "dull." Can be aroused, is unclear about what is happening, is disoriented, talks very little, is difficult to rouse but will talk (may give inappropriate responses), may have Biot's respirations.
LOC IV	Stuporous and not truly arousable but will respond to painful stimuli with defensive or organized movements or groans. Usually falls back into stupor at end of stimulus. May have Cheyne-Stokes respirations.
LOC V	Comatose and *not* arousable. May have reflexes or be decorticate, decerebrate, or flaccid, depending on the depth of coma. Neurogenic hyperventilation (apneustic) often seen (40-50/min).

Cardinal Signs and Symptoms

- An altered state of mentation with deterioration and changes in LOC
- Abnormal respiratory patterns
- Abnormal eye signs
- Abnormal body movements, reflexes, postures, and inappropriate responses to painful stimuli

Abnormal Eye Signs

Eye signs are probably the most crucial observations, other than the LOC, in comatose patients, observing for position and pupil response.

If there is no tumor or destructive lesion in the brain, anoxia, glutethimide (Doriden) overdose or hypoglycemia, the following eye signs will be seen in metabolic coma:

1. Pupils are *reactive* to light and may be small or large. Use strong light and look closely and carefully at reactivity. *Pupils will not be unequal in metabolic coma.*
2. Pupils are responsive to the ciliospinal reflex. (Pinch side of neck and pupil will decrease in size.)
3. Eyes are conjugate in midposition, roving, or still.

4. Doll's eye maneuver is normal.

5. Ice water in the ear produces conjugate deviation. The eyes will try to look away from the cold stimulus, and there will probably be *nystagmus*. The eyes will jerk away but drift back. This is a negative caloric test to be remembered with the mnemonic *COWS* (cold opposite, warm same).

6. The patient *can* have normal pupillary reflexes despite depressed respirations, no caloric responses, decerebrate rigidity or flaccidity.

7. The lid reflex can be assessed by gently touching the tips of the eyelashes. In light coma states or in those of a functional origin, the lids will blink involuntarily. *Absence of lid reflex is indicative of a deeper coma.*

Motor Systems Status

In evaluating body movements, reflexes, or postures, there are several concepts to aid in determining the depth of coma:

1. The patient's arm or leg may be raised and allowed to drop. In light coma, it will fall gradually. In deep coma the limb will drop suddenly in a limp fashion.

2. Any resistance to passive motion by the elbow or knee joints should be noted.

3. Any spontaneous movements of the limbs, whether unilateral or bilateral, should be noted, as well as increased or decreased muscle tone, if present.

4. Some early changes (nonspecific as to structural or metabolic origin) occurring during lethargy or stupor are:
   A. Paratonia or "lead-pipe" stiffness of extremities
   B. Grasping reflex
   C. Focal weakness or hemiplegia, as an inability to move one side

5. Some late changes (also nonspecific as to structural or metabolic origin) occurring with brain-stem depression are:
   A. Decorticate posture, with the arms rigidly flexed, hands rotated internally, and stiffened legs
   B. Decerebrate posture, with rigid extension of all extremities, abduction of the arms, arching of the back, and toes pointed inward.

6. Some specific movements of particular significance that should be accurately documented are:
   A. Tremors
   B. Myoclonic (multifocal) jerks and spasms
   C. Asterixis (liver failure, diabetic acidosis, uremia), a flapping tremor of the hand when the forearm is elevated to a 90° angle.

Diagnostic Drugs

Emergency nurses must be aware of the diagnostic drugs indicated for usage in the comatose patient and must understand the rationale for their use.

1. A dose of 50 cc 50% glucose IV push will reverse hypoglycemia.
2. Naloxone (Narcan) 1 ml IV push and repeated twice over 5 min will reverse coma caused by heroin, opiates, pentazocine (Talwin), or propoxyphene HCl (Darvon).
3. Thiamine, 100 mg IV (up to a total of 500 mg after glucose) for Wernicke's encephalopathy (seen in chronic alcoholism and manifested by nystagmus, ataxia, and mental changes ranging from deterioration to delirium tremens).
4. Steroids (Decadron or Solu-Medrol) are given to protect against swelling in the brain and the resulting hypoxia. Often the administration of these drugs in the ED is the lifesaving step in reversal of a descending lesion (mass).

These drugs should be readily available in the ED, and the EDN should be alerted to their need, knowledgeable in their usage, and ready to administer whatever the physician feels is indicated and orders.

Guidelines for Nursing Management

1. Secure an airway, ventilate with O_2.
2. Establish baselines on flowsheet with BP, heart rate, body temperature. Observe pattern of respiration. If shocky, look elsewhere for occult trauma. Record serial LOC, eye signs and posture.
3. Place a No. 17 or 18 venous intracatheter, start 500 cc D5/W. Push fluid if blood pressure is low.
4. Collect venous blood sample for:
   - Glucose
   - CBC, HCT
   - BUN
   - Creatinine
   - Bilirubin
   - SGOT
   - Sodium, potassium, calcium
   - Type, crossmatch, and sedimentation rate (5 cc unclotted blood)
   - Take 15 cc for drug/toxicology studies: diphenyhydantoin (Dilantin), salicylate, barbiturate levels, and blood alcohol. (Barbiturate coma accounts for one-third of all suicides in the United States.)
5. Administer drugs as indicated:
   - 50 cc 50% glucose, IV push (but not until venous sample for baseline studies has been drawn)
   - Naloxone (Narcan) 1.0 cc (0.4 mg) IV push (repeat twice over 5 min)
   - Thiamine, 100 mg IV push
6. Review physical examination:
   - Determine the level of consciousness.
   - Determine size and equality of pupils and reaction to direct light stimulus.

- Test for extraocular eye movements.
- Check respiratory pattern and note patient's color.
- Check extremities for reflexes.

7. Continue to document all findings on the neurological flowsheet. If stupor or coma continues, take the following steps:

   - Insert Foley catheter; send urine specimen to laboratory for urinalysis (UA) and toxicology study if indicated. Set up an output sheet.
   - Place endotracheal tube with inflatable cuff and bag or ventilate as necessary.
   - Place an Ewald tube into stomach and lavage with 4 liters of isotonic saline. Remove contents and save. Replace Ewald tube with NG tube connected to intermittent low suction.
   - Draw arterial blood gases for PaO_2, PCO_2 and pH.
   - Control body temperature, working for normothermic status.
   - Place ECG leads as necessary for monitoring cardiac status.
   - Remove contact lenses; begin physical survey, repeat the neurological examination. If signs of neurological deterioration develop, time will be the essence so immediately perform these procedures:

     A. Call a neurosurgeon.

     B. Hyperventilate patient with 100% oxygen.

     C. Prepare to give dexamethasone (Decadron) or methylprednisolone (Solu-Medrol) IV push on order.

     D. Prepare to start 500 cc 20% mannitol at maximum drip rate on order.

     E. Prepare patient for OR.

Mnemonics

Dr. Theodore Goldberg suggests the use of mneumonics when working through the differential diagnosis on comatose patients.* A mnemonic is a tool or device to help the memory recollect certain ideas, and in this instance, the word TIPS and the vowels (AEIOU) are used as follows:

T	Trauma
I	Infection
P	Psychosis
S	Syncope
A	Alcoholism
E	Encephalopathy
I	Insulin
O	Opiates
U	Uremia

---

*Goldberg T: Physicians in Hospital Emergency Departments. U.S. Department of Health, Education, and Welfare, Rockville, Maryland, 1971

TIPS would probably be the first checklist to rule out before proceeding to metabolic causes with the patient.

Trauma

An injury may be direct and obvious or may be indirect, with occult findings. Trauma may also precipitate other forms of coma and near-coma, such as Addisonian crisis or diabetic acidosis from the increased stress factor.

Infection

As a general rule, infection presents in older persons who may have meningitis or bacteremia, especially gram-negative, and does so without the classic picture of infectious disease. This patient may have had previous prostatic surgery followed by a personality disturbance and lowgrade fever. Acute bacterial endocarditis in the older patient may be minimal with no murmurs but with a personality disorder and fever. Pneumonia can also precipitate personality disturbances in the older patient.

Psychiatric Problems

These should be diagnosed by exclusion rather than jumping to the conclusion that the problem is psychotic in origin.

Syncope

Fainting due to reduced cardiac output is not uncommon, and a confused state or a depression of mental acuity may be seen in the patient with heart failure. Organic brain syndrome may be the result of a low cardiac output over a period of time.

After the TIPS have been checked, the AEIOU mnemonics should be investigated.

Alcoholism

The presence of alcohol on the breath does *not* mean that alcoholic intoxication is the cause of the coma or near-coma, as alcoholism masks many problems. Alcoholics are especially subject to other causes of coma, such as hypoglycemic reactions on the basis of liver disease (give 50 cc 50% glucose IV), subdural hematomas (to which they are particularly prone because of the many falls and associated head trauma, or because of coagulation abnormalities stemming from the hepatotoxicity), and a tendency to rapid intoxication from barbiturates and other forms of alcohol. Alcoholics are very commonly subjected to errors in judgment, and if the coma deepens instead of lightening, you should suspect an associated process or another cause for the coma.

Encephalopathy

Epilepsy is the most frequently seen form of encephalopathy and is generally well recognized; the problem is in recognizing the postictal state. These patients may also be victims of other causes of coma or near-coma, and head trauma is common, resulting in subdural hematoma. If the postictal state deepens instead of lightening, look for other causes. These patients have access to large doses of drugs and are frequently depressed. Ingestion of barbiturates or other drugs may well be the causative factor in the problem.

Intracranial hemorrhage is a serious and common problem. Spontaneous subarachnoid hemorrhage can be a deceptive diagnostic problem but must be ruled out in young adults with or without nuchal rigidity. Be careful this patient is not mistakenly labeled as "a stroke." In a young adult complaining of severe headache and restlessness, a subarachnoid hemorrhage must be considered, regardless of the circumstances or the way in which it presents.

The patient who has suffered a cerebrovascular accident (CVA) will usually present conscious and without nuchal rigidity, will rarely convulse, and may show calcification of the intracranial arteries, or a pineal shift from edema. There may be hemiplegia present with speech impairment and the typical puffing cheek with respirations. Immediate care of these patients frequently includes the necessity to suction the airway clear of mucus, to administer low-flow oxygen, and to carefully position to avoid pressure points. The skin must be kept clean and dry, so if necessary, a Foley catheter should be placed with a closed-system drainage bag before the patient is admitted to the floor. These patients are usually elderly and require a great deal of reinforcement and assurance from the nurse to help alleviate some of the tremendous apprehension.

Lumbar puncture is a helpful diagnostic maneuver in a patient with suspected encephalopathy but is not indicated with evidence of increased intracranial pressure, papilledema, or known head trauma *unless* it is done by a neurosurgeon.

Insulin

In this context, insulin is related to the problems of the diabetic patient—diabetic coma, hypoglycemia, and hyperglycemia. Diabetic problems account, by and large, for a very significant number of the comas and stuporous conditions seen in the ED, often presenting in bizarre ways and most frequently with patients using long-acting insulin or the more potent oral hypoglycemic agents. The average diabetic patient struggles with a surprisingly inadequate knowledge of the disease process. This population is one for whom the EDN is in a fine position to do some really constructive teaching.

Diabetes mellitus is found in 2% of the population and is said to be increasing. Eighty percent of diabetics are the adult type (mature diabetics) with an onset at over 40 years of age and are obese females. The patient's pancreas is still producing small amounts of insulin but cannot meet the demands of the overweight body requirements for insulin. Control is primarily by diet with caloric restrictions and the use of the oral hypoglycemic agents, which provide *no* insulin but do stimulate the pancreas to produce *more* endogenous insulin.

The so-called "juvenile" type diabetic is seen in approximately 5% of the diabetic population, with the onset *usually* appearing in childhood or adolescence. In this type of patient, the pancreas makes *no* insulin; therefore, insulin must be taken into the body from another source (exogenous). The onset of this disease is often precipitated by severe stress resulting from influenza, high temperatures, serious accidents, surgery, trauma, etc., and frequently manifests itself with severe dehydration, excessive thirst and urination, and an anxious flushed appearance. This patient is suddenly recognized to be in ketoacidosis.

Careful teaching and continued encouragement are essential to the well-being of these patients if they are to understand the disease process and care for themselves properly. Years of poorly controlled high blood sugars will accelerate the breakdown of the basement cell membrane of the capillaries, which will result in early circulatory problems, accelerated arteriosclerosis, persistent infections, poor healing capacity, gangrene, sensory loss in the periphery, renal pathology, and retinopathy.

Hypoglycemia

Hypoglycemia, or "insulin shock," as it is commonly called, is not confined to the overaction of insulin. Exogenous insulin is a hormone derived from beef and pork livers and is pure protein; therefore, it cannot be given orally since the digestive juices would immediately destroy it. Insulin must be given subcutaneously; there is no such thing as "oral insulin." The oral hypoglycemic agents—the sulfonylureas such as tolbutamide (Orinase), tolazamide (Tolinase), acetohexamide-(Dymelor), chlorpropamide (Diabinese),—are medications that help control blood sugar by either stimulating production of endogenous insulin in the mature-type diabetic or increase muscle utilization of glucose. These agents can cause problems much like insulin shock. Sulfonylureas such as chlorpropamide and tolazamide can drastically lower the blood sugar unexpectedly, but whether it is insulin or one of these potent oral drugs, the patient must deal with it once the dosage is aboard.

The following are some general points to remember about oral hypoglycemic agents:

1. Tolbutamide is the mildest of the hypoglycemic oral agents.
2. Tolazamide is the next strongest.
3. Acetohexamide is close to tolazamide in strength.
4. Chlorpropamide is the strongest of the sulfonylureas, and 750 mg/24 hours is the *maximum* safe dosage! The diabetic patient frequently cannot remember the name of his medication, but the pill shaped like a D and light blue in color is chlorpropamide (Diabinese) 250 mg. Three of

these in a 24-hour period represent the maximum dosage; the patient on this high a dosage must maintain adequate caloric intake to prevent severe hypoglycemia.

5. Phenformin (DBI and DBI-TD spansule) is highly irritating to the gastrointestinal tract and frequently causes severe nausea and vomiting and occasionally a severe lactic acidosis with sudden, sharp, steady adominal pain and hypoactive or absent bowel sounds.

6. Alcohol qualifies as an oral hypoglycemic agent, and diabetics should be advised that if alcohol is taken, it should be mixed with a fruit juice or mixer to offset glucose depletion. They should also be reminded that alcohol is a CNS depressant and can have a double-barreled effect on them.

Other common causes of hypoglycemia are decreased food intake, increased exercise without extra food, medication changes, concomitant illness with depleted caloric intake. There are also reactive or idiopathic hypoglycemia, insulinoma (rare) and other tumors, myxedema, adrenal insufficiency, and liver disease to be considered.

Recognition. The manifestations resulting from a *rapid* decrease in blood glucose (around 45 mg/100 ml is a dangerously low level; 60 mg/100 ml is low normal) are tachycardia, palpitations, diaphoresis, and tremulousness. A *gradual* decrease in the blood sugar manifests with fatigue and hunger, then headache, inappropriate behavior, poor mental acuity, seizures, coma, focal CNS signs, hypothermia (hypothalamic dysfunction), and occasionally hyperthermia.

Guidelines for Nursing Management

1. Take appropriate steps to insure airway and ventilation as necessary.
2. Draw blood to test for sugar.
3. If patient is conscious, give oral carbohydrate (15 g, or 3 tsp. sugar) *or give Instant Glucose* (manufactured and distributed solely by the Diabetic Association of Cleveland, Ohio). Instant Glucose can be placed into the buccal pouch of a relatively unresponsive hypoglycemic patient for immediate absorption and frequently reverses even severe hypoglycemia by the time the ambulance arrives. Many insulin-dependent and more severe mature-type diabetics carry Instant Glucose on their persons for emergency situations, and every ED and ambulance should have it available. (Diabetic Association of Cleveland, 2022 Lee Rd., Cleveland, Ohio 44118.)
4. If patient is unconscious or severely confused, give 50 cc 50% dextrose, IV push, or glucagon, 1 mg IM or SC (be aware that it will take 15-20 min to work).
5. If hypoglycemia is due to insulin, consider readjusting daily dose downward and observe patient carefully for at least 1 hour.
6. If hypoglycemia is due to chlorpropamide (Diabinese), hospitalize the patient and give IV D10/W at 150 ml/hour to keep the blood sugar level

at around 100 mg/100 ml until the half-life of chlorpropamide (36 hours) has ended.

HYPERGLYCEMIC STATES

Diabetic Ketoacidosis. Diabetic ketoacidosis is the initial manifestation of diabetes mellitus, precipitated by failure to increase the body's insulin requirements with stress (infection, trauma, surgery, etc.) as well as by discontinuation of insulin dosage as prescribed.

Signs and symptoms. The patient presents with polydipsia, polyuria, polyphagia, dehydration, weight loss, abdominal pain, nausea and vomiting. Kussmaul respirations (continuous, rapid, deep, and labored, with "fruity" odor of ketones), and stupor progressing to coma and shock.

Diagnosis. Laboratory analysis of the blood sugar, serum ketones, BUN, electrolytes, UA, CBC, and ABGs and a chest film confirm the diagnosis. Appropriate cultures are taken if the patient is febrile, and an ECG should be done if the potassium level is low.

Immediate treatment.

1. Intravenous fluids should be given—normal saline or 0.5 normal saline, usually 3-6 liters necessary to replace losses (10% of body weight).
2. Insulin—high dose bolus is given (100 units regular insulin, half IV and half subcutaneously, or continuous IV infusion at 6-10 units per hour; *i.e.,* 50 units regular insulin in 500 ml NSS at 1 ml/min; reduce to 0.5 ml/min when blood sugar is under 300 mg/100 ml).
3. Potassium—give 10-40 mEq/hour when urine output is established and decrease with correction of acidosis.
4. Bicarbonate—requires partial correction if pH is 7.2 or less.

Guidelines for nursing management. Some additional considerations in the management of the ketoacidotic patient are:

1. A flow sheet is essential to properly assess patient response.
2. A Foley catheter and NG tube should be placed if patient is comatose, and a CVP line initiated if the patient is in shock.
3. Initial fluid should be 0.5 normal saline unless shock is present, and switch to D5/0.5 NSS when blood sugar is les than 300 mg/100 ml.
4. Watch the potassium levels carefully. Initial potassium may be normal, but total body stores are depleted as a result of acidosis and huge solute diuresis.
5. Correction of acidosis reduces insulin resistance.
6. Cerebral edema can result from *too rapid correction of dehydration and hyperglycemia* with increased mental confusion progressing into coma while "chemically" the patient is improving. Watch the LOC closely!

Nondiabetic Ketoacidosis. This is a recently described complication of *chronic alcoholism,* with signs and symptoms of anorexia, nausea and vomiting, abdominal pain, disorientation progressing into coma, tachycardia, and Kussmaul respirations.

Laboratory analysis shows a normal blood sugar, increased ketone bodies—betahydroxybutyrate not measured by tests for acetone (Acetest)—and acidosis. Therapy involves administration of IV fluids and bicarbonate given cautiously if the pH is less than 7.20.

Lactic Acidosis. Lactic acidosis can occur spontaneously or secondary to *circulatory insufficiency,* hepatic disease, hematologic disorders, medications (phenformin), pancreatitis, and uremia.

Laboratory findings show acidosis *without* hyperglycemia or ketonemia, an elevated serum lactate, and a low P_{CO_2}. Therapy involves general resuscitation measures with bicarbonate given according to the computed method:

$$\text{mEq replacement} = \frac{\text{Base deficit} \times \text{Weight in Kg}}{5} \times \tfrac{1}{2} \text{ and recheck ABGs.}$$

Hyperosmolar, Hyperglycemic Nonketotic Coma. This is an entity commonly seen in *elderly* persons, mild or previously undiagnosed diabetes, consumption of large quantities of sugar solutions (iVs), associated illness (extensive burns, MI, CVA), and large doses of corticosteroids.

Signs and symptoms. These people often present in a confused state, which progresses into coma. Dehydration and polyuria result from osmotic diuresis, and there may be acidosis if shock is present. The *mortality* is 40-50%, and the onset can be very *insidious.*

Laboratory findings include a marked hyperglycemia (blood sugar frequently as high as 1500 mg/100 ml), no ketonemia, and no acidosis (unless shock is present).

Osmolarity is determined by the following formula:

$$\text{Osmolarity} = 2 \times Na^+ + \frac{\text{Blood sugar}}{18} + 10$$

Normal level is 280-300 mOsm/liter.

Management. The main problem is *hypovolemia,* and there may be fluid deficits as high as 6-14 units, with the patient in shock, for which saline is given IV; otherwise 0.5 NSS is given, correcting 50% of the deficit in the first 12 hours. Low dose IV insulin (6 units/hour infusion) is given, avoiding the high-dose bolus (greater then 100 units). Potassium is given at 10-40 mEq/hour. The patient must be monitored very closely with ECGs, cardiac monitor, and continuous O_2 at high liter flow.

Opiates

Included in the opiates are the sedatives and tranquilizers that comprise the high-abuse groups seen so frequently in the ED. Barbiturate intoxication may lead to serious airway problems, with laryngospasm; the treatment is covered in the chapter on drug abuse and toxicology. Phenothiazine reactions will present with what resembles a parkinsonian crisis: stupor, eyes rolled upward, and drooling from the mouth. This is rapidly reversed with IV diphenhydramine HCl (Benadryl) and caffeine sodium benzolate is also effective (see Chapter 26 on Drug Abuse and Toxicology).

Uremia

When no other diagnosis of coma has materialized, a BUN may be the deciding factor in establishing the problem as one of kidney function and uremia. This evaluation should be done routinely on all patients with serious medical problems, as well as the CBC, electrolytes, blood sugar, and urinalysis. The patient with uremia will probably complain of severe headache if responsive, and if convulsions develop, supportive treatment and admission are indicated, with perhaps small doses of sedatives in the interim.

ENDOCRINE EMERGENCIES

ADRENOCORTICAL INSUFFICIENCY

The patient with adrenocortical insufficiency will present with weakness, tachycardia, nausea, vomiting, diarrhea, dehydration, hypotension, and probably hypoglycemia. There will be a metabolic acidosis with increased serum potassium and decreased serum sodium. There will be a history of acute stress from surgery, pregnancy, etc., and predisposing factors such as steroid withdrawal, tuberculosis, or meningococcemia, with accompanying signs of increased pigmentation of the skin and weight loss.

The treatment is correction of electrolyte abnormalities, administration of corticosteroids, fluid challenge to correct the shock state, and probably administration of digitalis.

HYPERTHYROIDISM

Thyroid storm, as it is called (or thyrotoxic crisis), also follows trauma such as surgery, infection, and stress in patients with a history of hyperthyroidism. They will present in the ED with tachycardia, palpitations, severe weakness, a widened pulse pressure, diarrhea, a fever over 100° F, increased CNS activity followed by obtundation and coma, an enlarged thyroid gland with possible exophthalmos, and a history of hyperthyroidism. There is an associated mortality of 50%.

Immediate treatment involves administration of antithyroid drugs: methimazole (Tapazole) or propylthiouracil is given by mouth immediately to suppress synthesis of thyroid. If the patient is comatose or incoherent, an NG tube must be passed and the medication instilled by gavage. Thirty minutes after the antithyroid drugs have been given, sodium iodide or potassium iodide is begun, as well as steroids occasionally. The increased metabolic needs are met with IV glucose and B vitamins; supportive treatment is given for hyperpyrexia (cooling blanket) and dehydration, and the precipitating cause is isolated and treated.

MYXEDEMA OR HYPOTHYROIDISM

The patient with myxedema presents in the ED with slow mental responses, cool, thickened, dry skin, which has a yellow-orange tint, sparse hair and eyebrows, characteristic puffy facies, nonpitting edema, depressed respirations with CO_2 retention, bradycardia, hypothermia, possibly signs of pericardial effusion, and the presence of a thyroidectomy scar, with a history of cessation of thyroid replacement.

Laboratory requisitions should include CBC and electrolytes, blood sugar, ABGs, and thyroid function tests.

Nursing management and therapy include 1) a *slow* rewarming, if patient is hypothermic (submersion is not suggested, but if the patient is severely hypothermic, active internal warming with warmed saturated oxygen may be beneficial); 2) correction of hypoglycemia; 3) searching out the precipitating illness (MI, CHF, pulmonary emboli, infection, trauma); and 4) respiratory care to reverse CO_2 narcosis that is common. Secondary hypoventilation may require intubation and ventilation. Again, steroids may be given (hydrocortisone, 100 mg IVq24 hours), and in severe cases thyroid replacement is begun with levothyroxine (Synthroid), IV or PO, or L-triiodothyronine (Cytomel), PO. These patients require close observation and nursing care; *myxedema coma carries a 50% mortality!*

OTHER MEDICAL EMERGENCIES

ANAPHYLAXIS

Anaphylaxis is one of the most acute medical emergencies and requires immediate recognition and intervention. It should be suspected anytime a patient has received a systemic medication and begins to react in any way. Most commonly, the cause is an unusual or exaggerated allergic reaction of an organism to foreign protein or a specific medication, such as penicillin and related antibiotics, to allergens, local anesthetics, hormones, enzymes, and diagnostic agents such as BSP, dehydrocholic acid (Decholin), and iodinated contrast media. There is a mass outpouring of *histamine* and SRSA (a hormonal-type substance called the Slow Reacting Substance in Anaphylaxis) that cause profound vasodilatation, local edema, and hives due to the increased capillary permeability and bronchial constriction. This rapidly deteriorates into a shock state followed by collapse and sudden death unless effective intervention is instituted without delay.

Immediate treatment:

1. Manage airway with intubation or cricothyroidotomy if necessary and supplemental oxygen administration at high concentrations.
2. Epinephrine (Adrenalin) should be given to stimulate vasoconstriction, relax the bronchospasm, decrease the capillary permeability, and inhibit any further histamine release.

    A. A tourniquet should be applied above the site of entry if possible and 0.3 cc 1:1000 epinephrine infiltrated into the area.

    B. Epinephrine, 0.3-0.5 cc 1:1000 is given subcutaneously, *or*
0.1 cc of 1:1000 is given by slow IV push, *or*
1 cc of 1:10,000 is given by slow IV push, *or*
if veins are inaccessible because of peripheral collapse, epinephrine is given into the base of the tongue.

3. Diphenhydramine HCl (Benadryl) 50-75 mg is given parenterally.
4. Aminophylline or theophylline is given IV in doses appropriate to an asthmatic attack.
5. Steroids are recommended by some physicians.
6. Volume is replaced with rapid administration of crystalloid or colloid, as indicated, if there is a generalized vascular collapse and hypovolemia.
7. Continue close monitoring of the airway.
8. Admit patient.

Prevention of anaphylactic reactions is possible in a great many instances that involve the administration of medications. The following guidelines are excellent ones to follow:

1. Take a careful history of allergies and previous drug reactions *before* giving *any* medications.
2. Never give a drug without a good indication and avoid those with known antigenic potential.
3. Avoid the parenteral route if the oral route will do. Serious reactions are less likely to occur with oral agents.
4. Give parenteral injections far enough distally on extremities so that a proximal tourniquet can be applied if necessary.
5. After a parenteral injection, observe the patient for untoward reactions for *at least* 15 min. The reaction in most fatal cases begins in 1-2 min.
6. Be prepared for allergic reactions whenever you are using parenteral drugs. Keep a tray handy containing a tourniquet, epinephrine, syringes, and equipment for starting an IV.
7. Educate the patient concerning any possible drug reaction, and supply a written record for the patient to carry.
8. Tell the patient what drugs you are giving, and make an effort to have all prescriptions labeled with the name of the drug.

CONVULSIONS AND SEIZURES

Febrile convulsions in children are discussed in Chapter 23 on Pediatric Emergencies. Generally, seizures are characterized in one degree or another by 1) an aura, 2) the seizure state, and 3) the postictal state.

According to *Dorland's Medical Dictionary,* the symptoms of epilepsy are due to paroxysmal disturbance of the electrical activity of the brain and are divided clinically into four subdivisions: *grand mal* with subgroups of 1) generalized, 2) focal (localized) and 3) jacksonian, *petit mal, psychomotor seizure,* and *autonomic seizure,* with flushing, pallor, tachycardia, hypertension, perspiration, or other visceral symptoms.

The *grand mal* epileptic seizure is frequently preceded by an aura, in which a sudden loss of consciousness is immediately followed by generalized convulsions. *Jacksonian* epilepsy is characterized by unilateral clonic (alternate contraction and relaxation) movements that start in one group of muscles and spread systematically to adjacent groups, reflecting the march of the epileptic activity through the motor cortex. The seizures are due to a discharging focus in the contralateral motor cortex. *Petit mal* seizures are those with a sudden momentary loss of consciousness, with only minor myoclonic jerks, seen especially in children.

The history of a postictal patient is extremely important, and if the seizure occurs in the ED, it should be described in as much *objective* detail as possible. If not, get as much history as possible about the seizure from friends or relatives, asking them to describe the activity pattern. Avoid terms such as "grand mal" and "jacksonian," rather ask and note *where* the seizure started, where it spread, the duration, the type of movement or activity, and the immediate postictal behavior.

Physical assessment of these patients should include:

1. Inspection to see if the tongue was bitten. Look for the presence of blood on the teeth or in the mouth. Do *not* use the fingers!
2. Inspection for other injuries, in case the patient may have fallen and hit head or sustained abrasions.
3. Recording VS, including temperature (axillary is probably best).
4. Documentation of any "fruity" or alcohol odor on breath.
5. Auscultation of chest and heart.

If the seizure occurs in the ED, the immediate steps to be taken are protection of the patient from harm, maintenance of the airway with supportive O_2, use of suction if necessary, and administration of diazepam (Valium), diphenyhydantoin (Dilantin), or phenobarbital, according to the physician's orders.

Supportive follow-up care includes these steps:

1. Keep the patient protected.
2. If cause of seizure is unknown, the following may be indicated:
   CBC
   Blood sugar
   BUN
   Serum calcium
   Lumbar puncture
   ECG and EEG
   Blood cultures
   Skull series

3. Keep family and/or friends informed.

4. Use tepid baths, acetylsalicylic acid, etc., if indicated for treatment of febrile seizure.

5. Arrange for immediate home care and follow-up instructions to patient and family if findings do not warrant hospitalization.

SICKLE CELL DISEASE

Dorland's describes sickle cell anemia as a hereditary, genetically determined hemolytic anemia, one of the hemoglobinopathies occurring almost exclusively in the Black race, and characterized by elevated temperature, arthralgia, weakness, respiratory distress, acute abdominal pain with swelling, ulcerations of the lower extremities, and sickle-shaped erythrocytes in the blood.

The patient with sickle cell anemia is subject to depletion of bone marrow production when infection strikes and may present with increasing anemia accompanied by marked weakness, pallor, and icterus if hemolysis develops.

Treatment consists of *pain relief* with the lesser analgesics, administration of *fluids* to reverse dehydration and sickling, typing and crossmatching blood, with administration of blood products as indicated by CBC, and supplemental oxygen, as indicated by ABGs to offset hypoxia. Essentially, the therapy for sickle cell anemia is purely symptomatic; very few patients live beyond the age of 40.

Both young Black males and females may die suddenly from complications of the sickle cell *trait,* not the disease, and these may occur when the victim is exposed to decreased oxygen tension, which produces a massive sickling of almost the entire red blood supply of the body. For this reason, patients with this hemoglobin abnormality should be cautioned against high altitudes and unpressurized planes since lowered oxygen tension increases the sickling tendency, and several instances of splenic infarction and death following air travel have been reported.

HEADACHES

Until 1962 little or no classification had been developed for headaches, and they were considered a symptom of a great number of diseases and abnormalities. Since 1962 there has been the "Classification of Headache" table, which was developed by the Ad Hoc Committee on Classification of Headache.* Headache may be a symptom of intracranial or systemic disease, or it may indicate a stress reaction (as in migraine or tension headache). Although most patients suffer from the latter, emergency personnel must be aware of and alert to the potentially more serious causes of headache.

Physical signs are rare in the patient complaining of severe headache, and history is extremely important. There are several formats for gathering the patient's historical data, but essentially the most significant information is obtained by utilizing the following checklist.

---

*Classification of headache. JAMA, Vol 179, pp 717-718, 1962

1. Duration of illness (headache)
2. Age at onset
3. Frequency of attacks
4. Time of onset
5. Mode of onset
6. Quality of pain
7. Site
8. Associated symptoms
9. Precipitating factors
10. Relieving factors

The individual patient's history, with special reference to the pattern of the headache, is the best guide to the specific diagnostic procedures that should follow.

Some excellent axiomatic guidelines for the evaluation and management of headache are offered by Dr. Alan Friedman, Professor of Neurology at the University of Arizona Medical Center*:

1. Headaches recurring regularly for a number of years most likely represent some form of vascular headache.
2. A sudden onset of severe headache, particularly if followed by impairment of consciousness, suggests a serious illness.
3. Headache appearing for the first time in the aged is not likely to be due to migraine, muscle-contraction headache, or a primary psychiatric disorder.

BITES AND STINGS

Although bites and stings technically fall into the category of surface trauma, they will be considered here as medical emergencies and the four most serious types of envenomation will be briefly discussed.

Snake Bite

The majority of poisonous snake bites in the United States are those of *pit vipers,* so termed because of a deep "pit" between the eye and nostril as well as a triangular head. This group includes the cottonmouth, copperhead, and the rattlesnake; they are found in every state in the continental United States except Maine. Victims will experience early signs of burning pain, numbness and tingling, anesthesias about the tongue, lips, head, and extremities. Swelling, starting within minutes, will progress from the wound proximally and, if present, can be diagnostic. Systemic symptoms include malaise, sweating, and dizziness which are followed by vesiculations, petechiae, ecchymoses, thrombosis, tissue necrosis, fever, hypotension, and pulmonary edema.

The mainstay of treatment is *antivenin,* given as early as possible; it is probably of little use if started more than two hours postbite. Suggested doses

*Friedman AP: *In* Pain, Current Concepts on Pain and Analgesia. Vol 1, No 3, Burroughs Wellcome, New York, 1974

have increased steadily with an average dose being 10 to 20 vials. "Early" pro-phylactic fasciotomy which used to be the recognized standard treatment has become highly controversial.

The only indiginous *non-pit viper* that carries a threat is the coral snake. Its range is limited to the Southeast and Southwest United States. The bite pro-duces little pain with no necrosis or edema; the venom contains a highly neu-rotoxic component which primarily produces flaccid paralysis and death by respiratory failure, the onset of which occurs from 4 to 6 hours after the bite. Victims require three to six vials of specific coral snake antivenin and it must be given immediately since the neurologic abnormalities are difficult to reverse if the antivenin is administered late.

With both types of envenomation, the ED must be able to support the pa-tient's respiratory, circulatory, neurological, and immunologic systems. Shock, DIC, electrolyte imbalance, and respiratory arrest are the main threats to life.

Spider Bites

Two major types of reactions occur with spider envenomation; *black widow spider* venom causes systemic neurotoxic reactions, and *brown recluse* venom causes local tissue necrosis.

The black widow female is *shiny* black with a red *hourglass* on the abdo-men; its web is characteristic in that it appears completely disorganized and will be found in attics, garages, dark recesses, and cracks in cement walls. Calcium gluconate IV will help relax abdominal rigidity of victims, Valium IV may help sedate, and one injection of antivenin is usually sufficient in most cases.

The brown recluse spider, which is prevalent only in Arkansas, Oklahoma, and Missouri (but may occasionally be transported), envenomates and causes severe local necrosis. Initially, the bite causes little pain and is often overlooked until localized pain and erythema develop several hours later. A typical "bulls-eye lesion" develops subsequently and is followed in several days by a large necrotic area with a purple-black ulcerating center. This forms an eschar within about a week, followed by sloughing and tissue defect in another week or two.

Dexamethasone IM is given every 6 hours during the acute phase of the lesion, some physicians recommend excision of the bite area, tetanus pro-phylaxis is given, and secondary infection is treated, if it develops, with broad-spectrum antibiotics. Eventually, many of these cosmetically unacceptable lesions require excision and plastic repair.

REVIEW

1. List four criteria for treating fever as an emergency.
2. Describe three major mechanisms of fever production.

3. Define heat stroke and its symptoms.

4. Describe five steps in the management of temperature elevation.

5. Explain the difference between heat stroke and heat exhaustion.

6. Outline at least six steps for control of fever and febril convulsions in children.

7. Identify the five mechanisms of heat loss from the body.

8. Describe the signs and symptoms of a lowering core temperature as they correlate to the degree of hypothermia.

9. Identify the temperature range within which the heart beat becomes erratic.

10. Identify some widely used drugs that can contribute to hypothermia.

11. Define active internal warmth, external warmth, and active external warmth, as applied to management of the hypothermic patient.

12. Describe the nursing responsibilities in the management of rewarming a hypothermic patient.

13. Explain the drawbacks of using the tub immersion method of rewarming.

14. Describe the rationale for administration of warm saturated oxygen to a hypothermic subject.

15. Describe the management for frostbite of the extremities.

16. List at lest six reasons to suspect a metabolic cause for coma or near-coma.

17. Identify the mnemonics used when working through a differential diagnosis for the comatose or near-comatose patient.

18. Identify the two conditions that will produce flaccid paralysis and reactive pupils.

19. Describe the treatment for parkinsonian crisis secondary to phenothiazine ingestion.

20. Explain the physiology of an anaphylactic reaction and the immediate steps that must be taken.

21. Identify some nursing actions that may reduce the possibility of anaphylactic reactions.

22. Identify the three characteristics or phases of a seizure.

23. Describe a grand mal seizure.

24. Describe a jacksonian seizure.

25. Explain the way in which a seizure episode should be documented.

26. Describe the postictal assessment and supportive follow-up care of the seizure patient.

27. Explain sickle cell anemia and describe the basic management of a patient in sickle cell crisis.

28. Identify the important historical data to be gathered for the patient with severe headache.

29. List three axiomatic guidelines for the evaluation and management of patients presenting with severe headache.

30. Describe the recognition and management of diabetic patients with hypoglycemia and hyperglycemia with ketoacidosis.
31. Identify the key points in recognition and management of snake bite and spider bite victims.

BIBLIOGRAPHY

Alexy BJ: Problems due to cold. JEN, Vol 6, No 1, pp 22-24, January/February 1980

Auerbach P, Geehr E (eds): Environmental Emergencies, TEM. Aspen Systems Publications, Rockville, Maryland, Vol 2, No 3, October 1980

Barber, Budassi S: Management of the comatose patient (a decision tree). JEN, Vol 3, No 1, 1977

Brady WJ: Medical Investigation of Deaths in Oregon. State Health Division, Salem, Oregon, 1981

Brunner L, Suddarth D: The Lippincott Manual of Nursing Practice, 2nd ed. J.B. Lippincott Co., Philadelphia, Pennsylvania, 1982

Budassi SA, Barber JM: Emergency Nursing: Principles and Practice. C.V. Mosby Co., St. Louis, Missouri, 1981

Cain H: Flint's Manual on Emergency Treatment and Management. C.V. Mosby Co., St. Louis, Missouri, 1980

Canan J: Migraine headaches. JEN, Vol 6, No 2, pp 9-13, March/April 1980

Chaney R: Hypothermia: Rewarming methods and hazards. Seventh Annual Scientific Assembly, SeaTac, Washington State ACEP, 1977

Cosgriff J, Anderson D: The Practice of Emergency Nursing. J.B. Lippincott Co., Philadelphia, Pennsylvania, 1975

Dorland's Illustrated Medical Dictionary, 26th ed. W.B. Saunders Co., Philadelphia, Pennsylvania, 1982

Friedman AP: The headache patient. In Pain, Current Concepts on Pain and Analgesia. Vol 1, No 3, Burroughs Wellcome Co., New York, New York, 1974

Friedman B: Hyperpyrexic syndromes. Emergency Med, July 1973

Gephardt D: Anaphylaxis from insect stings. JEN, Vol 4, No 3, pp 19-23, May/June 1978

Glanzer E: Headache. Third Annual Rocky Mountain Emergency Conference, Keystone, Colorado, ACEP, 1977

Goldberg T: The unconscious patient. Physicians in Hospital Emergency Departments, US Department of Health, Education, and Welfare, Rockville, Maryland, 1971

Kolin M: A third diabetic shock syndrome: Hyperosmolar hyperglycemic nonketotic coma. JEN, Vol 3, No 1, pp 15-17, 1977

Kleid J, Heckman B: Handbook of Medical Emergencies. Medical Examination Publishing Co., New York, 1973

Martin P: Is it ketoacidosis? Jen, Vol 3, No 1, pp 11-14, 1977

Mafford E: Allergic reactions: Plan ahead! JEN, Vol 1, No 5, pp 36-40, 1975

Meeuwsen M: Near drowning. Emergency Highlights, Vol 2, No 3, Emanuel Life Flight, Portland, Oregon, October 1981

Merck Manual of Diagnosis and Therapy, 13th ed. Merck, Sharpe & Dohme Research Laboratories, West Point, Pennsylvania, 1977

Poward D, Lee S, Haywood J: What the emergency nurse needs to know about sickle cell disease. JEN, Vol 2, No 4, pp 15-21, 1976

Ravin M, Modell J: Introduction to Life Support. Little, Brown, & Co., Boston, Massachusetts, 1973

Siegel AM: Endocrine emergencies. Emergency Med, pp 114-117, July 1973

Speich P: Brought back to life: A case study in hypothermia. JEN, Vol 3, No 2, pp 9-12, 1977

Stevenson B: Anaphylaxis. Seventh Annual Scientific Assembly, SeaTac, Washington State ACEP, 1977

Treating cold exposure injury. Emergency Products Magazine, pp 30-33, November/December 1974

Warner C: Emergency Care: Assessment and Intervention, 2nd ed. C.V. Mosby Co., St. Louis, Missouri, 1978

Wingert WA: Poisoning by animal venom. Environmental Medical Emergencies, TEM, Vol 2, No 3, Rockville, Maryland, October 1980

Yocum RF, Bohler S: Heat stroke. JEN, Vol 7, No 4, pp 144-147, July/August 1981

PHARMACOLOGY REVIEW **25**

KEY CONCEPTS

The material in this chapter has been compiled to provide an opportunity for the EDN to review some areas of basic pharmacology and to develop an overview of some of the more frequently used drugs and combinations of drugs in the emergency department. The bulk of the chapter content was developed for presentation to emergency nurses by James Sanger, Director of Pharmacy at Good Samaritan Hospital and Medical Center in Portland, Oregon.

After reading and studying this chapter, you should be able to:

- Define some of the specific terms used with drug actions and interactions.
- Identify the known mechanisms of drug interactions.
- Identify some of the factors affecting the amount of drug absorbed by the body.
- List the major general guidelines pertaining to safe drug administration in the emergency department.
- Identify three major pharmacologic actions that influence the control of pain.
- List the major actions of morphine sulfate.
- Identify the major analgesics in use other than morphine sulfate.
- Identify the clinical uses, side effects, and toxic levels for barbiturates.
- Identify agents that intensify the actions of sedative/hypnotic drugs.
- Describe the management of a tricyclic antidepressant overdose.
- Identify the major groups of commonly used anti-anxiety agents.
- List the considerations in avoiding toxic reactions with local anesthesia.
- List the major groups of diuretic agents commonly used and their actions.
- Identify the groups of most commonly used antibiotics.
- Identify some of the commonly used steroids and their emergency applications.
- Describe the administration of medication in a hypertensive crisis.

Recent years have seen the introduction and widespread use of an incredibly large number of potent and highly effective pharmacologic agents. Simultaneously, there has been a trend developing to combine drugs into one medication, resulting in multiple drug therapy as a fact of life, a fact that every physician and nurse must be cognizant of. Total awareness must be developed toward the possibilities of drug interactions resulting in serious problems for the patient. For this reason it is incumbent upon every EDN to maintain a current knowledge of the major properties of individual drugs that are kept and used in the department as well as the ability to recognize cardinal untoward reactions which may occur if the wrong drugs are administered simultaneously. As one physician has put it, "Some of these drugs, although innoculous in solo, can be lethal in concert."

DRUG TERMINOLOGY

A review of some of the specific terminology applied to drug actions and interactions is appropriate:

Therapeutic effect: The main effect desired from the administration of a drug in a curative sense.

Secondary effects: Beneficial changes as a result of improvement of the primary condition for which the therapy was initiated; may include a sense of well-being in a person whose asthma has been relieved or a relief of mental anguish caused by pain, or an arthritic condition relieved by an anti-inflammatory agent.

Side effects: All effects seen as a result of drug use beyond the principal desired effect. *Example:* Morphine constricts the pupil of the eye.

Untoward effects: A harmful side effect. *Example:* Morphine can cause nausea and vomiting.

Intolerance: Excessive side effects in some, as in the postural hypotension occasionally seen with small doses of nitrites, well below the usual therapeutic dose.

Idiosyncrasy: An abnormal or unexpected effect of a drug peculiar to an individual. *Example:* Morphine or codeine may excite rather than sedate some persons.

Hypersensitivity: A reaction to a drug in excess of, or different from, the expected effect, as with an allergic response. May be annoying or even severely toxic. *Example:* agranulocytosis, serum sickness, urticaria, or anaphylactic shock.

Cumulative effect: The effect when a drug is absorbed more rapidly than it is excreted. Toxic effects may occur as a result of an accumulation of drug in the tissues.

Antagonistic effect: The effect of one drug opposing the other. This is the principle of many antidotes.

Synergistic effect: Joint action of drugs, each enhancing the effect of the other.

Potentiation: Much like synergism in that one drug enhances the effect of the other.

Addiction: A state of periodic or chronic intoxication produced by repeated consumption of a drug, characterized by 1) an overwhelming desire or need (compulsion) to continue use of the drug and to obtain it by any means; 2) a tendency to increase the dosage; 3) a psychological and usually a physical dependence on its effects; and 4) a detrimental effect on the individual (Dorland's Medical Dictionary, 25th edition) and on society.

FACTORS INFLUENCING
RESPONSE TO DRUGS

Numerous factors influence the body's response to any given drug, including environmental situations, genetic makeup, diet, other concurrent drug ingestions, age, sex, height, weight, tolerance, body temperature, diurnal variation, liver and kidney function, pathologic states, mode of administration, dosage level, and circulatory status. These are but some of the many and variable factors that are thought to have an effect on drug interactions as well. Generally, the known mechanisms of *drug interactions* involve one or sometimes a combination of alterations in absorption, distribution, metabolism, enzyme activity, or excretion of one drug by another.

Absorption is affected by the factors relating to the contents of the GI tract, such as pH of the gut, motility, bacterial flora, etc. *Example*: Acidic drugs such as aspirin and phenobarbital are more readily absorbed from a stomach that has a low pH, but absorption can be delayed or inhibited if antacid drugs that raise the pH of the stomach are administered.

Availability is affected by the extent to which the drug is bound to plasma protein. Most drugs are bound to the albumin portion, and there is a varying affinity between the drug and its binding site on the albumin molecule. The part bound to the plasma protein is pharmacologically inactive; the remaining portion is available to produce the pharmacologic effect.

Metabolism of large numbers of drugs occurs with enzymes located in the liver so that the drugs are changed into a chemical form more easily excreted by the kidneys, and the rate at which these enzymes metabolize drugs varies considerably. Many drugs delay the metabolism of other drugs by inhibition of the liver enzymes.

Excretion of one drug can be affected by the action of another drug, depending upon alteration of the urinary pH and occasionally on tubular excretion interference. Acidic drugs (phenobarbital, aspirin, the sulfonamides, etc.) are excreted more rapidly when urine is alkaline, while basic drugs (amphetamines, imipramine, meperidine, etc.) are more promptly excreted at an acid pH. The effects of a single dose of amphetamine can last for several days if the urinary pH is sufficiently alkaline.

Other factors such as alterations of electrolyte levels and sensitivity of enzyme system receptor sites have an effect as well on drug interactions.

All drug interactions should be viewed in their proper perspective. They are not all clinically significant, obviously, but we should be informed and aware of potential hazards, and we should know the drugs we use, employing the *Physicians' Desk Reference* or *National Formulary* as often as necessary, as well as any other drug references or evaluations that we may have ready access to.

GUIDELINES FOR
SAFE DRUG ADMINISTRATION

The following general guidelines pertain to safe drug administration in the ED setting:

1. Know the drugs you are giving! Do not give a drug unless you are certain of its indications, contraindications, dosage, how often it may be given, and the side effects and untoward effects that may be encountered.
2. Take a careful drug history, making it a part of your nursing history. Your patient may be on the wrong drug, too much drug, incompatible drugs, and the presenting problem may, in fact, be drug-related.
3. Check for a history of drug allergy or idiosyncratic reaction to drugs, being specific as to the manifestation of the "allergy" and remembering to chart allergies on *all* patients.
4. Know the preferred route of administration, since some drugs are poorly absorbed IM or PO, and some drugs should not be given IV. Know the factors influencing oral administration absorption, two examples of which are the interference of antacids in tetracycline absorption and the decreased absorption of many drugs by the presence of food, especially antibiotics.

EXAMPLES OF DRUG INTERACTIONS

A few examples of some of the more commonly prescribed drugs and their interactions are given in Table 25.1.

CONTROLLED DRUGS

In 1970 the old Harrison Narcotic Act (which dealt only with narcotics) and its amendments were superseded by the passage of the Comprehensive Drug

Table 25.1 Examples of Interactions of Some Commonly Prescribed Drugs With Other Drugs

DRUG	INTERACTING DRUG	RESULT
Alcohol	Barbiturates and Narcotics	Increased CNS Depression
Alcohol	Oral hypoglycemics	Antabuse reaction
Alcohol	Metronidazole (Flagyl)	Antabuse reaction
Neomycin	Furosemide (Lasix)	Ototoxicity
Oral hypoglycemics	Phenylbutazone (Butazoladine)	Hypoglycemia
Coumarins	Salicylates	Increased hypoprothrombinemia
Digitalis	Diuretics	Increased toxicity
Sodium diphenylhydantoin (Dilantin)	Antabuse	Dilantan toxicity
Tetracyclines	Iron, antacid, food	Decreased absorption
Probenecid (Benemid)	Salicylates	Decreased uricosuric effect

Abuse Prevention and Control Act, which created the Bureau of Narcotics and Dangerous Drugs (BNDD). During 1974 the BNDD was renamed and reorganized into what is now called the Drug Enforcement Agency (DEA).

Drugs subject to control by DEA have been regrouped and reclassified and are now divided into five schedules instead of what used to be "classes" of drugs. With the advent of the numerous groups of sedative/hypnotic/tranquilizer drugs that have come on the market in the last 10-15 years, the need for closer regulation and elimination of free access to these drugs has become very clear. For this reason the five categories or "schedules," as they are called, have come into existence, replacing the old classifications under the Harrison Act.

Schedule I   Substances that have no legitimate medical use and high addiction or abuse potential: heroin, LSD, marijuana, mescaline

Schedule II   Substances that have an accepted medical use and a high addiction and abuse potential: morphine, methadone, methaqualone (Quaalude), cocaine, amphetamines, alphaprodine (Nisentil), and others. Recent additions have been the short-acting barbiturates such as pentobarbital (Nembutal), secobarbital (Seconal) and amobarbital (Amytal), oxycodone HCl (percodan), and methylphenidate (Ritalin).

Schedule III   Substances that have an accepted medical use and a lower abuse potential than those listed in Schedules I and II: Glutethimide (Doriden), codeine phosphate (Empirin 3 Compound and Tylenol 3 Compound), etc.

Schedule IV   Substances that have an accepted medical use and a lower abuse potential than substances listed in Schedules I, II and

III: Meprobamate (Equanil), chloral hydrate, chlordiaze-poxide (Librium), diazepam (Valium), oxazepam (Serax), flurzepam (Dalmane), propoxyphane HCl (all Darvon prep-arations), and pentazocine (Talwin), although several states have independently moved Talwin to Schedule II because of its wide abuse potential.

Schedule V   Substances that have an accepted medical use and a lower abuse potential than substances in the preceding sched-ules. *Examples:* Diphenoxylate HCl with atropine sulfate (Lomotil). Some states include cough syrups containing co-deine and Tedral which contains ephedrine (stimulant).

ANALGESICS

It is important for the EDN to remember that assessment of the quality and nature of pain belongs to the one who experiences it, too often patients are given inadequate doses and too infrequently. It is the old story of too little, too late. If a narcotic has been ordered by the physician and if, in the best judg-ment of the nurse, the patient will not be harmed by administration of the drug it should be given as ordered for the relief of both pain *and* anxiety. Analgesics given in the ED are by nature short-term administrations, and the EDN need not fear that the patient will become addicted by doses commensurate with the level of pain he is experiencing.

The control of pain is influenced by three major pharmacologic actions:

1. Counteracting the cause of pain.
2. Blocking the peripheral pain impulses.
3. Modifying the central reception of pain.

Morphine sulfate is the standard of reference for all potent analgesic drugs. Named for the Latin god of sleep, Morpheus, it is a bitter white crystalline alkaloid of opium, which produces relief of pain and induces sleep; it is one of the oldest pharmacologic and therapeutic drugs used in "modern" medicine.

The actions of morphine are:

1. Depression of the CNS response to pain
2. Constriction of the pupils
3. Depression of the respiratory rate
4. Decrease in GI motility
5. Decrease in gastric, biliary, and pancreatic secretions
6. Peripheral vasodilatation with histamine release (never give to patients with head injuries or asthma)
7. Stimulation of the chemoreceptor trigger zone, with vomiting.

Some of the properties of morphine that should be kept in mind are:

1. Peak brain levels are achieved 45 min after subcutaneous administration.

2. Morphine is metabolized by the liver.
3. It is poorly absorbed from the GI tract.
4. Tolerance to the drug develops rapidly.
5. Dependence on the drug develops at a lower level than does dependence on heroin or hydromorphone (Dilaudid).

Morphine is used as an analgesic for severe pain and frequently as a preliminary medication before anesthesia, often with atropine. This combination promotes a relaxed state and aids with induction of anesthesia. It is the drug of choice for acute MI pain and is given IV in that instance to prevent "pooling," to give rapid analgesia, and to prevent an elevation of the CPK from IM administration. Morphine should be diluted out and given in small increments of 2-4 mg when it is given by IV push. It should be used with caution in 1) any potentially hypotensive state, 2) convulsive disorders, and 3) trauma with concomitant head injury because of the respiratory depression, increased PCO_2, and vasodilatation that it may cause, resulting in increased intracranial pressure. It must *never* be given during asthmatic attacks or to patients with acute cholecystitis (it is thought to cause spasm of the sphincter of Oddi).

Some general points of pertinent information regarding the strong analgesic agents are:

1. Morphine sulfate 10 mg is an equivalent dose to meperidine HCl (Demerol) 100 mg.
2. Codeine is less potent than morphine and is used for mild to moderate pain, has a low dependence potential, depresses the cough center, and the optimum dose for severe pain is 60 mg.
3. Meperidine HCl (Demerol), oxymorphone (Numorphan), and methotrimeprazine (Levoprome) are less antitussive than codeine.
4. Hydromorphone (Dilaudid) is more active than morphine but has a shorter duration of action.
5. Hydrocodone (Hycodan) is similar to codeine and is used to lessen coughing.
6. Meperidine (Demerol) is a synthetic substitute for morphine; it causes addiction at a slower rate, and withdrawal symptoms are not as severe. The respiratory depression produced is less than that of morphine.
7. Methadone HCl (Dolophine) is a synthetic analgesic at least as effective as morphine. It may be substituted for morphine for the drug addict and subsequent withdrawal will be less severe, although it may be more prolonged. Methadone is now one of our most abused drugs.
8. Levorphanol tartrate (Levo-Dromoran) is a synthetic about five times as analgesic as morphine.
9. Methotrimeprazine (Levoprome) has no dependence, gives marked sedation, and may induce postural hypotension.
10. Pentazocine (Talwin) has a low incidence of dependence and will precipitate withdrawal in patients on narcotics. It is a narcotic antagonist. It is also a poor drug for relief of MI pain since it increases myocardial oxygen consumption by elevating the blood pressure.

11. The *best* narcotic antagonist to use is naloxone (Narcan) because 1) it is not a partial agonist and 2) has no respiratory depression, unlike nalorphine (Nalline).

Two points of interest concerning the "milder" analgesics are that 1) it is generally acknowledged that no evidence exists to prove that one acetylsalicylic acid tablet is better than any other, and 2) that propoxyphene (Darvon) overdose is very serious and can precipitate hypotension worse than that caused by other narcotics. It should always be treated immediately with naloxone. Management of overdoses is discussed in Chapter 26.

The standards by which all analgesics are compared, by and large, are the doses that are given subcutaneously or orally to produce approximately the same analgesic effect as morphine sulfate, 10 mg, codeine sulfate, 60 mg, or aspirin, 10 gr. Therefore, morphine is at the top of the scale as follows:

Morphine sulfate   10 mg SC or PO—severe pain
Codeine sulfate   60 mg SC or PO—moderate pain
Aspirin   10 gr PO—mild pain

There are many drugs available for analgesia but these three remain the standards by which the potency of all others is adjudged. Both morphine and codeine retain most of their analgesic efficacy when given orally.

SEDATIVE/HYPNOTICS

Among the sedative/hypnotics are the barbiturates, bromides, chloral hydrate, scopolamine and glutethimide (Doriden). These drugs are CNS depressants, affecting the respiratory centers of the brain. Barbiturates are considered the standard by which to gauge all the others, and an example of the dose-related effects of barbiturates is shown with pentobarbital (Nembutal), in which the effects at various dosage levels are as follows:

30 mg   Tranquilization
60 mg   Sedation
100 mg   Sleep (hypnotic level)
500 mg   Coma
1000 mg   Death

With toxicity of barbiturates or any other sedative/hypnotics, the rule of thumb is that about *10 times the hypnotic dose* (sleep-producing) *is generally fatal.* In other words, an overdose of 10 × 100 mg pentobarbital capsules would be lethal unless intervention is initiated in time.

CLINICAL USES

The clinical uses of the barbiturates include 1) sedation, 2) preanesthetic medication, 3) anticonvulsant therapy, and 4) hypertension therapy. The side effects include drowsiness and impaired performance and judgment.

INTENSIFYING AGENTS

Agents that intensify and/or potentiate the actions of sedative/hypnotic drugs are *alcohol,* phenothiazine derivatives (Trilafon, Sparine, Stelazine, Thorazine), narcotics, and other sedative/hypnotics.

TERMINATION OF EFFECTS

The mechanisms for termination of the barbiturates are physical redistribution from the brain to other tissues (fat or muscle), metabolism (inactivation by enzymes in the liver), and excretion of the drug by the kidneys. With barbiturate intoxication, the urine should be alkalinized to speed excretion of the drug.

The difference between sedative/hypnotics and the antianxiety drugs is that the sedative/hypnotics affect the reticular activating system (RAS) of the cerebral cortex, producing symptoms much like those of alcohol ingestion, with ataxia, euphoria, drowsiness, and incoordination, while the antianxiety drugs effect the limbic system and the emotions. These include the phenothiazines such as Trilafon, Sparine, Stelazine, and Thorazine. Alcohol may *severely* enhance the depressive effect of all these sedative drugs and does, indeed, account for many of the profoundly potentiated barbiturate ingestions.

As hypnotics, chlorate hydrate 1 g, pentobarbital (Nembutal) 100 mg, secobarbital (Seconal) 100 mg, and diphenhydramine (Benadryl) 50 mg, are all effective; they all decrease rapid eye movement (REM) sleep. Flurazepam HCl (Dalmane) is one sedative/hypnotic that does not decrease REM sleep and is rapidly metabolized.

One major hypnotic agent responsible for many serious problems in the ED is glutethimide (*Doriden*). This is a very effective drug, especially with elderly patients, but produces an extremely serious overdose situation and is felt by many to be a drug that should be taken off the market because of the fatalities that have resulted from its availability and abuse. Doriden overdose will be discussed in Chapter 26.

PSYCHOTHERAPEUTIC AGENTS

PSYCHOLEPTICS

All the drugs in the major and minor tranquilizer groups are known as *psycholeptics,* meaning that they affect the psyche and emotional responses by action of the limbic system. Management of cumulative and toxic effects will be discussed in Chapter 26, Drug Abuse and Toxicology.

This group of antianxiety drugs is so widely used by the general public and becomes so confusing with the many categories and modes of action that their characteristics should be briefly discussed.

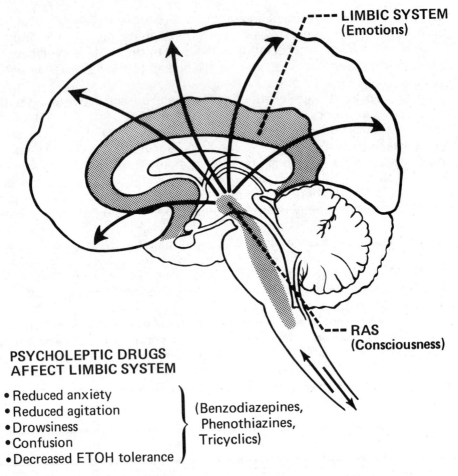

**SEDATIVE/HYPONOTIC DRUGS
AFFECT RAS↓**

- Ataxia
- Euphoria
- Drowsiness
- Incoordination
- Decreased ETOH tolerance

(Barbiturates,
Bromides
Chloral Hydrate,
Doriden)

---- **LIMBIC SYSTEM**
(Emotions)

---- **RAS**
(Consciousness)

**PSYCHOLEPTIC DRUGS
AFFECT LIMBIC SYSTEM**

- Reduced anxiety
- Reduced agitation
- Drowsiness
- Confusion
- Decreased ETOH tolerance

(Benzodiazepines,
Phenothiazines,
Tricyclics)

Figure 25.1. Drugs affecting the CNS.

The *minor tranquilizers* are the *benzodiazepines* which include chlordiaze-poxide (Librium), diazepam (Valium), oxazepam (Serax), and chlorazepate (Tranxene). They may cause frequent drowsiness, confusion, ataxia, tolerance and physical dependence, with an occasional case of hypotension and extra-pyramidal symptoms occurring with chlordiazepoxide. Blood dyscrasias and jaundice are rare.

The *major tranquilizers* include the *phenothiazines* such as prochlorpera-zine (Compazine), proxmazine (Sparine), fluphenazine (Prolixin), pro-methazine (Phenergen), trifluoperazine (Stelazine), thioridizine (Mellaril), chlorpromazine (Thorazine), and triflupromazine (Vesprin) and the *butyro-phenones* such as haloperidol (Haldol), droperidol (Inapsine), and fentanyl/droperidol (Innovar). These drugs sedate the psychotic patient and reduce anxiety and agitation. During administration of these drugs, however, the patient should be warned that:

1. All CNS depressants, such as alcohol and barbiturates, must be avoided.
2. The drugs may reverse the effects of epinephrine to produce a lowered blood pressure, may mimic alcoholic drunkenness in their effect, and may cause dermatitis, anorexia, and jaundice.

PSYCHOANALEPTICS

Drugs that exert a stimulating effect on the mind are called *psychoanaleptics*. This group is comprised of both *MOA inhibitors* and the *tricyclic antidepressants*.

Monoamine oxidase (MAO) inhibitors are drugs that elevate the mood, reduce fatigue, and increase vigor, some of them also lower blood pressure. They include tranylcypromine (Parnate), phenelzine (Nardil), and pargyline (Eutony). When patients are given these drugs, they must be warned as follows:

1. Avoid any other MAO inhibitors concurrently; avoid amitriptyline (Elavil), imipramine (Tofranil), ephedrine, and all sympathomimetic amines and nasal decongestants, cold and sinus remedies.
2. *Acute hypertension* may be produced by the concurrent use of alcohol, broad beans, cheddar cheese, pickled herring, and chicken livers, which are all *tyramine-containing* foods. Tyramine is a breakdown product of metabolism that is closely related structurally to epinephrine and norepinephrine and has a similar but weaker action. It is found in decayed animal tissue, ripe cheese, and ergot.

The *tricyclic antidepressants* include the amitriptyline hydrochlorides (Elavil, Etrafon, and Triavil) and imipramine hydrochlorides (Tofranil and Presamine) and are *not* MAO inhibitors.

Elavil and Tofranil are the two most commonly used of this group and may cause a mild CNS stimulation but may also produce oversedation with high doses, which manifests with CNS disturbances, hypotension, and arrhythmias. These drugs should not be taken concurrently with barbiturates, other CNS depressants, or MAO inhibitors. Management of overdoses with these drugs is discussed in Chapter 26.

Two other commonly used sedatives are the hydroxyzines (Atarax and Vistaril) and diphenhydramine (Benadryl). Benadryl has a strong antihistamine effect, is an antiemetic, and an effective sedative. When administered parenterally, Benadryl should be given deep IM or IV but never SC.

Atarax is given orally with either tablet or syrup, while Vistaril is given PO or IM. Vistaril is a rapid-acting true ataraxic, capable of producing a detached serenity without depression of mental faculties or clouding of consciousness, as well as having antihistaminic and antiemetic effects. Vistaril *potentiates* narcotics and barbiturates, and concurrent doses must be adjusted accordingly. *Never* give Vistaril SC or IV; it must be given deep IM to avoid local discomfort to the tissues.

The pharmacist who dispenses, or the physician or nurse who administers, any of these sedative/hypnotic medications has an obligation to the patient to warn him or her of the sedative properties and their effect on *decreased alcohol tolerance, driving ability, and the overall coordination required to operate any other machinery.*

Diazepam

A word of warning about diazepam (Valium), since it is used so frequently in the ED for intervention in seizure states, preparatory to cardioversion and closed reduction of fractures, and for reversing hypersensitivity response to lidocaine. When diazepam is given IV, the solution should be injected *slowly,* directly into the vein, taking at least 1 min for each 5 mg (1 cc) given. *Do not mix or dilute injectable diazepam with other solutions or drugs and do not add to IV fluids.* When diazepam is injected via a running IV line, it should be preceded and followed by an alcohol flush (absolute alcohol 1 ampule in 30 cc distilled water) to prevent precipitation in the IV line.

Extreme care must be used in administering diazepam by IV line to the elderly, to very ill patients, and to those with limited pulmonary reserve because of the possibility that *apnea and/or cardiac arrest may occur.* Resuscitative equipment, including that necessary to support respiration, should be readily available.

When diazepam is used with a narcotic analgesic, the dosage of the narcotic should be reduced by at least *one-third* and administered in *small increments.* In some cases the use of a narcotic may not be necessary.

Butyrophenone

The butyrophenones droperidol (Inapsine) and fentanyl/droperidol (Innovar) should be reviewed here as well since droperidol is being increasingly used in highly disturbed patients and have some specific guidelines that must be followed for safe administration.

Innovar contains fentanyl (Sublimaze) as well as droperidol (Inapsine), both of which have different pharmacologic actions with widely differing durations of action.

Fentanyl (Sublimaze) is a potent narcotic analgesic (Schedule II) with a rapid onset and short duration of activity. It is similar to morphine but is 60 times more potent; drug-induced bradycardia from fentanyl is blocked or reversed by atropine and most of fentanyl's effects including analgesia are reversed with naloxone (Narcan).

Droperidol (Inapsine), the other component part of Innovar, is administered separately as a potent neuroleptic agent (having an antipsychotic action affecting principally psychomotor activity and generally without hypnotic effects). Other CNS depressant drugs (e.g., barbiturates, major tranquilizers, narcotics, and general anesthetics) will have additive and potentiating effects with droperidol. The administration of other CNS depressants and droperidol should be monitored carefully to avoid excessive CNS depression. When the patient has received other CNS depressants, the effects of which will overlap with those of droperidol, the dose of the latter that is required may be less than usual. Postprocedure narcotics and other depressants should be given in *reduced doses, as low as 25% or 33% of those usually recommended!* A patient in the ED who has received droperidol should have a recording of dose and time given taped to his forehead until transferred out of the department, and an appropriate report should be given to the unit receiving the patient, as well as the documentation on his or her emergency record.

DIURETICS

Diuretics are agents that increase the rate of urine flow. The action of *any* diuretic depends upon functionally active kidneys. Most diuretics interfere with reabsorption of electrolytes by the kidneys, promoting water loss secondarily.

Diuretics can be classified as:

- Naturetic—increases sodium loss
- Diuretic—regulates loss of water, sodium, and chloride
- Saluretic—increases excretion of sodium and chloride

A normal man filters approximately 170 liters of fluid through his kidneys in 24 hours and produces approximately 1.7 liters of urine.

The nephron of the kidney, through which blood is filtered to produce urine, contains the proximal convulution or tubule, which reabsorbs approximately 80% of the sodium, the loop of Henle, which reabsorbs approximately 5-10% of the sodium, and the distal convulution or tubule, which reabsorbs approximately 10-20% of the sodium.

Diuretics are administered for several clinical conditions and the most important among them are:

1. Edema of cardiac origin
2. Sclerosis of the liver
3. Nephrotic edema
4. Essential hypertension
5. Problems relating to chronic fluid retention without essential pathology
6. Emergency situations

THIAZIDES

The thiazide diuretics are the most widely used and act in the proximal tubules to inhibit sodium, chloride, and water reabsorption. The commonly used thiazides include Diuril, HydroDiuril, and Esidrix.

Some of the side effects of the thiazides are 1) potassium depletion, 2) increased uric acid in the blood (prevents urea excretion into the urine), 3) elevated glucose tolerance, and 4) allergic reactions.

OTHER DIURETICS

Other types of diuretics are the *sulfonamide derivatives,* which include quinethazone (Hydromox) and chlorthalidone (Hygroton), and the *mercurial diuretics,* which are not used frequently since the advent of the thiazides but are given to severely dyspneic or massively edematous patients when the thiazides have been ineffective. The mercurials must be given deep IM.

The potent diuretic which is most frequently employed in the emergency setting is furosemide (Lasix) which blocks the reabsorption of sodium and water in the proximal tubule and interferes with sodium reabsorption in the loop of Henle and the proximal portion of the distal tubule. Furosemide given IV is rapid-acting and usually produces profuse diuresis. If given in excessive amounts, it may produce profound diuresis, with water and electrolyte depletion, and therefore, the dosage must be carefully adjusted to the patient's needs.

Ethnacrynic acid (Edecrin) is also a potent diuretic and has much the same mode of action as furosemide. It, too, may produce profound diuresis with water and electrolyte depletion. Sodium ethacrynate (Sodium Edecrin) occasionally causes local irritation and pain after IV administration.

Mannitol is an obligatory osmotic diuretic, which is a commercially prepared sugar alcohol and is virtually inert metabolically. It induces diuresis by elevating the osmolarity (the concentration of osmotically active particles in solution) of the glomerular filtrate, thereby hindering tubular reabsorption of water. The excretion of sodium and chloride is also enhanced. Mannitol is indicated in:

1. Prevention or treatment of the oliguric phase of acute renal failure before irreversible renal failure becomes established.
2. Reduction of intracranial pressure and brain mass.
3. Reduction of high intraocular pressure when the pressure cannot be lowered by other means.
4. Promotion of urinary excretion of toxic materials.

Solutions of mannitol may crystallize when exposed to low temperatures; concentrations of greater than 15% have a greater tendency to crystallization. If crystals are observed, the bottle should be warmed to 50° C (112° F) in a water bath, then cooled to body temperature before administration. When 20% mannitol is infused, the administration set should include an in-line filter for safety.

ANTIBIOTICS

As a general rule, all antibiotics should be taken 1 hour before meals and at bedtime since food decreases absorption of the drug, especially with lincomycin, tetracyclines, and penicillins. Antibiotics given out from the ED should have these instructions written out and explained verbally, as well, to the patient or family.

Any infectious process should be cultured before antibiotics are administered or prescribed for the patient, and every patient should be instructed carefully to continue taking the medication until the entire prescription is gone or to continue medication at least 48-72 hours after the temperature has returned to normal, whichever occurs first.

PENICILLIN

The penicillins (bacteriocides) are among the most effective and least toxic of the available antimicrobials and are excreted by the kidneys.

Pencillin was discovered in 1929 by Sir Alexander Fleming. Some original problems were with penicillin G in crystalline form, which was short-acting, destroyed by stomach acid, led to development of resistant strains, and had a limited spectrum of activities. Since 1929 several longer-acting forms of penicillin have been developed, two of which are a procaine penicillin (Wycillin), having an effective blood level of 12-24 hours, and benzathine penicillin (long-acting) with blood levels from IV injection lasting 48-72 hours.

All the penicillins are effective against gram-positive organisms, although there are many complicating factors. Penicillinase-producing organisms will be most effectively treated by penicillinase-resistant agents. Ampicillin and carbenicillin, while having some activity against gram-positive organisms, are reserved for gram-negative organisms, e.g., *E. coli* and other enterobacters.

1. Acid-labile penicillins are those destroyed by stomach acid:
   A. Penicillin G
   B. Methicillin (Staphcillin)

2. Acid-stable penicillins, not destroyed by stomach acid are:
   A. Phenoxymethyl penicillin (Pen Vee K, V-Cillin K)
   B. Ampicillin (Polycillin, Omnipen)
   C. Oxacillin (Prostaphlin)
   D. Cloxacillin (Tegopen)
   E. Nafcillin (Unipen)

3. Penicillinase-sensitive agents:
   A. Penicillin G
   B. Phenoxymethyl penicillin (Pen Vee K, V-Cillin K)
   C. Ampicillin

4. Penicillinase-resistant agents:
   A. Methicillin (Staphcillin)
   B. Oxacillin (Prostaphlin)
   C. Nafcillin (Unipen)

5. Extended-spectrum penicillins:
   A. Ampicillin (effective against *E. coli* but ineffective with *Staph. aureus*)
   B. *Carbenicillin (Geopen, Pyopen) has resistance problems, is effective against Pseudamonas and Proteus, and is incompatible with gentamicin (Garamycin) in IV solution.*

Penicillin is used widely today against *Streptococcus* and pneumococcus since there are still no resistant forms, and it is used on nonresistant strains of *Staphylococcus*. The toxicity from penicillin ranges from allergic reactions in the form of rashes and diarrhea from ampicillin to anaphylaxis, requiring supportive measures as previously discussed.

Penicillinase (Neutrapen) is an enzyme obtained from cultures of *B. Cereus*, which specifically destroys penicillin G. Penicillinase effectively lowers blood levels of penicillin G in a matter of hours.

CEPHALOSPORINS

The cephalosporins are a group of bacteriocidal agents that have an advantage over pencillin in that they are resistant to hydrolysis by penicillinase. They, too, are excreted primarily by the kidneys and are effective against gram-negative organisms (*E. coli, Proteus,* and *Klebsiella*) and are often substituted in cases of penicillin allergy.

Some of the more commonly administered cephalosporins are cephalothin Keflin (which is painful given IM), cephazolin (Kefzol), cephalexin (Keflex-oral cephalosporin), and the third generation cephalosporin, cephataxime (claforan), which has an extended gram negative spectrum.

The Macrolide antibiotics and lincomycin, used to treat patients allergic to penicillin, include the following:

1. Erythromycin (Ilosone), which develops rapid resistance and may cause jaundice but is drug of choice in *Mycoplasma pneumonia*.
2. Lincomycin (Lincocin) which can cause colitis.
3. Clindamycin (Cleocin) which has fallen into relative disuse because it has been found to cause severe pseudomembranous colitis. It should be used only for severe staphylococcal infections in patients allergic to penicillin and in anaerobic infections, especially bacteroides. It should never be used as routine treatment of otitis media, respiratory infections or UTIs.

Vancomycin (Vancocin) is an antibiotic effective against gram-positive cocci. *Rifampicin* (Rimactane, Rifadin) is an effective antituberculosis drug.

TETRACYCLINES

The tetracyclines are broad-spectrum antibiotics and are bacteriostatic. They are known to discolor the teeth of babies, if given in the last trimester of pregnancy, and of young children, as well as causing frequent cases of photosensitivity. Monilial overgrowth is common following a course of tetra-cycline administration. These drugs are most valuable in mixed infections such as chronic bronchitis and peritonitis. Their intestinal absorption is interfered with by milk; antacids taken to offset frequent toxic responses of nausea, vomiting, and diarrhea will build up toxic levels in patients with poor kidney function.

The commonly prescribed tetracyclines include:

1. Tetracycline (Achromycin and Sumycin), which is effective especially with acne
2. Oxytetracycline (Terramycin)
3. Chlortetracycline (Aureomycin)
4. Demeclocycline (Declomycin) which is particularly prone to causing photosensitivity
5. Methacycline (Rondomycin)
6. Minocycline (Minocin) which may cause dizziness and tinnitus.
7. Doxycycline (Vibramycin) and doxycycline II are the best tetracycline for treatment of gonococcal infections. They should not be used for urinary tract infections (UTIs) because of low urine levels of the drug.

CHLORAMPHENICOL

Chloramphenicol (Chloromycetin) is a broad-spectrum antibiotic that has a high toxicity level and can cause nausea, diarrhea, severe aplastic anemia, and death if given over an extended period of time. It should never be used when another antibiotic will work, but it is considered the drug of choice for typhoid fever, bacteroides, rickettsial infections, tears in the dura because of its ability to cross the blood-brain barrier and *Hemophilus* (organisms that grow best in the presence of hemoglobin) influenza.

AMINOGLYCOSIDES

The aminoglycosides include streptomycin, kanamycin, gentamicin, and neomycin and are used in gram-negative infections because of their spectrum. Their toxicity limits their use with gentamicin (Garamycin) being especially nephrotoxic and ototoxic, affecting the auditory and vestibular branches of the eighth cranial nerve. They are poorly absorbed from the intestinal tract and consequently are frequently used for a bowel prep. Kanamycin and gentamicin are most often used parenterally to combat *Pseudomonas*.

PEPTIDES

The peptide antibiotics include bacitracin (Baciguent), which is used topically against gram-positive organisms, and polymyxin (Aerosporin), which is used against gram-negative organisms. Bacitracin used in large amounts can be nephrotoxic.

SULFONAMIDES

The sulfonamides are coal-tar derivatives that are bacteriostatic and inhibit the bacterial synthesis of folic acid. Sulfonamides are excreted by the kidneys and are used primarily in urinary tract infections, with the usually susceptible organisms being *E. coli, Klebsiella, Staph. aureus,* and *Proteus.* There may be toxicity with prolonged use of large amounts, causing crystallization of the drug in kidney tubules, and nausea, diarrhea, a photosensitivity rash, and hemolytic anemia.

Patients taking any of the sulfa drugs should always be instructed to force clear liquids as long as the medication is being taken. The most common sulfa drugs in use are sulfadiazine, sulfisoxazole (Gantrisin), sulfamethoxazole (Gantanol), triple sulfa mixtures, succinylsulfathiazole (Sulfasuxidine), and mafenide (Sulfamylon cream).

Methenamine mandelate (Mandelamine) is a urinary antibacterial agent and is the chemical combination of mandelic acid with methenamine. It is readily absorbed but remains essentially inactive until it is excreted by the kidney and concentrated in the urine. An acid urine is essential for antibacterial action; therefore, it is given with ascorbic acid, 500 mg/day to lower the pH of the urine.

NURSING GUIDELINES CONCERNING INFECTIONS IN THE EMERGENCY DEPARTMENT

1. When pharyngitis presents, always take a culture, especially with children.
2. Gonococcal pelvic inflammatory disease is a complication of gonorrhea, and it is essential that it be treated for 7-10 days with ampicillin, 500 mg every 6 hours. Patients must be carefully counseled as to its severity and consequences if it is untreated.
3. Always take a culture and sensitivity swab before starting antibiotics on any patient.
4. When pediatric suspensions are mixed and given out from the ED, the nurse must carefully instruct the parent on times of administration (1 hour before meals and at bedtime) and to keep the mixture refrigerated until it is used. Stress that the entire course of medication must be taken as prescribed until the patient is afebrile for 48-72 hours. You may have to explain that afebrile means without fever.
5. Penicillin injections should not be given in the ED unless it is an absolute necessity in the physician's judgment. If given, the patient should be kept under constant surveillance for at least 30 minutes and preferably longer with epinephrine and oxygen ready and at hand. All allergy injections should be monitored in the same careful fashion.
6. EDNs should take the time to explain, when necessary, that viral infections should not be treated with *antibacterial* agents unless a secondary

infection has established itself. The majority of consumers of health care have been led to believe that "a shot of pencillin" will cure anything.

CORTICOSTEROIDS

The use of corticosteroids (corticoids) is discussed here only insofar as it relates to EDN applications. Steroid production and release in the normal human being follows a 24-hour pattern or rhythm, which is referred to as circadian or diurnal. A normal "day" person will have a high corticoid level at 8 A.M., which dips to a low point at 8 P.M. and returns to a high point again at 8 A.M. If steroids are given therapeutically beyond a 2-week period, there may be suppression of the normal circadian rhythm, and there will be a serious interference with the body's process of gluconeogenesis, or conversion of protein to glucose. When steroids are to be administered for a period of time, they should be given as alternate-day therapy to preserve the adrenal activity and prevent interference with the normal circadian rhythm.

The use of corticoids in the treatment of various types of shock and other selected emergencies has been, and probably will remain, a controversial issue. One reason for this might well be that in the past, whenever corticoids were used, the doses were much smaller than those currently being recommended; additionally in many cases they may have been used too late in the course of shock. Current work utilizing Solu-Medrol in massive pharmacologic doses (initial doses ranging as high as 30 mg/kg) has elaborated a variety of mechanisms by which steroids may help increase the survival rates in septic shock. The following hemodynamic effects have been reported following massive pharmacologic doses:

1. Vasodilation
2. Increased tissue perfusion
3. Increased venous return
4. Tendency to normalize peripheral resistance and cardiac output
5. Increased urine flow
6. Tendency to preserve the integrity of capillaries in the face of anoxia
7. Tendency to stabilize the cellular and lysosomal membranes
8. Apparent facilitation of pulmonary shunt closure (shock lung)
9. Reduced lactic acid accumulation
10. Apparent antiendotoxic effect

Corticosteroids are found often to be very effective in the short-term treatment of allergic reactions (urticaria), asthma, anaphylactic reactions, contact dermatitis, acute lupus erythematosus, acute rheumatic fever, esophageal burns, serum sickness, and moderately severe and severe croup.

There are no ill effects, even in high doses, if given for a brief period (less than 1 week). These drugs can be stopped without being tapered off if they are given for less than 21 days, or if the dosage has not exceeded 15 mg of prednisone (or its equivalent) in a 2-week period.

ANTIHYPERTENSIVES

Hypertensive crises may be managed with either diazoxide (Hyperstat), hydralazine hydrochloride (Apresoline, Apresoline-Esidrix, Ser-Ap-Es, Serpasil-Apresoline), or sodium nitroprusside (Nipride).

DIAZOXIDE (HYPERSTAT)

Diazoxide (Hyperstat) 300 mg (one ampule) is given IV bolus and must be given *rapidly* (within 30 sec) and *only* into a peripheral vein. Hyperstat produces a prompt reduction in blood pressure by relaxing smooth muscle in the peripheral arterioles. Cardiac output is increased as blood pressure is reduced, coronary and cerebral blood flow are maintained, and renal blood flow is increased after an initial decrease. The average duration of action is 30 min.

Diazoxide (Hyperstat) IV injection is a *potent* antihypertensive agent requiring close monitoring of the patient's blood pressure at frequent intervals. Its administration may occasionally cause severe hypotension, requiring treatment with sympathomimetic drugs, such as norepinephrine (Levophed), and therefore the capability to deal with such untoward reactions must be immediately available.

Diazoxide is *highly* alkaline (pH is adjusted to approximately 11.6), and it is *extremely* irritating to the vein. Extravascular injection or leakage should be avoided and the bolus delivered *within 30 sec!*

HYDRALAZINE

Hydralazine, (Apresoline, Ser-Ap-Es, Apresoline-Esidrix), unlike diazoxide, given 10-20 mg IV *slowly* for intervention in the hypertensive crisis is slower acting than diazoxide. It is given in severe essential hypertension when the drug cannot be given orally and there is an urgent need to lower the blood pressure.

SODIUM NITROPRUSSIDE (NIPRIDE)

Nipride is a potent, immediate-acting, intravenous, hypotensive agent which acts directly on the blood vessels, independent of autonomic innervation, causing peripheral vasodilitation. Nipride is *never* given as a direct injection; it is *always infused* after mixing with D5/W.

Sodium nitroprusside is indicated for immediate reduction of blood pressure in hypertensive crisis and should be infused at rates of up to 10 mcg/Kg/min; however, if blood pressure reduction is not achieved within 10 min at this rate the infusion should be stopped.

Once diluted for administration, the drug should be protected from light by wrapping it in foil, not kept or used longer than 4 hours, not employed as a vehicle for simultaneous administration of any other drug, and discarded if it becomes highly colored.

If possible, an infusion pump should be employed for administration to assure precise measurement of the flow rate. Continuous monitoring of the blood pressure (every 5 minutes) during administration is essential; BP must not be allowed to drop too rapidly or the systolic pressure to fall below 60 mm Hg.

REVIEW

1. Define the following: therapeutic effect, secondary effects, side effects, untoward effects, intolerance, idiosyncrasy, hypersensitivity, cumulative effect, antagonistic effect, synergistic effect, potentiation, addiction.
2. Identify the chief factors affecting the body's response to any given drug.
3. Describe the variable factors that affect drug interactions.
4. Identify four general guidelines for safe drug administration in the ED.
5. Explain the origin of the Controlled Drugs program and the five schedules now employed, with examples of each.
6. Identify the three major pharmacologic actions in the control of pain.
7. Describe the chief actions and properties of morphine sulfate.
8. Identify the best narcotic antagonist available for use and explain why it is preferred.
9. List the drug groups that are included in the sedative/hypnotic category.
10. Explain the rule of thumb concerning lethal doses of medication.
11. Identify some of the most common agents that potentiate the actions of the sedative/hypnotics.
12. Explain the basic difference between the sedative/hypnotic drugs and the antianxiety drugs.
13. Identify the drug groups that fall within the general category of psychotherapeutic agents.
14. Explain the difference between the psycholeptic and the psychanaleptic drugs.
15. Identify some of the commonly prescribed MAO inhibitor drugs and describe the warnings which should be given.
16. Describe the action of hydroxyzine HCl (Vistaril) singly and when combined with narcotics.
17. Describe the precautions that must be observed when diazepam is given IV.
18. Describe the precautions that must be observed with droperidol administration and the reasons.
19. Identify at least seven major analgesics in common use other than morphine.
20. List three classifications of diuretics.

21. Identify the most commonly used thiazide diuretics and describe some of their side effects.
22. Identify the most commonly used potent diuretic in the emergency setting and describe the side effects if given in excessive doses.
23. Describe the mode of action of mannitol and the indications for its use.
24. Identify at least eight groups of commonly used antibiotics.
25. Identify the toxic effects of chloromycetin and the clinical indications for its use.
26. Explain the instructions a patient should be given when taking sulfonamides.
27. List at least five nursing guidelines concerning management of infections in the ED.
28. Define the circadian or diurnal rhythm.
29. Identify some of the effects that have been reported following administration of massive doses of corticoids.
30. Describe the indications and method of administration of diazoxide.

BIBLIOGRAPHY

Beckman H: Pharmacology, 2nd ed. W.B. Saunders Co., Philadelphia, Pennsylvania, 1961
Brunner L, Suddarth D: The Lippincott Manual of Nursing Practice, 2nd ed. J.B. Lippincott Co., Philadelphia, Pennsylvania, 1982
Cosgriff JH, Anderson DL: The Practice of Emergency Nursing. J.B. Lippincott Co., Philadelphia, Pennsylvania, 1975
Current Drug Therapy—Barbiturates. American Hospital Formulary Service, Vol 33, pp 333-339, 1976
Dorland's Illustrated Medical Dictionary, 26th ed. W.B. Saunders Co., Philadelphia, Pennsylvania, 1982
Goodman LS, Gilman A: The Pharmacological Basis of Therapeutics, 6th ed. The Macmillan Co., New York, 1980
Hussar DA: Recently introduced drugs and anti-infectives. In Drug Therapy, Biomedical Publishing Co., New York, April 1976
Meyers FG, Jawetz E, Goldfein A: Review of Medical Pharmacology, 5th ed. Lange Medical Publications, Los Altos, California, 1976
Miller R: Drug therapy review. Am J Hosp Pharmacol, Vol 31, pp 990-995, 1974
Morreli HF, Melmon KL: Clinical Pharmacology, Basic Principles in Therapeutics, 2nd ed. The Macmillan Co., New York, 1978
Physicians' Desk Reference, 36th ed. Medical Economics Co., Oradell, New Jersey, 1982
The Role of Corticoids in Selected Emergencies. The Upjohn Co., Kalamazoo, Michigan, 1970
Sanger J: Pharmacology Review for Emergency Department Nurses. Good Samaritan Hospital & Medical Center, Portland, Oregon, 1981
Van Horne R: A Brief Review of Practical Pharmacology. Oregon State Health Division, Portland, Oregon, 1974
Zupko AG: Drug interactions. Pharmacy Times, September/October 1969

DRUG ABUSE AND TOXICOLOGY 26

KEY CONCEPTS

This chapter has been developed to familiarize emergency personnel with the various types of commonly abused drugs and the cardinal points of management with the overdosed patient. The section on toxicology deals with drug groups that act upon the CNS, blood alcohol evaluations, and the administration of antidotes. Portions of these materials have been presented to EDNs by Michael McCullock, M.D., psychiatrist, of the Portland Metropolitan Area; John Aitchison, Ph.D., Assistant Professor of Clinical Pathology, and Marc Bayer, M.D., Associate Director of Emergency Medical Services, both of the University of Oregon Health Sciences Center, Portland; and Keli Keliikoa, EMT-P, of Coos Bay, Oregon.

After reading and studying this chapter, you should be able to:

- Identify the categories into which the abused drugs fall.
- Define habituation, addiction, physical dependence, and drug dependence.
- Identify the classic symptoms and immediate steps of management with the opiate overdose.
- Describe the other possibilities that are always suspect with an overdose.
- Identify the stages of the abstinence syndrome in alcohol abuse.
- Describe the treatment for management of a severe alcohol abstinence case.
- List the principles of treatment and support in a barbiturate overdose.
- Describe the management of a barbiturate abstinence problem and the withdrawal procedure that should be followed.
- Describe the specific treatment for an overdose of amitriptyline.
- Identify the specific hazards associated with methylphenidate abuse.
- Describe the management of patients with amphetamine abuse.
- Explain the serious hazard involved with acetaminophen overdose.
- Describe the EDN's role in the management of overdosed patients.
- Describe the necessary equipment and procedure for performing a rapid and effective gastric lavage in an overdosed patient.

- Define *poison* and *adverse effect.*
- Identify the common groups of drugs that act on the CNS.
- Describe the progressive effects of alcohol on the CNS and as they relate to performance.
- Describe the proper procedure for obtaining a blood alcohol sample.
- Explain the hazards of having salt, vinegar, and mineral oil on a poison cart.
- Identify the essential antidotes that should be available in every ED.
- Explain the proper dosage and administration of ipecac.
- List the equipment and medications which should be aboard a poison cart.

DRUG ABUSE

Drug abuse as it relates to the overdose situation is the topic at hand. Toxicology as it relates to other poisonings will be discussed later in the chapter. The line is a fine one to draw, but for the sake of discussing drug abuse and its management, this portion will be confined to the drugs in specific categories of abuse most frequently seen.

Drug abuse is a prevalent problem in this country and emergency departments see a good percentage of the results. Depending upon the catchment area of the hospital, overdoses (ODs) can account for between 5% and 10% of hospital admissions. It is a known fact that most overdosing occurs in the home since *more prescription drugs* are being abused than are "street drugs," and findings released from a Dade County Miami Treatment Program study show that *diazepam with alcohol* is first among all drug emergency crises (approximately 38%) although diazepam is considered a safe drug, with no recorded deaths from diazepam taken *singly.* Barbiturates ranked fourth and aspirin ranges fifth; heroin was the only illicit drug in the top ten rankings.

Drugs are poisons. When taken in mild clinical amounts, drugs are therapeutic, but any taken in excess, from aspirin to opiates to alcohol, can kill.

DRUG DEPENDENCE

The general terms applied to the abuse of drugs are habituation (low-dose habit), addiction (physical dependence), psychological dependence, and drug dependence. *Drug dependence* is the term now used by the American Psychiatric Association to cover all of these outdated terms.

CATEGORIES

Drugs that fall into abuse categories may be divided as follows:

| I | Opiates: | Morphine, meperidine (Demerol), hydromorphone (Dilaudid), pentazocine (Talwin), etc. |

| II | Alcohol/barbiturates: | Same type of addiction as that of all psycho-therapeutic drugs |

| III | Amphetamines: | Dextroamphetamine (Dexadrine), methyl-phenidate (Ritalin), methamphetamines (Desoxyn, Fetamin, Phelantin Kapseals), co-caine, etc. |

| IV | Hallucinogens: | LSD, ketamine (Ketalar), etc. (Ketamine is a short-acting IV anesthetic) |

V   Marijuana

Physical dependence, psychological dependence, and tolerance of these categorized drugs can be broken down further to reveal the patterns that develop as a result of prolonged use (Table 26.1).

Table 26.1 Drug Dependence Patterns From Prolonged Use

CATEGORY	PHYSICAL DEPENDENCE	PSYCHOLOGICAL DEPENDENCE	TOLERANCE
Opiates	++++	++++	++++
Alcohol/barbiturates	+ to ++++	+ to ++++	++
Amphetamines	0	++ to ++++	++++
Cocaine	0	++++	0
Hallucinogens	0	+	+
Marijuana	0	+	0

Opiates (Schedule II Drugs and Heroin)

These highly addictive agents are the greatest cause for concern, but the abstinence syndrome is *not* lethal and, although serious in appearance, is not a medical emergency. The addict believes he or she will die in withdrawal and makes urgent demands in the ED, as opposed to the barbiturate abuser who will underestimate his or her load. The opiate addict exaggerates the situation and need for medication. Do not respond to the addict's level of escalation and be alert for one who is feigning other illnesses and begging for medication. The addict in true withdrawal will be yawning, perspiring, lacrimating, and will exhibit mydriasis, tremors, and piloerection ("goose flesh"). Remember that all of these manifestations can be faked one way or the other—all that is, except the piloerection! The patient who *is* suffering withdrawal should be referred to the closest alcohol and drug center for screening and treatment.

Opiate overdose is a severe problem because opiates on the market (particularly in unskilled hands) will often overdose the victim when they are taken even in small amounts because of unexpected potency. The commonly abused agents in these situations are heroin, methadone, morphine, oxyco-done HCl (Percodan), morphine suppositories, high doses of codeine and methaqualone (Quaalude, newly moved to Schedule II).

The symptoms of opiate overdose are classic:

- Pinpoint pupils
- Respiratory depression
- Needle tracts

The immediate intervention and treatment indicated with an opiate overdose is establishment of the airway and reversal of the narcotic effects. Naloxone (Narcan) is the drug of choice for the following reasons:

1. It reverses the opiate effects, including all degrees of opiate-induced respiratory depression.
2. It will reverse the narcotic-like effects of other antagonists.
3. Administration of naloxone can be diagnostic as well; failure to obtain significant respiratory improvement after repeated IV doses given at 2- to 3-min intervals suggests a nonopiate cause for the crisis.
4. The onset of action is generally apparent within 2 min following IV administration.
5. It may be repeated at 2- to 3-min intervals (usual dose, 0.4 mg—1 cc) for 2 or 3 doses.
6. It has no narcotic-like properties of its own.
7. It exhibits virtually no pharmacologic activity in the *absence* of narcotics.

Naloxone does not interfere with resuscitative procedures, such as the maintenance of the airway, artifical ventilation, cardiac massage, or vasopressor agents. It should be administered cautiously in known or suspected narcotic dependence since abrupt and complete reversal of narcotic effects may precipitate acute withdrawal symptoms. The patient should be kept under continued close surveillance in the unit and given repeat doses if necessary, since the duration of action of some narcotics may exceed that of naloxone (glutethimide [Doriden] and methadone [Dolophine] being prime examples).

Heroin stabilizes faster than many of the other opiates, but the degree of OD, or how much is "on board," must be determined. Remember that the patient may have ingested combinations of other medications as well, so obtain barbiturate, salicylate, and routine laboratory levels provided in the toxicology screen.

ALCOHOL/BARBITURATE/ PSYCHOTHERAPEUTIC DRUGS

ALCOHOL

Alcohol represents the number one drug problem in the country, except for the overuse of prescription tranquilizers (predominantly diazepam), which is iatrogenic in origin (physician-caused). In the ED we see three different presentations of alcohol (ethanol) abuse: *intoxication, overdose,* and *abstinence.* Beware of masking the neurologic problems and other disease states in the alcohol-troubled patient. Do not accept denial of pain in the injured alcoholic, and *always* look further in screening for other symptoms and evaluations such as salicylate and barbiturate levels. Remember too that the alcoholic is "anesthetized" and may not feel the pain.

Intoxication is defined variously by statute according to the blood level of alcohol found in laboratory determinations and will be discussed fully in the toxicology section. Alcohol is addictive, and the alcoholic can be walking and talking with blood alcohol levels of 0.25% and as high as 0.3% and 0.345%.

Overdose level is achieved at 0.5% (or 500 mg/100 ml) and is usually fatal.

Abstinence is seen manifested in four stages of withdrawal from alcohol; these patients must be carefully observed and managed.

Stage I   Acute withdrawal begins within 6 to 12 hours or even 12 to 24 hours, with agitation called "the shakes." Mild hypertension and tachycardia are seen, and there may be lateral nystagmus.

Stage II   May or may not be bypassed. There are early hallucinations (auditory, visual, and tactile), and a searching, picking behavior. Agitation is prominent, but the sensorium is gradually blunted.

Stage III Disorientation Delusional with an altered sense of time, increased agitation, progressive paralysis, evidence of malnutrition, and serious electrolyte imbalances. (This patient often arrives by ambulance.)

Stage IV   Seizures, generally the grand mal type, status epilepticus, and death! Acute abstinence can kill just as effectively as acute poisoning.

Treatment of the patient in acute withdrawal or delerium tremens requires admission to the hospital following initial intervention as follows:

1. Draw a blood sugar sample and start an IV with D5/NSS.
2. Give 50 cc 50% glucose IV since hypoglycemia secondary to the alcoholic state *may* contribute to the problem.
3. Give thiamine, 100 mg/liter of IV fluid, to replace the deficiency, which is usually a contributory factor to delerium tremens.
4. Manage agitation and seizure activity with the following drugs:
   A. Hydroxyzine (Vistaril), 100 mg IM every hour, is the first choice for agitation.
   B. Magnesium sulfate, 50% 2 cc IM, is often given for motor agitation.
   C. Paraldahyde (old standby) is effective with the "shakes," but is hepatotoxic and should be avoided when possible.
   D. Diphenylhydantoin (Dilantin), 200 mg IM, works well in alcoholic seizure states when it is combined with other management techniques.

E. Chlorpromazine (Thorazine) and droperidol (Inapsine) are less effective with alcoholics. They lower the seizure threshold and may produce a marked drop in BP.

Remember that mortality is as high as 15% when this condition is untreated; these patients must be hospitalized and evaluated further.

BARBITURATES

Barbiturates and the psychotherapeutic drugs are the next group causing concern, with or without the additional potentiating effects of alcohol. Barbiturates are classified according to their duration of action (Table 26.2).

Table 26.2 Barbiturates Classified by Duration of Action

TYPE OF ACTION	DRUG	DURATION OF ACTION	COMATOSE LEVELS (mg/100 ml)	LETHAL LEVELS (mg/100 ml)
Ultra short	Thiopental (anesthesia)	min.	—	—
Short (put to sleep)	Pentobarbital (Nembutal)	2-4 hr	> 0.5	> 1
	Secobarbital (Seconal)	2-4 hr	> 0.5	> 1
Intermediate	Amobarbital (Amytal)	4-6 hr	> 1	> 2
Long (keep asleep)	Phenobarbital	6 hr	> 5	> 10

The symptoms of barbiturate overdose are nystagmus, ataxia, and slurred speech, followed by coma if intervention is not initiated rapidly. The findings in a study done in Denmark show that a mortality of 12-15% in barbiturate overdoses was reduced to 1% by simply supporting the patient's cardiovascular status on a respirator while his liver and kidneys metabolized and excreted the drug. The following protocol was observed:

1. Continuous close observation with respiratory support
2. Prevention and/or treatment of shock with IV fluid maintenance
3. Careful screening for blood levels of alcohol, other barbiturates, and salicylates
4. Maintenance of renal function, increasing rate of excretion by alkalinization of the urine, using sodium bicarbonate
5. Penicillin prophylaxis against hypostatic pneumonia
6. Intensive nursing care with continual turning and suctioning of mucus
7. Restriction on use of stimulants

8. No lavage! The average amount of drug recovered with lavage was about one therapeutic dose (100 mg), and it was not felt to be worth the medicolegal risk since questionable ECG disturbances were associated with the procedure.

The following points present information to keep in mind when dealing with a possible barbiturate abuse:

1. Intoxication in a nonaddicted person can be caused by a very small dose.
2. Tolerance to barbiturates develops to *very high levels.*
3. The alcohol/barbiturate abuser will always *underestimate* intake.
4. If barbiturate overdose is suspected, investigate *all* medications the patient may be taking for barbiturate ingredients (Belap, Fiorinal, etc.).
5. Always suspect mixtures of medications and/or alcohol.

In the hospital, watch where the "barbs" go (*all* barbiturate-containing medications). Hospital personnel are known to take significant amounts of medications from their hospitals regularly, and this is a widespread problem.

The barbiturate abuser who has developed an enormous tolerance for the drug cannot be withdrawn "cold turkey" without a crisis being precipitated. Improper management may result in the patient having seizures and even a full-blown psychosis. For this reason, barbiturate abstinence must be treated as a serious withdrawal problem; these patients must be "re-addicted," which involves a rather complicated in-hospital procedure.

Treatment consists of challenging the patient with 200 mg of pentobarbital (Nembutal) every 6 hours until there is slurred speech, ataxia, and nystagmus. For example, a patient may require a total ingestion of 900 mg/day before the signs of intoxication develop, at which time the dosage is gradually decreased 100 mg/day until the patient is completely withdrawn. This regimen requires *close* medical management by a psychiatrist and qualified nursing personnel.

PSYCHOTHERAPEUTIC DRUGS

Minor Tranquilizers

The benzodiazepines (such as Valium, Librium, and Serax, among others) cause little concern alone, even though they are the most widely used. The problem develops when they act in concert with other drugs that may exert a CNS depressant effect, most frequently alcohol.

Major Tranquilizers

The phenothiazines such as prochlorperazine (Compazine), chlorpromazine (Thorazine), fluphenazine (Prolixin), trifluoperazine (Stelazine), promazine (Sparine), promethazine (Phenergan), and thioridizide (Mellaril), when taken in excess, tend to have a cumulative effect, which produces a state of hypotension, possible ECG changes and arrhythmias, and *extrapyramidal effects,* resemblig the parkinsonian syndrome, with the neck arched, eyes rolled back, and the patient staring and drooling. The immediate first step in management are to insure the airway, ventilate effectively, and administer diphenhydramine (Benadryl) 25-50 mg IV by slow push to reverse the symptoms.

Methaqualone (Quaalude)

This sedative/hypnotic is unrelated to others in this large group. Methaqualone has euphoric and lightening qualities and is a popular, highly abused, street drug; this has resulted with it being placed in Schedule II. (The street slang for it is "soper" for soporific.) Users with overdoses of Quaalude present with delirium, coma, convulsions, spontaneous vomiting with the danger of aspiration, pulmonary edema, shock, and respiratory arrest. Most of the fatalities linked to Quaalude have occurred when the overdose was *accompanied by alcohol ingestion.*

Tricyclic Antidepressants

These drugs are nonaddictive in therapeutic dosage but are often taken in combination with other minor tranquilizers or alcohol, again resulting in an overdose situation (OD). The most frequently abused in this group are amitriptyline (Elavil) and imipramine (Tofranil); others are doxepin (Sinequan), perphenazine (Etrafon), and desipramine (Norpramin). These patients may present in delirium or coma with significant arrhythmias noted on the ECG. The specific treatment for an amitriptyline OD is IV administration (slow push) of 1-3 mg (1 mg/cc) of physostigmine (Antilirium) for rapid reversal of symptoms. It may be helpful to remember that physostigmine will also reverse the toxic effects of the belladonna alkaloids. The dose may be repeated in 20 min and every 30-60 min prn. Diphenylhydantoin (Dilantin) is also effective with these patients in treatment of arrhythmias and CNS disturbances.

Glutethimide (Doriden)

A fast-acting nonbarbiturate hypnotic, which has been effective with elderly patients and the chronically ill, glutethimide (Doriden) is a controlled substance (Schedule III), which has become the source of many severe OD management problems. The patient with a glutethimide overdose will present with CNS depression, including coma, respiratory depression, dilated pupils fixed at midpoint, cyanosis, and a tendency to apnea following the manipulation of gastric lavage or endotracheal intubation.

The immediate management requires stabilization of the airway with effective ventilation and supportive measures as indicated including administration of naloxone. The patient will have recurrent episodes of drifting in and out of coma (sometimes for several days, *even after lavage*), since the low degree of water solubility of the drug and the high degree of fat solubility contributes to a redistribution phenomenon (recirculation through the biliary tract). Severe management problems result. Some investigative studies have indicated that possibly lavage with a *1:1 mixture of castor oil and water* is capable of removing larger amounts from the stomach than a plain water or saline lavage. Lavage must be done as soon as possible but *not until* a cuffed endotracheal tube is in place and the patient is being adequately ventilated. Following lavage, an activated charcoal "slurry" should be instilled into the stomach since the charcoal has a propensity to absorb large amounts of the drug and assist in its continued excretion.

Amphetamines

These very commonly abused drugs include methylphenidate (Ritalin), dextroamphetamine (Dexedrine), methamphetamine, and cocaine. Although they are not considered addicting, there is a tremendous psychological drug dependence developed by the user.

These drugs are predominantly used on the "street" and are available as "cross-tops," "bennies," etc., taken every 3-4 hours to get a "high." Once the "high" has been achieved, the person experiences a letdown and then a rebound. Complete exhaustion, irritability, sleep, extreme depression, and fatigue result; this is a cyclic use with "highs" and "crashes." Treatment of patients with amphetamine abuse involves the use of phenothiazines to decrease anxieties and bring the user "down"; promazine (Sparine), trifluoperazine (Stelazine), chlorpromazine (Thorazine), thioridazine (Mellaril) and dextromethorphan (Phenergan) are all effective, as a rule. These patients should be hospitalized for observation and support with psychiatric counseling available.

Methylphenidate (Ritalin) is a popular amphetamine on the street although it is a controlled drug (Schedule II) and theoretically difficult to obtain. The drug is used effectively as an antidepressant in senile patients and does not have the long-term effect of the tricyclics.

The blood pressure and all body processes elevate with methylphenidate ingestion, and heroin is frequently combined to "mellow out" the high effects. The injection of crushed tablets of methylphenidate mixed with talc causes microabscesses in the lungs, deposits in the eyes, and skin abscesses at injection sites; patients with emphysema and asthma are especially prone to respiratory arrest with the abuse of methylphenidate. Chronic abuse in users leads to acute psychotic episodes which are often paranoia resembling paranoid schizophrenia *with* awareness and insight into the problem, and abrupt withdrawal may lead to cardiovascular collapse. There is no laboratory test that will define the presence of methylphenidate in serum, but a specialized procedure can be done to quantify its presence in the urine.

Hallucinogens

LSD has been the most widely used of the hallucinogens but there seems to be a trend toward a decreasing use of LSD among drug users and abusers. The LSD user on a "bad trip" usually presents with acute psychosis, often with bizarre hallucinations, and unless carefully managed can progress to a highly agitated state. There are several approaches to management of this situation, but it should always be treated as an acute psychosis; 4 cc of droperidol (Inapsine) are effective given IV, but occasionally an LSD tripper can be "talked down" successfully without use of adjunctive drug administration. Another backup method that has demonstrated effective results in administration of Thorazine 50 mg IM followed by diazepam (Valium), 10-20 mg IV.

Mescaline and peyote are variants of the hallucinogens and may account for LSD-like behavior, but regardless of what the patient has ingested or what bizarre behaviors are manifested, the first responsibility is protection of the patient with as quiet surroundings as possible and documentation of cogent and objective observations for the physician.

"Blotter acid" which is LSD sprinkled on blotter paper and cut into small squares for sale on the street, can account for a wide variety of responses with idiosyncratic reactions, and because it is highly impure with no quality control, there can be a variance of 1-250 times in potency.

Phencyclidine (PCP), originally marketed as a surgical anesthetic and subsequently discontinued for human beings because of severe adverse side effects, has become a widely abused hallucinogen with many serious ramifications. PCP is ingested, injected, inhaled as smoke, and "snorted;" it is said to "actually breed violence," that "users end up playing hallucinogenic Russian roulette," and that, according to law enforcement agencies, "a physical encounter with a suspect under the influence of PCP is as potentially dangerous as confronting an armed suspect."

PCP abuse manifestations are dose related. Low dose abuse results in communication difficulty, blank stare, time-place disorientation apprehension, aggressive or self-destructive behavior. Moderate dose abuse results in comatose or stuporous condition with eyes open, response only to deep pain stimuli, period amnesia, and coma/stupor. High dose abuse produces a patient who is comatose, responds only to noxious stimuli, and has a long recovery period of alternating sleep and waking illusion and hallucination with amnesia.

Vital signs are accelerated, motor function varies from catatonia to seizures; nystagmus is present in all directions.

Management is difficult and dangerous and ED personnel should *exercise all caution.* The best approach is to reduce *all* verbal, tactile, and visual stimulation; sensory isolation is key with close physical observation and readiness to adminster Valium or Librium for seizure control, high flow oxygen, and possibly naloxone HCl (Narcan) 0.4 mg IV to reverse effects of a possible narcotic mixture.*

Marijuana

Cannabis is generally thought to be harmless and nonaddictive, but syndromes have developed with chronic use of the weed (grass, pot, hash, Mary Jane, etc.). The drug is not totally benign; it does alter perception of the environment and amplify sensory perception. Heavy users can develop chronic

*Scarano SJ: Field Response to the PCP Emergency. Emergency Medical Services, p 22, January/February 1979

apathy, withdrawal, inattentiveness, and the inability to "get started"; this may tend to be irreversible in some people, and there may be an atypical psychosis, paranoia, or "bad trip." There is no known associated CNS, cardiac or respiratory depression, however.

Salicylate and Acetominophen Intoxications

Salicylate ingestion is one of the commonest forms of drug abuse, and children seem to be more sensitive to its effect, consequently getting into disproportionate problems. Blood levels of salicylate should always be requisitioned in cases of questionable abuse, and the following are some guidelines for the EDN:

1. Up to 2 tablets taken, for instance, for headache will give a blood level of 5 mg/100 ml.
2. Up to 10 tablets per day (150 grains) for arthritis will produce a serum level of about 25 mg/100 ml (30 5-grain tablets).
3. The toxic serum level develops at about 50 mg/100 ml (60 5-grain tablets).
4. The lethal serum level of salicylates is over 100 mg/100 ml.
5. Excretion begins after 3-4 hours.
6. Treatment is symptomatic and supportive. The patient should always be lavaged for stomach content *even up to 10 hours* after ingestion.

Acetominophen (Tylenol) ingestion has become a problem, and *severe liver toxicity,* which is compounded by the ingestion of other drugs such as the sedative/hypnotics, frequently turns out to be the underlying cause of death. An overdose of Tylenol is considered to be any amount in excess of 7.5-10 g orally (24-30 325-mg tablets).

Oral aminstration of Mucomyst as an antidotal agent in acetominophen toxicity is not currently approved by the FDA, but is widely used in the United States, as an antidotal agent under strict protocol from Poison Control Centers across the country.

TOXICOLOGY

Toxicology is the study of poisons. A poison is defined as a chemical agent that produces an adverse effect on living organisms; the effect can be relatively minor, or it may be fatal. An adverse effect is a state of toxicity produced by too much of anything. It is estimated that there are more than 1 million compounds in the world that will kill you if you take enough, and this tends to present problems in trying to define specific agents responsible for a specific toxicity. Fortunately, the offending compounds tend to group into a "frequency" pattern and can be generally identified.

It is recommended that every ED have reference material to identify toxic substances; two such volumes are suggested here:

Meyers FH, Jawetz E, Goldfein A: *Review of Medical Pharmacology*, 7th ed. Lange Medical Publications, Los Altos, California, 1980

Gosselin R, Hodge H, Smith R, Gleason M: *Clinical Toxicology of Commercial Products*, 4th ed. Williams & Wilkins Co., Baltimore, Maryland, 1976

The latter text provides the following information:

1. An ingredient index with toxicity rating including lethality
2. An index of general formulations of most commercial compounds according to use
3. Brand names with ingredients of each and indications of the degree of toxicity.

Clinical pathology laboratories that provide analytical services in toxicology are maintained in most states and the larger metropolitan areas. The services of these laboratories are made available, as a rule, for toxicology studies on samples submitted from EDs, monitoring of blood levels on samples submitted from outlying areas, medicolegal evaluations for law enforcement agencies, and postmortem toxicology studies for the state medical examiner or coroner.

These laboratories employ a highly sophisticated methodology based largely on gas chromatography and mass spectrometry techniques by which they are able to separate individual drug components from submitted samplings, identify them, and quantitate their presence.

One of the chief services rendered is the computation of blood alcohol samples, which are submitted as evidentiary material in drunk driving cases.

BLOOD ALCOHOL

Blood alcohol is a complicated subject with a peculiar medicolegal significance.

Alcohol is a small molecule and, once it is ingested, 25% is absorbed directly from the stomach, with the balance absorbed from the small intestine. Alcohol is widely distributed and follows water, appearing anywhere in the body where there is water—in the organs, muscle, brain, and can be measured in blood, urine, saliva, and perspiration. Once absorbed into the bloodstream, it is eliminated to the extent of 5% via saliva, urine, and sweat. The other 95% is eliminated via oxidation in the *liver*.

Blood alcohol is a "picture" of the extent to which the body's capacity to get rid of alcohol has been exceeded. A single drink (1 oz) is absorbed in about 20 min, and the drug remains in the body for approximately 1 hour, oxidizing at the rate of 15 mg/100 ml/hr. One drink an hour should not result in measurable levels of blood alcohol.

A 150-lb male, given 1 oz of 80-proof whiskey, will show a blood alcohol level equivalent to 0.02% or 20 mg/100 ml (1 oz of 80-proof whiskey is equivalent to a blood alcohol level of 20 mg/100 ml, proportionately, depending to a greater or lesser extent upon body weight). A 12-oz can of beer will show a blood alcohol of 25 mg/100 ml and the rate of oxidation, or disappearance from the blood, will be about 15 mg/100 ml/hr like the 80-proof.

Rule of Thumb: 50-80 mg/100 ml (0.05-0.08%), a cocktail party level.
450-500 mg/100 ml (0.45-0.50%), *toxic and lethal!*

The effects of alcohol are an irregular, progressive, descending depression of the CNS. Low doses decrease attentiveness to the task at hand (an example is careless driving after two or three drinks) although chronic alcoholics currently drinking may tolerate higher blood levels before deteriorating.

The first things affected are the higher centers of the brain, the most skilled task abilities, and the most recently learned tasks. As the level climbs higher, more of the brain's functions become depressed, and the effects become obvious. Alcohol does tend to be a self-limiting overdose with coma or sickness limiting further intake, and for this reason lethality from alcohol alone is rare.

Most states now have an implied-consent law, whereby, as a condition of accepting a driver's license, the applicant agrees to give a sample of blood or breath if an officer of the law has reasonable grounds to suspect the person has been drinking and driving a car irresponsibly. The option is either to submit a sample or to accept a 6-month suspension of the driver's license if cooperation is refused.

The trend is to bring the legal levels of blood alcohol down. A level of 80 mg/100 ml (0.08%) has been adopted by England and Canada, and at this time Germany and Scandanavia observe a legal limit of 50 mg/100 ml (0.05%). Most states recognize the legal limit at around 100 mg/100 ml (0.1%), and if there has been a negligent homicide involving a MVA, an alcohol blood level must be obtained to submit essential proof to a jury. Therefore, it is necessary to get a blood alcohol sampling if at all possible; otherwise there may not be any enforcement action available.

Interpretation of the statutes relating to obtaining blood alcohol levels for evidentiary purposes varies from state to state, but some basic guidelines are given that can well apply anywhere:

1. For the evidence to be admissible, the blood alcohol determination must be done by a qualified laboratory duly authorized by the state jurisdiction.

2. Hospital policy should clearly articulate the procedure for obtaining blood alcohol samplings and the conditions of consent.

3. The consent of the patient is necessary, and it should be *informed* consent.

4. If blood is drawn, it should be drawn in the police officer's presence so that he can so testify, eliminating the need for other witnesses to appear and testify.

5. Blood drawn must be given to the officer requesting it, and he then takes it to an authorized laboratory, preserving the chain of evidence.

6. A notation of blood drawn, by whom, and the time, must be documented in the ED record of the patient, and the blood so labeled before it is sealed with tape, cross initialed, and given to the officer.

7. If a blood alcohol determination is needed for medical purposes, draw separate samples.

8. The skin prep for drawing a blood alcohol sample should be done with aqueous benzalkoninum (Aqueous Zephiran) and *never* with alcohol.

9. Draw 10 cc, and label with name, date, time drawn, and your initials. If it is a case of negligent homicide, draw *two* samples, 1 hour apart, to demonstrate the curve as firm legal evidence. Either the blood alcohol level will have peaked and started down, or it will be higher, indicating that the subject took more alcohol immediately prior to the incident. It is estimated that the blood level will fall 15-20 mg/100 ml/hr, so if, for instance, a blood alcohol is drawn 4 hours after an arrest and tests at 0.18% (180 mg/100 ml), it can be legally assumed that the subject's blood level at the time of arrest was 0.26% or 260 mg/100 ml.

By way of interest and to clarify much confusion, *methanol* (C-1) is used in the laboratory, chafing dish burners, and anti-freeze; *ethanol* (C-2) is used for drinking; and *isopropyl alcohol (C-3) is used for rubbing alcohol, sterilization, etc.*

SUMMARY OF POINTS OF GENERAL MANAGEMENT FOR OVERDOSES AND TOXICITIES

Treat the patient, not the poison!

A. Establish airway and maintain adequate ventilation.
B. Evaluate state of coma:
   • Response to verbal commands
   • Response to painful stimulus
   • Presence or absence of reflexes
   • Cardiorespiratory status
C. Examine patient carefully.
D. Initiate IV line with large-bore needle.
E. Identify the poison or drug and obtain an accurate history.
F. Get rid of the poison:
   • No emesis should be elicited if 1) the patient is comatose, convulsive or without the gag reflex, 2) the patient has ingested a strong base or acid, and 3) the ingestion has been a petroleum distillate.
   • Otherwise induce emesis (test gag reflex first) with *ipecac*, 30 cc (adults), or 15 cc for children. Follow ipecac with several glasses of

warm water or 7-Up, ambulate the patient if possible, and if there are no results in 15-20 min, stimulate the pharynx.

- Gastric lavage is used if the patient is comatose, except with petroleum products. A cuffed endotracheal tube *must* be in place if a comatose patient is to be lavaged. Use a large Ewald tube (34 mm), place the patient on left side, in a head-down position to prevent aspiration and promote better drainage, and lavage with saline. Use 300 cc per tidal wash for adults and 10 cc/kg of body weight per wash for children until the return is clear.* This procedure is effective after 4-6 hours and up to 12 hours with acetylsalicylic acid, meprobamate (Equanil), and anticholinergic agents. Lavage samplings should be saved for possible laboratory analysis. A "slurry" of activated charcoal is frequently instilled to absorb many drugs and it marks intestinal transit time as well. The dose is 20-30 g mixed with saline and instilled at the end of the lavage. Sometimes magnesium sulfate is instilled (10-20 g) as a cathartic.

G. Place a Foley bladder catheter with closed drainage system and calibrated receptacle. Force diuresis for acetylsalicylic acid, barbiturates, and isoniazid (antitubercular drug), and monitor output carefully.

H. Initiate hemodialysis or peritoneal dialysis if indicated.

I. Send urine to laboratory for toxicology screening (analgesics including salicylates, opiates, amphetamines, tricyclics, and phenothiazines).

I. Counteract the toxic effects of specific poisons as indicated (Table 26.3).

Emergency nurses are responsible for remaining aware of the changing methods of management and for seeking current knowledge independently to recognize and manage overdoses and toxic states. Be fully capable of airway management, including intubation and the use of ventilatory equipment, remembering that the *best* ventilator is the bag/mask unit. Document adequately before the patient leaves the ED for transport to the ICU and see that the patient is always accompanied by respiratory support equipment, including oxygen. Have standing orders in your department for administration of naloxone, intervention in respiratory arrest, arterial blood gases, gastric lavage, initiation of IVs, etc., and be alert to the hazards of management, such as aspiration, catheter contamination, overhydration, and further respirator problems.

TEACHING THE PATIENT

The ED is an excellent spot for teaching the public, and poison prevention is a critically important area, especially in light of studies showing that children

---

*Jensen G: The Initial Management of Acute Poisoning. JEN, Vol 3, No 4, pp 13-16, 1977

Table 26.3 Agents That Counteract the Toxic Effects of Specific Poisons

POISON	AGENT
Arsenic or mercury	British antilewisite (BAL)
Tricyclics and Phenothiazines	Physostigmine (Antilirium)
Coumarin	Vitamin K
Cyanide	Sodium nitrite (Lilly cyanide kit)
Fluoride	Calcium
Iron	Deferoxamine (Desferol mesylate)
Methanol	Ethanol
Nitrites	Methylene blue
Opiates (including propoxyphene-Darvon)	Naloxone (Narcan)
Organic phosphates	Atropine
Oxalic acid	Calcium
Carbon monoxide	Oxygen (100% or hyperbaric chamber)

who have had a toxic ingestion stand a 25% chance for a *repeat* ingestion in the next year, while their siblings have a 56% chance. Ask parents, while they are in the ED, where they keep the Drano, insect sprays, rodent poisons, cleaning fluids, and medications of *all* kinds, and suggest special locked storage areas for all these hazardous materials. Start people thinking!

THE POISON CART

A well-organized and logically equipped poison cart can save untold and unnecessary mileage during the management of an overdose or toxic ingestion since it can be taken directly to the patient's stretcher and worked much like a code cart.

The old standby antidotes of vinegar, olive oil, and salt have fallen into great disrepute, and it is recommended that they be removed from the department before damage is done. If vinegar or citrus juice is given to counteract caustic material ingestion, it will generate chemical activity and burn the esophagus further. Ingested caustics should be diluted with copious amounts of water or milk.

Instillation of olive oil or vegetable oil may lead to aspiration pneumonia and will certainly prevent effective endoscopy if that procedure is indicated.

Salt water ingestion (administered as an antidote) can cause severe hypernatremia and may rapidly result in death in children.

The small-wheeled cart with three drawers and a bottom compartment is recommended for the Poison Cart, preferably the molded plastic type with rounded corners and large quiet casters. The suggested inventory is given in Table 26.4.

Table 26.4 Recommended Contents of Poison Cart

Top Drawer

60-cc Asepto syringes
Y Connectors
Utility tubing sections—standard size
Lubricant (water-soluble)
Straws
2 Forceps for clamping tubing
Alcohol wipes
Medicine cups
Spoons

Second Drawer

Assorted NG tubes including 32-mm
  red rubber Ewald tubes (or equivalent)
Paper cups
Disposable lavage bags (6)

Third Drawer

Injectable medications:
  • Mucomyst
  • Physostigmine (Antilirium)
  • Naloxone (Narcan)
  • Diphenhydramine HCl (Benadryl)
  • Epinephrine
  • Atropine
  • Methylene blue
  • Lilly cyanide kit
Pitchers
Activated charcoal (30-g doses)
Ipecac (30-cc doses)
Magnesium Citrate
Topical anesthetic spray

Bottom Shelf

Supply of normal saline irrigant (1500-
  cc bottles)
Cover gowns or aprons for personnel

REVIEW

1. Define the terms *drug dependence, habituation,* and *addiction.*
2. Identify the categories of abused drugs.
3. Identify the classic signs of opiate addiction and describe the immediate steps in management of the patient overdosed on opiates.
4. Describe the stages of the abstinence syndrome seen in patients in withdrawal.
5. Describe the management of the patient in alcohol withdrawal.
6. Explain the classifications of barbiturates and give examples of each.
7. Describe the recommended protocol for management of the barbiturate OD.
8. Describe the recommended procedure for withdrawing a barbiturate "addict."
9. Describe the specific treatment for an overdose of amitriptyline (Elavil).
10. Explain the problems involved with the glutethimide (Doriden) OD.
11. Explain the purpose of instilling a charcoal slurry after lavage.
12. Explain why naloxone is diagnostic in opiate addiction.
13. Identify the specific problems seen with methylphenidate (Ritalin) abuse.
14. Describe the patterns of abuse with amphetamine drugs.
15. Identify the drugs employed in management of amphetamine abuse.

16. Describe three methods of dealing with a "bad trip" resulting from LSD.
17. Identify the combination of drugs that causes most ED crises.
18. Explain why Narcon should be given in preference to Nalline in the OD patient.
19. Identify the only symptom that an opiate addiction cannot fake in claiming withdrawal.
20. Define poison and adverse effect.
21. Describe the function of a clinical pathology laboratory that specializes in toxicology.
22. Describe the absorption rate of alcohol in the body.
23. Describe the progressive effects of alcohol on the CNS.
24. Describe the basic guidelines that should be observed in drawing blood samples for evidentiary blood alcohol analysis.
25. Identify the underlying philosophy in the management of overdoses and toxicities.
26. Identify the circumstances under which two blood alcohol samples would be drawn 1 hour apart on the same patient.
27. List three circumstances in which emesis should not be induced.
28. Describe the procedure which must be done before lavaging a comatose patient.
29. Describe the method employed to increase the rate of urine excretion with phenobarbital, aspirin, and isoniazid OD.
30. Identify the specific antidotes for opiates, carbon monoxide, organic phosphates, nitrites, methanol, cyanide, tricyclics, and phenothiazines.
31. Identify the most effective means of ventilating a patient who is intubated.
32. Identify the important areas of teaching that can be done in the ED with regard to drug abuse and toxic ingestions.
33. Describe the hazards involved with the use of vinegar or citrus juice, olive oil, and salt in treating toxic ingestions.
34. Describe the inventory that should be available in a portable poison cart.

BIBLIOGRAPHY

American Hospital Formulary Service: Current Drug Therapy—Barbiturates. Vol 33, pp 333-339, 1976

Bayer M, Rumack B (eds.): Poisonings and Overdose, TEM. Aspen Systems Publications, Rockville, Maryland, Vol 1, No 3, October 1979

Beckman H: Pharmacology, 2nd ed. W.B. Saunders Co., Philadelphia, Pennsylvania, 1961

Bradley NV: The alcoholic and the ED. JEN, pp 14-18, January/February 1975

Brunner L, Suddarth D: The Lippincott Manual of Nursing Practice, 2nd ed. J.B. Lippincott Co., Philadelphia, Pennsylvania, 1982

Budassi SA, Barber JM: Emergency Nursing: Principles and Practice. C.V. Mosby Co., St. Louis, Missouri, 1981

Cosgriff JH, Anderson DL: The Practice of Emergency Nursing. J.B. Lippincott Co., Philadelphia, Pennsylvania, 1975

Czajka PA, Duffy JP: Poisoning Emergencies: A Guide for Emergency Medical Personnel. C.V. Mosby Co., St. Louis, Missouri, 1980

Doweiko H: Identifying street names of drugs. JEN, pp 41-47, November/December 1979

Elston PL: Management of methaqualone overdose. JEN, Vol 6, No 5, pp 17-19, September/October 1980

Goodman LS, Gilman A: The Pharmacological Basis of Therapeutics, 6th ed. Macmillan Co., New York, New York, 1980

Gosselin R, Hodge H, Smith R, Gleason M: Clinical Toxicology of Commercial Products, 4th ed. Williams and Wilkins Co., Baltimore, Maryland, 1976

Holtman DJ: Acetaminophen overdose. JEN, Vol 4, No 3, pp 50-52, May/June 1978

Ilo E: Charcoal: Update on an old drug. JEN, Vol 6, No 4, pp 45-48, July/August 1980

Jensen S: The initial management of acute poisoning. JEN, Vol 3, No 4, pp 13-16, 1977

McElroy C: Alcohol withdrawal syndromes. JEN, Vol 7, No 2, pp 195-198, September/October 1981

Metz V, Hanenson I: Management of drug overdose in the adult. JEN, Vol 1, No 6, pp 8-15, 1975

Meyers FH, Jawetz E, Goldfein A: Review of Medical Pharmacology, 7th ed. Lange Medical Publications, Los Altos, California, 1980

Morreli HF, Melmon KL: Clinical Pharmacology, Basic Principles in Therapeutics, 2nd ed. Macmillan Co., New York, 1978

Physicians' Desk Reference, 36th ed. Medical Economics Co., Oradell, New Jersey, 1982

Rumack B: Managing the poisoned patient in the ED. Third Annual Rocky Mountain Emergency Medicine Conference, Keystone, Colorado, ACEP, 1977

Van Horne R: A Brief Review of Practical Pharmacology. Oregon State Health Division, Portland, Oregon, 1974

Watkins RN: Overdose in the emergency department. Sixth Annual Scientific Assembly, SeaTac, Washington State ACEP, 1976

Zupko AG: Drug Interactions, Part I. Pharmacy Times, September/October 1969

PSYCHIATRIC AND EMOTIONAL CRISES

27

KEY CONCEPTS

This chapter provides some brief but pertinent material relating to assessment and intervention in emotional crises, with some simple guidelines on management of psychiatric emergencies, the rape victim, patients presenting with pain and anxiety, the dying patient, and staff stress. It is hoped that the chapter will familiarize the EDN with the essentials of management for the various stressful situations and near-crises that arise daily and to help the patient through with the knowledge that someone cares.

The content offered here is based on lecture material presented to emergency nurses, predominently by other nurses with expertise in these areas: Joanne Hazel, R.N., psychiatric emergencies; Terry Moldanado, R.N., and Sherry Heying, R.N., the rape victim; Marilyn Hogrefe, R.N., pain and anxiety; Myra Lee, R.N., on death, dying and grief, and Jack J. Crawford, Ph.D., on psychiatric emergencies and stress.

After reading and studying this chapter, you should be able to:

- Identify the general categories of psychiatric emergencies and outline the significant areas of assessment.
- Identify the components necessary to an effective approach in dealing with a severely disturbed patient.
- Describe the cardinal signs and symptoms of depression.
- Describe the general physical management of the acute paranoid patient.
- Identify the groups of psychotherapeutic agents commonly used.
- Describe the significance of auditory hallucinations as opposed to the implications of visual hallucinations.
- Identify the important management techniques in conducting the patient interview with a rape victim and identify three goals that should be achieved.
- List the contents of a representative crime detection laboratory chain-of-evidence examination kit, and describe the simplicity, workability and effective results in using such a kit.

- Identify the areas in which the rape victim must have follow-up attention or at least access to attention if necessary.
- Understand the ways in which the nurse can reinforce the dying patient or families of deceased patients.
- Recognize the stress patterns that develop in the emergency department as the result of interaction between patients and staff.
- Identify some workable solutions to personal stress.

PSYCHIATRIC EMERGENCIES*

The Emergency Department is becoming the point of entry into mental health services for an increasing number of people. The EDN can look forward to more psychiatric emergencies in the future. Deinstitutionalization, the drastic discharge of patients from state hospitals, and the growing emphasis on community services rather than residential treatment, places the chronically mentally ill in the community served by the ED. The ED is also impacted by an accelerating number of younger patients with emotional, behavioral, and alcohol/drug related problems.

A psychiatric emergency arises when anyone comes into the ED for immediate relief from distress that is obviously of a psychiatric nature, or when anyone is brought in by family, friends, or neighbors, stating that the patient was acting in a bizarre, dangerous, or ominous fashion.

Psychiatric emergencies can be placed into general categories as they are most commonly encountered:

1. Depression and attempted suicide
2. Panic-stricken patient
3. Manic episode
4. Paranoid disorder
5. Schizophrenic disorder
6. Depressive episode
7. Alcohol/drug abuse or dependence

The general principles of management with these patients involves a careful assessment with an attempt to obtain pertinent information in five key areas: 1) The chief complaint or reason for being brought to the ED; 2) the patient's general behavior as you observe it and the impression you derive (frightened, angered, inappropriately responding, catatonic, etc.); 3) the history or as much as you can get from the patient or whoever accompanied him; 4) the physical examination with every effort made to obtain accurate baseline information and full vital signs if possible; and 5) an observation period, during which time the situation can be objectively evaluated.

There are several components to an effective approach with a psychiatrically disturbed patient, and it is important to realize that if you can exhibit a

---

*Suggested reading: Soreff SM: Management of the Psychiatric Emergency. John Wiley & Sons, New York, 1981

calm and confident manner at the outset you may be able immediately to reduce the patient's anxiety level. Let the patient know you are interested and care about helping as well as offering hope for a short-term solution that is reasonable. Try to draw the patient out by sometimes sharing your observations with him and elicit enough information that you can prepare the physician for the general problem.

Depression and Suicide

Depression and suicide are the tenth cause of death annually in the United States; 30,000 die annually, and 10 times that number attempt self-destruction. Depression accounts for 70-80% of all psychiatric referrals. To understand a depression, you must gain an understanding of all the patient's feelings and areas of energy that are expelled daily. We all have essential areas of biologic, social, vocational, avocational, intellectual, and emotional activity, and when one or two are chronically neglected there may be manifestations of depression. These feelings of deprivation are difficult for the patient to verbalize or describe and sometimes are not even recognized, and this makes depressions a most difficult clinical state to deal with.

The symptoms of depression in adolescents may present as detachment and a cynical lonely attitude, with the child acting out sexually. These patients are frequently involved in reckless driving, drug abuse, and delinquency problems. The depressed adult exhibits careless dress, a slow gait, slumpy posture, a monotonous whiny voice, ruminating thought processes, and loss of social interest, with decreased sexual activity. Physically, they frequently complain of backache, headache, GI upset, chest pains, and vertigo. A good way to spot the depressed patient is to remember that depression begets depression in the nurse, and ask yourself: "How do I feel? How does this patient make me feel?"

Once you have identified a severely depressed patient, you must determine how severe the depression really is. The best approach in dealing with the *severely* depressed patient is to talk about the situation and discuss suicidal thoughts with the patient. Ask: "How's life treating you?" "How do you feel about life?" "Do you feel like harming (killing) yourself?" Explore whether the patient has a plan and if so when, how, has the plan been rehearsed and practiced? Ask: "Do you feel hopeless about the future?" "Has there been any recent loss (a loved one, job, social position, etc.)?" "Have you tried suicide before?" The chances are twice as great if a family member has made an attempt. Ask about the use of alcohol or drugs that produce suicidal tendencies. Frequently the sociopathic personality who manipulates the environment, gets away with it, and makes others angry *does* commit suicide!

The suicide rate increases between ages 48 and 60 and then decreases up to age 72. Find out if your patient suffers from any physical illness that may be contributing heavily to the depression, such as cancer, rheumatoid arthritis, peptic ulcer disease, hypertension, anticipation of disfiguring surgery or urogenital surgery. Is there social withdrawal and is the patient putting his or her affairs in order? These are all, of course, indicative of deep problems, and the patient has a need to ventilate. Talking with someone who is interested, empathetic, and warm can be both diagnostic and therapeutic for that patient. Depression may be symptomatic of organic illness such as brain tumor (organic brain syndrome), hypothyroidism, or a manifestation of long-term cortisone therapy.

If the patient is sent home, it must be to a responsible person who can administer medication, which must be *well labeled*. The tricyclics take 2 weeks to achieve effect, and sedatives are unsafe to send home with an already depressed patient, so diphenhydramine (Benadryl), 50 mg PO, is frequently prescribed. There must be clearly arranged plans for patient referral and follow-up.

The Panic-Stricken Patient

This patient identifies a crisis situation, which in reality is often a common, garden-variety, anxiety attack. Frequently, the patient demands immediate attention because of terrible fear that he/she or a family member is going to die or is going crazy. Give these patients time to unwind by talking to you, and this is best done when the family is not present. The patient may need a minor tranquilizer like diazepam (Valium), 10 mg, or chlordiazepoxide (Librium), 50 mg. Most often the problem can be talked out, the patient calmed and reassured, and sent home with a follow-up appointment for the mental health clinic or a psychiatrist.

MANIC EPISODE

The manic patient is sometimes difficult to separate from the schizophrenic patient who is exhibiting peculiar behavior with bizarre gestures, inappropriate behavior, and odd postures. The schizophrenic person may also be hearing voices. The important point is to determine whether this patient is dangerous to self or to others. The key, as one physician points out, is not "which patient do I have to be afraid of," but "which patient is afraid of me?" The fearful patient becomes destructive and assaultive because he or she feels trapped and "cornered like a rat."

The most useful guide is the patient's expression and manner. If the patient's eyes are shifting around looking for the nearest exit or for something to grab to protect himself or herself, be ready for a potential "acting out."

1. If you can determine the person is not assaultive, sit down to talk.
2. Leave the door open during your interview; do not place your chair between the patient and the door.
3. Avoid talking about the patient's delusional symptoms, talk rationally to the patient.
4. The patient may need major tranquilizers, hospitalization, or a follow-up appointment. If assaultive, sedate immediately! The psychotic patient who may erupt should be restrained either physically or effectively with medication like droperidol (Inapsine), 2-4 cc IM.

The true manic is not usually a threat in the ED, but the main problem is that the patient will exhaust himself or herself and indeed, may finally die of exhaustion. A manic patient must be hospitalized and placed on medication. Starting lithium in the ED is a very controversial practice, and a patient who has never received lithium needs a complete medical workup before being placed on the medication, as well as being closely monitored for blood levels on a follow-up basis.

Paranoid Disorder

The acute paranoid is an extremely dangerous person, who must be dealt with very carefully and taken very seriously. There are four types of ideation: 1) jealousy, 2) eroticism, 3) grandiosity, and 4) persecution. There is a total lack of ability to conform to the society around them, and all activity around and toward them is turned into a personalization.

The management of the acute paranoid patient includes the following considerations:

1. Have a psychiatrist there as soon as possible.
2. Do not be offhand with the patient; be definite about his or her reception.
3. Minimize the paranoid deviation.
4. Look him or her in the eye, sit on the same level, minimize interruptions.
5. Let him or her sit close to the door.
6. Encourage him or her to talk; do not add credence to ideations of persecution, but hear the patient out.
7. Explain your movements so as not to alarm the patient.
8. Evaluate patient's rigidity.
9. *Be calm.*
10. *Do not probe* into the patient's delusional system.
11. Remember that venting reduces agitation.
12. Notify whomever necessary to protect others.

You will want to ask this patient some general reality-oriented questions, such as: "Where do you work?" "Who makes up your family?" "What type of work do you do?" "Where were you raised?" "Where were you born?" These questions will test his orientation to reality. As the patient vents paranoid ideations, he or she will frequently "come down" enough to realize that the magnitude of the problem is less than he or she thought, and often then the patient is able to talk about what mode of therapy might be best.

Depressive Episode

Agitated depression is often seen in the older person who is pacing up and down, wringing the hands, and exhibiting ruminative thought processes. The treatment is to administer a minor tranquillizer and send the patient home with a responsible person. Some of these patients may be in need of electric shock therapy, but hospital admission should be avoided if possible. Be wary of the family's trying to "dump" a confused elderly relative in the ED, because an unwarranted hospital admission may break the established routine of daily life for this patient and cause him or her to lose contact with reality.

Alcohol/Drug Abuse or Dependence

This is a real problem and a complex one, which takes up a great deal of time in the ED. The greatest problem is that there is no really effective way of dealing with an alcoholic (or other substance abuser) in the ED. If the alcoholic can be motivated adequately, Alcoholics Anonymous may be a path to pursue. If not, the patient should be directed to the closest referral agency in the community for further care. The alcoholic who presents complaining of "the jitters" and asking for medication may be a candidate for delirium tremens within 24 hours. This patient should be sedated at once and admitted; if he or she refuses, you must obtain an AMA release and make every effort to notify family or friends of the patient's dangerous situation. (See Chapter 26 for management of drug abuse.)

PSYCHOTHERAPEUTIC AGENTS

The specific medications used for psychiatric emergencies fall into the two major categories of tranquilizers and antidepressants.

The tranquilizer drugs (ataractic agents) are given to decrease psychotic behavior and are comprised, for the most part, of phenothiazines and synthetic phenothiazines including the major tranquilizers, the piperazine group, the piperadine group, and minor tranquilizers.

The antidepressant drugs comprise monoamineoxidase (MAO) inhibitors and tricyclic compounds:

1. Monoamine oxidase inhibitors (psychic energizers) are isocarboxazid (Marplan), pargyline (Eutonyl), tranylcypromine (Parnate), and phenylzine (Nardil).
2. Tricyclics amitriptyline (Elavil), desipramine (Norpramin), imipramine (Tofranil), nortriptyline (Aventyl).

A drug that should be mentioned singly is droperidol (Inapsine), which has potent neuroleptic activity and is indicated in psychiatric emergencies for sedation or tranquilization, for anti-anxiety activity, and as a general aid in producing tranquility and decreasing anxiety and pain. Other CNS depressant drugs (e.g., barbiturates, major tranquilizers, narcotics, and general anesthetics) will have additive or *potentiating* effects with droperidol. The administration of other CNS depressants following droperidol should be carefully monitored to avoid excessive CNS depression. Caution should be exercised in administration to patients with known Parkinson's disease.

Some side effects generally seen from the prolonged use of the tranquilizing drugs are hypotension (especially with chlorpromazine [Thorazine] and thioridizine [Mellaril]), blood dyscrasias and leukopenia (WBC and differential should be done every month), obstructive jaundice, photosensitivity, retinopathy, a lowered seizure threshold, potentiation of analgesias and depression, and akathisia (the inability to sit down from nervous fear) from Stelazine and Prolixin administration, for which diphenhydramine (Benadryl) is an effective treatment.

Administration of the minor tranquilizers has essentially the same effect as "a shot of booze" for most patients. Alcohol, Librium, and diazepam (Valium) are all minor tranquilizers, and there may be ataxia, drowsiness, hypotension, and after the long term use of diazepam (Valium), depression.

SOME MISCELLANEOUS POINTS

1. Always do *vital* signs on psychiatric emergencies, if at all possible. Problems that produce psychological changes but are *organic* in nature can often be picked up with complete vital signs. Examples are CVA (aphagia, etc.), diabetes, cerebral arteriosclerosis, azotemia (BUN elevated in renal failure), postictal states, systemic or CNS infections, decompensated hepatic disorders (cirrhosis), brain tumors, barbiturate withdrawal, clavus hystericus (the sensation as if a nail were being driven into the head), and toxic conditions.
2. When talking with a psychiatric patient:
   A. Listen to the patient.
   B. Try to remember that at any given time a person is doing the best he can at *that* time and under *those* circumstances.
   C. Relate to the here and now with the patient.
   D. Paraphrase during the interview and when necessary, briefly intercede with the rambling patient.
   E. In nonverbal behaviors, label the patient's reactions, i.e., "You seem to be . . . ."
   F. Evaluate how that patient makes *you* feel.
   G. Ask for help from the patient in interpreting his words.
   H. Trust your own initial feelings toward the patient.

Remember that the schizophrenic patient has allowed his fantasy world to become a dominant part of his life and that *auditory* hallucinations are a manifestation of a schizophrenic psychosis. Visual hallucinations should *always* suggest organic problems such as toxic reactions, LSD, encephalitis, overdose, or delirium tremens.

THE RAPE VICTIM

Most victims of rape will present to the ED through their own volition or be brought by law enforcement personnel for the purpose of obtaining evidence to sustain criminal proceedings against the suspect. This is a frightening and often humiliating experience for the woman involved and is a deeply traumatic emotional crisis. It is a situation in which the understanding of the ED personnel can be invaluable.

Victims of rape can be all ages, all races, and from all walks of life. Rape can occur any time of the day or night and any place. In the United States it is estimated that a *reported* rape occurs every 12 min. Many rapes go unreported, so the incidence is probably higher than stated. By law in some states only females can be raped; there are laws that cover males but not under the definition of rape. For our purposes here, the definition of rape is unlawful sexual intercourse by force and against a female person's will.

The book *Rape, Victims of Crisis,* by Ann W. Burgess and Lynda L. Holstrom, published by the Robert J. Brady Company, deals to the full extent with all the ramifications of rape and its consequences and problems; we defer to that publication. Our purpose here is to outline very simply the goals that should be sought in ED management of the victim and the chain-of-evidence examination that must substantiate the victim's plight if the case goes to court.

The three goals in management of the rape victim are:

1. Provision of privacy.
2. Return of control to the victim.
3. Medical and chain-of-evidence examination within the confines of the first two goals.

Regardless of how the rape victim presents in the ED or by what means she arrived, complete privacy should be afforded her, with immediate attention to medical needs, if any, and a supportive attitude toward her *emotional status* with a very carefully conducted examination following a protocol designed to provide a comprehensive physical examination of the victim as well as the chain-of-evidence (COE) for use in criminal proceedings against the alleged assailant. The victim should be taken directly to an examining room for complete privacy, and no questions should be asked at the admitting desk. The nurse accompanies the victim to the examining room and stays with her through the COE examination, which may take as long as an hour. The nurse should introduce herself, carefully explain the questions that have to be asked and why, and make an effort to establish a rapport with the patient by showing concern for her needs and treating her with respect.

The medical examination requires little historic documentation; too much information will result in the physician and nurse having to testify in court; therefore, obtain only medical information pertaining to the patient's physical status.

Police procedure may vary from community to community insofar as interviewing and investigational follow-up are concerned, but the nursing protocol should be established and followed at every hospital according to the same format to protect the patient, provide the medical care necessary, and produce a COE for legal proceedings. During any police interviews, the patient should be attended by the EDN or another person capable of functioning in the role of the patient advocate. In many communities volunteer groups are forming to act as "rape victim advocates," and in this situation individuals are on call as necessary to provide emotional and situational reinforcement to the victim of assault.

INTERVIEWING THE VICTIM

It is important for the patient to be treated as though the ED personnel care about her personal situation, and this is accomplished to a great extent by the manner in which the patient interview is conducted. There are a few little techniques which should be employed, including the following:

1. Introduce yourself.
2. Explain the procedure.
3. Treat the patient with an air of respect and concern for her situation.
4. Avoid using "yes" or "no" questions if possible.
5. Try to draw the patient out into free-flow conversation without intimidating her.
6. Do not force or rush the questions.

There are some "stalls" and "warnings" in interviews, for which the nurse should try to be on guard and to deal with as necessary:

1. The nurse feels something is wrong.
2. There is a change of attitude by the nurse or the victim.
3. The nurse becomes judgmental.
4. The nurse begins to feel ambivalent, with positive and negative reactions.
5. The nurse must beware of labeling responses or attitudes.
6. The nurse must beware of offering false assurances.

The EDN can avoid some of the pitfalls in listening by maintaining eye-to-eye contact and by avoiding talking too much (let the patient talk) or making decisions for the patient (let *her* make the decisions), changing the subject (let the patient finish her responses), and using emotionally charged words. Try to stay with clinical terms.

POLICIES AND PROCEDURES

One goal of every ED should be the development of policies and procedures for the management of the sexually assaulted person, to provide the level of care that is frequently critical to the patient's future emotional well-being, as well as to obtain a valid chain of evidence. Some guidelines follow:

Purpose

- To provide the patient with an optimal amount of privacy
- To examine the patient for determination of the presence of physical and/or emotional trauma, to initiate the necessary appropriate treatment and to refer the patient to the necessary follow-up services as indicated.

- To provide a chain of evidence to sustain criminal proceedings against the alleged assailant

Procedure (Sample)

1. Each patient brought to the ED for an examination for alleged rape shall be accompanied directly to the ED by the admitting clerk on duty. If the patient is accompanied by a law enforcement official, he and/or she shall be directed to the waiting room in the ED to await completion of the chain-of-evidence (COE) examination. No interviews will be made at the outpatient admitting desk.
2. The EDN will accompany the patient to the private examination area. The first priority will be to reassure and calm the patient. When the patient is able, the nurse will obtain her written permission for "Release of Information" (to the police). The EDN will then interview her to complete the preliminary portion of the form for Medical Examination for Alleged Rape.
3. The EDN will, at this point, notify the admitting clerk that the patient may be interviewed for required information. This can generally be done before the physical examination is carried out.
4. The COE examination will be done by the ED physician, using a pre-scribed form according to the local jurisdiction.
5. Instructions are to be given for follow-up care if there is need for a pregnancy test, if signs and symptoms of pregnancy present, and the availability of abortion referral services if needed.
6. Actual treatment of the patient will consist of careful medical description of findings and the treatment of local and/or general trauma.
7. Prophylactic doses of penicillin are no longer given.
8. The patient should be informed of available psychiatric services even if the need for these is not apparent at the time of treatment. If the patient does not have a private physician, referral should be made for follow-up care.

CHAIN-OF-EVIDENCE EXAMINATION

Purpose

To properly obtain an evidentiary specimen and document cases of possible sexual assault.

Procedure

1. The patient must either be accompanied by police, or the nurse must obtain a police request (either verbal or written) for COE examination. If the patient does not wish to have the police notified, a COE exam will be done, dated, sealed, and initialed by the nurse, and the evidence placed

in the refrigerator for 1 week, in the event that the patient should decide to contact the police and file a criminal complaint. Explain the procedure carefully, since this may be the patient's first vaginal examination.

2. The patient's clothing worn at the time of the alleged assault is to be held for scientific examination. Generally, only the panties and any clothing that may be stained are desired for examination. The panties must be bagged separately in a small plastic bag and may be placed in a larger bag with any other clothing to be examined. These bags must be labeled with the date, time, and patient's name. If the clothing has spots of seminal fluid, mark these spots for certification by circling with marking pen and attach a piece of tape with date, time, and initials of person obtaining the evidence.

3. While removing the patient's clothing, check the entire body for bruises, abrasions, etc., and note on the ED patient's chart.

4. Prepare the patient for vaginal examination. Most areas have a COE "kit" with varying degrees of elaboration on gathering of evidence. To a great extent this eliminates the necessity for every ED to maintain an extensively equipped assault examination tray, although it is necessary for every ED to maintain a ready supply of extra slides, marking pens, plastic evidence bags, etc.

5. In simplest form the kit is a cardboard mailer container with a sealing flap. The kit contains:
   - 1 comb
   - 3 small marked envelopes for pubic and head hair
   - 1 test tube with cork for saliva-soaked swabs
   - 1 Vacutainer blood tube for specimen to be typed
   - 1 slide mailer container with:
       1 sectional slide marked for vaginal, cervical, and rectal smears
       1 plain slide for wet mount or oral smear if appropriate
   - 1 test tube with cork and 2 swabs for vaginal content

6. Be certain to initial and note patient's name and date on each specimen taken!
   A. Comb pubic area with comb provided and place any loose hair or debris in the envelope and seal it.
   B. Place at least five (5) *pulled* pubic hairs (for identification of hair follicles) into an envelope and seal it. Place at least five (5) *pulled* head hairs into an envelope and seal it.
   C. Have the victim deposit two (2) saliva-soaked applicators into the tube provided. At this time add approximately 1 cc of NSS and bring solution to a boil. Cool and seal.
   D. Obtain from the victim, if possible, 1 cc of whole blood, using the Vacutainer provided.
   E. The slide mailer contains two slides. One is marked "V-C-E."
       - Place the vaginal smear on section marked V.
       - Place the cervical smear on section marked C.
       - Place the rectal smear on section E.

The extra slide is to be used for the wet mount or oral smear if appropriate.

F. Obtain two vaginal swabs, place in the large culture tube and seal.

G. The wet mount must be sealed by drying around the edges of the cover slide carefully, gently pressing out any air trapped under the cover slide, and when surface is dry, seal edges around the cover slide with clear nail polish and allow to dry.

H. Place all materials into the container, seal envelope, and label with patient's name, date, and initials of collector.

To preserve the evidentiary value of this COE collection, the container must be closed and sealed with a cross-taping which extends the tape ends well down onto the envelope by 2 inches on each side. The nurse then initials the tape, writing half on the tape and half on the envelope, to insure a tamper-proof closure. The entire envelope and contents, after being sealed and labeled, are to be kept in a refrigerator until turned over to the police officer who has signed the property receipt form.

All specimens and articles of clothing given to the investigating officer are to be listed. The investigating officer is to give the nurse a receipt for the itemized materials, and this is to be attached to the patient's medical record. The receipt should note the time, date, and the name of the officer. A copy of form for Medical Examination for Alleged Rape should also be sent with the investigating officer; the original stays with the patient's medical record.

The investigating officer or agency may require pictures to be taken of the victim. Since this is an evidentiary procedure, it is not necessary for the hospital to obtain consent of either the patient or the parents. It is to be noted on the patient's ED record that pictures were taken, however. A nurse must be in attendance during picture-taking procedures.

It is suggested that every ED have a tray available to the pelvic examination area to augment the supplies found in the kit which may be supplied by the local jurisdiction. Some suggestions would be:

1. Slides (with one frosted end for marking indelibly) premarked for vaginal, cervical, rectal, and plain
2. Slide covers and a bottle of clear nail polish
3. Marking pens with fine indelible points for marking frosted slides.
4. Dropper bottle of NSS
5. Transgrow culture media
6. Sterile cotton-tipped applicators
7. Small plastic bags for dried slides
8. Small plastic bags for underclothing
9. Supply of small-toothed combs
10. Small specimen tubes for receipt of vaginal contents for acid phosphotase test.

Philosophy

When medical evidence is offered in court for cases of alleged rape, it is essential that the district attorney be able to demonstrate that he is using the same evidence that was collected during the medical examination of the complainant. He must, therefore, be able to identify all those who handled the evidence and account for each step in the process of collection, storage, transportation, and delivery. In order that this "chain of evidence" be completely traceable, it is essential that as few people as possible actually touch the evidence.

For hospital procedures, then, it seems most reasonable to have the person collecting the evidence hand it directly to the nurse, who, after sealing the envelope, deposits it with "security" (either the police or the refrigerator). Proper chain-of-evidence sealing consists of placing all evidence in the provided container and sealing it with tape: the date, time, and name of the person sealing the container should be affixed in such a manner that the information covers both the container itself and the sealing tape. This should then be refrigerated and remain as is until handed over to the proper authority.

ON DEATH, DYING AND GRIEF

In the past few years a great deal of controversy has arisen regarding the definition of death. Death is not the final stage of life that it once was; it has become more uncertain, thereby creating an atmosphere of both hope and despair.

To cope with this recent phenomenon, nurses must 1) learn to accept death according to their own individual beliefs, 2) accept the cultural, ethnic, or religious beliefs relating to death of people they are caring for, and 3) recognize that everyone deals with death in his or her own unique way. Surviving family or friends must be allowed the right to express their grief in any way that is not harmful to others or themselves.

The type of death most often encountered in the ED is sudden and unexpected, usually resulting from trauma or heart attack. Because of this, the survivors are faced with the sudden onset of a process they neither understand nor wish to accept. This is the process of grief. It is encountered by peoples of all cultures and has several recognizable stages.

These stages, as outlined by Dr. Elisabeth Kubler-Ross, are apparent in the dying patient, in the dying patient's survivors, and in the survivors of the person who has died a sudden death. To help both patients and survivors, it is important to understand and recognize these stages: 1) denial, 2) anger, 3) bargaining, 4) depression and 5) acceptance.

To prevent the inappropriate support of any of these stages, nurses must also recognize these same stages within themselves. It is easy and dangerous for a nurse to promote any or all of these stages; this can undoubtedly lead to unnecessary feelings of guilt of both the survivors and the nurse who has helped this process along. Most importantly, it can leave the dying patient without the critical support of the family at a time it is most needed.

Every effort should be made to contact the family of someone who is dying from an unexpected cause. If this cannot be done, the nurse must provide as much support as possible to the dying person. It is generally not necessary to confirm or deny that one is dying. Instances in which the patient is conscious of the efforts to save his or her life may also afford the patient the awareness that he or she is dying. Even though the activities are hectic and often impersonal, it is imperative that the person be made to feel that he or she *is* still alive. The nurse has the best opportunity to accomplish this, since it is the nurse who spends more continuous time with the patient and can reassure him/her that he/she will not be left alone; and indeed, this should be the case.

Since death is hard on everyone, there is a tendency to avoid allowing the family to be with the loved one who has just died. The tendency, moreover, is to send the family home with condolences and sedatives; however, this simply delays the grief process and in some cases seriously inhibits it.

If the family wishes to see the deceased person, they should be allowed, even encouraged, to do so, and in fact should be asked if they would prefer to be alone with the person for a short period of time. If they decline, they are providing an indication of their method and capacity for dealing with the death. Nurses should never let their own feelings interfere with the normal bereavement process of the family.

Events surrounding death in the ED happen so quickly that personnel have very limited time to initiate the healthy first stages of grief. The more understanding a nurse has of death, dying, and grieving, the better able to provide appropriate support and assistance. However, not all the questions related to these issues can be answered in a matter-of-fact manner. With a greater realization of their involvement with death, nurses frequently have the singular opportunity of providing understanding, comfort, and support in a meaningful fashion.

Nurses must realize that they are not impervious to the same feeling shared by the patient and the family and that they may be able to offer the only rational focal point from which others can gain perspective and stability.

COMMUNICATION WITH PATIENTS AND FAMILIES

The quality of the communication that the ED staff establishes and maintains with patients, and their families, is a crucial factor in dealing with all psychiatric and emotional crises. The importance of communication with the trauma victim is often unrecognized, yet the trauma patient and family are frequently in an incapacitating emotional state, not unlike the psychiatric crisis.

The ED staff needs, first of all, to be constantly aware of the depth of patient anguish, and that these anguished emotions are "normal" human responses to severe crises. Emotional responses to traumatic events often follow a sequence not dissimilar from death and dying. A typical pattern is 1) numbing; 2) anger and, in particular, outbursts of anger at the "helper;" 3) disbelief and denial; 4) guilt; 5) searching and yearning for restitution; 6) disorganization and despair; and 7) depression and loneliness. These are all *normal,* rather than pathological, responses of humans in physical/emotional trauma states. ED staff must anticipate this "venting" process verbally, as well as non-verbally, and be prepared to interact professionally and supportively.

Although one can enumerate a bewildering variety of emotional and psychiatric entities, there are some common communication strategies that are appropriate across the entire spectrum of emotionally "charged" situations:

1. Be aware of the intense emotions, and their probable sequence, that are engulfing your patient;
2. Introduce yourself as early and as warmly as you can, both by name and as a professional;
3. Recognize and treat the patient as a person, not a clinical entity. Address them by name and start supportive communication immediately, e.g., reassurance, personal warmth, and professional confidence;
4. Be aware that patients hear and sense what is said and felt by staff. They are particularly sensitive to emotional implications.
5. Assure the preservation of your patient's dignity and privacy;
6. Listen, actively and responsively, but as a professional and not as a fellow victim;
7. Monitor your own reactions and comments; know your own emotional biases and/or hang-ups and your early warning signs;
8. Presenting and maintaining an organized, confident, and assertive but caring manner will provide the setting for a therapeutic climate;
9. Allow and encourage the patient and family expression of feelings. You can help them start "working through" the involved patterns of response to crisis and irretrievable loss;
10. Plan and allow time and space to explain and re-explain procedures, what to expect next, and options and resources available. People in distress need more explanation than may seem logically sufficient. Repeated efforts in explanation are an important part of the EDN's therapeutic intervention.
11. Remember always that the nurse is the only "constant" in the patient's environment and bears the responsibility of being the patient's advocate, an especially important role in times of crisis.

STRESS

More is being written all the time about stress factors in nursing, and consideration of the emotional aspects of emergency nursing and the resulting stress levels seems entirely appropriate.

Every nurse entering the emergency nursing field should be totally aware of the emotional highs and lows that will be encountered in the course of daily assignments and challenges; a reorientation to this reality would be excellent each time a new employee joins the department staff.

Stress is an essential component of healthy function, but when demands on physical and emotional stamina exceed the individual's "buffering" capacity, stress becomes "dis-stress" and manifests itself with what could be called the "overloaded circuit syndrome" that sooner or later (if not unloaded) blows fuses! One of the easiest places in the world to acquire the syndrome is a busy ED where patients present for care and bring with them a host of personal complexities that must be dealt with, compounded by mounds of paperwork and documentation, jangling telephones, ambulance radio calls, attending physicians bustling in and out with individual requests, communication foul-ups, sudden unexpected death, broken equipment, short staffing, interpersonal misunderstandings, back-to-back codes, and more patients than you can find stretchers and wheelchairs for!

It is the rare individual who has not stood in the midst of all this, fighting back hopeless frustration in the seeming futility of it all, trying desperately to clear the thought processes to determine priorities, while struggling to maintain equilibrium and the ability to *respond* to the situation rather than blindly *reacting*.

The demands of patient care may trigger so many feelings of inadequacy in the nurse (due to the sheer fact that one person can move only so fast and do just so many things correctly in a given period of time) that suddenly responses to patients and coworkers take on a different and very terse note. Realize that if you work in ED, you *will* be subject to stress, crises, and emotional peaks and valleys that occasionally take their toll in extreme physical as well as mental and emotional fatigue. For this reason, emergency personnel must pay special attention to their own well-being in order to cope with demands on the job, and should protect their physical and mental health by getting enough rest and insuring a sound nutritional status to provide required energy levels.

All of us encounter potentially stressful events each day of our lives no matter what we do. These external situations are *stressors*. Our reaction to these constitutes the *stress*. Stress is our own response; Dr. Hans Selye, probably the leading authority on stress research, defines stress as "the non-specific response of the body to demands made upon it." Stress is not always harmful; some is helpful, energizing, and positive. In fact, complete absence of stress is impossible; only the dead are totally without stress. When stress is pleasantly exciting, the "roller coaster" effect, our response is often referred to as *eustress*. In contrast, the unpleasant pressure level response is called *distress*.

The major misconception about stress is that it is all bad and that the effects are always destructive. This distorted view is reinforced by large scale commercial enterprises promoting tranquilizers, alcoholic beverages, varied therapies, relaxation aids, etc. In contrast, Selye (1976) points out that stress is "the spice of life." In the right amount for you, it enhances the flavor of life. Too low a level may be bland and boring. If the level is too high, it becomes unpalatable and upsetting.

The key is not to eliminate stress, an impossible task, but to manage it and to find the appropriate level—your personal "just right" cruising range.

Almost all of us have experienced traumatic events—major changes, personal disasters, painful experiences—in our lives. Holmes and Rahe (1967) developed a Social Readjustment Scale which identifies the mean stress impact of each of 43 generally representative events, the top ten of which are rated as follows:

LIFE EVENT	MEAN VALUE
1. Death of spouse	100
2. Divorce	73
3. Marital separation	65
4. Jail term	63
5. Death of close family member	63
6. Personal injury	53
7. Marriage	50
8. Fired at work	47
9. Marital reconciliation	45
10. Retirement	45

Not everyone would consider *all* of these events as negative. However, some people even have difficulty coping with "positive stressors." All of us probably carry scars from old or recent personal disasters, but most stress isn't caused by explosive dramatic catastrophies; it builds day to day from the relatively minor but *chronic* wear and tear pressures.

Some stress-producing events are *episodic,* others are chronic, occurring continually. The work life in an ED involves an abundance of both episodic and chronic stressors, some of which typically include:

EPISODIC	CHRONIC
• Sudden changes in the pace of work	• Coworkers seem unclear about what my job is
• Another reorganization in the department	• Conflicting demands for my time
• Transferred to new shift or position against my will	• Expected to interrupt my work for new priorities
• Frequent changes in policies and procedures	• Receive feedback only when something is wrong
• Transfer, resignation, or termination of a valued coworker/colleague	• Decisions/changes affecting me are made without my knowledge

Sound familiar? These were *not* derived from emergency nursing surveys but came from a range of studies across business, professional, and industrial work areas. A complete set of work and non-work stress scales with comparable scores from a large sample is contained in the review by Adams (1980).

Stress management doesn't mean avoiding all stressors. It means attending to your own reactions to stressors, identifying the stressors, and finding better ways to cope. Most of us have favorite ways of coping with our stress and keep using them whether they work or not. There is probably no "one right" way of coping with *all* stressors. Most of us can profit in significant terms, however, from assessing our present coping styles and deciding where/when we need to try new strategies.

The whole point is to keep yourself healthy and be aware that 1) your emotions will be affected strongly by what goes on around you in a busy department, and, conversely, 2) your response will certainly have its own unique effect on both patients *and* coworkers. Whether the patient has a serious emergency or something that can be seen as a lesser priority should have no effect on the manner in which the emergency nurse responds to the request for help. The patient is entitled to a courteous and, hopefully, concerned reception on entering the department (which will automatically help reduce the *patient's* stress level and anxiety). In actuality, the nurse who manages the patient skillfully in this regard reaps a double bonus: the personal satisfaction goes a long way toward offsetting the personal stress load, making for a happier situation all the way around.

The problem of stressful situations must be handled realistically. It may be helpful, when the going gets rough, to break the pace as soon as possible with a breath of fresh air, a cup of coffee, or perhaps just a quiet moment *alone* for a brief period of meditation to "get it all together." Most of us take ourselves too seriously too much of the time, but a wonderful way to offset this tendency is to look for the humor in a situation and develop the ability to laugh at yourself, smile at your patients and coworkers and *mean it!* There is a lot of truth in the old saying "laughing just to keep from crying," and it is pure fact that a warm smile can break a tense situation. So as you evaluate your own response to heavy stress, realize that stressful situations *cannot always be prevented* but *can* be reversed before the dominoes start falling, *if* healthy, aware attitudes prevail.

Basically, there are four major clusters of coping strategies. Within each cluster you can select and develop specific stress management skills.* The basic approaches are:

1. *Reorganize yourself*

    Manage the way you spend time and energy—take more control of your day. Coping skills in this cluster include:

    A. Managing time

    B. Pacing—develop a tempo that is right and consistent for you

    C. Value and goal setting—get in touch with what's really important and develop a daily program that invests more time for you

2. *Change your relations with people*

    A. Developing support groups—contact others and develop some sharing and accepting relationships

---

*See reference to Tubesing in Suggested Readings, page 532

  B. Listening—tune in and respond to the feelings of others

  C. Learning to say "no"—express your own preferences and reduce the pressures of others' requests and expectations but in a considerate way

  D. "Fleeing the scene"—find suitable ways to retreat, take a legitimate time-out

 3. Change your own perceptions

  A. Relabeling—discover other meanings in each experience; find out that every event has many possible meanings and learn to select those that are helpful

  B. Imagining and laughing—creativity and humor allow you access to the most powerful "high" known

  C. Speaking gently to yourself—learn to give *yourself* the positive, considerate messages you often choose to give to others.

 4. *Build up strength and resistance*

  A. Exercise

  B. Diet

  C. Relaxation techniques

Each strategy is appropriate some of the time with some of the stressors in each individual's daily life. Often, however, we keep repeating *one* favorite technique just like the little boy with the hammer looking for *anything* to hit.

The destructive effects of too much stress are immense. Recent research attributes to stress an even larger role in arteriosclerotic heart disease, vascular lesions, cirrhosis, breast cancer, lung cancer, auto accidents, diabetes, and on and on. Daily responses of coping with daily stressors, multiplied thousands of times, becomes our life style, and often a terribly destructive one.

Since we are each solely responsible for our actions and behaviors, we each have the opportunity to change and develop healthy coping patterns by identifying stressors, reorganizing or planning a personal stress management approach, and putting it into daily action. Investing this personal thought and time can be one of the most productive activities, both short and long-term, for the EDN, her family, patients and last but not least, of course, co-workers.

Many good references and guidebooks are available; several of the better works are referenced here for your enrichment.

SUGGESTED READINGS ON STRESS

Adams J: Understanding and managing stress: A workbook in changing life styles. University Associates, San Diego, California, 1980

Applebaum S: Stress management for health care professionals. Aspen Systems Publications, Rockville, Maryland, 1981

Greenberg S, Valletutti P: Stress and the helping professions. Paul Brooks, Baltimore, Maryland, 1980

Holmes TH, Rahe RH: The social readjustment rating scale. Psychosom Res, Vol 11, pp 213-218, 1967

House J: Work stress and social support. Addison-Wesley, Menlo Park, California, 1981

Selye H: The stress of life. McGraw Hill, New York, 1976

Tubesing D: Kicking your stress habits. Whole Person Associates, Duluth, Minnesota, 1981

REVIEW

1. Identify the general categories of psychiatric emergencies that are seen in the emergency department.
2. Identify the chief areas of assessment required for the psychiatric patient.
3. Identify four components of an effective approach to the psychiatric patient.
4. Describe some of the cardinal signs and symptoms of depression.
5. Describe the areas that should be questioned with a severely depressed patient.
6. Describe the general physical management of the acute paranoid patient.
7. Identify the groups of psychotherapeutic agents commonly used.
8. Describe the significance of auditory hallucinations as opposed to the implications of visual hallucinations.
9. Describe the three cardinal goals in the management of a rape victim.
10. Identify the techniques that should be employed in conducting the patient interview with a rape victim.
11. Explain the purpose of the chain-of-evidence examination.
12. Describe the correct procedure for handling clothing that is evidentiary.
13. Describe the basic items that should be present on a sexual-assault examination tray.
14. Identify three areas in which the rape victim must have access to follow-up.
15. List the community resources available in *your* community to a rape victim.

BIBLIOGRAPHY

Bellack J, Woodward P: Improving care for the rape victim. JEN, Vol 3, No 3, 1977

Budassi SA, Barber JM: Emergency Nursing: Principles and Practice. C.V. Mosby Co., St. Louis, Missouri, 1981

Burgess AW, Holmstrom LL: Rape: Crisis and Recovery. The Robert J. Brady Co., Bowie, Maryland, 1979

Caldwell MM: Staff stress: What you can do about it. JEN, Vol 2, No 2, 1976

Cauthorne C: Coping with death in the ED. JEN, Vol 1, No 6, 1975

Cohen F, Chappell D, Geis G: Changes in hospital care for rape victims. JEN, Vol 2, No 6, 1976

Cosgriff J, Anderson DL: The Practice of Emergency Nursing. J.B. Lippincott Co., Philadelphia, Pennsylvania, 1975

Dealing with Death and Dying: Nursing Skillbook. Intermed Communications, Jenkintown, Pennsylvania, Nursing 77 Books

Fordyce WE: Operant conditioning: An approach to chronic pain. In Pain, Current Concepts on Pain & Analgesia, Vol 1, Current Concepts for Burroughs Wellcome Co., New York, 1973

Fulton R, Bendiksen R: Death and Identity. The Charles Press Publishers, Inc., Bowie, Maryland, 1976

Gaffney K: Helping grieving parents. JEN, Vol 2, No 4, 1976

Glick R, Meyerson A, et al: Psychiatric Emergencies. Grune & Stratton, New York, 1976

Grant H, Murray R: Emergency Care, 2nd ed. The Robert J. Brady Co., Bowie, Maryland, 1978

Halpern M: Treating pain with drugs. Minnesota Med, Vol 57, pp 176-184, 1974

Johnson D: Crisis intervention training for emergency medical personnel. JEN, Vol 3, No 4, 1977

Jones WH, Buttery M: Sudden death: Survivor's perceptions of their emergency department experience. JEN, Vol 7, No 1, pp 14-17, January/February 1981

Kashoff S: Nursing your stress. JEN, Vol 2, No 2, 1976

Kess RC: Victims of rape—how can we help? JEN, Vol 6, No 6, pp 21-24, November/December 1980

Koenig R: Handling grief in the emergency department. Emergency Medical Services, pp 18-22, July/August 1975

Margolin CB: Assessment of psychiatric patients. JEN, Vol 6, No 4, pp 30-33, July/August 1980

Margolin CB: Evaluating suicide potential in the ED. JEN, Vol 3, No 4, 1977

Melzack R: The Puzzle of Pain. Basic Books, Inc., New York, 1973

Meyers FH, Jawetz E, Goldfein A: Review of Medical Pharmacology, 7th ed. Lange Medical Publications, Los Altos, California, 1980

Resnik HL, Beck AT, Lettieri DJ: The Prediction of Suicide. The Robert J. Brady Co., Bowie, Maryland, 1974

Resnik HL, Ruben HL: Emergency Psychiatric Care. The Charles Press Publishers, Inc., Bowie, Maryland, 1975

Reynolds JI, Logsdon JB: Assessing your patient's mental status. Nursing 79, Vol 9, No 8, pp 26-33, August 1979

Schultz CA: Cultural aspects of death and dying. JEN, pp 24-27, January/February 1979

Schultz CA: The dying person. JEN, Vol 5, No 3, pp 12-16, May/June 1979

Schultz CA: The dynamics of grief. JEN, Vol 5, No 5, pp 26-30, September/October 1979

Sherman J: The Crisis Management of Depression. Phenomenology and Treatment of Depression. Spectrum Publications, Inc., Vol 3, No 5, p 314, 1977

Skodol A, Karasu T: Emergency Psychiatry and the Assaultive Patient. American Journal of Psychiatry, Vol 135, No 2, pp 202-205, February 1978

Sletten I, Barton J: Suicidal patients in the emergency room: A guide for evaluation and disposition. Hospital & Community Psychiatry, pp 407-411, June 1979

Smith MJT, Selye H: Reducing the negative effects of stress. AJN, Vol 79, No 10, p 1953

Speich PL: Taking a psychosocial stress "pulse." JEN, Vol 5, No 3, pp 37-43, May/June 1979

Tishler CL, Lent WJ, McKenry PC: Assessment of suicidal potential in adolescents. JEN, Vol 6, No 2, pp 24-26, March/April 1980

Warner CG: Emergency Care: Assessment and Intervention, 2nd ed. C.V. Mosby Co., St. Louis, Missouri, 1978

Warner CG (ed.): Rape and Sexual Assault: Management and Intervention. Aspen Systems Corporation, Gaithersburg, Maryland, 1980

SECTION III

MANAGEMENT AREAS

LEGAL IMPLICATIONS IN EMERGENCY DEPARTMENT NURSING **28**

KEY CONCEPTS

The aim of this chapter is to promote an understanding and awareness of the duties and legal responsibilities of emergency department nursing, adapted from lecture materials presented to emergency department nurses by Peter Fleissner, J.D., and Ray Mensing, J.D., Oregon Association of Hospitals; W. Stanley Welborn, M.D., J.D., Portland, OR, and James E. George, M.D., J.D., FCLM, publisher, *The Emergency Nurse Legal Bulletin*.

After reading and studying this chapter, you should be able to:

- Identify the common denominators in statutory provisions regulating hospitals and the practice of nursing, regardless of state.
- Identify the three types of law falling within the realm of American law, which is based essentially on English common law.
- Define malpractice, negligence, tort.
- Identify and define the four basic elements of negligence that must all be alleged and proved in a court case.
- List three defenses employed in negligence actions that are by and large statutory.
- Define technical battery.
- Identify and define three types of consent.
- List three rules of thumb dealing with the drawing of blood to determine alcohol levels and obtaining consent.
- Define the "borrowed servant" doctrine.
- List the types of cases that have mandatory report requirements in your state.
- Identify two very common types of intentional torts.
- Describe the importance of upholding the patient's right to privacy and the guidelines for allowing photographs to be taken in the ED.
- Name the one certain way of preventing the loss of foreign material into the patient's tissues, as with the use of catheters, sponges, needles, etc.

Across the United States, the role of the emergency nurse is being expanded, concomitant with development and expansion of emergency medical services systems and the advent of life-support capability and transport in areas where it was previously unknown. Emergency departments today are busy places with ever-increasing patient loads and commensurate demands upon the skilled personnel who staff these departments. The EDN is expected to be qualified, competent, highly skilled, and knowledgeable in the basic areas concerning legal implications as they apply to emergency nursing.

Until recently little emphasis was placed on a nurse's being knowledgeable in legal matters, but today there is much being written and taught relating to the subject. Statutory provisions regulating hospitals and the practice of nursing vary from state to state, but the nurse's moral and legal obligation to the patient does not vary and may be considered the "law of the land." The nurse is expected to exercise common sense, judgment, and empathy at all times, protecting the patient's welfare, and adhering to the tenet *primum non nocere* (first, do no harm).

RESPONSIBILITIES OF THE HOSPITAL

Most hospitals today provide some degree of emergency service to the public although there is no law requiring *every hospital* to maintain an emergency facility. State laws and regulations demand that certain requirements be met by hospitals, and those wishing to participate in health insurance programs for the aged (Medicare) must comply with the federal "conditions of participation," which are administered at the state level if the hospitals wish to realize fiscal solvency. The standards of the Joint Commission on Accreditation of Hospitals (JCAH) are not statutory but may be compulsory if the particular state requires it within its licensing regulations. Noncompliance on the part of a hospital may well result in liability for negligence and may even disqualify it for governmental reimbursement and relicensure.

Essentially, if a hospital holds itself capable of providing emergency service, it must provide that service according to the standards set forth by the state, Medicare, and/or JCAH. These standards and their interpretations are discussed in Chapter 32, Emergency Department Management.

TYPES OF LAW

American law is based on elements of English common law in an extremely abbreviated way. There are a number of types of law that relate to medical and nursing practice and guarantee a means by which the patient is treated safely and within his rights as a free citizen.

Statutory law is the result of a bill passed by a State legislature, with *administrative rules and regulations* promulgated pursuant to those laws, which have the force and effect of law but are more easily changed than a statute. Licensing laws fall into this category.

Case law is an interpretation by the courts on statutes, administrative rules, and the underlying common law.

Constitutional law determines the validity of both statutory decisions and case law with the provisions of the Fourth Amendment (the right of the individual to be protected from illegal search and seizure), the Fifth Amendment (the right of the individual to be protected from self-incrimination), and the Fourteenth Amendment, which provides the right to due process of law.

STANDARD OF CARE

Standard of care is an important term. In the past each community has had its own level of care, which followed custom. Courts across the country have abandoned that concept, and it is now being held that a similarly trained person should function at the same level or standard of care as a person operating in the same capacity elsewhere. The amount of training and/or expertise does have implications in establishing the standard of care and many times this is the factor that prolongs a court case. Generally, you will be held to the *ORPP* standard of care—the *ordinary, reasonable, prudent person* with like or similar training in like or similar circumstances standard of care. It is each EDN's responsibility to stay current educationally and in practice and to know what the accepted standards of nursing practice are, as well as adopting improved standards as they develop.

NEGLIGENCE AND MALPRACTICE

There seems to be a general feeling among hospital personnel that any kind of incident that occurs in a hospital may result in a lawsuit. This may be true in broad terms; however, most incidents do not lead to lawsuits. Even if you were named to a court action for malpractice or negligence, there are certain things that must be proved to the jury and to the court before you will be held liable. There are many occurrences in hospitals where blame cannot be attributed to any one person and certainly not every instance of mishap is a malpractice situation.

Negligence and *malpractice* are terms often used interchangeably, but there is a difference. *Negligence* is the omission or commission of an act that should or should not have been performed, coupled with unreasonableness or imprudence or both on the part of the doer. This is a general definition that can apply to any sector of the public, be it parents in the home or the professional nurse on duty. *Malpractice,* on the other hand, is negligence on the part of a professional, who is licensed to practice in a specific field, and is applied to that professional when his misconduct, lack of skill, omission, misjudgment in the commission of duty causes harm to the person or property of the recipient of the services. A *tort* is an unintentional negligent act upon the person of another which results in injury to that person.

There are four basic elements of negligence that must all be alleged and proved. They are 1) *duty,* 2) *breach of duty,* 3) *proximate causation,* and 4) *damages or injury. Duty* means to perform in such a manner that your patient receives skilled care used by other nurses in like circumstances. *Breach of duty* is the failure to carry out that which is implied in the definition of duty. *Damage* must be proved before an award is made, even though there may have been gross negligence. *Proximate causation* is more difficult to prove, and it must be shown that there was a causal relationship between a breach of duty and the resulting damages. A break in the chain of causation makes it difficult for the plaintiff to prevail.

There are several defenses in negligence actions that are, by and large, statutory. One is *assumption of risk,* which is injury when instructions are ignored. Another is *contributory negligence,* wherein the injured person has contributed to the injury. Information of this sort should be carefully documented and made available for use in the defense. *Comparative negligence* determines whether there was negligence on the part of the defendant or the plaintiff, and if there was on both parts, what percent or extent. It must be proved that the defendant was *at least 51% negligent* for an award to be made, and the award is made according to percentage. Several states now have this statute.

Remember, however, that the jury finds the facts, and the court (judge) determines the law!

CONSENTS*

Since *battery* is the unlawful touching of another person without consent, any treatment given a patient without consent can be construed as technical battery, unless the treatment was required to save the patient's life, in which case the consent is implied.

There is no law requiring written consent from a patient before treatment, and when a patient voluntarily presents for treatment, the consent is generally considered to be *implied.* It is considered essential practice, however, to document the consent for the protection of everyone involved, and this written consent should be an *informed* consent, with the patient participating, if at all possible. Many hospital attorneys feel that the patient should be required to write out the consent in his or her own words and sign it with a date, time, and witness. The patient must be advised of the contemplated course of action, the alternatives, if any, and the degree and kind of risk involved with the proposed treatment. In the ED, in particular, where time is the essence, all too often it may be helpful to explain the procedure or plan of treatment to the patient in *the same way you would want it explained to you and in simple layman's terms* to avoid confusion and misunderstanding of what was said.

When a patient has expressed his consent directly, either orally or in writing, and has been informed fully of the procedure, alternatives, risks, etc., he has

*George JE: Consent in the ED. Emerg Nurs Legal Bulletin, Vol 1, No 4, 1975

given his general consent to subsequent treatment and has established the voluntary physician/patient relationship. This is generally adequate for the usual procedures involving physician examination, X-rays, injections, laboratory samplings, and so forth. There are medicolegal experts, however, who advocate a more specific additional consent form for further specific diagnosis procedures, such as *lumbar punctures, intravenous pyelograms,* and others, which carry a higher risk factor.

When intervention is instituted to sustain life and prevent further damage, consent is secured after the fact, if necessary, from the patient or from the family. Under these circumstances, *emergency doctrine* prevails, and consent is implied. Remember, however, that a patient can always withdraw consent at any time and that intoxication can invalidate a signed consent form. Generally, it is felt that if an intoxicated person cooperates with the procedure the consent is implied.

When the EDN is involved with obtaining blood alcohol specimens, there are many misgivings and the EDN is frequently caught in a dilemma. While consent requirements may vary widely from state to state, a good rule of thumb is as follows:

1. Only draw blood if the patient expressly consents. If an intoxicated person holds out his arm to be drawn without restraint, this consent is adequate.
2. When police have a search and seizure warrant, draw blood without the patient's consent, but use *no* physical force.
3. If there is no consent and the patient refuses, *do not* draw blood.

Valid consents can be given only by competent adults, and the age of majority varies from state to state. Most states now observe 18 years as the age of majority, and some states allow persons as young as 14 and 15 to consent to their own treatment. Some special situations require their own consent procedures and are as follows:

1. Never accept a consent form for an abortion from parents unless the girl also *signs* an *informed* consent.
2. A consultation should be called for emergency treatment of a child if parents are absent and the next-of-kin cannot be reached.
3. In the case of Jehovah's Witnesses, a court order can be obtained to give blood to a child but *not* to an adult.

DOCTRINE OF
RESPONDEAT SUPERIOR

The various functions of the EDN are governed not only by state law, as it affects professional (Nurse Practice Act) as well as hospital licensure, but by hospital policy as it specifically relates within its own institutional walls to that which the nurse may perform and that which the nurse may not perform. How binding is hospital policy on the nurse? This is a problem that frequently surfaces.

The doctrine of *respondeat superior* (let the master answer) holds that the employer is vicariously (or secondarily) liable for acts of its employees and has a shared legal responsibility for negligent acts. The nurse, as a licensed professional, has a duty to respond to hospital policy as well as to the patient. Any decision must be carefully weighed before hospital or physician judgment is overridden, with the realization that respondeat superior requires that the employer be responsible for the acts of a professional employee. Ordinarily, decisions of such weight are not within the nurse's province.

LIABILITY AND MALPRACTICE INSURANCE

There is also a doctrine of law known as the *borrowed servant*. The classic example of this is the nurse who is employed by the hospital but is under the exclusive control of a surgeon at the operating-room table. That person is deemed to have been "borrowed" by the surgeon and technically becomes the employee of the physician while at the operating-room table. The hospital will not be secondarily liable for the negligent acts of that employee. The circulating nurse in the operating room is *not* deemed to be a borrowed servant, but rather is doing clerical and/or administrative work in the surgery that is ordinarily embraced within the scope of her employment. She remains the employee of the hospital even though she also responds to the surgeon's needs.

Many hospitals carry insurance for "all named employees," which is the same as *all* employees. If the hospital policy so states, the nurse is covered by the hospital's insurance, and there is not necessarily a need for the nurse to carry personal malpractice insurance. However, unless the hospital insurance policy is so written, it may not insure him or her, and the nurse named as a defendant would then be obliged to retain and pay his or her own defense counsel. This status of the employed nurse should be investigated, and if not covered, the nurse should arrange coverage under the hospital policy or obtain personal insurance coverage. Generally, the hospital liability coverage will protect the employee only while he or she is acting within the scope of employment. If a nurse is performing nursing acts outside of hospital employment, personal liability insurance should be carried. The prevalent belief among nursing personnel to the effect that having no significant assets makes them "suit-proof" is a highly erroneous conclusion. They are foolhardy in overlooking the unhappy fact that if they are married, commonly held assets are in jeopardy, since a judgment can be collected many years later when the husband/wife joint assets are sufficient to satisfy the claim.

Essentially, most who are in a position to counsel professional personnel warn them that as professional persons, they are responsible for their own acts of wrongdoing or acts of nursing negligence, whether shared with other parties (be they hospital and/or physician) or not.

LEGAL IMPLICATIONS IN DISPENSING MEDICATIONS

Medications are not only administered in most emergency departments, they are also dispensed. Dispensing (identifying, counting, packaging, labeling, etc.) is the responsibility of the pharmacist, but many state laws are extremely conflicting in this area. Most state laws provide for licensed nursing personnel to administer drugs and to withdraw any drug from the drug room, if the pharmacist is not on the premises, in the amount needed to treat a patient with a "starter" or "carry-over" dosage, but *not* to dispense.

The ED presents a unique situation in that the nurse faces obligations that do not exist in the inpatient hospital setting. Generally speaking, there should be a tray or cupboard in the ED containing precounted, prepackaged, prelabeled medications of the types most likely to be given out to patients. Most state laws provide that a physician may dispense from the ED in an emergency situation and may go to the pharmacy for any medication needed to send with the patient.

In reality, the nurse is the one who performs this function for the physician, and great care must be taken to carefully verify the medication with the physician to be very certain the medication(s) is properly identified with the date, name of patient, doctor, and instructions for taking the medication before the patient receives it to take home. Most state hospital associations now make available a publication on "Guidelines for Hospital Pharmacy," which contains an ED section with suggestions for the handling of packaged and labeled drugs most likely to be given out in the ED. These guidelines are approved by most state boards of pharmacy and would be extremely supportive, should a case go to court on "dispensing" drugs from the ED. Guidelines should be carefully followed on labeling, and these are included in the publication.

LEGAL OBLIGATIONS OF THE NURSE REGARDING PRIVILEGED COMMUNICATIONS

Ethically and legally, the nurse has an obligation to hold confidential anything communicated by the patient. This is known as the *nurse-patient relationship of privileged communication.* You cannot be required to testify in court to a private confidential communication between the patient and you, but it is the *patient's right*—not yours! Therefore, if the patient files suit and brings out the confidential matter, it is deemed to be a waiver on the patient's part of the right of confidentiality, and you then can testify. In most states this statute applies to physicians and nurses in civil cases only. The lawyer-client relationship applies to both civil and criminal cases, as does the clergy-parishioner relationship.

INTENTIONAL TORTS

Intentional torts are legal wrongs intentionally perpetrated. *Defamation of character* is an intentional tort and includes both *slander* (the spoken word) and *libel* (the written word) generally, although this is not always true. Defamation of character is a defamatory remark made by one person about another person in the *presence of a third party*.

The theory is that the defamatory remark has damaged that person's reputation in the community, and there are certain things for which punitive damages can be awarded if the plaintiff prevails: 1) damaging one's business reputation, 2) the inference of the presence of a dread disease such as VD, Hansen's disease (leprosy), etc., and 3) derogatory remarks about a woman's chastity, or lack thereof. The only defense available to a defendant is to be able to prove that everything said to the third party is truth, and the *burden of proof is on the defendant*. There is no requirement for the plaintiff to prove that any damage actually occurred.

THE PATIENT'S RIGHT TO PRIVACY

The right to privacy is a problem that frequently presents itself in the ED, and the most frequent problem is that of photographing patients. Everyone has the right to withhold himself from public scrutiny, and this must be upheld. If a patient is to be photographed, a consent form should be obtained, and the use to which the photograph will be put must be clearly explained. If the patient's knee is to be photographed, without any identification, you probably do not need a consent. If, however, you are going to photograph a patient's face for a scientific reason and identify the pictures only by number as before and after photographs, the patient should be informed of the reason and be asked to consent to *both* before and after photographs. The patient then has the right to withdraw his or her consent for either or both of the pictures if he or she wishes to do so, at any time up to the time the picture(s) will be used or published. In short, written permission is needed for any photograph in which there is a possibility that the patient may be identified.

The press has a right to photograph a patient in the public areas of the hospital (parking lot, corridors, lobby) without consent. Once inside the ED, however, the press *does not* have the right to photograph without consent or even to be in the department. News personnel do not have access to patient areas without permission. Police officers *do* have the right to photograph in the ED, *in pursuit of duty only,* and the nurse has an obligation to assist the officer in doing so.

The patient has the right to hold himself from public scrutiny, with a few exceptions (as, for instance, a holder of public office) even though the nurse's responsibility is to the patient and to prevent, if possible, the invasion of the patient's right to privacy.

OTHER LEGAL CONSIDERATIONS

Report to Authorities

Certain cases and situations are required by law in *most* states to be reported to the proper authorities (although requirements may vary widely). Such reporting is required even though it might be deemed to be a breach of the confidential relationship. These cases are as follows:

1. Gunshot wounds (self-inflicted or otherwise)
2. Stab wounds (self-inflicted or otherwise)
3. Anything that appears to have been the result of violence, including MVAs
4. Communicable diseases
5. Child abuse (now mandatory for physicians and nurses in most states)
6. Any death occurring in-hospital within 48 hours of admission (including DOAs) when not previously treated by a physician
7. Drug abuse
8. Poisonings
9. Seizures
10. Fetal deaths

Self Defense

In any ED situation, the nurse has the right to self defense, but only to the extent of avoiding or escaping grave bodily harm. There is no right to reprisal, except as a defensive maneuver.

Determination of Death

Determination of death in an institutional setting is a medical judgment, and the nurse does not have the right to "pronounce" death. The nurse does, certainly, in most instances have the ability to recognize or decide that a person is dead, but it is the physician who must *certify* the death; this involves deciding the cause of death and filling out the death certificate. Usually, DOAs have been recognized as such before being brought into the hospital ED, but not always. If a patient expires shortly after arrival, it is the responsibility of the ED physician to determine death (pronounce) and sign the death certificate.

Reports of Incidents

Incident reports must be made out *by the one who observes the incident,* and should *never* become part of the medical record and must be kept confidential. Nurses have the obligation to *know* the specific requirements of the insurance carrier for the hospital in which they work. The form should be taken directly to the administrator or his designee, who should review the incident report and send it directly to the hospital attorney. This then becomes confidential information since the chain of confidentiality has been maintained (and is more credible if a case develops and is taken to court), and becomes inadmissible (privileged) evidence. The nurse should put what is *medically* relevant to the incident into the patient's chart and what is *legally* relevant into the incident report.

Statute of Limitation

In a medical malpractice situation, the statute of limitation is 2 years, unless a foreign body has been left in the patient, or unless the patient had no reason to know or could not have known that the untoward incident occurred. In these cases, the term would run from 2 years from the discovery up to 5 years, and if fraud is involved, the statutes usually provide that the time may be extended further.

Presence of Foreign Bodies

As an all-around protection against the loss of foreign bodies in patients' tissues (needles, catheters, gauze sponges), the nurse and physician should be absolutely certain to check that no item is put into a patient's body or through the tissues which is not *radiopaque*. (This should include materials like infant feeding tubes frequently used for cutdowns.)

Consent Questions

Whenever the EDN has consent questions about a life and death matter or serious harm, the administration should be involved as soon as possible, in order to pursue every available legal avenue.

Witnesses

Two witnesses are required for attesting to the signature on a last will and testament.

Record Accuracy and Completeness

Accurate times and dates are essential on ED records, both for the statute of limitations and for establishing the *order of death* in settling estate questions, should one spouse predecease the other by a matter of a few moments.

In a court of law, a medical record can be very damaging if it is incomplete and does not accurately reflect the treatment given a patient. Medical records must be concise, complete, and properly signed. To all intents and purposes, *if it was not documented, it was not done!*

Patient Consent

Treatment cannot be instituted against a patient's will, and generally speaking, a conscious adult or emancipated minor has the right to refuse medical treatment. When such a situation arises, it is essential that the refusal of treatment be documented and that the patient sign the hospital's form for leaving "against medical advice" (AMA). If the patient is a child and the parent, guardian, or next-of-kin refuses treatment for that child, a child's AMA form should be signed by the responsible adult. These situations demand cool thinking and as much common sense as can be mustered. Generally, it is felt that the safest guidelines are to err on the side of patient safety and to do everything possible to convince the patient to remain for treatment, arguing gently and cajoling all the way.

If a patient leaves the hospital premises without signing the AMA form, the incident should be *carefully* documented and signed by the personnel involved.

When a life-and-death situation presents itself and the patient refuses consent, it is wise to involve the hospital administration as rapidly as possible.

REVIEW

1. Identify the common denominators in statutory provisions that regulate hospitals and the practice of nursing, regardless of state.
2. Identify the three types of law that fall within the realm of American law.
3. Define malpractice.
4. Define negligence.
5. Define tort.
6. Identify and define the four basic elements of negligence that must all be alleged and proved in a court case.
7. List three defenses employed in negligence actions that are by and large statutory.
8. Define technical battery.
9. Identify and define three types of consent.
10. Give three rules of thumb dealing with consent forms for blood alcohol determinations.
11. Identify the two factors governing the various functions of the EDN.
12. Define the "borrowed servant" doctrine.
13. Define the role of the nurse as opposed to the role of the pharmacist in management of ED take-home medications.
14. List the types of cases or situations that are required by law in your state to be reported.
15. Identify two very common types of intentional torts.
16. Explain the statute of limitation in your state in a medical malpractice situation.

17. Describe one very certain way of preventing the loss of foreign bodies into a patient's tissues.
18. Why are accurate dates and times important on ED records?
19. Explain why thorough and concise documentation is important on a medical record if it is taken to court.

BIBLIOGRAPHY

Anderson DL, Cosgriff JH: The Practice of Emergency Nursing. J.B. Lippincott Co., Philadelphia, Pennsylvania, 1975

Budassi SA, Barber JM: Emergency Nursing: Principles and Practice. The C.V. Mosby Co., St. Louis, Missouri, 1981

Cazalas MW: Nursing and the Law, 3rd ed. Aspen Systems Corporation, Gaithersburg, Maryland, 1979

Fleissner P: Legal Aspects of Registered Emergency Nurse Training Program. Oregon Association of Hospitals, Portland, Oregon, 1974

George JE: Consent in the ED. Emerg Nurs Legal Bull, Vol 1, No 4, 1975

George JE: Malpractice insurance and the ED nurse. Emerg Nurs Legal Bull, Vol 1, No 3, 1975

George JE: Malpractice insurance—law and the emergency room nurse. JEN, March/April 1975

George JE: Nursing procedures in the ED—legal or not? Emerg Nurs Legal Bull, Vol 1, No 2, 1975

George JE: The legal limit. JEN, Vol 2, No 1, 1976

George JE: The Law and Emergency Care. The C.V. Mosby Co., St. Louis, Missouri, 1980

Hemelt MD, Mackert ME: A nursing 79 handbook: Your legal guide to nursing practice. Nursing 79, Vol 9, No 10, pp 57-64, October 1979

Mancini MR, Gale AT: Emergency Care and The Law. Aspen Systems Corporation, Gaithersburg, Maryland, 1981

Miller M: Consent forms: Who does what? When, where, and why? JEN, Vol 7, No 1, pp 33-34, January/February 1981

Warner CG: Emergency Care: Assessment and Intervention, 2nd ed. The C.V. Mosby Co., St. Louis, Missouri, 1978

THE ROLE OF THE MEDICAL EXAMINER

29

KEY CONCEPTS

The contents of this chapter are based on materials presented to emergency nurses in lectures by William J. Brady, M.D., Chief Medical Examiner for the State of Oregon, who feels strongly that emergency personnel must understand the function and jurisdiction of the medical examiner and the responsibilities that EDNs have in the management of DOAs and ED fatalities. It is hoped that this chapter will help to clarify some areas of doubt and confusion.

After reading and studying this chapter, you should be able to:

- Explain who may determine that a person is dead and who must certify to that fact.
- List the deaths that are generally reportable to the medical examiner or coroner.
- Name and differentiate the personnel levels in *your* county medical examiner program.
- Explain the management of a DOA.
- Describe the proper environment for examination of a possible DOA.
- Describe the recommended manner in which family and friends should be handled.
- Explain the importance of obtaining a thorough history for the medical examiner.
- Describe the recommended procedure for notification of death.
- Describe some of the factors relating to sudden infant death syndrome.
- Explain the guidelines to follow when an autopsy may be indicated.
- Describe the recommended methods of handling evidentiary materials.
- Describe the policies applying to drawing blood samples of a dead person.
- Describe the policies that should govern the release of the body.
- Describe the safest policy for protecting the valuables of the deceased.

The medical examiner system has evolved from the days of the Roman legions, when a physician was assigned to determine death and the causes of death among members of the legions. The first medical examiner system was established in the United States in the 1890s; many states now have a medical examiner system which functions within the framework of that state's statutory provisions. There are still other states, however, that operate under a coroner system, in which the office is elective, with no prerequisite medical background, as opposed to the medical examiner system which requires that the medical examiner be a licensed physician in that state. The term "coroner" dates back into early English times, when the Crown sent a man to claim the estates and holdings of slain knights. The term *Crown's man* was applied, later becoming colloquially known as the *crowner* and then as the *coroner*.

Whether your state and/or county functions under the jurisdiction of a medical examiner or a coroner, there are responsibilities that fall to emergency department personnel and should generally be handled along well-established lines of policy, employing common sense and judgment at the same time.

DETERMINATION OF DEATH

Deciding or determining death means merely that one is able to ascertain that death has occurred by the absence of vital signs. *Pronouncing* death, a term frequently used, means little or nothing, since death must first be *determined* and then must be *certified*. The determination of death can be made by any person under appropriate circumstances, but the certification of a death must be done by a licensed physician, either the medical examiner or the coroner, in that particular jurisdiction. The death certificate is documentation of the date, time, cause of death, contributing cause of death (if indicated) and manner of death, including details of burial. This certificate is a document that will be filed with the bureau of vital statistics of the state, along with birth certificates, marriage licenses, etc.

The frequent use of the term *pronouncing* applies mainly to the formality of having the physician confirm or verify the death when it occurs in hospital, and this is a requirement of the hospital's policies and procedures, notwithstanding the fact that the nurse is usually capable of recognizing the fact that death has, indeed, occurred.

REPORTABLE DEATHS

Particular types of deaths are of such general importance to society that for centuries a government agency (the medical examiner or coroner) has assumed jurisdiction of these deaths:

1. Deaths involving criminal activity (homicides or suspicious deaths) which may include unlawful use of dangerous or narcotic drugs or the use or abuse of chemicals or toxic agents

2. Cases of self-destruction
3. Traumatic deaths, including those that are apparently accidental or that follow an injury
4. Persons dying without medical attention during the period immediately prior to death or not under the care of a physician during the period immediately prior to death.

   The terminology *immediately prior to death* was intentionally left vague. A person seen by a physician in a small, remote town within a week of death may well be under closer care than a person seen in a clinic setting in a large metropolitan area the day of demise. The time definition of an "unattended death" is left to the individual physician's discretion and good judgment.

Many jurisdictions require that all deaths of persons admitted to a hospital or institution for less than 24 hours be immediately reported to the medical examiner, but need not always be investigated and certified by the medical examiner or coroner.

The person DOA from natural causes, under the care of a private physician who is in attendance, while reportable, will generally *not* be a medical examiner case. Once this natural death is reported to the medical examiner by phone, the latter generally will "release" the body, which simply means that there is no further need for a governmental agency to be involved, since the private physician will complete the death certificate. This body then can be removed to the funeral establishment.

Reportable deaths should be made known to the medical examiner, his or her deputy, or the coroner immediately. If this becomes difficult and time-consuming in the ED, the problem should be turned over to the supervisor on duty for follow-up. Your county medical examiner or coroner should provide your ED with names and telephone numbers of the on-call personnel for their offices at all times.

MANAGEMENT OF THE DOA

The person who arrives by car or ambulance "dead on arrival" frequently presents a problem of jurisdictional responsibility. The EDN must be aware of the local lines of authority, realizing that two possibilities exist. The person DOA becomes the responsibility of either 1) the county in which the death was discovered, or 2) the county from which the body has been transported, since exact time and place of death are uncertain during transport. This area *must* be clarified for proper reporting and subsequent release of the body.

EXAMINING FOR DETERMINATION OF DEATH

When DOAs arrive at the ED or patients die while in the department, a careful examination must be made to determine death and the absolute cessation of vital functions. The following are guidelines that *must* be observed to avoid extremely embarrassing errors in judgment:

1. Do *not* allow the examination to be conducted in the ambulance or other vehicle.
2. *Always* remove the body to an area with adequate space and adequate *light* for a thorough and complete examination.
3. Remove or open enough clothing to clearly expose the precordium, neck, and head for the physician to examine.
4. Expect the ED physician to do a thorough and careful examination to determine death. If there is any doubt, record a single ECG lead.

EMERGENCY DEPARTMENT PROCEDURES ON ALL FATALITIES

A written policy on notification of the medical examiner or coroner should be readily available in your department. The details of the notification procedure will vary with the local situation, but definite written policies should exist to insure that a medical examiner's or coroner's representative knows of the death as soon as possible.

Whether or not there exists a statutory requirement, notification should be made immediately and directly. Do not depend on police agencies unless the officer with whom you talk is a deputy medical examiner or deputy coroner.

Your county examiner may prefer to work through a deputy, so make an effort to know the county policy and determine who will respond to your call.

When relatives and friends accompany the body of a DOA, make every effort to provide them with a private area, and ask that they remain at the emergency room until the medical examiner is contacted. Ask the medical examiner or coroner for his or her expected time of arrival and ask if he or she wishes the family detained. If an unreasonably long time ensues, or if the family has insisted on leaving, *always* find out the address or telephone number where they can be reached. Families frequently do not return home and may be unavailable when it is vitally important to reach them. The information obtained from these people is often the most important part of the death investigation. If they are gone and cannot be reached for interview, significant problems frequently arise.

The EDN can participate in a very constructive role by obtaining and recording as much information as possible from the ambulance or fire attendants, including their names and a telephone number where they may be reached. Their story is often crucial in arriving at judgments concerning disposition of the case. Any information that can be obtained from family or friends that may have a bearing on the medical history of the deceased person should be recorded objectively and accurately.

In some states the person investigating the death has a right to review the hospital chart, and it is extremely helpful to have this readily available to expedite the proceedings. If a deputy medical examiner or deputy coroner responds, explain the examining physician's observations, treatment, and diagnoses. Better yet, if the ED physician is available, have the physician talk directly with the deputy. If diagnostic tape, venipunctures, or cutdowns were done, be certain this is explained to the deputy so that these are not misinterpreted as wounds.

If the family has accompanied the body, notification in the ED depends on the particular circumstances of this death and may be handled by the physician who has made the determination in the ED, or the medical examiner or coroner or deputy. Preferably a physician should be the person to notify the family members since the physician is in the best position to explain the preliminary impressions as to cause and to render supportive care as necessary. If the family has *not* come to the ED, ask the medical examiner to notify them. An individual policy for your hospital has probably been establishd, but generally it is best to avoid phone notification. Grieving relatives are best handled at home or at a funeral home rather than having them respond to the ED, where there may not be personnel or space available to support their emotional and physical needs.

SUDDEN INFANT DEATH SYNDROME (SIDS)

The disease known as sudden infant death syndrome (crib death) is a condition causing the sudden death of a normal, generally healthy 1- to 6-month-old infant during sleep, with no apparent cause. Statistics reflect that there are 10,000-15,000 of these deaths annually in the United States. Sudden infant death syndrome (SIDS) is the most common cause of infant death after the first week of life and is second only to accidents as a cause of death between 1 week and 15 years of age. The incidence is 1:300 live births.

Some further studies reveal that it occurs most frequently in babies from 2 to 4 months of age, with 1-6 months considered the usual range. It occurs less commonly in summer months and occurs in cluster patterns during the winter among populations with "colds." The incidence among premature infants is higher than that among infants with a normal birth weight. Most studies show that 60% of the victims are male. The SIDS is generally more commonly seen in the lower socioeconomic groups but is also routinely seen in more affluent population groups; almost all of these babies die while asleep, a fact suggesting that sleep has something to do with the causation of this obscure syndrome.

Three common theories regarding SIDS have been unequivocally disproved in recent years. It is now well known that

1. The victims *absolutely do not* smother or suffocate in their pillows or bedclothing.
2. The victims *do not die* from vomiting or choking on their milk.
3. The victims *are not* battered children.

As Dr. Brady* points out, untrained investigators all too often consider the death "suspicious" and react accordingly. A pathologist can easily and rapidly

---

*Brady WJ: Medical Investigation of Deaths in Oregon, 2nd ed. Oregon State Health Division, Salem, Oregon, 1976

differentiate a case of child abuse from a crib death at autopsy, and before any serious consideration of parental interrogation occurs, an autopsy should be immediately ordered.

The SIDS is a common and complex medical problem but is also a tragic situation for the parents and family, who frequently blame themselves until someone with knowledge of the syndrome explains the disease. Frequently, too, older children are psychologically devastated by the loss of the sibling, and all too often other family members (in-laws, grandparents, and even neighbors) may become suspicious and accusative.

Everything possible should be done in the ED to support and comfort the parents of the SIDS victim and to provide counseling through a public health nurse or someone equally knowledgeable on the subject.

A 1974 National Institute of Health grant in excess of $5 million was given for development of a national program to deal with explaining the disease to bereaved parents and alleviating guilt feelings. Several states and cities have pilot programs underway as a result of this funding.

SPECIAL SITUATIONS

The following are guidelines for management of some of the special situations that may arise in the ED, all of which should be applied with common sense and judgment:

Autopsies

Generally speaking, the medical examiner, coroner, district attorney, or their designees have the authority to order an autopsy. The family need not give permission for this autopsy, and in fact, if the autopsy is clearly indicated, they will not be asked. This is the medical examiner's, coroner's, or district attorney's decision alone.

In some instances the EDN will be faced with indecision as to whether permission for autopsy should be requested of the family by hospital personnel. The nurse's involvement with this dilemma should be predicated on the qualifications of persons responsible for the local death investigation program; it is important to be aware of the level of professional competence of the medical investigators in any community, and if the local system performs adequately, hospital personnel should leave the job of obtaining autopsy permission to the medical investigators.

Handling Evidence

A general rule for handling *any* evidence in a criminal case is "the less handling of evidence, the better." If the case goes to court and you are involved in the "chain of evidence," excess handling of evidence may create an awkward and time-consuming procedure for you and the prosecution.

Clothing Removal

Do not cut the victim's clothing unless absolutely necessary. If an immediate examination of the wound is necessary, try to either unbutton or pull up the clothing. If cutting or ripping the clothing is not a lifesaving necessity, spend a few seconds and try to avoid tearing or cutting through either a bullet wound hole or a knife slash in the clothing. Always remember that some other persons (hours, days, or weeks later) must carefully reconstruct this clothing, matching knife wounds and bullet holes. Please do not make their task more difficult; always save clothing for the investigators and never discard any articles that accompany the victim, since this is often important evidentiary material. Think through the consequences of your act! If clothing is wet (blood, water, etc.), hang it to dry for as much time as possible (in the patient's area), carefully fold and bag (preferably brown paper shopping bag which "breathes"), and identify with name, date, time, and your initials before it is turned over to the death investigator. Do not cram wet, soiled clothing, from a person who is a candidate for medical investigation, into a bag to sit at room temperature and "vegetate"—not that this alters the evidentiary merit, but it certainly makes for unpleasant working conditions.

If bullets or fragments of any significance are found in, around, or beside the body, save them for the investigators along with the clothing and accord them the same careful identification.

Valuables accompanying the deceased person are a source of never-ending grief to everyone involved unless very carefully handled. The best policy is to entrust rings, watches, wallets, money, credit cards, and other valuable items to safe-keeping in the hospital vault, following whatever policy is standard. The rightful survivors may claim the belongings, subsequent to establishing their identity, and this will avoid untold problems for the hospital, nurses, medical investigation personnel, undertakers, and the survivors themselves. We urge common sense here, citing an example of a man who accompanies his wife to the ED by ambulance and waits quietly while she is coded and determined to be without vital signs. Certainly, no sensible personnel would lock this woman's engagement and wedding rings in the valuables vault; they would be given to the husband and so documented on the ED record. Common sense and judgment must prevail.

Drawing Blood Samples

Generally the medical examiner's authority applies only to bodies of deceased persons. There is nothing in the statutes, by and large, that relates to living patients or living suspects insofar as the medical examiner or coroner is involved; i.e., an injured but living driver who may be charged with a DOA as a result of a negligent homicide.

The medical examiner or coroner does have the authority, however, to draw postmortem blood or urine samples without an autopsy order, since this becomes the handling of evidence post mortem. The deceased individual no longer has any rights of protection under the Fourth Amendment of the U.S. Constitution.

Multiple Homicidal Gunshot Injuries

X-ray films, both AP and lateral, of a body shot several times are generally of great help to the pathologist. If films of this sort can be obtained before the body is removed, you may be able to help expedite the death investigation and will earn the pathologist's gratitude.

Releasing the Body

The body should be released to a funeral home only after the medical examiner or his or her representative has specifically authorized that it be released. When the body *is* released, *always* be certain that notation is made on the identification that this is a medical investigation case. The undertaker appreciates having this information since he should then contact the medical examiner or coroner before embalming the body.

REVIEW

1. Explain the origin of the medical examiner system in this country.
2. Explain the origin of the coroner system in this country.
3. Explain who may make a determination of death and who must certify death.
4. Identify the categories of death that are generally reportable to a medical examiner or coroner.
5. Describe the jurisdictional responsibility for a DOA.
6. Describe the proper environment for examination of a DOA and explain the reasons.
7. Identify one of the most important pieces of information that should be obtained from the family if they leave the hospital.
8. Explain the reasons you think a well-documented history is important.
9. Explain why ambulance personnel should be questioned for information.
10. Explain the reasons for the recommended notification-of-death procedure.
11. List the statistical findings relating to SIDS.
12. Identify some of the frequency patterns in SIDS that have been documented.
13. List three common theories regarding SIDS which have been unequivocally disproved in recent years.
14. Describe the proper method of removing clothes and preserving evidentiary materials.

15. Explain the underlying legal principle that allows the medical examiner to draw body fluids post mortem without an autopsy order or search warrant.

16. Explain the circumstances under which the body may be released to the funeral home.

17. When the body is a case for the medical examiner or coroner, describe the action that should be taken before releasing the body as ordered.

BIBLIOGRAPHY

Brady WJ: Medical Investigation of Deaths in Oregon, 3rd ed. Oregon State Health Division, Salem, Oregon, 1981. (Available from the Oregon State Medical Examiner's Office, Portland, Oregon 97227)

Fatteh A: Handbook of Forensic Pathology. J.B. Lippincott Co., Philadelphia, Pennsylvania, 1973

Helpern M, et al: Legal Medicine, Pathology and Toxicology, 3rd ed. Appleton-Century-Crofts Inc., New York, 1954

Miles M: SIDS: Parents are the patients. JEN, Vol 3, No 2, 1977

Nakushian C: The other victims of SIDS. JEN, Vol 2, No 3, 1977

Spitz W, Fisher R: Medico-Legal Investigation of Deaths. Charles C. Thomas, Publisher, Springfield, Illinois, 1973

COMMUNICATIONS IN THE EMERGENCY DEPARTMENT 30

KEY CONCEPTS

This chapter should develop an awareness of the processes involved in effective communication and the importance of *accurate* communication processes in the Emergency Department, as well as communication between the department and emergency services provided in the pre-hospital phase of patient care, utilizing both telephone and radio communications.

Much of this material is based on lectures presented by Joan Henkel, R.N., Emergency Department Supervisor at Providence Hospital and Medical Center, Portland.

After reading and studying this chapter, you should be able to:

- Identify the basic factors involved in communication.
- Identify the most common ways in which miscommunication develops.
- Describe the levels of communication.
- Describe the chief factors that affect the message sent and the message received.
- Identify the forms of communication that are employed on a daily basis in every ED.
- Describe the emergency medical services cycle.
- Explain the 911 system concept and describe its advantages.
- Describe the importance of ambulance-to-hospital communication capability.
- Describe the procedure for the correct use of the hospital-to-ambulance radio and the FCC regulations that affect transmission.

Some very pertinent thoughts on the effectiveness of the communication process are presented by Delbert W. Fisher, Ed.D. (Director of Education and Training at the Veterans Administration Hospital in Battle Creek, MI) in Ethicon's journal *Point of View.* Portions are condensed here as they relate to the general topic.

FACTORS IN COMMUNICATING

Communication involves two factors: 1) the ability of a person to make his or her thoughts, feelings, and needs known to others, and 2) the ability to be receptive to the attempts of others to impart similar information in return. Simply stated, communication is a two-way process: the sending and receiving of a message.

However, in every transaction between two people, several levels of communication take place at the same time. A portion of the communication is in the words that are used, another in the tone of voice, and another is nonverbal—in the actions of the people while the words are being exchanged. Once one realizes that different levels of communication exist, the more able one is to control the communication process.

COMPLICATIONS OF COMMUNICATING

In considering the verbal portion of the communication process alone (or the words spoken), one can find six ways in which miscommunication develops. For example, consider that I am the sender and you are the receiver of a message. In sending a message, three important things can differ:

1. What I say
2. What I meant to say
3. What you heard me say

The process is parallel in receiving the reply. Three more possible meanings exist:

4. What you say
5. What you meant to say
6. What I heard you say

Only when all six interpretations are the *same* is the communication totally successful. Verbal communication becomes more complex with the addition of each person in the transaction. Three people in a transaction increases the number of possible meanings to 18, thereby tripling the possibility of misunderstanding.

LEVELS OF COMMUNICATING

Communication can be viewed from two distinct vantage points: the *content level* and the *feeling level.* The content level is the surface communication—the who, what, when, and where of the message. Content level communication is important, but frequently it is not so powerful or meaningful as the *feeling* level of the message. The tone of voice one uses is part of the feeling level of communication. The tone of voice may confirm, deny, or confuse the words that are used. For example, a person who uses a cold and remote tone of voice while saying, "Well, you did the best you could," conveys a message that changes the meaning of the words.

Nonverbal communication takes place at the feeling level. What is not said can be more powerful than what *is* said. Hunches often are built on the feelings aroused in astute individuals.

Communication or understanding breaks down more frequently at the feeling level than at the content level. For example, management and union negotiators may discuss a contract and not hear a word that is said until the feeling level of communication is heard. Once the negotiators develop a feeling of trust in the people on the opposite side, the words begin to have meaning. People who have trouble understanding each other probably communicate at the feeling level, and the nonverbal communication blocks the understanding of the verbal communication.

BREAKDOWNS AND BLOCKS

Preoccupation blocks communication. A person who is occupied with other matters will not be able to listen at the feeling level of the transaction. The words will be heard and a decision might be made, but the person attempting to communicate will leave with the feeling, "I don't believe he was listening to me."

Hostility creates misunderstanding. When one has hostile feelings, whether they are toward the person speaking or derive from some recent experience, one is too preoccupied with those feelings to listen to the feelings of another. For example, if a charge nurse has hostile feelings, whatever that charge nurse hears or says will be distorted; therefore a charge nurse must be aware when experiencing hostile feelings, for a staff nurse then will only hear the hostile feelings and not the intended message. The staff nurse will leave the conversation wondering why the charge person is so upset.

Stereotyping because of past experience creates a block to effective communication. Once a person's expectations are set, the other person will usually live up to them. This is called the *fulfillment* prophecy. When a person expects above-standard performance and reliable information from a coworker, it usually will be forthcoming. However, if a person expects below-standard performance and false information, this also will happen.

Other factors that are likely to contribute heavily to obstacles in good communication are an *uncomfortable physical environment, fatigue* (instructions given a few minutes before quitting time will frequently have to be repeated the following day), *insecurity,* and *status* (which may bring out feelings of hostility, envy, power worshipping, or stereotyping). All of these complicate the communication process.

As in the parlor game, when one person tells a story that must be passed from person to person, the last story is usually quite different from the original. Communication from a staff person to a head nurse or supervisor, to an administrator, and then to the board of directors can become quite distorted. As each person hears the words, past experience and feelings condition that person to hear those words in his or her own interpretative manner.

FACTORS AND FEEDBACK

Remember then, communications in the emergency department on a verbal plane involve a sender (mouth) and a receiver (ear), and many factors affect the message sent and the message heard. In addition to the factors discussed previously, general environment, background, education, experience, mood, facial expression, purpose, and use of vocabulary may also be included. The receiver must understand the sender's *symbols;* written messages must be clear and phrased in commonly understood terms.

A breakdown in communication occurs when the idea of the receiver does not match the idea of the sender, and the communication process is not complete until the message from the sender is fed back. Communication is *always* most effective on a one-to-one basis with the *message paraphrased* and, again, *fed back.*

FORMS OF COMMUNICATION WITHIN THE EMERGENCY DEPARTMENT

The ED is a critical care area, and when primary care is given in a critical care setting, there is an absolute need for highly skilled personnel who are capable of effective communication on a continual basis.

The department employs many systems in communicating with staff, patients, other departments, the consumer public, and the media. A full awareness and working knowledge of all these areas is the responsibility of the EDN, and some examples of everyday lines of communication are given here as they have been outlined by Joan Henkel, R.N., Emergency Department Supervisor in Portland, OR:

1. Hospital policy book
2. Emergency department policy and procedure book
3. Employee contracts with hospital
4. Orientation procedure within department (with proficiency list)
5. Department "communication book" with all pertinent information recorded from shift to shift
6. Drug alert book
7. Social service referral procedures and documentation
8. Call list within the department for on-call physicians' roster
9. Medic-Alert tags worn by patients for allergies, diabetes, coumadin, etc.
10. Accounting log for long-distance telephone calls
11. Attendance book for staff development programs
12. Emergency department log with time of entry, name, number, treatments, doctor, disposition, and time for each patient treated

13. Statistic sheet

14. Phone messages and telephone orders (these are legal dynamite, and only the charge nurse should accept telephone orders)

15. Bulletin board for posting schedules, meetings, jobs, social functions, EDNA notices, staff development functions, new memos, and new procedures. Bulletin board contents should be handled in the following manner:
    A. When read, all bulletins should be initialed.
    B. All posted material should be dated and remain posted for 2 weeks.
    C. All retrievable information should be filed after 2 weeks.

16. Intradepartmental communications (every effort must be made to maintain these at the highest level)

17. Posting of CPR and burn charts and tetanus schedules, as required by the Joint Commission on Accreditation of Hospitals

18. Shift report with continuity (the change of shift is the *most* vulnerable part of the day and is when *most mistakes are made*). All members of the oncoming shift and the charge nurse of the off-going shift should review:
    A. The doctor on duty
    B. The status of patients (how many and where) with a summary of each patient in the department
    C. The emergency capacity inventory and the critical bed status
    D. The narcotic count

19. The patient chart forms

20. Hospital-to-ambulance radio network system

THE EMERGENCY MEDICAL SERVICES CYCLE AND RADIO COMMUNICATION

Prehospital communication requirements for emergency medical care are similar whether there is a single case of sudden illness or injury, or a disaster involving large numbers of victims. The normal emergency medical services EMS cycle consists of the following stages and functions:

1. *Incident:* The occurrence that generates the need for emergency services—patient(s) with acute illness or injury

2. *Detection:* The action that determines that the incident took place

3. *Notification:* The action that informs the emergency resource control agency where and when the incident took place and the nature of the incident

4. *Dispatch:* The act that orders emergency resources to the scene of the incident

5. *Closure:* The process that transports emergency resources to the scene of the incident

6. *Action:* The necessary acts that correct or alleviate conditions generated by the incident, including both immediate care and transport to a medical facility

7. *Return to station:* The return of all emergency resources to a state of readiness for a new cycle.

Once the incident is detected, *communications* are necessary complements to each successive stage of the EMS cycle, from initial detection and notification of the incident to the return to station, so that the dispatching center knows immediately when an ambulance is ready to begin a new cycle.

The use of two-way radio equipment is by no means limited to the dispatching-center—ambulance—emergency-department relationship. Other advantages of the two-way radio system are 1) having an operable communication system when the local telephone network is severely damaged or overloaded during a major disaster, 2) having the fastest mechanism for coordinating emergency medical activities with other disaster services in the community, 3) providing rapid intercommunication among hospitals about distribution of casualty loads, and 4) effectively alerting medical manpower to report to meet emergency needs.

TELEPHONE AND THE 911 CONCEPT

In January, 1968, the American Telephone and Telegraph Company announced the establishment of nine-one-one (911) as the single emergency telephone number for use in the United States. The single emergency number concept is not new; it has been used in England for more than 30 years.

The *911-system* can be described as an easy-to-remember, three-digit telephone number used to provide the general public with an immediate and direct access to emergency service resources. The system eliminates the need for the caller under stress to make decisions for which he may be ill prepared, particularly when outside his home community. There are 911-systems in existence today in jurisdictions that range in population from several thousand to several million, and the area, to be efficient, does have some size limitation but does not have to conform to any geographic or jurisdictional boundaries although it *will* normally coincide with those boundaries.

The public, as the user of the 911-system, has a major role in its successful operation. The term *emergency* is highly subjective; it defies precise definition. The public, however, must be educated to use the 911-system correctly and intelligently and the number must not be used as an information service or as a means of airing grievances. When the public is properly educated, the 911-system can be used effectively by the young, the old, the handicapped, the illiterate, and by those with limited knowledge of English to report an emergency, allowing almost every citizen quick access to the EMS agencies to receive fast and effective emergency care.

AMBULANCE-TO-HOSPITAL RADIO

Two-way radio communication between ambulance and hospital is necessary during the action stage of the EMS cycle if optimum emergency medical care is to be provided. The voice channel to the emergency room from the scene of the incident enables the emergency medical technician on the ambulance to request advice to aid in stabilizing the condition of the casualty prior to transport. Communities should consider equipping ambulances with portable communication units for use where victims are beyond the point where the ambulance can travel. Ideally, the portable unit should tie into the vehicle's communication system so that the vehicle system can function as a relay station. The need for two-way radio communication between hospital emergency room and the emergency medical technician in the ambulance is important for the care of casualties during transport to the medical facility. It also permits the ambulance crew to advise the treatment facility of the patient's condition, special requirements if any, estimated time of arrival, and other pertinent information.

This communication capability provides the direct line of contact between ambulance personnel and hospital ED personnel who will receive the patient. It is the vital link necessary to provide optimum prehospital medical intervention with essential continuity of care once the patient has been delivered to the ED. A department that has been alerted to the needs of a critical patient in transit can be ready and on standby to receive the patient with minimal loss of precious time. All too often time *is* of the essence.

GOVERNMENT REGULATIONS AND USE OF THE RADIO

The radio frequency spectrum is a national and international resource in the public domain. Since 1906 international administrative radio conferences have controlled the orderly development of this vital resource through carefully planned frequency allocations to various radio services.

The Federal Communications Commission (FCC), established by act of Congress in 1934, controls frequency allocations in the United States to various nongovernment radio services and licenses individuals. The FCC has set aside specific radio band assignments for very high frequencies (VHF) that are available to the Special Emergency Radio Service, which *includes* hospitals, ambulances, and rescue organizations.

All of these frequencies are subject to FCC regulations, some of which are given here:

1. Hospital radios, except for test transmissions, may be used only for the transmission of messages necessary for the rendition of an efficient hospital service.
2. Ambulance operators and rescue organizations, except for test transmissions, may use these frequencies only for the transmission of messages pertaining to the safety of life or property and urgent messages necessary

for the rendition of an efficient ambulance or emergency rescue service.

3. Test transmissions may be conducted by any licensed station as required for proper station and system maintenance, but such tests shall be kept to a minimum and precautions shall be taken to avoid interference to other stations.

Further, strict rules of the FCC prohibit the use of profane or abusive language by either party on the air. If such language is used, transmission will be immediately cut off and service discontinued. It is also illegal to repeat or divulge to anyone any information heard on the air and superfluous, false, or deceptive messages are prohibited.

GUIDELINES FOR CORRECT USE OF RADIO

Most hospital EDs across the country now have or will have an emergency radio base station at the ED desk with hospital-to-ambulance radio capability. There are several console models in use and the operating particulars will vary slightly from manufacturer to manufacturer. However, the basic general guidelines to follow when using the radio do not vary and some of the key points are included here.

1. Time

Time is a very important factor in two-way radio communication since only one person can talk on a frequency at any given time. When a message is interrupted, the receiving station will not be able to receive the transmission and this prolongs air time for clarification, as well as adding confusion and the chance for error. Therefore, always be certain the air is clear before initiating a message and always listen first to be certain no one else is talking on the air. Keep your message as brief as possible and pronounce words slowly and distinctly; numbers should be transmitted first as individual numbers and then repeated reading the number as a whole. The number 729 Bed 2, for example, would read: "Seven, two, nine—bed two—729 bed 2." The possibility of error can be minimized by reading numbers in this fashion. Messages longer than 30 sec should be broken at 30 sec intervals and wait for 2-3 sec before resuming transmission in order to allow another station which might have an emergency message to go ahead without waiting when minutes could be valuable.

2. Receiving Call

When receiving a call, wait until the signal tone has stopped, press the transmit bar or button and say, "This is (name of hospital) emergency. Go ahead." Release the transmit bar and listen to the message.

3. Recording Message

Keep a pad and pencil at the radio desk at all times and write messages down with time "cleared." Many departments keep a permanent log, on which they record the time of transmission, ambulance identification by company or number, message (age, sex, chief complaint, vital signs, ETA), length of air time, and initials of person receiving call. Although the FCC does not require that such a log be kept, it is considered good practice to do so.

4. Transmitting

When transmitting, relax and speak in a normal and clear manner with your mouth close to the microphone or handset. There is no need to shout since the radio takes care of amplification, and speaking too loudly may distort the voice and make the message unintelligible. Emotion will also lend to distortion, so attempt to speak in a monotone and remain as emotionless as possible. Courtesy is understood, and there is no need to say "please" or "thank you," since time is of the essence on the air. Be impersonal and do not use the name of the person to whom you are speaking or "I," since stations in Emergency Radio Service are not licensed for person-to-person communications.

5. Checking

When the message is completed, be certain you have understood the content. Do not guess at transmissions; check any doubtful portions with the sending operator and do not acknowledge a message until you are certain you have received it accurately. If the message is clear and you have no questions, simply acknowledge receipt of message by pressing the transmit bar, and saying "Roger" or "10-4" (commonly understood radio terms) and then identify with your call number, clear at (time of day), and release the transmit bar. *Example:* "10-4, this is KRI-998, clear at 0715."

Since the use of numeral codes (the "10 code" and the "12 code") varies in meaning from locale to locale, the EDN should be familiar with the codes utilized in the region of employment.

REVIEW

1. Identify the two key factors involved in effective communication.
2. Identify the six ways in which miscommunication can develop.
3. Describe the two basic levels of communication.

4. List eight factors that affect the message sent and the message received.
5. Identify at least 10 systems employed in the ED for communicating essential information.
6. Identify the specific times of day when most mistakes are made in the ED.
7. Identify the seven functions or stages that comprise the normal emergency medical services cycle.
8. List the advantages of two-way radio capability in the emergency application, other than ambulance-to-hospital communications.
9. Explain the concept of the 911-system.
10. Explain the FCC regulations regarding use of the emergency radio service.
11. Describe the important steps to observe when talking on the emergency radio network.
12. Describe the one component that completes the communications process.

BIBLIOGRAPHY

American Hospital Association: Emergency Services: The Hospital Emergency Department in an Emergency Care System. American Hospital Associatoin, Chicago, Illinois, 1972

Barber JM, Dillman PA: Emergency Patient Care. Reston Publishing Co., Reston, Virginia, 1981

Boyd DR, Flashner BA, Ogilvie RB, Yoder FD: The Critically Injured Patient. Department of Public Health, Chicago, Illinois, 1971

Budassi SA, Barber JM: Emergency Nursing: Principles and Practice. The C.V. Mosby Co., St. Louis, Missouri, 1981

Cosgriff J, Anderson D: The Practice of Emergency Nursing. J.B. Lippincott Co., Philadelphia, Pennsylvania, 1975

Fisher DW: Communication—a key to hospital supervision. Point of View, Vol 13, No 2, pp 4-5, 1976

Ford JD: Planning depends on analysis of capabilities. Hospitals, May 16, 1973

Joint Commission on Accreditation of Hospitals: Manual on Standards of Accreditation of Hospitals, JACH, Chicago, Illinois, 1981

Munn HE, Metzgar N: Effective Communication in Health Care. Aspen Systems Publications, Rockville, Maryland, 1981

Pfeiffer JW: Conditions which hinder effective communication. In The 1973 Annual Handbook for Group Facilitators, University Association Press, pp 120-122, 1973

Reid HV: Communications improve care. Hospitals, Vol 47, p 32, 1973

Shabozian D: Mobile intensive care unit nurse. JEN, Vol 1, No 4, pp 20-22, 1975

US Department of Health, Education, and Welfare: Emergency Department Policy and Procedure Guidelines. USDHEW, Rockville, Maryland, 1972

US Department of Health, Education, and Welfare: Emergency Medical Services Communications Systems. USDHEW, Rockville, Maryland, Publication No. (HSM) 73-2003, 1972

US Department of Health, Education, and Welfare: Hospital Outpatient and Emergency Activities. USDHEW, Rockville, Maryland, Publication No. (PHS) 930-H-1, 1971

Warner C: Emergency Care: Assessment and Intervention, 2nd ed. The C.V. Mosby Co., St. Louis, Missouri, 1978

DISASTER MANAGEMENT 31

KEY CONCEPTS

This chapter has been developed to provide an overview of some general aspects and problems consistent with those that might easily be encountered in a disaster situation and for which every ED should be prepared well in advance with supplies, personnel, and a carefully worked-out disaster plan to follow. The materials presented were compiled by Myra Lee, R.N., Disaster Coordinator for Multnomah County, Oregon.

After reading and studying this chapter, you should be able to:

- Define disaster and the types of disaster that occur.
- Describe the realities of disaster nursing.
- Describe the public health aspects of disasters.
- Discuss the supply and space problems that are encountered in hospitals.
- Identify the resource personnel in a community who can and should be utilized.
- List the elements of a disaster plan.
- Describe effective methods of identifying both patients and personnel during disaster situations.
- Identify some of the commonly recurring problems seen during disaster management.
- Identify the areas that should be covered on a preparedness checklist.

Disaster is an unpredictable unknown. No one knows where it may hit, how it will occur, or the extent of damage it may cause. We do know that disaster usually brings the tragedy of death and injury, destruction of homes, disruption of family life and of the established patterns of community organization. We also know that in every disaster there is a need for someone to help care for the victims.

It is realistic for nurses to recognize that they will be expected to assume leadership roles in disaster situations and important to visualize the conditions under which they will be expected to function.

DEFINITION OF DISASTER

What is a disaster?

Disaster has been defined by some as a *sudden and massive disproportion between hostile elements of any kind and the survival resources which can be brought into action in the shortest possible time.*

Disaster does not necessarily mean that the situation is of mammoth disruptive proportions, involving numerous dead and injured. In a small community, disaster may consist of a two-car accident involving five seriously injured people. Each community and its medical facilities must define what constitutes a disaster for them. Most disasters, as we think of them, involve victims who have need for food, clothing, shelter, medical and nursing care, and other necessities of life.

TYPES OF DISASTER

There are many types of disaster and all deliver their impact with a uniqueness of their own. Disasters are usually divided into two categories:

1. Natural (violence of nature) such as tornadoes, hurricanes, earthquakes, blizzards, epidemics, conflagrations, etc.
2. Man-made (human error) such as fires, explosions, transportation accidents, civil disorders, and nuclear incidents.

These vary in degree of suddenness of onset, the degree of preparation possible immediately before disaster strikes, and the problems created that require emergency health services response. Persons providing medical and nursing service must be prepared to serve in a variety of capacities and should realize that each disaster situation will pose a widely varying complexity of problems.

Tornadoes, fires, explosions, major or even minor transportation mishaps, and other disasters all tend to produce more illnesses and health problems; communicable disease is usually a lurking public health threat, and there is a sudden demand for short-term provision of special care for the aged, the chronically ill, infants, young children, and expectant mothers.

DISASTER MEDICINE

Disaster medicine is that which is practiced when the number of casualties outbalances the possibilities of treating them as usual with the available means. The basic principles of medical care administered during disaster situations are no different from those administered under ordinary circumstances, but their application requires special organization in order to be effective. In full disaster conditions, with large numbers of casualties, all available physicians must immediately be summoned, as well as the maximum possible number of nursing staff, medical assistants, and first-aid and hospital volunteers. These personnel must know their roles in certain aspects of emergency care which were not necessarily included in their professional training and must be ready to improvise when necessary, following a carefully worked out master plan for the hospital and community, known as the Disaster Plan.

FACTORS IN EFFECTIVE MANAGEMENT

One major key to success in meeting disaster situations is training not only of physicians and nurses but of all the paramedical and ancillary personnel who will be drawn into the situation. This training *must* be followed up by refresher courses and exercises every year to maintain levels of proficiency and to update the master plan on a regular basis.

Another key factor is organization, and this can never be stressed too much. Each disaster situation is different in some respects from every other one and by nature disasters are chaotic. If disaster management is to be effective to any degree, order must be developed out of chaos, and in many instances this responsibility will fall to nurses since they are the primary people available to control the immediate situation in the hospital ED.

By implication, emergency nursing connotes organizational ability. Nurses must be, therefore, resourceful, flexible, and able to recognize the problems that accompany disaster and particularly those that may have a direct effect on provision of emergency medical care and supportive services. The compounding problems will include disruption of transportation, communications, and electrical power; destruction of or damage to other utility services, such as water and sanitary facilities; disruption or overburdening of public services, such as fire, police, emergency medical and civil defense services; inability of emergency personnel to respond because of weather conditions, accumulation of debris, confusion, etc. The list of problems can go on and on. However, it is essential that emergency personnel be able to cope with the reality of mass casualties, effective triaging, and traffic control, and the most effective utilization possible of whatever resources *are* available.

DISASTER NURSING

In addition to the obvious, the EDN must be alert and maintain a high index of suspicion toward illnesses, injuries, and health problems of a less obvious nature, for which the disaster forces may be indirectly responsible. These problems may not be apparent in the immediate emergency but may be lessened or prevented to some degree by early recognition of the probability and provision for the eventuality. Physical damage is generally fairly apparent. However, the nurse must also be alert to the additional signs and symptoms of emotional shock and trauma. Remember that in a disaster many people have undergone extremely stressful circumstances and may be disoriented, confused, withdrawn, exhausted, hyperactive, angry, or frankly hysterical. They must be given emotional support and the opportunity to express their feelings if they wish. Of necessity, nurses are often unable to provide the necessary support, but there are many professional and volunteer groups that are trained to this. Utilize them! Willing participants include clergymen, social workers, mental health workers, professional counselors, and church groups. They can and will offer their services, thus relieving nurses of an overwhelming and time-consuming responsibility.

SPECIFIC PROBLEMS ENCOUNTERED

There are many communicable diseases that can surface during a disaster, and although it would be impossible to immunize against all of them, the public can certainly be informed of the precautions they should take to minimize the danger.

The national Center for Disease Control (CDC) in Atlanta has advised that in flood disasters, there is no necessity to vaccinate against typhoid, but rather the most practical preventive strategy in a natural disaster is to advise the population to boil water before drinking it or to take other appropriate measures to insure a safe supply of drinking water. This approach provides immediate protection against typhoid and other water-borne diseases. A massive vaccination campaign would not provide protection at the time of greatest risk or add to the protection already achieved by water purification measures. It would also be an unnecessary expenditure of sometimes scarce emergency health resources, and it would not likely affect transmission, particularly in areas of low endemicity. Regardless of what other measures are taken to prevent an outbreak of typhoid following natural disasters, however, it is very important to maintain disease surveillance.

Another problem that arises is the shortage of whole blood, blood expanders, and plasma when large quantities are needed. Prior arrangements and written procedures should be developed to obtain these supplies when they are badly needed. Written agreements should be made with the local blood bank and/or the Red Cross.

RESOURCES

Extra supplies should be readily available to the emergency and critical care units from sources both within and outside the hospital. Emergency and key hospital personnel should be well informed of the resource agencies, with contingency plans in writing.

Space in which to locate patients will be at a premium. Any area can be used for this purpose that is not already dedicated to patient care, such as waiting rooms, hallways, and even parking areas adjacent to the emergency entrance. These areas can be cleared of *all* people not needing medical attention and can be declared patient areas and kept off limits to the press and onlookers.

Families can be referred to Red Cross shelter facilities to wait for word on the injured. A well-coordinated communications system should be established and maintained between the medical facilities and the Red Cross shelter facilities.

One person, usually the hospital administrator or his designee, should be responsible for maintaining liaison with the press. If there is no available space in the medical facility, the press should have extremely restricted access to patient care areas and should never be allowed to interfere with disaster operations.

Volunteer personnel can be effectively utilized to carry messages from the patient care areas to waiting family members or to other areas of the hospital, thus sparing the more qualified personnel for direct patient care.

Many people will not leave their homes to seek medical attention, and therefore, when it is feasible, medical personnel or Red Cross workers are permitted access to disaster areas to render medical assistance. There may be times when people must be forcibly removed from their property by the appropriate authorities; if this occurs, there will frequently be anger and hostility exhibited toward the personnel who are attempting to render assistance. Nurses must be prepared to cope with this eventuality and understand that it is cause and effect.

Usually Red Cross or Civil Defense personnel attempt to help people locate missing friends or relatives, and they are trained to assume this responsibility, thereby removing another time-consuming burden from medical personnel. If people inundate the hospital looking for missing persons, they should be referred to the appropriate agencies.

DISASTER READINESS—THE PLAN

Even with pictures, charts, and discussions, it is hard to visualize the overwhelming stress that disaster brings to a community. Until one has actually witnessed a disaster, it is also hard to imagine that "it can happen here." However, real-life disasters prove that no community or segment of our society is immune; they also prove that the public expects the nurse to function with know-how in the emergency.

Nurses should be alert to this expectation and at the same time recognize their own right to react with the same anxieties and feelings of inadequacy as others do.

The demands may be greater and the circumstances unusual, but the nursing fundamentals practiced in smaller crises will be applicable. Disaster nursing involves the adaptation of professional skills in recognizing and meeting the medical and nursing needs evolving from a disaster situation *as they evolve*. To respond in a rational manner to the demands of a disaster situation, it is *essential* that every hospital have a disaster plan in writing and available to every department. This plan must:

1. Provide for admission, disposition, discharge, and transfer of patients into and out of the hospital
2. Include provision for calling personnel back and notifying administrative people (Every ED should have a *direct* outside telephone line to insure this.)
3. Include a means of securing supplies and services from other areas with a list of suppliers, addresses, and telephone numbers
4. Define the specific area for the triage center
5. Provide for two drills a year. Remember that whatever is planned will have to be lived with in a disaster!

DISASTER TAGS

Disaster tags are an essential adjunct to disaster management in the ED. An adequate supply of tags should be available in the department and ready to use if needed, along with numbered plastic or paper sacks for belongings. There are several types of disaster tags available, but whatever is utilized should contain at least the following:

1. Sufficient space for patient identification
2. Sufficient space for allergies or current medications
3. Space to record VS, medications given, treatments, X-ray films, etc.
4. Space to record disposition of patient.

IDENTIFICATION

Identification for emergency personnel should be provided to gain admission through police lines and hospital security during disasters and large-scale emergencies. If your hospital does not provide employee identification, perhaps this is a good time to start thinking about how to acquire it. Provisions should be made with the appropriate local authorities for acceptance of the employee ID cards during a disaster to assure ready access to the facility where they will be working.

COMMON PROBLEMS IN DISASTER

An analysis of disasters within the United States since 1900, involving 100 or more deaths and suggesting several common problem areas, was presented to the Southern California Chapter of Disaster Associations by Dr. O.L. Gericke, Medical Director of Patton State Hospital in California.

Dr. Gericke points out, among many other areas, the following recurring problems:

1. Fast driving caused additional injury to many transported victims, and sightseers and volunteer vehicles invariably converged in the disaster zone and clogged the roads.

2. In spite of efforts at traffic control, the general pattern was that the nearest hospital was overwhelmed and the hospitals more remote received fewer than their reasonable share.

3. Where no previous plans for control of traffic were developed, an uncontrolled flood of traffic seriously handicapped operations and overloaded access roads and parking areas of the hospitals.

4. The vast majority of injured received medical care at hospitals and not in homes or physicians' offices.

5. Hospitals with more highly developed disaster planning and longer periods of warning have been successful in establishing medical control over admission of the injured.

6. Triage was possible only when certain key posts were manned, facilitating the flow of the injured. This success appears to depend absolutely upon arrangements made before disasters occur. Records can be started by a system of tagging at this point although no hospital has successfully improvised a *spur-of-the-moment* record or tagging system.

7. Misuse of personnel occurred frequently in the absence of planning.

8. Surprisingly, there has been a sufficient supply of blood usually, since there seems to have been a tendency to use less blood and plasma volume expanders under confused conditions than normally would be used.

9. Communications between hospitals and other agencies presented serious problems, with poor central control of telephone traffic, heavily overloaded switchboards that eventually became jammed, and the necessity to closely monitor the use of radio transmission since the volume of traffic that can be accommodated is extremely limited.

10. Notification of responsible officials and call-in staff was seriously hampered because of haphazard preparation for the eventuality.

11. The analysis showed that adequate record-keeping can be accomplished only when a high degree of preplanning and organization has been accomplished at the hospital. An effective system is to start the record by preplanned tagging at the triage point with specific designation made to continue maintenance of the record after the patient has left the triage point.

DISASTER PREPAREDNESS CHECKLIST

It is hoped that the areas that have just been enumerated will help point up some weaknesses of a disaster plan that may be considered functional until the time comes. Although the Joint Commission on Accreditation of Hospitals has outlined a policy calling for disaster drills twice a year, there is too great a tendency to simply go through the motions and not pay close enough heed to some of the details that can seriously hamper patient flow and effective treatment if they are not worked out ahead of time.

Where would your hospital start if a local school bus in your community slid on an icy road and rolled into the river at 7:45 in the morning with 30 grade-school children aboard? If you can activate that sort of tragic occurrence in your thought processes, perhaps you should start looking at your own department and its state of preparedness and capabilities, applying the following checklist:

1. What is the chain of command in your hospital?
2. Do you have radio transmission capability?
3. Do you have a direct outside telephone line?
4. Do you have a written procedure and call list for notifying off-duty personnel (to be carried out by nonmedical personnel)?
5. Do you have numbered disaster tags with numbered clothes bags ready to use?
6. Do you have a written procedure for appropriating nonpatient areas of the hospital for medical use?
7. Do you have a formal triage system with a written protocol?
8. Do you have written procedures for requisitioning blood, drugs, and food from outside the hospital?
9. Do you have employee identification that will allow you through police lines at your hospital?
10. Do you have job descriptions for volunteers in the nonmedical areas?
11. Do you take your disaster drills seriously enough?

Disasters can and do happen and always unexpectedly, but advance preparation can prevent chaos and provide delivery of the necessary emergency medical care if there is enough motivation on the part of those *doing* the advance preparation. Disaster preparedness is a real challenge and a very worthwhile effort that pays *big* dividends when it pays!

REVIEW

1. Define a disaster.
2. Identify at least six major effects upon a community struck by disaster.
3. Describe some of the realities of disaster nursing and the problems that should be anticipated.
4. Identify the resource personnel in a community who can and should be utilized.

5. List the essential provisions of a disaster plan.

6. Describe the essential areas for documentation that must be provided for on a disaster tag.

7. Describe at least six common problem areas found to be common among disaster situations in the United States.

8. Identify at least eight key areas that should be provided for and taken into consideration on a disaster preparedness checklist for your emergency department.

BIBLIOGRAPHY

American Hospital Association: The Hospital Emergency Department in an Emergency Care System. The American Hospital Association, Chicago, Illinois, 1972

Budassi SA, Barber JM: Emergency Nursing: Principles and Practice. The C.V. Mosby Co., St. Louis, Missouri, 1981

Cosgriff J, Anderson D: The Practice of Emergency Nursing. J.B. Lippincott Co., Philadelphia, Pennsylvania, 1975

Ford JD: Planning depends on analysis of capabilities. Hospitals, May 16, 1973

Joint Commission on Accreditation of Hospitals: Manual on Standards for Accreditation of Hospitals. JCAH, Chicago, Illinois, 1981

US Department of Health, Education, and Welfare: Emergency Department Policy and Procedure Guidelines. USDHEW, Rockville, Maryland, 1972

US Department of Health, Education, and Welfare: Emergency Medical Services Communications Systems. USDHEW, Rockville, Maryland, Publication No. (HSM) 73-2003, pp 14-15, 1972

US Department of Health, Education, and Welfare: Hospital Outpatient and Emergency Activities. USDHEW, Rockville, Maryland, Publication No. (PHS) 930-H-1, 1971

Warner CG: Emergency Care: Assessment and Intervention, 2nd ed. The C.V. Mosby Co., St. Louis, Missouri, 1978

EMERGENCY DEPARTMENT MANAGEMENT

32

KEY CONCEPTS

This chapter provides an overview of the evolving hospital emergency department, its role and that of the EDN within the system. The standards of the Joint Commission on Accreditation of Hospitals affecting EDs are discussed, as well as the housekeeping matters of ED management, including staffing patterns and job responsibilities, with some thoughts on the functions of EMTs and continuing education for EDNs.

After reading and studying this chapter, you should be able to:

- Identify the government agencies which developed and funded the EMS system.
- Identify the responsibilities of the emergency department physician.
- List the types of contractual emergency department physician coverage available.
- Identify the role and responsibilities of a well-qualified emergency department nurse.
- Outline briefly the eight JCAH standards that apply to emergency services.
- Explain the benefits that can be realized by supporting the standards.
- Identify some key areas that should be reinforced with written policies and procedures.
- Describe some variations of routine staffing patterns that can be effectively utilized in the emergency department.
- Identify some effective methods of expediting patient flow in the department.
- Describe the prehospital functions of the basic emergency medical technician (EMT).
- Explain the position taken by the Emergency Department Nurses Association regarding EMTs in its 1974 paper.

- Identify some specific areas of professional interface between EMTs and EDNs.

- Discuss the merits of the ED technician job description.

Since the advent of national interest and congressional emphasis on emergency medical services in the early 1970s, after the National Academy of Sciences released statistics identifying trauma as the killer of 155,000 Americans each year, emergency departments have taken on a new stature, along with an increasing complexity of roles.

Emergency medical services (EMS) projects have been funded in their various aspects since the early 1970s by regional medical programs (communications systems, research and evaluation, cardiac telemetry, and ambulance personnel training), Hill-Burton programs (expansion of emergency departments) and the Division of Emergency Health Services, DHEW (National Emergency Medical Stockpiles, Medical Self-Help Training Courses, Development of EMS Criteria, and EMS staff assignments at the state level).

With all the emphasis on EMS, there has been a concurrent increase in the utilization of emergency departments all over the United States, although this utilization can be attributed to *many* other factors, which include 1) ease of physical and financial access to immediate medical care, 2) lack of availability of private physicians, 3) the decrease in the number of general practitioners, 4) increasing physician specialization, 5) an increasing acceptance and confidence in emergency department facilities, and 6) the reimbursement policies of health insurance groups that cover treatment in emergency departments but will not reimburse for office calls or house calls.

Annual ED visits have increased to well over 80 million per year, an increase greater than any other single measure of hospital utilization and continue to burgeon at a rate of 10% a year. There has been a similar increase in the proportion of ED visits that are nonemergency in nature and repeated surveys of urban hospital EDs indicate that probably two-thirds of patients presenting at emergency departments represent nonemergent or clinic-type problems.

Many qualified observers candidly point out that the ED should be considered the key entry point to the health delivery system and that hospitals and ED personnel should demonstrate a willingness and a readiness to provide the comprehensive and continuous services needed by the population area which the hospital serves. Patients will continue to utilize emergency facilities at increasingly greater rates with the realization that doctor's offices are frequently inaccessible or inconvenient; that funding and/or reimbursement for office visits and nonhospital ambulatory care centers is declining; and that emergency departments provide service, convenience and quality medical care. These observers suggest that EDs cease to despair at the volume of nonemergencies arriving at their doors but, rather, meet the need by responding with appropriate services.

THE ROLE OF THE EMERGENCY DEPARTMENT PHYSICIAN

When a hospital indicates, in any way, that it has an ED, the public will expect just that. When the patient presents with what he believes to be a problem, he expects to be taken care of; he does not necessarily care about the internal operational problems of the hospital or the staffing problems and the expense of operating the ED. He does care, however, about whether he receives prompt attention and treatment with courtesy and respect shown to him as an individual and, indeed, as a paying customer. He expects to be seen by a physician who is knowledgeable, competent, and thorough.

To this end a new medical specialist has emerged—the emergency physician—who is the patient's advocate in the ED and responds quickly to acute needs by providing initial care, directing the emergency team in its function (both prehospital and in the department), and referring the patient on to definitive care and follow-up. In 1969 the American College of Emergency Physicians was established to develop standards of practice with certification of competency; currently, residency programs and specialty boards in emergency medicine are recognized.

If career emergency physicians are not available, the medical staff of the hospital frequently provides full-time or on-call coverage, with staff members rotating call, while some hospitals rely on coverage by house staff with a medical staff member supervising.

There are, however, four basic types of contractual arrangements possible to furnish physician coverage to EDs, and all have been successfully employed in many hospitals. The plans include 1) the Pontiac Plan, 2) the Alexandria Plan, 3) a combination of these, and 4) full-time salaried physicians.

The Pontiac Plan originated at Pontiac General Hospital in Pontiac, MI, in 1961 and involves full-time coverage of the ED by a relatively large number of physicians who still retain their individual practices but contractually agree to spend varying amounts of time in the hospital ED. The group may be small or as large as 50-60 physicians and is usually incorporated wherever the state law allows.

The Alexandria Plan, named for its city of origin in Alexandria, VA, was begun in 1961 with physicians providing coverage to the ED without outside practice. These are usually small groups of four physicians who form a partnership or corporation and hire substitutes as necessary from time to time.

Some combinations of the Pontiac and Alexandria plans have been utilized according to the needs of the individual hospital, and full-time salaried physicians have been employed in facilities where there is the responsibility for teaching and supervising as well as patient care, making it difficult to establish a fee system.

Whatever system is employed, the reality is that the demand far exceeds the supply of willing and qualified emergency physicians.

THE ROLE OF THE EMERGENCY DEPARTMENT NURSE

In the not-too-recent past the nurse in the "receiving ward" or "ambulance entrance" was one who merely logged patients in on their way to bed or was expert with Bandaids and phone calls. For that matter, the emergency room or "first aid room" was generally a small, poorly lighted, and shabbily equipped area, which was stocked with leftovers and castoffs that had fallen into disuse in other areas of the hospital. There was little to work with and less incentive to even try.

Since 1970 a group of nurses whose chief concern and driving interest was the improvement of quality of care to ED patients has evolved and formed the Emergency Department Nurses Association (EDNA), the sister organization to the American College of Emergency Physicians (ACEP). With EDNA has come the emergence of new roles and responsibilities for EDNs and an awareness of the need for educational standards and opportunities that were nonexistent until relatively recently with the publication of the *Journal of Emergency Nursing* (JEN), the development of the EDNA Core Curriculum, and other programs emerging all over the country to teach emergency nursing and expand the capabilities of the EDN.

National certification is now a reality for emergency nurses, with a certification examination available which validates and documents the nurse's mastery of a body of knowledge in emergency care, covering clinical assessment and priority setting, care of critical patients, care of noncritical patients, and roles and responsibilities *in* that patient care.

Emergency department nurses who have had specialized training and are assigned to the ED as their primary responsibility are becoming accomplished in primary assessment and effective triage and generally will be found to be those nurses who are looking for a challenge in their work. They participate in expediting patient flow, providing rapid response and hands-on care, establishing and maintaining airways, obtaining vital signs, initiatiing IV lines, maintaining adequate circulation and perfusion, executing the physician's orders, teaching and counseling patients and families, providing accurate documentation and any further support that is indicated. Patient care, incidentally, has been found to be expedited significantly in situations where the EDN is allowed to requisition certain laboratory tests, ECGs and X-ray films when appropriate, making the preliminary reports available to the physician in considerably less time.

The EDN must be expected to be totally accountable and responsible for cardiopulmonary resuscitation, including the use of drugs and their dosages, and physiologic responses, defibrillation procedures, and the full gamut of airway-management techniques, including endotracheal intubation, as endorsed in the Standards on Advanced Life Support of the American Heart Association.

The ability to assess life-threatening situations resulting from trauma, neurologic damage, cardiopulmonary distress, and arrhythmias is a skill that must be developed in every nurse participating in emergency care, since frequently the EDN is called upon to make a decision of priority before the physician ever sees the patient, and when time is crucial, the nurse's assessment is often critically important to the patient's outcome. Less obvious complaints not infrequently turn out to be life-threatening, and the ability to carefully assess and screen for occult problems makes that nurse a very valuable member of the patient care team. These skills do not just happen; they must be developed and employed daily to achieve the desired level of competency and reliability. For this reason it is urged that EDNs be recognized as specialized personnel and, wherever possible, permanently assigned to the ED. This can be achieved in the small hospital as well, by assigning the ED to *qualified* nurses as their *primary* responsibility, even though they may occasionally have to be drawn into the units during staffing shortages.

STANDARDS

Every nurse who works or expects to work in the ED has the obligation to be familiar with the Standards for Accreditation of Hospitals, specifically the Standards for Emergency Services in Hospitals, as developed by the Joint Commission on Accreditation of Hospitals (JCAH).

The Joint Commission evolved from the Hospital Standardization Program, which had been established by the American College of Surgeons in 1918 to encourage the adoption of a uniform medical record format that would facilitate accurate recording of a patient's clinical course.

The founding sponsors of JCAH were the American College of Surgeons, the American College of Physicians, the American Hospital Association, the American Medical Association, and the Canadian Medical Association, which participated until 1959 when the Canadian Council on Hospital Accreditation was established.

Through the years the standards have been revised and updated to meet the rapid pace of change which has occurred, and the Joint Commission has developed its own full-time field staff, which now surveys over 2000 hospitals a year. A survey fee was established in 1964 to make the field program self-supporting.

Although the standards were aimed initially at minimal achievement in terms of the necessary supportive elements of hospital life, voluntary accreditation was offered as a yardstick to progressive institutions that wished to attain a level of care set by a professional and nationally recognized group. In the absence of legal and other regulatory requirements, the accreditation program was the only benchmark by which to identify those hospitals.

In 1965 Medicare was enacted, and written into the Medicare Act was the provision that the hospitals participating in that program were to maintain the level of patient care that had come to be recognized as the norm. The standards of JCAH were cited in the law as reflecting that norm and were incorporated into the law by reference. The "Conditions of Participation for Hospitals," subsequently promulgated and published by the Social Security Administration, reflected the 1965 standards of the Joint Commission. These conditions of participation as updated periodically are administered at the state level through the licensing and certification divisions of most state governments for all hospitals that are not accredited by JCAH, to assure safety and quality care.

Most nurses know very little about the standards, and the same applies no less for EDNs. They know only that "before JCAH comes around" all of the policy and procedure books disappear from the department and are nowhere to be found for several weeks, only to reappear again "shining and golden," newly updated and jacketed the very day before JCAH arrives.

The Standards for Emergency Services should in reality be a working tool for EDNs because they clearly spell out the components that must be present to maintain an effectively operating department, provide safe surroundings, and promote high quality care to insure patients optimum benefit. The standards deserve your attention; they are on your side and should be your tools.

Currently, the Standards have been expanded from five basic standards to eight and are spelled out in greater detail in ways that should generate even more interest among emergency nurses. The basic principle states "any individual who comes to the hospital for emergency medical evaluation or initial treatment shall be properly assessed by qualified individuals, and appropriate services shall be rendered within the defined capability of the hospital." The new standards follow.

Standard I

> *A well-defined plan for emergency care, based on community need and on the capability of the hospital, shall be implemented by every hospital.*

This standard spells out specific and general requirements which have been established for four levels of emergency services (Levels I, II, III and IV) with specific requirements for essential areas including patient transfers, directional hospital signs on highways, disaster plans, and external communications capabilities.

Standard II

> *The emergency department/service shall be well organized, properly directed, and staffed according to the nature and extent of health care needs anticipated and the scope of services offered.*

This speaks to the qualifications of the physician director and his authority and responsibilities, defining the method of providing medical staff coverage for the department, specific requirements for nursing service personnel, and the specifically defined functions of emergency medical technicians or other allied health personnel when used.

Standard III

> *The emergency department/service shall be appropriately integrated with other units and departments of the hospital.*

The interpretation of this standard relates to specific services to be provided by laboratory, radiology, operating suite, and other special care units.

1

2

Standard IV

All personnel shall be prepared for their emergency care responsibilities through appropriate training and educational programs.

This standard is of highly significant interest to emergency nurses since it outlines required orientation and training specifically to include the following:

- Recognition, interpretation, and recording of patients' signs and symptoms, particularly those that require notification of a physician
- Initiation of cardiopulmonary resuscitation and other related life-support procedures
- Parenteral administration of electrolytes, fluids, blood, and blood components
- Wound care and management of sepsis
- Initial burn care
- Initial management of injuries to the extremities and central nervous system
- Effective and safe use of electrical and electronic life-support and other equipment used in the emergency department/service
- Prevention of contamination and cross infection
- Recognition of, and attention to, the psychological and social needs of patients and their families.

This standard continues to give definitive substance to the increasingly important area of continuing education for personnel as follows: "All emergency department/service personnel shall participate in relevant in-service education programs. The director, or his qualified designees, shall contribute to the in-service education of emergency department/service personnel. In-service education shall include the safety and infection control requirements described in this *Manual*. Cardiopulmonary resuscitation training shall be conducted as often as necessary for all physicians, nurses, and specified professional personnel who work in the emergency care area.

The hospital administration shall assure that there are opportunities for physicians, nurses, and, as required, other personnel to participate in emergency department/service continuing education programs outside the hospital, as needed. Education programs for emergency department/service personnel shall be based at least in part on the results of the review and evaluation of the quality and appropriateness of emergency care. The extent of participation shall be documented and shall be realistically related to the size of the staff and to the scope and complexity of the emergency care services provided.

Standard V

Emergency patient care shall be guided by written policies and procedures.

Specific requirements for policies and procedures covering all aspects of patient care are spelled out in detail in this standard.

Standard VI

The emergency department/service shall be designed and equipped to facilitate the safe and effective care of patients.

The physical layout of the department is defined in terms of basic requirements, as well as provision for observation beds, internal communication, special provisions, and minimal equipment and drugs.

Standard VII

A medical record shall be maintained on every patient seeking emergency care and shall be incorporated into the patient's permanent hospital record. A control register shall adequately identify all persons seeking emergency care.

This standard specifies what information is to be included in the patient's medical record, as well as information to be recorded in a control register, or as it is sometimes called the Emergency Department Log.

Standard VIII

The quality and appropriateness of patient care provided in the emergency department/service shall be continuously reviewed, evaluated, and assured through establishment of quality control mechanisms.

Specific quality control mechanisms are outlined here to be established with reference to the Quality Assurance section of the *JCAH Manual*.

Obtain a Copy. It is strongly suggested that if you do not have access to the full standards in your department, send for a copy of your own with the full interpretations. The new standards now include special care units, infection control, quality assurance and can be obtained from the Joint Commission on Accreditation of Hospitals, 875 North Michigan Avenue, Chicago, IL 60611.

POLICIES AND PROCEDURES

An updated and workable policies and procedures book is essential to a smooth-running department, providing answers to questions when personnel are in doubt as to specific management approaches, and preventing errors in judgment when a situation arises that the person may never have had to cope with. Policies are guidelines by which to function, and policies that have been established and approved by administration, the medical staff, and the nursing staff have the full weight of authority when quoted. Policies and procedures should be used for the purposes they have been designed to serve; emergency personnel should pay close heed to what their policy books outline.

One of the *most* helpful policies is that which distinctly defines authorized procedures and unauthorized procedures for the ED, thereby eliminating tie-up of the department for minor surgery, general anesthesia, contaminated (dirty) cases, and elective sigmoidoscopy and endoscopy when time, space, and personnel are unavailable to cope with these procedures. Enemas and removal of fecal impactions likewise have no place in the ED, which is primarily an acute care area and usually has neither staff nor space for these procedures.

Some of the other important policy areas, most of which the new JCAH standards include, involve the following situations and should have well-defined written interpretation in your policy books:

1. Child abuse
2. Treatment of a minor child with/without that child's consent
3. Consent in absentia for minors
4. Management of the press
5. Blood alcohol procedure
6. Procedure for DOA
7. Transfer procedure*
8. Release from responsibility for transfer
9. Release from responsibility for leaving against medical advice (AMA)
10. Handling pathology specimens
11. Helicopter landings
12. Decontamination after radiation exposure
13. Management of sexual assault victim
14. Expiration times on sterile supplies
15. Reporting of contagious disease, acts of violence, overdoses, etc.
16. Management of the emotionally ill patient
17. Management of patients under the influence of drugs or alcohol
18. Activation of the Disaster Plan
19. Housekeeping and linen guidelines
20. Infection control and management of communicable diseases
21. Personnel policies with complete job descriptions for every department employee

STAFFING PATTERNS

To arrive at the number of nurses needed to staff an emergency department and to schedule them in the most appropriate time slots, EDs should carefully analyze their patient loads during weekday and weekend hours. There is no

---

*ACS Committee on Trauma, ATLS Program; Appendix C-1, Inter-Hospital Transfer of Patients.

hard-and-fast rule requiring staffing schedules in the ED to correspond to staffing schedules elsewhere in the hospital, nor is it necessary for all members of a shift to change at one time. It may well be that one nurse would be most valuable spanning two shifts, for instance 11 A.M. to 7 P.M., or 2 P.M. to 10 P.M., providing not only continuity between shifts but augmenting the staff capability during the usually heavier patient-load hours.

In most EDs, three day nurses, three or four evening nurses, and two night nurses per shift with an ED technician each shift can handle up to 30,000 patients per year, with additional fill-in personnel available to cover for vacations and sick-time. Some EDs may require additional personnel on weekends to accommodate their patient loads.

Because of the unique demands of emergency nursing, many departments are testing various staffing patterns, and one hears frequently of arrangements such as 1) the "7-70" (7 shifts in a row for 10 hours a day with the next 7 days off), which requires two crews to alternate; 2) regular 10-hour shifts (4 shifts in a row with 3 days off); 3) 10-hour shifts with a 2-week cyclic pattern (OO-SSM-O-WT-OOO-MTW) which gives 3 days off every other weekend; and even 4) 12-hour shifts in various patterns. The distinct advantage of all these extended shifts (aside from more scheduled time off) is the shift overlap of coverage, which provides a greater continuity of care in the department.

PATIENT FLOW

The triage nurse is generally the key person who carries the responsibility for management of patient flow, utilizing the most appropriate area at the most appropriate time for the care of specific patients. The triage nurse expedites patient care, assigns nurses and patients to specific areas, keeps the physician advised of the status of patients in the department and even, at times, encourages him to "move a little faster."

To shorten the elapsed time in the department for patients, it is good practice to ready them for discharge as soon as the physician has finished instructing them, helping them dress, and allowing them to wait for medications or family members while sitting in a wheelchair in a nontreatment area of the department. This allows preparation of the patient area for the next admission and significantly accelerates the patient flow, increasing the number who can be treated in a given period of time.

Departments that are fortunate enough to have "holding" or observation beds are able to utilize this means of freeing up acute care areas for incoming patients. Unless your department has facilities for providing adequate extended observation when necessary, the patient should either be admitted or transferred to an institution that *can* provide the necessary observation.

EMERGENCY MEDICAL TECHNICIANS

The emergency medical technician training program, initiated in 1970, was the direct result of studies done in 1968 by the National Academy of Sciences and the Department of Transportation, which pointed up the dire need for a standardized training program to train persons already involved in emergency rescue and ambulance work to the higher level of emergency medical technician.

Now, eight years later, with proper training and experience, ready availability of equipment and supplies, radio communication, and a vehicle designed to meet the needs of the injured or sick with life-support capability, the emergency medical technician (EMT) is able to serve as the most valuable lay member of the medical care team outside the hospital.

Standards for the training of EMTs have varied widely from state to state and in some states, from county to county, although most jurisdictions have recognized the basic 81-hour Dunlop curriculum as the standard. Depending on the state or city program in effect, there are gradations over and above the basic training, some of which approach well in excess of 1000 hours of didactic and clinical time and qualify the technician as a "paramedic." Unfortunately, there are still many "levels" of paramedic qualification across the country, and the term becomes relative.

A 1974 position paper was issued by the EDNA board of directors relating to the "Roles, Responsibilities and Relationship of EDNA to Emergency Medical Technicians and the System of Prehospital Emergency Care." Some excerpts* from this paper are as follows:

Some EMTs will also need to have additional training and experience in all the sophisticated and advanced techniques they will need to utilize in a given geographical area (e.g., IV therapy, electrocardiograph monitoring, defibrillation, endotracheal intubation or other such skills as accepted and potentially needed). Such advanced training should be based on the behavioral objectives for applying such skills, and care should be taken not to overtrain these persons. EDNA urges the adoption of national standards for training, testing, certification, and evaluation of these advanced emergency medical technicians or "paramedics."

In the day-to-day operation of the Emergency Health Services System, it is the emergency department nurse to whom EMTs most directly relate. It is, therefore, vital that a close working relationship exist between emergency department nurses and EMTs. This EMT-to-nurse relationship is vital to the continuity of care of each patient involved. It is critical to the patient's well being that the emergency department staff pay close attention to the information the EMTs convey concerning the prehospital condition of the patient and the care administered. A written record of each patient's prehospital condition and emergency care rendered should be prepared by the emergency medical technician and a copy should be made part of the patient's permanent hospital record.

The EMT-nurse interaction has other benefits as well. It provides a sort of "checks and balances" system whereby the emergency health providers involved can constructively criticize or question each other's actions, thereby

---

*EDNA Board of Directors, JEN, p 29, January/February 1975

reducing the likelihood of repeated inappropriate action. Also, such interactions frequently result in learning experiences from the advice or explanations nurses can offer EMTs on patient care, anatomy, and physiology or pathophysiology; and EMTs can offer nurses on prehospital care techniques and actions.

When possible, joint emergency care training programs should be held on topics and skills common to both groups. Systems for joint case audits should be established and every opportunity should be utilized to foster professional growth and working relationships.

In some parts of the country, EDNA recognizes that emergency nurses may be called upon to take a more direct role in emergency ambulance services by actually delivering or assisting in the delivery of sophisticated prehospital emergency care. In such cases, EDNA urges these nurses to complete such specialized training programs as needed before assuming these duties.

The professional interface between EMTs and the ED nursing staff includes, but is certainly not limited to, the following premises:

1. The EMT provides valuable and accurate baseline data (VS, history of accident or illness, emotional status of patient, evidence of ingestion, such as pill bottles, etc.).
2. The EMT can give valuable assistance in the ED with patient management problems.
3. The EMT is capable of life-support en route to the ED and can communicate the patient status prior to arrival. Conversations on the emergency radio must be kept to a minimum so only pertinent information should be given or requested, but should include running code (1, 2, or 3), number of patients aboard, sex and age of each and whether "up" (sitting) or "down" (stretcher), possible diagnosis or chief complaint, VS and LOC, and ETA (estimated time of arrival).

A close rapport and team spirit between ED staffs and EMTs will assure continued learning experiences and optimal continuity of care for the patient and will provide the EMT with opportunities to critique situations, benefit from experience, and become an increasingly capable and contributing member of the emergency medical care team.

THE EMERGENCY DEPARTMENT TECHNICIAN

With the increasing number of qualified EMTs available and the many experienced corpsmen seeking employment in emergency departments, a need has developed to define a job description for emergency department technicians who can function in a productive role without assuming the RN's responsibilities and violating the nurse practice acts in most of the 50 states.

Such a job description is given here in a basic format, which can easily be adapted to individual department needs:

JOB DESCRIPTION

Rationale

There is a need for skilled emergency department technicians to assist the professional nursing and medical staff of the emergency department in providing the highest quality medical care possible to emergency patients, with every due consideration for the personhood, privacy, and safety of the patient.

A formally structured educational program of sufficient depth with a minimum core curriculum of 15 hours will be administered to define standards of performance as well as to assure competence consistent with the responsibilities delegated to the emergency department technician.

Basic Qualifications

Intelligence, the ability to relate to people, a capacity for calm and reasoned judgment in meeting emergencies, and an orientation toward service are essential attributes of the emergency department technician.

The candidate must be a high-school graduate with

1. Two years' prior experience in emergency department work, or
2. Military training with designation as a specialist in the medical field, or
3. An intensive on-the-job training period given by an accredited hospital.

The EMT must have the ability to meet and deal with the public with understanding and empathy.

Skill Areas

The technician will demonstrate competence and current knowledge in the following areas:

1. Airway management
2. Oxygen administration
3. Suctioning techniques
4. Bag/mask techniques
5. Cardiopulmonary resuscitation (must qualify for current state Heart Association certification)
6. Obtaining and recording vital signs, including visual acuity
7. Gross neurologic examination, including pupil size, equality, and reaction to light and accommodation (PERL-A)
8. 90-second trauma evaluation
9. Documentation procedures
10. Nasogastric intubation
11. Male catherizations (optional skill)

12. Surgical preparation of wounds
13. Sterile technique
14. Orthopedic procedures as outlined
15. Surgical setups for lacerations, minor repairs, Crutchfield tongs, chest tubes, lumbar punctures, and pin insertions
16. Obtaining specimens
17. Medicolegal aspects of the emergency department, including limitations on the job, as defined by state statues.

Duties and Responsibilities

The emergency department technician is responsible for performing assigned duties within his or her capabilities and under the direct supervision of a registered nurse.

Emergency department technicians shall not assume any responsibility of the physician and shall not mislead patients or visitors as to their identity, shall not accept verbal orders for medications, nor shall they administer medications, and all such matters shall be referred to the registered professional nurse on duty.

Basic Routine Duties

1. Maintain and stock supplies in
   A. Surgery rooms
   B. Wards
   C. Cast room
   D. Utility rooms
2. Maintain linen supply in all rooms
3. Clean up after procedures
   A. Make up stretches after discharges
   B. Clean, wrap, and resterilize instruments and trays as used
   C. Clean up rooms
   D. Maintain utility workroom in orderly fashion
4. Be current and familiar with the use and location of all surgical instruments and supplies
5. Dispose of trash and linen during and at end of each shift.
6. Practice clean technique at *all* times and have a working knowledge of formal precaution, isolation, and sterile techniques, employing them as indicated.

Emergency Procedures

1. Establish airway, inserting plastic oropharyngeal airway as necessary
2. Breathe patient with bag/mask until, if necessary
3. Initiate and maintain CPR until relieved

4. Apply monitor electrodes for cardiac monitor and ECG machine
5. Suction patient as necessary
   A. Oral
   B. Nasal
   C. Endotracheal
6. Apply direct pressure to control bleeding or employ arterial pressure points if necessary
7. Immobilize injuries on multiple trauma patients

Assistance With Nursing Procedures

1. Assist in admitting and discharging patients (*all* trauma patients must be fully disrobed for examination)
2. Perform primary evaluation of the patient in the absence of a RN by obtaining vital signs on every patient, including temperature, pulse, respirations, and blood pressure, and recording on the patient's chart
3. Check neurologic signs (if indicated) and record as necessary
   A. Level of consciousness and degree of orientation
   B. Condition of PERL-A
   C. Postures and/or position
4. Provide bedpans and urinals as needed
5. Assist in obtaining specimens and transporting them to the lab as necessary
   A. Urine by way of
      • Catheter
      • Clean catch
   B. Stool
   C. Sputum
   D. Throat culture
   E. Wound culture
6. Chart observations
7. Perform clinitest, acetest, guaiac, etc.
8. Apply heat or cold packs
9. Position patients rapidly, as indicated for coma, seizures, shock, dyspnea, combativeness
10. Restrain patients as necessary in the safest and most effective fashion
11. Lift and move patients as necessary, being aware of and using precautions for possible injuries
12. Transport patients
    A. To X-ray department
    B. To and from automobiles
    C. To bed following admission
    D. To morgue
13. Lend general support to the nursing staff in whatever areas are indicated that fall within the scope of the technician's training and capabilities

Assistance With Physicians' Procedures

1. Employ sterile technique at all times when indicated
2. Carry out sterile prep and irrigation for minor surgeries as necessary.
3. Assist in minor surgeries as necessary and as directed
4. Set up for sterile procedures
   A. Chest tube insertions
   B. Laceration repairs
   C. Elective minor surgeries
   D. Lumbar punctures
   E. Chest and abdominal taps (thoracentesis and paracentesis)
   F. Bone-marrow taps
   G. Orthopedic pin insertions and Crutchfield tongs
5. Apply Steri-strip skin closures
6. Apply dressings
   A. Surgical dressings
   B. Compression dressings for control of bleeding
   C. Burn dressings
7. Set up traction as directed by physician
8. Assist in cast application
9. Perform cast cutting
   A. Removal of cast
   B. Windowing and bivalving of casts
10. Apply Buck's extension traction as directed by physician
11. Apply forearm splints and finger cages, ace bandages, Manchu compression dressings, and traction splints
12. Fit crutches and instruct in crutch walking
13. Insert urethral catheters in male patients as ordered
14. Irrigate eyes for chemical injuries as directed

Other Out-of-Department Responsibilities (Optional)

On call to rest of house for 1) male catheterizations, 2) lifting and moving patients

Core Curriculum for Emergency Department Technicians

A formal 15-hour education program following general orientation should consist of a minimum of the following:

3 hours   *AIRWAY MANAGEMENT*
Airway placement (nasopharyngeal, oropharyngeal), oxygen administration (mask, catheter, prongs, liter flow gauge), capability and oxygen concentrations, bag/mask techniques and suctioning techniques

3 hours	*CARDIOPULMONARY RESUSCITATION*
	Standards I and II of basic life support
3 hours	*VITAL SIGNS*
	TPR, blood pressure and the sounds of Korotkoff, visual acuity, gross neurological assessment with PERL-A, Doll's eyes, LOC, orientation postures
3 hours	*TUBES, SPECIMENS AND TECHNIQUES*
	Naso-gastric tubes, urinary catheters, chest tubes and the Pleurovac or three-bottle underwater seal, epistaxis setups
	Specimens—urine, stool, throat cultures, sputum, wound cultures
	Techniques—precaution, sterile, isolation
3 hours	*COMMUNICATION*
	Interpersonal skills, interdepartmental skills, emergency radio (HEAR system, Med-Net, etc.), telephone techniques

SUMMARY

For a multitude of reasons, today's emergency department finds itself in the position of providing the general public access to the health-care delivery system of this nation, while simultaneously functioning as the interface between the hospital and an increasingly sophisticated level of prehospital care made possible by development of EMS system capabilities.

The emergency department has become the "face" of the hospital, which is seen by the public, and impressions made on patients and their families linger long after the fact. Emergency nurses find themselves standing right in the doorway, receiving patients, dealing with families and friends, and contributing heavily to the lasting impressions made.

The complexities of these responsibilities require a highly skilled and well-educated group of dedicated people who take pride in their abilities to effectively manage the patient loads and deliver quality care with total accountability and concerned provision for follow-up care as necessary.

Many existing factors can be put to advantage in emergency department management resulting in efficient, economical, and consistent levels of performance, which hospital administration and the public has the right to expect.

The JCAH standards exist and are there to be used as working tools, assuring the operation of a safe, well-staffed, and well-equipped department. Staffing patterns can be tailored to patient load demands, with shift overlaps scheduled appropriately for the busiest hours. An intelligent triage system can be formulated to meet department needs and utilize personnel and space in the most productive fashion. Ambulance personnel can be made a part of the emergency team and included in joint training programs with ongoing critiques and provision for feedback that will build morale and contribute significantly to improved performance and quality of care. Emergency department technicians can be recruited from the ranks of interested EMTs and excorpsmen and trained for utilization in numerous areas to release the EDN for the primary nursing responsibilities of assessing, evaluating, intervening where necessary, and teaching patients.

Effective management of an efficient and patient-oriented emergency department will depend heavily on the quality and accountability of leadership, the philosophy of patient care that is established, proper utilization of personnel who have been carefully qualified for their responsibilities, and the continued pursuit of educational opportunities appropriate to the field of emergency medical care, all of which ultimately insure the patients' access to competent emergency assessment and intervention by skilled caring professionals.

REVIEW

1. Identify the three major responsibilities of an emergency department physician.
2. Describe the expanded role of the emergency department nurse.
3. Identify the eight JCAH standards that apply to emergency services.
4. Explain the benefits that can be realized by supporting the standards.
5. Identify some specific key areas that should be reinforced with written policies and procedures in every emergency department.
6. Describe some of the staffing pattern variations which can be employed to advantage in ED scheduling.
7. Identify some effective methods of expediting patient flow in the department.
8. Explain the position taken by EDNA regarding EMTs in its 1974 position paper.
9. Identify some of the specific areas of interface between EMTs and EDNs.
10. Outline the advantages to be realized by staffing every shift with an ED technician.
11. Identify the groups that would be most qualified to train as ED technicians.
12. Describe the advantages that the EDN would realize if released from specific responsibilities by an ED technician.
13. Describe the benefits that can be realized if the ambulance personnel are made a part of the emergency team.

BIBLIOGRAPHY

American College of Emergency Physicians: Emergency Department Organization and Management. The C.V. Mosby Co., St. Louis, Missouri, 1978

American College of Surgeons, Committee on Trauma: Guidelines for Design and Function of a Hospital Emergency Department. Chicago, Illinois, 1978

American Hospital Association: Emergency Services: The Hospital Emergency Department in an Emergency Care System. Chicago, Illinois, 1972

American Medical Association: Emergency Department: A Handbook for the Medical Staff. Chicago, Illinois, 1967

American Medical Association: Proceedings, Conference on Emergency Medical Services. Chicago, Illinois, 1967

Boyd RD, et al: The Critically Injured Patient. Illinois Department of Public Health, Chicago, Illinois, 1971

Brown BJ: Nurse Staffing: A Practical Guide. Aspen Systems Corporation, Gaithersburg, Maryland, 1980

Budassi SA, Barber JM: Emergency Nursing: Principles and Practice. The C.V. Mosby Co., St. Louis, Missouri, 1981

Cosgriff J, Anderson DL: The Practice of Emergency Nursing. J.B. Lippincott Co., Philadelphia, Pennsylvania, 1975

Cronin J, Benson R, Rogers W: First aid and emergency care training. Its effect on prehospital emergency care. JACEP, Vol 4, pp 309-312, 1975

Gibson G: EMS: A facet of ambulatory care. Hospitals, Vol 47, 1973

Grubb RD: Hospital Manuals: A Guide to Development and Maintenance. Aspen Systems Corporation, Gaithersburg, Maryland, 1981

Hannas RR: Staffing the emergency department. Hospitals, Vol 47, May 16, 1973

Jelenko C, Frey CF: Emergency Medical Services: An Overview. The Robert J. Brady Co., Bowie, Maryland, 1976

Joint Commission on Accreditation of Hospitals: Manual on Standards for Accreditation of Hospitals, Chicago, Illinois, 1981

Kirz H: The greening of an emergency department nurse. Point of View, Vol 11, No 7, pp 3-6, 1974

Payne JT, Kranz JM, Eade GG: A survey of hospital emergency rooms in the state of Washington. Bull Am Coll Surg, September 1973

Romano T: The future of nursing in emergency care. JEN, pp 19-21, January/February 1975

Smith L: From ambulance driver to EMT. Hospitals, Vol 47, 1973

US Department of Health, Education, and Welfare: Hospitals Outpatient and Emergency Activities. USDHEW, Rockville, Maryland, Publication No. (PHS) 930-H-1, 1971

Warner CG: Emergency Care: Assessment and Intervention, 2nd ed. The C.V. Mosby Co., St. Louis, Missouri, 1978